Foundations of Chiropractic
Subluxation

Foundations of Chiropractic
Subluxation

Second Edition

Edited by

Meridel I. Gatterman, MA, DC, MEd

Consultant, Oregon Board of Chiropractic Examiners
Portland, Oregon

Former Dean, Chiropractic and Clinical Sciences
Western States Chiropractic College
Portland, Oregon

Former Director, Chiropractic Sciences
Canadian Memorial Chiropractic College
Toronto, Ontario, Canada

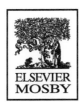

ELSEVIER
MOSBY

ELSEVIER
MOSBY

11830 Westline Industrial Drive
St. Louis, Missouri 63146

FOUNDATIONS OF CHIROPRACTIC: SUBLUXATION   0-323-02648-6
Copyright © 2005, 1995 by Mosby, Inc.

International Standard Book Number 0-323-02648-6

Publishing Director: Linda Duncan
Managing Editor: Christie Hart
Publishing Services Manager: Patricia Tannian
Project Manager: Kristine Feeherty
Designers: Gail Hudson, Jyotika Shroff

Printed and bound by CPI Group (UK) Ltd, Croydon, CR0 4YY

Transferred to digital print 2012

To the memory of

A. Earl Homewood
A respected friend whose vision of the neurodynamics of
the vertebral subluxation predicted much of the work
reported in this book

Contributors

THOMAS F. BERGMANN, DC, FICC
Professor
Chiropractic Methods Department
Northwestern Health Sciences University
Bloomington, Minnesota

PATRICIA C. BRENNAN, PhD
Dean of Research
National College of Chiropractic
Lombard, Illinois

BRIAN BUDGELL, DC, MSc.
Associate Professor
School of Health Sciences
Kyoto University
Kyoto, Japan

PETER CAUWENBERGS, DC, PhD
Director
Department of Anatomy
Canadian Memorial Chiropractic College
Toronto, Canada

GREGORY D. CRAMER, DC, PhD
Professor and Dean of Research
National University of Health Sciences
Lombard, Illinois

SUSAN A. DARBY, PhD
Associate Professor
Department of Anatomy
National University of Health Sciences
Lombard, Illinois

DOUG DAVISON, DC
Chiropractic Physician
Department of Musculoskeletal Medicine
Belmont Medical Associates
Cambridge, Massachusetts

BRIAN A. ENEBO, DC, MS
Chiropractor
Department of Integrative Medicine
University of Colorado Hospital
Aurora, Colorado

GLENN R. ENGEL, DC
Professor of Clinical Science
Department of Clinical Education
Canadian Memorial Chiropractic College
Toronto, Canada

L. JOHN FAYE, DC, FCCSS (HON.)
Private Practice
Los Angeles, California

DONALD FITZ-RITSON, BA, DC
Vice President
Physical Rehabilitation
International Managed Health Care
Toronto, Canada

RICHARD G. GILLETTE, MS, PhD
Professor of Neurophysiology
Division of Basic Sciences
Western States Chiropractic College
Portland, Oregon

ADRIAN GRICE, DC, FCCS
Professor
Division of Chiropractic Sciences
Canadian Memorial Chiropractic College
Toronto, Canada

MITCHELL HAAS, DC, MA
Professor and Dean of Research
Division of Research
Western States Chiropractic College
Portland, Oregon

CHARLES N.R. HENDERSON, DC, PHD
Associate Professor
Research Department
Palmer Center for Chiropractic Research
Davenport, Iowa

JOHN K. HYLAND, DC, MPH, DACBR,
DABCO
Research Associate
Parker Research Institute
Parker College of Chiropractic
Dallas, Texas

ROBERT D. MOOTZ, DC, DABCO
Associate Medical Director for Chiropractic
Department of Labor and Industries
State of Washington
Olympia, Washington

JOHN P. MROZEK, BA, DC, FCCS(C)
Dean
Undergraduate Programme
Canadian Memorial Chiropractic College
Toronto, Canada

DAVID M. PANZER, DC, DABCO
Adjunct Professor
Chiropractic Science Division
Western States Chiropractic College
Portland, Oregon

CYNTHIA K. PETERSON, RN, DC, DACBR,
M. MED, EDD, FCCR(C)
Professor, Chairperson
Department of Radiology

Canadian Memorial Chiropractic College
Toronto, Canada

REED B. PHILLIPS, DC, PHD
President
Southern California University of Health
Sciences
Whittier, California

DAVID R. SEAMAN, MS, DC
Assistant Professor
Palmer College of Chiropractic
Port Orange, Florida

ZOLTAN T. SZARAZ, DC, FLACA
Associate Professor
Division of Chiropractic Sciences
Canadian Memorial Chiropractic College
Toronto, Canada

JOHN A.M. TAYLOR, DC, DACBR
Professor of Radiology
Department of Radiology
New York Chiropractic College
Seneca Falls, New York

ALLAN G.J. TERRETT, DIPAPPSC, BAPPSC,
MAPPSC, FACCS, FICC
Associate Professor
School of Health Sciences
Royal Melbourne Institute of Technology
Bundoora, Australia

JOHN J. TRIANO, DC, PHD
Research Professor
Joint Biomedical Engineering Program
University of Texas at Arlington
Arlington, Texas

HOWARD VERNON, DC, FCCS(C)
Professor, Director
Centre for the Study of Spinal Health
Research
Canadian Memorial Chiropractic College
Toronto, Canada

Foreword

Nearly a decade after the publication of Dr. Gatterman's first edition of *Foundations of Chiropractic: Subluxation,* we are facing a virtual avalanche of new data that has propelled our concepts of the term *subluxation* into a new environment. No longer is it possible for the term, which has been most closely associated with chiropractic health care in recent generations, to be regarded as a chimera devoid of physical attributes. As in all productive scientific inquiry, these important new observations lead to the development of greatly expanded models, which in turn guide our further explorations into the nature of the nervous system and how its integrity is an essential—arguably the primary—component of overall health.

With our ever increasing awareness of preventive health care, chronic illness, cost issues, and side effects of many conventional treatments, it is virtually a foregone conclusion that the appearance of this second edition of Dr. Gatterman's book is not only welcome but necessary. In these pages we are presented with a broad range of new perspectives on subluxation, based upon a triad of approaches involving the systematic recording of more precise evidence, the development of more comprehensive theories that accommodate this new evidence, and the crafting of consensus statements that encompass the whole and ensure both comprehension and acceptance by the greater community.

Among its many attributes, this new edition indicates to us the power of basic research in that more recent observations with animal models have produced a series of unambiguous anatomical and biomechanical benchmarks that amply demonstrate the consequences of spinal fixation, which from several points of view is in fact a subluxation. Perhaps even more dramatic is the fact that these sequelae to spinal fixation become more pronounced with time and may eventually become irreversible. Elsewhere in this new edition, we find that in a discussion of headache, we are given more precise tools for diagnosis and find that correction of a subluxation as a presumed causative agent may be associated with symptom relief; indeed, discrete anatomical structures in the cervical spine appear to play a role in headache development.

Yet in other sections of this new edition are new models of subluxation. From a biomechanical viewpoint, spinal buckling is proposed as a new theoretical construct. And from a biochemical stance we gain a fresh perspective by means of a comprehensive discussion of the roles of the cell membrane, free oxidative radicals, and energy production as they relate to the joints, muscles, ligaments, and disc in the spine—ultimately presenting a more tangible construct of the subluxation complex than what had been proposed previously.

Depending on one's point of view, the term *subluxation* represents either a unique crossroads or a tug-of-war in our society. On one hand, to paraphrase Oliver Wendell Holmes, Jr., the term should not be regarded as crystallized and immutable, because it encompasses a living thought that therefore will shift according to the time and place in which it is used.[1] On the other hand, some degree of precision in self-expression is required, for as Mark Twain once suggested:

The difference between almost the right word & the right word is really a large matter—it's the difference between the lightning bug and the lightning.[2]

And so it is with "subluxation." Despite its history of usage, which has markedly exceeded that of chiropractic health care, it has sometimes been held up for derision by detractors of chiropractic as an opaque, inaccessible, or—even worse—unscientific or cultist term. Even more problematic is the fact that the term *subluxation* has been chastened at chiropractic research conferences,[3] is not being used by all researchers in recent scientific journals,[4] and is even suspected to be shunned by practicing chiropractors in their discussions with their own peers.[5] On the other hand, the term remains the basis by which several public entities, such as the U.S. government through its Medicare program, recognizes chiropractic care.

How is the dilemma surrounding "subluxation" therefore to be resolved? Clearly, the need to further explore and explicate this term remains acute. This book fulfills a major portion of that demand by attempting to refocus our attention on the term *subluxation* and its importance in our grasp, understanding, acceptance, and perhaps even embrace of chiropractic care.

Particularly noteworthy is the principle that subluxations exist in both manipulable and nonmanipulable forms, such that the terminology is not at all the discontinuous entity with its predecessor as often regarded by allopathic physicians. In its clinical presentations, this volume offers the reader discussions of cervicogenic headache and sympathetic syndromes; whiplash; thoracic outlet syndrome; and facet, intervertebral disc, sacroiliac, and coccygeal subluxation syndromes.

Yet the clinical presentations in and of themselves cannot be construed to indicate that the term *subluxation* is a finished work—a physical reality without the circumstantial attributes to which Oliver Wendell Holmes had alluded above.[2]

To do so would presume a certain arrogance, to say nothing of liability. Like Freud's evolving concept of the unconscious, subluxation has required and will likely continue to require many transformations and modifications before its full emergence into a new, holistic branch of health care. We must remember that, in its current state, the subluxation model *guides* rather than confines chiropractic and remains a useful concept with which to approach both future research and the patient. In other words, the subluxation remains a work in progress that, like any good scientific theory, must remain open to discussion and modifications as new evidence is accumulated in both further research and clinical observation.

Maintaining such an essential dialogue has been admirably achieved by the new findings presented in this book.

Given the facts that (1) subluxation cannot be defined uniquely by imaging[6]; (2) intraexaminer and interexaminer reliability of identifying motion or end feel restriction at specific segmental levels has been reported to be moderate to poor[7] although its validity was found to be excellent[8]; and (3) both animal models and more circumstantial observations in humans provide the best current evidence linking what we call "subluxation" with pain and/or dysfunction,[9] we need to maintain an open mind and sustain a vigorous dialogue rather than slink away in silence when faced with the *s* word. This work of Dr. Gatterman's serves as an important reminder that the term *subluxation* has a wealth of new information to support its continued usage and development in our understandings of health and health care.

Anthony L. Rosner, PhD, LLD (Hon.)
Director of Research and Education
Foundation for Chiropractic Education and Research
Brookline, Massachusetts

References

1. Gatterman MI. What's in a word? In: Gatterman MI, editor. Foundations of chiropractic: subluxation, 2nd ed. St. Louis: Mosby; 2005.
2. Twain M. Letter to George Bainton, October 15, 1888.
3. Research Agenda Conference IV. Arlington Heights, IL: July 23-25, 1999.
4. Wenban AB. Subluxation research: a survey of peer-reviewed chiropractic scientific journals. Chiropractic Journal of Australia 2003;33:122-30.
5. Haldeman S. Grand Rounds [Chair], Sixth Biennial Congress, World Federation of Chiropractic. Paris, France: May 24, 2001.
6. Van Schaik JPJ, Verbiest H, Van Schaik FDJ. Isolated spinous process deviations. A pitfall in the interpretation of the lumbar spine. Spine 1989;14(9):970-6.
7. Haas M, Panzer DM. Palpatory diagnosis of subluxation. In: Gatterman MI, editor. Foundations of chiropractic: subluxation. St. Louis: Mosby–Year Book; 1995. p. 56-67.
8. Jull G, Bogduk N, Marsland A. The accuracy of manual diagnosis for cervical zygapophyseal joint pain syndromes. Medical Journal of Australia 1988;148:233-6.
9. Rosner A. The role of subluxation in chiropractic. Arlington, VA: Foundation for Chiropractic Education and Research; 1997.

Preface

The second edition of *Foundations of Chiropractic: Subluxation*, like the first edition, is designed to provide a foundation textbook for the chiropractic profession. The idea for the first edition originated from a conference titled "Subluxation Revisited," held at Canadian Memorial Chiropractic College in Toronto. The **Consortium for Chiropractic Research (CCR)** terminology consensus process stimulated this conference, and many of the original presenters were members of the panels that developed and agreed to the terminology used in this book. Directed by the Standards of Care Committee of the CCR, this study was undertaken for the purpose of developing chiropractic nomenclature through consensus in the hope that clearer communication would be fostered. To facilitate nomenclature consensus, a model in the form of an algorithm was developed. Moving from small working groups that agreed to contentious terms, nominal and Delphi groups were struck that involved larger numbers and wide geographical and political representation. It is paramount that these terms and definitions not be cast in stone but rather be a platform for discourse and study of the issues important to the chiropractic profession. In time, some terms and definitions will no doubt evolve further, but it is equally important that the standardized terms and definitions be adopted and used as part of the daily dialogue of chiropractic practitioners, chiropractic educators, and chiropractic students.

Subsequent to the publication of the first edition, the topic of "subluxation revisited" was again discussed through a panel format at the **Research Agenda Conference** in 2003. As was the case with the first edition, panel members became contributors to the second edition. The ongoing debate in the chiropractic profession with regard to naming the primary lesion treated by chiropractors continues to spark much controversy. In 2004 the **European Chiropractic Union** included a presentation titled "Subluxation: Science or Science Fiction" that summarized much of the evidence included in this book. Failure to resolve the issues surrounding the use of the term *subluxation* continues to be a barrier to communication and fans the flames of disunity that continue to engulf the chiropractic profession. Those who would abandon the term *subluxation* in the hopes that the problems surrounding the term will be solved miss the point that a "subluxation" by any other name is still a "subluxation." Calling it a "spinal boo boo" or defining it as "an adjustment-seeking lesion" does not resolve the issue presented in Chapter 1.

Readers of this book are encouraged to keep an open mind, objectively evaluate the evidence, and examine and address the issues and theories presented in the second edition. If we are to move ahead as a unique profession, we must cease the song sung by the chorus that keeps adding to the synonyms for subluxation that has grown from the original 100 identified in 1995 to more than 300 in 2004. From a clinical perspective, it is essential that we address and document the evidence that is observed daily in chiropractic practice that describes the variety of syndromes that accompany subluxations in the patient's interest.

Meridel I. Gatterman

Acknowledgments

A second edition comes about because of the acceptance and popularity of the first edition. I am grateful therefore to the many students, chiropractic educators, and doctors of chiropractic who have found the first edition of *Foundations of Chiropractic: Subluxation* useful and valuable. I wish to acknowledge with thanks the assistance of the many people who have aided in the production of this book, particularly Alan Adams, Daniel Hansen, Henry Morrison, and Herbert Vear, who provided stimulus for the terminology study that initiated this work. This study was greatly helped by William Meeker and by the members of the **Consortium for Chiropractic Research** and the **Advisory Council to the Technique Committee of the American Chiropractic Association.** Without the participation of varied panel members who continued with the process through the multiple panel rounds, consensus would not have been achieved.

I am grateful to the contributors of the first edition and to those who provided revisions and new chapters to the second edition, making it even more comprehensive than the first. I wish also to thank librarians Lynn Attwood and Carol Lynn Webb, who provided valuable assistance in obtaining essential reference material.

I would like to acknowledge the editorial assistance provided by Christina Peterson for the Cervicogenic Headache chapter, Jennifer McClurkin for her research assistance for the Whiplash chapter, and the students and faculty of the Colorado Chiropractic College, who made subluxation syndrome problem solving a fruitful endeavor.

I would like to thank Donna Manello for serving as a chiropractic model and Robin Waterbury for serving as a patient model.

Gratitude is expressed to the staff of Elsevier for assistance in bringing this book to publication. I offer special thanks to Christie Hart for her patience and support and to Kristine Feeherty and Nicole Chilton, who have seen this project through to successful completion.

Finally, my love and appreciation go to my husband Mike for his continued support, understanding, and patience.

Contents

Part ONE

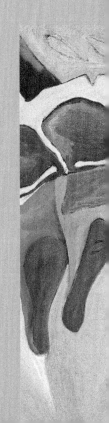

Subluxation
The Articular Lesion

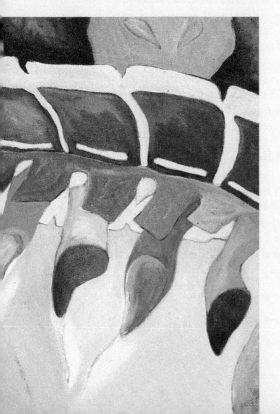

Central to the philosophy, science, and practice of chiropractic is the vertebral subluxation. Part One of this book discusses the fundamentals of subluxation, the primary articular lesion treated by chiropractors. Long one of the most controversial concepts of the principles of chiropractic, the enigmatic subluxation will be discussed in Part One through the reductionistic model of mechanical joint dysfunction. Palmer's early concept of the subluxation applied a mechanical model whereby the body part, that is, the spinal articulation, is not working, and the chiropractor fixes or adjusts it. The subluxation as a mechanical breakdown is like a carburetor that must be adjusted. A reductionistic practitioner might be satisfied with this analysis and send the car out of the shop after an adjustment. Following this model, Part One presents evidence of subluxation as mechanical joint dysfunction and establishes the foundation for the more complex theories presented in Part Two and the clinical manifestations of subluxation discussed in Part Three.

Chapter 1 "What's in a Word?" presents the terms and definitions related to subluxation, based on the nomenclature agreed to through nominal and Delphi consensus methods. These terms have been adopted by the Consortium for Chiropractic Research and the American Chiropractic Association House of Delegates. Issues related to subluxation that have generated semantic confusion and much heated debate during the past century are discussed.

Chapter 2 "Chiropractic Paradigms" discusses the development of a chiropractic model based on the subluxation concept agreed to through consensus by the Association of Chiropractic College Presidents. The process and historical sequence of events are presented.

Chapter 3 "Anatomy Related to Spinal Subluxation" describes the structural relationships associated with subluxation. This chapter describes the components of the spinal motion segment, the three-joint complex that forms the functional unit of the spine. An understanding of the structural relationship of the intervertebral disc with the two posterior facet joints is necessary for understanding of the mechanical interaction of the spinal joints. Pain that accompanies loss of articular function characteristic of subluxation is only comprehended with a thorough knowledge of the anatomic relationships of the spinal joints.

Chapter 4 "Animal Models in the Study of Subluxation and Manipulation: 1964-2004" discusses studies of animal models with experimentally induced vertebral misalignments, a component of subluxation. The methodology and findings of these studies are reviewed individually with comments on their methodology and findings. The models then are examined collectively, and their implications are synthesized into a coherent set of conclusions.

Chapter 5 "Palpatory Diagnosis of Subluxation" examines palpatory diagnostic criteria used to identify subluxation. Palpatory techniques have been used to diagnose and differentiate subluxations since the beginning of the art of manipulation. From the Renaissance and later, emphasized by Flexner, medicine has scorned the use of touch as being less reliable than visual and auditory procedures. Chiropractors have refined palpatory techniques, the diagnostic mainstay of manual therapy, along with the development of therapeutic manual procedures.

Chapter 6 "The Role of Radiography in Evaluating Subluxation" evaluates radiographic procedures used by the chiropractic profession to diagnose and differentiate spinal subluxation. Predominantly used by the medical profession to detect pathologic conditions, radiography has been used by chiropractors to detect mechanical as well as pathologic lesions. Methods used by the chiropractic profession to differentiate mechanical lesions are presented.

Chapter 7 "Chiropractic Technique" provides an outline of manual techniques used by chiropractors in the treatment of subluxations. Perfected to a sophisticated level, these procedures have been demonstrated to be safe and effective and serve as the primary therapeutic procedures used by chiropractors. Adjustive techniques used to treat subluxations through reflex mechanisms are included.

Chapter 8 "The Nonmanipulable Subluxation" discusses the diagnosis and treatment of subluxations that are not amenable to manipulative procedures. Motion segments that are unstable or ankylosed are not appropriately treated by thrust procedures, and in these cases spinal manipulation is contraindicated. Radiographic evidence of nonmanipulable subluxations is stressed.

A word is not a crystal, transparent and unchanged; it is the skin of a living thought and may vary greatly in color and content according to the circumstances and time in which it is used.

Oliver Wendell Holmes, Jr.

What's in a Word?

Meridel I. Gatterman

Key Words Adjustment, manipulable subluxation, manipulation, manual therapy, mobilization, subluxation, subluxation complex, subluxation syndrome

After reading this chapter you should be able to answer the following questions:

Question 1 Did the term *subluxation* originally come from the chiropractic profession?

Question 2 What is the definition of the word *subluxation*?

Question 3 Is more than one definition of *subluxation* practical?

Question 4 Explain the following issues related to the use of the word *subluxation*:

A) Historical D) Clinical

B) Philosophical E) Research

C) Political F) Economic

The word *subluxation* has been daubed in a kaleidoscope of colors and embodied with a multitude of meanings by chiropractors during the past 100 years. To some, it has become a holy word,[1] to others, an albatross to be discarded.[2] Currently, subluxation continues to be the most loved and hated, hotly debated, and consecrated term used by chiropractors. To add to the confusion, more than 100 synonyms for subluxation have been used (Table 1-1). If the term has become so "overburdened with clinical, political, and philosophical meaning and significance for chiropractors, that the concept that once helped to hold

Table 1-1

Subluxation Synonyms to 1993

Synonym	Author	Year	Synonym	Author	Year
Aberrant motion	Gatterman	1992	Fanning of interspinous space	Pate	1993
Abnormal joint motion	Lantz	1989			
	Gatterman	1992	Fixation	Homewood	1963
Acute cervical joint lock	Haas, Peterson	1992	Functional block	Dishman	1985
	DeBoer, Hansen	1993	Functional spinal lesion	Crawford	1992
Acute locked back	Wark	1831		Slosberg	1993
	Lantz	1989	Hyperemic subluxation	Hill	1949
Apophyseal subluxation	Hadley	1936	Hypermobility	Gatterman	1992
Articular derangement	Dishman	1985	Hypomobility	Brantington	1988
Articular dyskinesia	Slosberg	1993		Gatterman	1992
Blockage	Kunert	1965	Incomplete articular dislocation	Hubka	1990
Blocking	Kunert	1965			
	Good	1985	Instability of the posterior ligament complex	Pate (Cheshire)	1992
Cervical joint dysfunction	Salem Indust.	1992			
Chiropractic subluxation	Biedermann	1954			
	Brantingham	1988	Intersegmental instability	Pate	1993
	Chapman-Smith	1993	Intervertebral blocking	Brantingham	1988
Chiropractic subluxation complex	Dishman	1985	Intervertebral disrelationship	Watkins	1968
	Brantingham	1988	Joint aberration	Hubka	1990
Delayed instability	Pate	1993	Joint bind	Good	1985
Derangement	Collings	1960	Joint dysfunction	Northrup	1975
Dysarthritic lesion	Dalgleish	1960	Kinetic intersegmental subluxation	Haldeman	1975
Dysarthrosis	Dishman	1985			
Dysfunctional joint	Slosberg	1993	Kinetic subluxation	Watkins	1968
Dystopia	Gongal'skii, Kuftyreva	1992	Less than a locked dislocation	Watkins	1968
Erratic movement	Watkins	1968	Liga tights	Watkins (Smith)	1992
Facet joint dysfunction	Darrer	1993	Locked facet	Wood	1984
Facet syndrome	Mooney, Robertson	1976	Locking	Brantingham	1988
			Manipulable lesion	Haldeman	1979
Facet synovial impingement	Collins	1951	Manipulable joint lesion	Brantingham	1988
			Manipulable lesion	Hubka	1990
Facilitated segment	Dishman	1985	Mechanical disorder	Dishman (Suh)	1985

Table 1-1—cont'd

Subluxation Synonyms to 1993

Synonym	Author	Year
Mechanical musculoskeletal dysfunction	Boissonault, Bass	1990
Metameric dysfunction	Lohse-Busch	1989
Misalignment	Haas, Peterson	1992
	Sinh	1993
Motion restriction	Hubka	1990
Motor unit derangement complex	Vance, Gamburg	1992
Neuroarticular dysfunction	—	—
Neuroarticular subluxation	—	—
Neuroarticular syndrome	—	—
Neurobiomechanical (lesion)	Dishman	1985
Neurodysarthritic (lesion)	Dalgleish	1960
Neurodysarthrodynic (lesion)	Dalgleish	1960
Neurofunctional subluxation	—	—
Neurologic dysfunction	Watkins	1968
Neuromechanical lesion	—	—
Neuromuscular dysfacilitation	Slosberg	1993
Orthospondylodysarthritics	Dalgleish	1960
Osteologic lesion	Collins	?
Osteopathic articular lesion	Halliday	1936
Osteopathic lesion	Brantingham	1988
Osteopathic spinal lesion	Collins	?
Paravertebral subluxation	Haldeman	1975
Partial fixation	Watkins	1968
Posterior facet dysfunction	Haldeman	1975
Primary chiropractic lesion	Gatterman	1990
Pseudosubluxation	Pate	1990
Reflex dysfunction	Salem Indust.	1992
Restriction	Good	1985
	Slosberg	1993

Synonym	Author	Year
Sectional subluxation	Haldeman	1975
Segmental dysfunction	Pate	1993
Segmental vertebral hypomobility	Dishman	1985
Simple joint and muscle dysfunction without tissue damage	Mootz	1993
Slipping sacroiliac joints	Trostler	1938
Soft tissue ankylosis	Watkins	1968
Somatic dysfunction	Northrup	1975
Spinal boo boo	Rearing	1992
Spinal hypomobilities	Innes	1993
Spinal irritation	Wark	1831
Spinal joint blocking	Good	1985
Spinal joint complex	Dalgleish	1960
Spinal joint stiffening	Bourdillon	1982
Spinal kinesiopathology	Johnson	1985
Spinal subluxation	Haldeman	1975
Spondylodysarthritic lesions	Dalgleish	1960
Sprain	Palmer	1910
Stable cervical injury of the spine	Pate (Harris)	1993
Static intersegmental subluxation	Haldeman	1975
Structural disrelationship	Watkins	1968
Subluxation	Hieronymus	1746
Subluxation complex	Faye	1986
Subluxation complex myopathy	Peterson	1993
Subluxation syndrome	Gatterman	1992
Total fixation	Watkins	1968
Vertebral displacement	Kunert	1965
Vertebral dysfunction	Littlejohn	1992
Vertebral dyskinesia	Dishman	1985
Vertebral locking	Stoddard	1969
Vertebral subluxation complex	Faye	1976
Vertebral subluxation syndrome	Lantz	1989

Modified from Rome P, Terrett A.

The names in parentheses are original authors cited by others.

Note: Subsequent to publication of this table in 1995, Rome has identified 296 synonyms for subluxation. (Rome PL. Usage of chiropractic terminology in the literature: 296 ways to say "subluxation." Chiropractic Technique 1996;8:49-60.) Do I hear 500?

a young besieged profession together"[1] now divides and keeps it quarreling over basic semantics, why do we persist in using it? The obvious answer is provided by Terrett[3]: The concept of vertebral subluxation is central to chiropractic.

The notion that changing the word *subluxation* to another term will somehow change the clinical, political, and philosophical connotations is simply not rational. Changing the term used for the articular lesion treated by chiropractors (subluxation) does not eradicate the clinical, political, and philosophical issues that surround the construct—it evades them.[2,3] We have found it expedient to clearly and simply define the term *subluxation* and to objectively address issues surrounding the construct. The conceptual definition of subluxation has been the foundation on which chiropractic science has stood. It is time to provide an operational definition of subluxation by identifying the testable components of misalignment, aberrant motion, and dysfunction included in the definition. With these components delineated, we can examine current data and further study the topic of our discourse.

Defining Subluxation

The definitions of *subluxation* and related terms used in this book were developed by consensus methods that used an algorithm developed by Gatterman and Hansen[4] (Figure 1-1). These terms were agreed on through both nominal and Delphi methods that included broad geographic, philosophical, and political representation. This project was funded and supported by the Consortium for Chiropractic Research (CCR). Included in the 60-member Delphi panel were members of the American Chiropractic Association (ACA) Council on Technique, which adopted the terms in 1993. Subsequently, the House of Delegates of the ACA endorsed the terms that are now included in a number of leading chiropractic textbooks.[5-9] The field of terms includes *subluxation,* the articular lesion that is less than a dislocation; *manipulable subluxation,* a lesion amenable to chiropractic manipulation; *subluxation complex,* the theoretical model that describes the widespread effects of subluxation; and *subluxation syndrome,* the clinical manifestations that include the associated symptoms and physical signs of a subluxation.

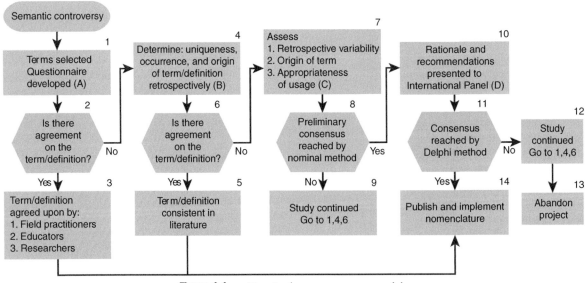

Figure 1-1   Terminology assessment model.

Each term is expanded on in relation to the principles of chiropractic, and support for these principles is the subject matter of this text. Essential for the definition of subluxation has been clarification of the terms *motion segment* and *spinal motion segment*. Definitions of therapeutic procedures used by chiropractors include the terms *manual therapy, manipulation, mobilization,* and most important, *adjustment*. To arrive at consensus for terms commonly used by chiropractors, the origin of each term was examined relative to the concepts that underlie the profession. (See Figure 1-1.)

Origin of the Word *Subluxation*

The root words for the term *subluxation* come from a combination of the Greek *sub* and *lux*, meaning "less than a dislocation." In 1746 Hieronymus[10] identified characteristics of a subluxation, stating the following:

> ...subluxation of joints is recognized by lessened motion of the joints, by slight change in position of the articulating bones and pain...

His characterization does not differ significantly from the consensus definition of the nominal and Delphi panels of the CCR that defined subluxation as follows:

subluxation   a motion segment in which alignment, movement integrity, and/or physiologic function are altered although contact between the joint surfaces remains intact.

Subsequent to the conclusion of the CCR consensus process, Swere[11] suggested that the word "partially" be added for clarity:

subluxation   a motion segment in which alignment, movement integrity, and/or physiological function are altered although contact between the joint surfaces remains *partially* intact.

The CCR definition of subluxation allows for physiologic dysfunction, which was described in 1821 by Harrison[12] as follows:

> When any of the vertebrae become displaced or too prominent, the patient experiences inconvenience from a local derangement in the nerves of the part.

He, in consequence, is tormented with a train of nervous symptoms, which are as obscure in their origin as they are stubborn in their nature....

Harrison considered both alignment and motion when describing subluxations. In 1824 he wrote the following:

> The articulating extremities are only partially separated, not imperfectly disjoined...
> and
> ...the articular motions are imperfectly performed, because the surfaces of the bones do not fully correspond.[13]

Although Palmer focused on vertebral displacement or misalignment in his early definition of chiropractic,[14-16] he also wrote extensively on the neurologic effects produced by subluxation.[16] In perhaps the earliest published chiropractic text, *Modernized Chiropractic,*[17] authors Smith, Langsworthy, and Paxson wrote the following:

> In the case of a simple vertebral subluxation, the vertebra is not lodged in a fixed and permanent abnormal position like a displaced brick in the wall; to consider it so is preposterous for it is a moveable bone in a flexible and moveable column. A simple subluxated vertebra differs from a normal vertebra only in its field of motion, but because of its being subluxated, its various positions of rest are differently located than when it was a normal vertebra....its field of motion may be too great in some directions and too small in others.

Within a decade of its inception, those in the chiropractic profession were arguing over the definition of subluxation, the primary focus of chiropractic treatment. Was it misalignment, altered motion, or joint dysfunction? Why not any one, two, or all three?

Manipulable and Nonmanipulable Subluxations

Not all subluxations respond to manipulation; those subluxations that can be seen on radiographs are often nonmanipulable pathologic subluxations that cannot be reversed or that require surgical repair. (See Chapter 8.) It is important that the definition of subluxation be broad enough to include the medical concept of subluxation severe enough to be visible on radiograph as well as the subtler manipulable subluxation detectable by palpation. The manipulable subluxation is further defined as follows:

manipulable subluxation a subluxation in which altered alignment, movement, or function can be improved by manual thrust procedures.

The term *subluxation complex* is used when addressing the complex of neurologic effects theorized to be caused by articular subluxation. This complex has been defined as follows:

subluxation complex a theoretical model of motion segment dysfunction (subluxation) that incorporates the complex interaction of pathologic changes in nerve, muscle, ligamentous, vascular, and connective tissues.

Faye[18] first described the subluxation complex in the mid-1970s. Building on the work of Illi,[19] Gillet,[20] Homewood,[21] and Janse,[22] Faye[18] formulated a theory that the chiropractic spinal adjustment (manipulation) restores normal joint motion, which in turn normalizes physiologic function. The subluxation complex has been developed further[23,24] and is discussed in Chapter 9.

Leach[25] has noted that the CCR definition lacks the central Palmerian concept that subluxation may affect organ function and general health. In response to this he has defined *subluxation complex* as follows:

subluxation complex a theoretical model of articular spinal lesions that incorporates the complex interaction of inflammatory, degenerative, and pathologic changes in nerve, muscle, ligamentous, vascular, and connective tissues and *may influence organ system function and health.*

Subluxation syndrome is the term used to describe the clinical manifestations of subluxation (i.e., articular lesion) and is defined as follows:

subluxation syndrome an aggregate of signs and symptoms that relate to pathophysiology or dysfunction of spinal and pelvic motion segments or to peripheral joints.

Most widely recognized of these syndromes are mechanical back pain, neck pain, and cervicogenic (vertebrogenic) headache. Chiropractic practitioners are familiar with other syndromes such as sacroiliac, rib, and facet joint subluxation. Each has its own aggregate of signs and symptoms characteristic of different spinal regions. The clinical manifestations of subluxation syndromes are discussed in Part Three of this text.

The terms *subluxation complex* and *subluxation syndrome* are used to broaden the idea of the effects of subluxation without attaching untested theories to the description of the articular lesion that responds to manipulation.

Why Different Definitions of Subluxation?

In a guest editorial[26] published in the *Chiropractic Journal of Australia* following the 2003 Chiropractic Research Agenda conference, it was noted that "a single definition fits all" for subluxation is not pragmatic. Nonetheless, different expressions of the same concept must be consistent across cultural domains. What is useful to the researcher may not be entirely appropriate for the educator. Similarly, what expresses the focus of the chiropractic clinician may be inappropriate for the orthopedic surgeon. Politicians may prefer to use a different term altogether, one that has greater colloquial familiarity or lacks political or legal coloring. The premise that "different expressions of subluxation are needed with relevance to different cultural domains" was central to the consensus process used to develop chiropractic nomenclature published in 1994.[4] Examples of terms relevant to the specific interests of different cultural domains are presented in Table 1-2.

Politicians are interested in widely accepted terms that carry little or no political or legal baggage. Consequently, *motion segment dysfunction*, a common-currency term, might be preferred. Much misunderstanding by the medical community arises from the medical use of the term *subluxation* to indicate an unstable segment that is less than a dislocation. Chiropractors would agree that nonmanipulable subluxations, some of which may require surgical repair, are not appropriate

Table 1-2

Terms Relevant to the Specific Interest of Different Chiropractic Domains

Term	Characteristics	Domain
Subluxation	Articular lesion	Researchers
Subluxation complex	Theoretical model	Educators
Subluxation syndrome	Signs and symptoms	Practitioners
Motion segment dysfunction	Common currency	Politicians
Medical subluxation	Unstable segment	Surgeons

From Gatterman MI. Guest editorial: subluxation revisited. Chiro J Aust 2003;33:41-2.

targets for forceful thrust procedures. (See Chapter 8.)

The Functional Unit of the Spine

In any definition, words or phrases that need clarifying must be clearly stated. So it is with the term *motion segment*. The need for a term that can be applied to peripheral joints as well as to spinal joints fostered the following definition:

motion segment a functional unit made up of two adjacent articulating surfaces and the connecting tissues binding them to each other.

The following definition is more specifically related to the joints of the spine:

spinal motion segment two adjacent vertebrae and the connecting tissues binding them to each other.

The idea of the three-joint spinal motion segment as a functional unit originated with Junghanns,[27] who coined the term *bewegungssegment*. The inaccurate translation[28,29] of the German word to *motor segment* in the English edition of the book printed in 1971 was clouded further when the term was modified to *motor unit* and popularized through the proceedings of the NINCDS mono-

graph, *The Research Status of Spinal Manipulative Therapy,* published in 1975.[30] The longtime use of "motor unit" by physiologists in reference to a single motor neuron and the group of muscle fibers that it innervates has precipitated the need for clarification of the original concept of *motion segment* as well as standardization of the term.

Defining Chiropractic Treatment Methods

Chiropractic treatment has been directed traditionally toward restoration of function and has not been designed solely to relieve pain. Just as the primary lesion treated by chiropractors has been subluxation, the primary chiropractic technique has used manual procedures to treat the body. As with the term *subluxation,* much confusion and controversy have surrounded the use of terms and definitions that describe chiropractic treatment methods. To clarify the procedures used by chiropractors, the terms *manual therapy, manipulation, mobilization,* and *adjustment* were subjected to the consensus process. The definitions arrived at are as follows:

manual therapy procedures by which the hands directly contact the body to treat the articulations or soft tissues.

This term generated little controversy but is included because it has been used synonymously with the terms *manipulation* and *spinal manipulative therapy.* If terms that include manual procedures are used interchangeably, mobilization may inadvertently be considered a form of manipulation. It is necessary to differentiate manipulation from mobilization because recent studies have indicated the greater effectiveness of thrust procedures (manipulation) in the treatment of back pain. Early studies did not make this distinction, which may explain equivocal data regarding the effectiveness of manipulation. As more studies are undertaken, significant differences between thrust and nonthrust procedures may emerge, making this distinction even more critical. When mobilization is considered a form of manipulative therapy, unknowing patients may assume that they have received manipulation when they have not. They are therefore denied the possible benefits of thrust techniques.

In 1991 a RAND Corporation study[31] of appropriateness of spinal manipulation for low-back pain defined manipulation as a thrust procedure. Using this study as a basis for their deliberations, those participating in the consensus process defined *manipulation* as follows:

manipulation   a manual procedure that involves a directed thrust to move a joint past the physiologic range of motion without exceeding the anatomic limit.

To differentiate manipulation from mobilization (a nonthrust procedure), the following definition was agreed on:

mobilization   movement applied singularly or repetitively within or at the physiologic range of joint motion, without imparting a thrust or impulse, with the goal of restoring joint mobility.

Next to the term *subluxation,* the use of the word *adjustment* has sparked the most heated debate. Participants in the consensus process agreed that when chiropractors apply an adjustment, there is intent to influence more than joint mechanics and related pain. They incorporated a reference to changes in neurophysiologic function in the definition. Although some proposed that *adjustment* should be restricted to mean specific short-lever, high-velocity, low-amplitude thrust techniques, a broader definition emerged. It includes procedures routinely used by chiropractors that fall outside this narrow category. The resulting definition is as follows:

adjustment   any chiropractic therapeutic procedure that uses controlled force, leverage, direction, amplitude, and velocity directed at specific joints or anatomic regions. Chiropractors commonly use such procedures to influence joint and neurophysiologic function.

Although reference to neurophysiologic function is omitted in the definition of *manipulation,* this is not to say that such neurophysiologic effects do not occur. On the contrary, it may be demonstrated that manual thrust procedures through reflex mechanisms produce widespread effects. These mechanisms are the subject of Part Two, in which data are presented that support Palmer's later contention that the body is not a simple machine but rather a complex interaction of systems mediated by the nervous system.[16] To those traditionalists who want chiropractors to use the term *adjustment* instead of *manipulation,* it should be noted that Palmer used the term *manipulation* to describe his early techniques; not until later in the twentieth century was the term *adjustment* used for Palmer's unique style of manipulation.[14]

Issues of Chiropractic Terminology

Unfortunately, when it comes to the word *subluxation,* too many chiropractors act quite like Humpty Dumpty in Lewis Carroll's *Through the Looking Glass:* "'When I use a word,' Humpty Dumpty said, in rather a scornful tone, 'it means just what I choose it to mean—neither more nor less.'"[32]

Such an attitude toward the use of the word *subluxation,* as with any term, does not facilitate communication. Lawrence[33] stated that "...one of the greatest challenges facing the chiropractic profession today is simply to learn how to communicate with one another." He emphasized the seriousness of miscommunication for the chiropractic profession because of semantic confusion by stating that "semantic difficulties have hampered our overall development."

Oppositional Thinking

Much of the controversy surrounding the use of the term *subluxation* has involved dualism or oppositional thinking by which the phenomenon is "one or the other" but not both. If a subluxation is *A,* it therefore cannot be *B.* Dualism handed down from the ancient Greeks is the enemy of compromise and, in the end, consensus. Dominance is the foundation of dualism. If I am right, you must be wrong.

Examples of such thinking include views that subluxation is an alteration of motion in which the misalignment component is nonexistent or unlikely or it is a medical term to describe displacement without joint dysfunction.[34] It seems probable that subluxation refers to impaired mobility with or without positional alteration. In many cases, the misalignment component is not discernible by current technologic methods and cannot be used as the sole criterion for subluxation detection. Slight misalignment cannot be accurately ascertained by analysis of radiographs; in those cases where misalignment is gross enough to be detected by plain film radiographs, manipulation may be contraindicated because of the potential for excessive motion in the compromised joint. Howe and Phillips[35] have both noted the following:

Any method of spinographic interpretation which utilizes millimetric mensurations from any set of preselected points is very likely to be faulty, because structurally asymmetry is universal in all vertebrae.

Does this mean that to be identifiable, a subluxation must be gross enough to be detected on radiographs? Some consider that the term *subluxation* should be reserved for radiographically measurable disrelationships of joint surfaces. Others suggest that subluxation should be reserved for static positional relationships measured by in vitro investigations.[36] For 100 years, have chiropractors been treating a lesion detectable only in vitro? Still others claim that subluxation has not been measured in any case. At the extreme, if a subluxation is a misalignment, then it is not motion restriction but rather a vertebra out of place.

Alternatively, the subluxation is viewed as motion restriction and no component of malposition should be considered. This is attractive to some, given the current lack of methods available to consistently detect spatial disrelationships. Logic leads us to conclude that we are dealing with a functional entity involving restricted vertebral movement, because it is the movement-restriction component of manipulable subluxation that responds to thrust procedures. As yet, reliable measurement of motion segment movement remains as elusive as radiographic detection of subtle misalignment. Does this mean that pain is the sole reliable criterion for detection of subluxation? What of the nonmanipulable subluxation

with excess motion and instability? Is it not painful? To properly identify and define the subluxation, consideration should be given to all three components:
1. Misalignment or spatial relationship
2. Excessive or restricted motion
3. Dysfunction with or without pain

One component should not be used to describe or detect a subluxation to the exclusion of any other, nor must all three components be present. Similarly, we saw that the prechiropractic use of the word *subluxation* included slight change in position of the articulating bones, lessened motion of the joints, and pain. Why must we now narrow the scope of the term *subluxation* to a lesion with only one of the early distinguishing features?

Issues Surrounding the Use of the Word *Subluxation*

Historical Issues
Early chiropractic terminology became distinct to differentiate the new profession from both osteopathy and medicine. Whereas the osteopath manipulated the osteopathic lesion, the chiropractor manipulated (and later adjusted) the subluxation. Palmer sought to differentiate chiropractic from osteopathy, probably in response to charges of having stolen ideas from the founder Still.[37] The distinction is that chiropractors do not diagnose symptoms and treat disease; rather, they analyze the spine and adjust subluxations, although a successful legal defense against early charges of practicing medicine without a license has led to much isolation and great misunderstanding of the chiropractic profession. Cleveland has noted that adding to the controversy is the concept put forth by B.J. Palmer that clinically relevant subluxation is restricted solely to displacement of the upper cervical vertebrae.[7]

Philosophical Issues
The use of the word *subluxation* as a metaphor has created a philosophic issue whereby it becomes like the medical use of the word *disease*,

the eradication of which restores homeostasis of the body and eliminates all human ailments.[38] Although it is yet to be conclusively demonstrated that, as Harrison wrote in 1821, "an almost infinite variety and endless complication of nervous symptoms"[12] may result from subluxation, this theory must be kept in perspective, examined, and tested. Criticism of this basic premise's validity must not be automatically rejected as an attack on the chiropractic profession but viewed instead as a challenge to be met. Evidence supporting the validity of Palmer's theory[16] that subluxations cause functional changes in the nervous system is presented in the following chapters. Emotional and unbending adherence to this construct without critical evaluation has polarized the profession. The notion that subluxation is the cause of all disease is not rationally defensible; much derision of the chiropractic profession has been brought on by dogmatic proponents of this theory.[39] Evidence must be evaluated and integrated to support the principles of chiropractic theory.

Political Issues

Political controversy surrounding the use of the word *subluxation* stems from the medical caveat that to qualify as a subluxation, visual evidence must be demonstrated on radiographs.[40] This is not stated, however, in the following dictionary definitions of subluxation:

1. Subluxation: A partial dislocation[41]
2. Subluxation: Partial dislocation (as of one of the bones in a joint)[42]
3. Subluxation: An incomplete or partial dislocation[43]
4. Subluxation: A partial or incomplete dislocation[44]
5. Subluxation: An incomplete luxation or dislocation; though a relationship is altered, contact between joint surfaces remains[45]

Radiographic visualization of a subluxation was the initial criterion for reimbursement of subluxation treatment by chiropractors under the United States Medicare and Medicaid Acts. Because the reliability of radiographic detection of manipulable subluxations has been questioned, some believe that by abandoning the term this

issue can be sidestepped. What then of Medicare and Medicaid coverage for chiropractic patients when the government recognizes detection and correction of subluxation as the primary functions of the doctor of chiropractic? The emotional responses to this political issue by some members of the chiropractic community stem from those who deny the existence of manipulable lesions on the grounds that they are not consistently seen on radiographs. Rather than falling prey to this political ploy, we must clearly determine and agree on criteria that can be used to detect manipulable subluxations, the primary issue surrounding the subluxation as a clinical entity.

Those who wish to abandon the term in the face of medical territoriality and those who cling to dogmatic philosophic beliefs once again polarize us. A more reasonable solution seems to be a classification of subluxation in which the most severe lesions are seen on radiographs and are not always amenable to manipulation. The less extreme lesions, still subluxations but of lesser degree, are nonetheless articular lesions; they are just less severe than dislocations. In many cases they are manipulable subluxations.

Medical use of the term *subluxation* for the lesion that responds to manipulation (as we have noted) existed before the advent of radiographs.[3] It continues to be used in this manner by modern practitioners. Examples include the following:

"Sacroiliac subluxation" implies that ligamentous stretching has been sufficient to permit the ilium to slip on the sacrum. An irregular prominence on one articular surface becomes wedged upon another prominence of the other articular surface, the ligaments are taut, reflex muscle spasm is intense, and pain is severe and continuous until reduction is effected. The displacement is so slight that it cannot be recognized in roentgenograms....The pain of subluxation is often relieved dramatically and suddenly by manipulation.[46]

and

Subluxated Facet Joint: The facet syndrome, which can cause severe back pain, consists of a subluxation or partial dislocation of a lumbar vertebral facet joint. This is the condition most likely to be relieved when a chiropractor manipulates the spine.[47]

It is apparent that medical use of the term *subluxation* when referring to the lesion treated by manipulation does not require radiographic evidence to support the existence of this clinical entity.

Another important political reason to maintain the use of the term *subluxation* is that a number of state statutes specifically identify the practice of chiropractic either directly or implicitly with subluxation or the elements of the subluxation complex. Included are Arizona, Connecticut, Delaware, Florida, Idaho, Maine, Massachusetts, New York, and the District of Columbia.[7] The Federal Workers' Compensation Program identifies and defines chiropractic services as follows:

> The term "physician" includes chiropractors only to the extent that their reimbursable services are limited to treatment consisting of manual manipulation of the spine to correct a subluxation.

Is it any wonder that physical therapists are eager to adopt the term *subluxation* so that they, too, can be reimbursed for treating the ubiquitous subluxation.

Clinical Issues

As previously noted, detection is the primary clinical issue surrounding the subluxation concept. It is ironic that an effective method of treatment has existed for centuries, yet there is no agreement on the criteria for detecting the lesion to be treated. Various palpation procedures, the traditional means used to detect subluxation, have been developed; these methods are under attack despite studies that have demonstrated both reliability and validity.[48-51] Difficulty arises in describing palpatory procedures because we use one-dimensional language to conceptualize a three-dimensional abstraction. Diagnosis of the manipulable subluxation is dependent on the kinesthetic perception of the palpating chiropractor, something akin to reading Braille because it is three dimensional and difficult to translate verbally. This phenomenon, which may account for the greater intrarater reliability than interrater reliability, must be better understood if we are to improve the chiropractor's diagnostic predictability. (See Chapter 5.)

The dogmatic irrationality exhibited by some regarding the detection of subluxation is embodied in the following quotation: "A chiropractic case is one with a subluxation.... We take a case even though our instrumentation doesn't show a subluxation because we know it's there."[52] It is more reasonable to determine objectively the most valid and reliable method for detection of subluxations than to argue over which method of detection is most effective. The detection of subluxations has given rise to a multitude of technique systems that apply a cookbook approach to diagnosis of chiropractic disorders. These include muscle testing, leg length checks, and finite radiographic-marking procedures. The medical community's use of pain syndromes as the criteria for manipulative therapy is not specific enough to be widely useful in chiropractic diagnoses and analyses of mechanical disorders of the spine. As the primary diagnostic criterion, the existence of pain does not aid the chiropractor in differentiating between manipulable and nonmanipulable subluxations and pathology.

Research Issues

Wenban[53] documented the absence of the term *subluxation* and, in some cases, the associated concepts in a survey of peer-reviewed scientific journals. He found that only 6.3% of the original research published in seven leading scientific journals during the period from 1990 to 1999 included the term *subluxation* in titles, abstracts, or clinical trials. He identified several possible explanations for this, including the following:

- Chiropractic researchers did carry out subluxation-related research but chose to publish it somewhere other than the seven peer-reviewed journals included in the survey.
- The body of an original research article may have contained the term *subluxation* and information pertaining to subluxation, but such an article may not have included the word in its title, abstract, or index terms.
- The title, abstract, or index terms included the term *subluxation,* but the text of the original research article did not contain information pertaining to subluxation.

- The chiropractic research community may have conducted subluxation-related research but abandoned the term.
- Except for a handful of chiropractic researchers who seemed to publish predominantly in the *Chiropractic Research Journal*, most largely abandoned research of the entity that many practicing chiropractors choose to call subluxation.

In discussing the possibilities Wenban does not discount any one. Many chiropractic researchers have stopped using the term *subluxation*, preferring a term less clinically, politically, and philosophically charged. This is understandable when the investigator seeks funding from external agencies that can have a bias against the term *subluxation*. A show of hands at a research agenda conference (RAC) demonstrated a preference for abandoning the term; just one researcher eloquently made a case for its continued use. (See Chapter 4.)

Those who want medical recognition at the expense of the use of terminology unique to the chiropractic profession may be throwing the baby out with the bath water. The irony is that if the chiropractic community chooses to divest itself of unique terminology, there is the risk of being relegated to the position of second-rate physical therapists allowed to treat mechanical back pain with some headaches and neck pain (if we are lucky), while first-rate physical therapists will be the ones treating subluxations.

Economic Issues

Perhaps the most damaging of all issues, considering today's economy and the escalating cost of health care, is the overtreatment of subluxations charged to third-party payers. Ongoing treatment of subluxations attributable to work-related and personal injuries that, in most cases, have long since healed strains the credibility of the chiropractic profession. It is imperative that chiropractors differentiate the subluxation leading to joint dysfunction from tissue abnormalities. Simple subluxations that exhibit only restricted motion respond rapidly to manipulation, usually in one or two treatments. More seriously injured joints with injured holding elements and damage to sur-

rounding soft tissue take much longer to heal. It is essential that the chiropractor make two types of assessment. The first is a biomechanical analysis to assess the site and nature of the subluxation. This determines where and whether manipulation and other adjustments are appropriate. The second is a diagnosis to ascertain the extent of damage and to determine the type of adjunct therapy that will hasten the healing process. The first diagnosis (biomechanical analysis) is necessary to determine the functional component of the patient's condition, including identification and description of any subluxation that is present. The second diagnosis gives the patient's prognosis based on pathologic changes that affect healing time. Both the functional and pathologic diagnoses must be noted in the name of ethical and legal recordkeeping, and both are necessary when seeking insurance reimbursement.[54]

Conclusion

The establishment of any profession requires terminology unique to that profession. Unless chiropractors would become ancillary to medicine in the same way that physical therapists and dentists are (akin to going from sharecroppers to slaves),[55] it is imperative that the chiropractic profession continue to develop and maintain its distinctive nomenclature. This is not to say that chiropractors should cling to outdated concepts and ambiguous terms. It is incumbent on the chiropractic profession to come to consensus whereby key terms used to describe chiropractic procedures and practices are used universally. The chiropractic profession has long enjoyed clinical legitimacy. If we are to move into the realm of scientific legitimacy, we must operationally define the terms we use for the methods we employ and, most importantly, the concepts and hypotheses that we investigate. Chiropractors do not have to be adversarial to medicine nor do they have to give up their principles to a hegemonic health care system dominated by treating disease as opposed to promoting health.

Chiropractic science is considered a poorly organized science by many. The first step in the organization of any science is the establishment of nomenclature that is widely recognized and accepted. What is in the word *subluxation?* The chiropractic subluxation is a subtler lesion than the radiographically recognized medical subluxation. For thousands of years before the advent of radiography, manipulation was employed to alleviate pain and loss of function from joint lesions less than a luxation or complete dislocation. For more than 100 years, chiropractors have successfully diagnosed and treated manipulable subluxations, thereby relieving much human suffering. A foundation of the chiropractic profession is the primary lesion treated with manual therapy—the subluxation.

References

1. Keating J. Science and politics and the subluxation. AJCM 1988;1:107-9.
2. Haldeman S. In: Inglis BD, Fraser B, Penfield BR. Chiropractic in New Zealand: report of the Commission of Inquiry. Wellington, New Zealand: PD Hesselberg, Government Printer; 1979. p. 55.
3. Terrett A. The search for the subluxation: an investigation of medical literature to 1985. Chiropr Hist 1987; 7:29-33.
4. Gatterman MI, Hansen D. Development of chiropractic nomenclature through consensus. J Manipulative Physiol Ther 1994;17:302-9.
5. Gatterman MI, editor. Foundations of chiropractic: subluxation. St. Louis: Mosby; 1995.
6. Peterson DH, Bergmann TF. Chiropractic technique. 2nd ed. St. Louis: Mosby; 2002.
7. Cleveland CS. Vertebral subluxation. In: Redwood D, Cleveland CS. Fundamentals of chiropractic. St. Louis: Mosby; 2003. p. 129-53.
8. Gatterman MI. Chiropractic management of spine-related disorders. 2nd ed. Baltimore: Lippincott, Williams & Wilkins; 2004.
9. Leach RA. The chiropractic theories: a textbook of scientific research. 4th ed. Baltimore: Lippincott, Williams & Wilkins; 2004.
10. Hieronymus JH. De luxationibus et subluxationibus [thesis]. Jena; 1746.
11. Swere J. Personal communication. 2004.
12. Harrison E. Observations respecting the nature and origin of the common species of disorders of the spine: with critical remarks on the opinions of former writers on this disease. London Med Phys J. 1821;45:103-22.
13. Harrison E. Observations on the pathology and treatment of spinal diseases. London Med Phys J 1824;51:350-64.
14. Palmer DD. Chiropractic workshop. The Chiropractic 1897;17:4.
15. Palmer DD. Chiropractic. The Chiropractic 1899;26:1.
16. Palmer DD. The chiropractor's adjuster: the science, art, and philosophy of chiropractic. Portland, OR: Portland Printing House; 1910.
17. Smith OG, Langsworthy SM, Paxson MC. Modernized chiropractic. Vol. 1. Cedar Rapids, MI: Lawrence Press; 1906. p. 26.
18. Faye LJ. Spinal motion palpation and clinical considerations of the lumbar spine and pelvis [lecture notes]. Huntington Beach, CA: Motion Palpation Institute; 1986.
19. Illi FW. The spinal column: lifeline of the body. Chicago: National College of Chiropractic; 1950.
20. Gillet H. The anatomy and physiology of spinal fixations. J Natl Chiro Assoc 1963;33:22-4,63-6.
21. Homewood AE. The neurodynamics of the vertebral subluxation. 3rd ed. St. Petersburg, FL: Valkyrie; 1977.
22. Janse J. History of the development of chiropractic concepts: chiropractic terminology. In: Goldstein M, editor. The research status of spinal manipulative therapy. Bethesda, MD: Government Printing Office; 1975. p. 25-42.
23. Dishman R. Review of the literature supporting a scientific basis for the chiropractic subluxation complex. J Manipulative Physiol Ther 1985;8:163-74.
24. Lantz CA. The vertebral subluxation complex. ICA Int Rev Chiropractic 1989;(Sept/Oct):37-61.
25. Leach RA. The chiropractic theories. 4th ed. Baltimore: Lippincott, Williams & Wilkins; 2003. p. 8.
26. Gatterman MI. Subluxation revisited. Chiropractic J Australia 2003;33:41-2.
27. Schmorl G, Junghanns H. Beseman EF, trans-ed. The human spine in health and disease. 2nd ed. New York: Grune and Stratton; 1971. p. 35-9.
28. Gatterman MI. Lost in translation. JCCA 1978; 22:131.
29. Oestreich AE. Inaccurate translation can cause a multitude of problems in medical communication. AMWAJ 1992;(July):2-4.
30. Goldstein M, editor. The research status of spinal manipulative therapy. Bethesda, MD: NINCDS; 1975. US Department of Health Education, and Welfare publication no (NIH) 76-988 (NINCDS monograph no 15).
31. Shekelle PG, Adams AH, Chassin MR, Hurwitz EL, Phillips RB, Brook RH. The appropriateness of spinal manipulation for low-back pain: project overview and literature review. Santa Monica, CA: RAND Corporation; 1991. RAND document no R4025/1-CCR/FCER.
32. Carroll L. Through the looking glass. New York: Alfred A. Knopf; 1992. p. 254 (originally published in 1865).
33. Lawrence D. Toward a common language [editorial]. J Manipulative Physiol Ther 1988;11:1-2.
34. Brantingham JW. A survey of literature regarding the behavior, pathology, etiology, and nomenclature of the chiropractic lesion. ACA J Chiropractic 1985;19:8.
35. Phillips RB. The use of x-rays in spinal manipulative therapy. In: Haldeman S, editor. Modern developments in the principles and practice of chiropractic. East Norwalk, CT: Appleton-Century-Crofts; 1979. p. 189-208.

36. Hubka MJ. Another critical look at the subluxation hypothesis. Chiro Technique 1990;2:27-9.

37. Brantingham JW. Still and Palmer: the impact of the first osteopath and the first chiropractor. Chiro History 1986;6:19-22.

38. Keating JC. The evolution of Palmer's metaphors and hypotheses. Philosophical Constructs for the Chiropractic Profession 1992;2:9-19.

39. Keating JC. Toward a philosophy of the science of chiropractic. Stockton, CA: Stockton Foundation for Chiropractic Research; 1992. p. 25-49.

40. Watkins RJ. Subluxation terminology since 1746. JCCA 1968;4:20-4.

41. Urdan L, editor. Mosby's medical and nursing dictionary. St. Louis: Mosby; 1983. p. 1032.

42. Pease RW, editor. Webster's medical desk dictionary. Springfield, MA: Merriam-Webster; 1986. p. 685.

43. Taylor EJ, editor. Illustrated medical dictionary. 27th ed. Philadelphia: WB Saunders; 1986. p. 1599.

44. Davis CL, editor. Tabor's cyclopedic medical dictionary. 16th ed. Philadelphia: FA Davis; 1989. p. 1772.

45. Hensyl WR, editor. Stedman's medical dictionary. 25th ed. Baltimore: Williams & Wilkins; 1990. p. 1494.

46. Turek SL. Orthopaedics principles and their application. 3rd ed. Philadelphia: JB Lippincott; 1977. p. 1469.

47. Keim HA, Kirkaldy-Willis WH. Low back pain. Clin Symp 1980;32:1-35.

48. Jull G, Bogduk N, Marsland A. The accuracy of manual diagnosis for cervical zygapophyseal joint pain syndromes. Med J Aust 1988;148:233-6.

49. Jull G, Zito G, Trott P, Potter H, Shirley D. Interexaminer reliability to detect painful upper cervical zygapophyseal joint dysfunction. Aust J Physiother 1997;43:125-9.

50. Jull G. Manual diagnosis of C2-3 headache. Cephalalgia 1985; 5 Suppl 5:308-9.

51. Jull G, Trott P, Potter H, Zito G, Niere K, Shirley D, et al. A randomized controlled trial of exercise and manipulative therapy for cervicogenic headache. Spine 2002; 27:1835-43.

52. Wardwell WI. Chiropractic: history and evolution of a new profession. St. Louis: Mosby; 1992. p. 271.

53. Wenban AB. Subluxation research: a survey of peer-reviewed chiropractic scientific journals. Chiropractic J Aust 2003;33:122-30.

54. Gatterman MI. Chiropractic management of spine-related disorders. Baltimore: Williams & Wilkins; 1990; p. 397.

55. Rosner A. In support of alternative medicine. Presented at: Assembly of the World Federation of Chiropractic; June 5, 1997; Tokyo, Japan.

Chiropractic Paradigms

Reed B. Phillips and
Meridel I. Gatterman

Key Words   Paradigm, patient-centered care, chiropractic paradigm, diagnosis

After reading this chapter you should be able to answer the following questions:

Question 1   What is the importance of paradigm to a profession?

Question 2   How are the characteristics of vitalism, holism, humanism, naturalism, conservatism, and rationalism applied to patient-centered care?

Question 3   What is the significance of the ACC paradigm to the chiropractic profession?

Within the Western health care system there are two basic paradigms, the dominant reductionist medical worldview found among mainstream health care practitioners, and the holistic perspective characteristic of practitioners of alternative medicine. Each paradigm provides a set of scientific and metaphysical beliefs, a theoretical framework in which scientific theories can be tested, evaluated, and applied. The vocabularies of the two frameworks comprise different languages, not easily translatable. These paradigms are what members of each scientific community share.[1]

A paradigm provides a framework or way of looking at the results of empirical inquiry. Paradigm is as important to solving puzzles in the practice of a discipline as it is to researching a discipline. It provides a disciplinary matrix based on worldview, habits of mind, and webs of belief. Science is conducted within a worldview that provides a disciplinary matrix, the glue that holds the discipline together. The power of any dominant paradigm is enormous and health conceptions are related to existing worldviews. Health care research and treatment practices are directed by the prevailing reductionist paradigm, thereby limiting the understanding and advancement of holistic models. Integration of chiropractic practice with mainstream medicine can be promoted through application of knowledge borrowed from a reductionist paradigm without abandoning a holistic worldview.

Paradigm Defined

According to Kuhn,[1] who articulated the concept, a paradigm is a constellation of group commitments that encompasses the following components:
1. Symbolic generalizations that encompass laws of nature and **common language and definitions**
2. Shared commitments to beliefs that include **explanatory models, analogies, and metaphors** (Communication and integration of chiropractic practice with mainstream medicine can be promoted through application of knowledge based on a reductionist paradigm without abandoning a holistic worldview.)

3. **Shared values** based on social need (and in the case of health care, patient need)
4. **"Exemplars"** consisting of "concrete problem-solutions that students encounter from the start of their disciplinary education" (Seeing the problem as similar to a problem already encountered solves new problems.)

Two Chiropractic Paradigms

Two chiropractic paradigms, both holistic in perspective, are presented in this chapter. The first is a patient-centered paradigm that discusses the traditional approach to patients observed primarily by non-doctors of chiropractic. The second is an educational model developed in 1996 by consensus of the presidents of all existing North American chiropractic colleges. The first paradigm is not unique to the chiropractic profession but accurately describes the characteristics of chiropractic practice as described by observers of the chiropractic profession (e.g., medical anthropologists, sociologists, psychologists). The second model is unique to the chiropractic profession and embodies traditional chiropractic principles. These models are not competing paradigms and both are useful for chiropractic practitioners, educators, and researchers.

A Patient-Centered Paradigm for Chiropractic Practice

A paradigm is useful as both a plan of action and a lens through which the doctor of chiropractic views the patient. The doctor of chiropractic is thus provided with a worldview by which the science of chiropractic can advance in the patient's interest. Paradigm or worldview is a central issue in the understanding of a patient-centered model for chiropractic practice as it is for the integration of reductionist research into a holistic model. Phillips and Mootz[2] noted in 1992, "The chiropractic model is a patient-centered hands-on approach intent on influencing function through structure."

Chiropractic practice has traditionally been patient centered with anthropological and sociological

BOX 2-1 ■ Characteristics of Patient-Centered Care

Recognition and facilitation of the innate organization and adaptation of the person

Recognition that care should ideally focus on the total person

Acknowledgment and respect for the patient's values, beliefs, expectations, and health care needs

Promotion of the patient's health through a preference for drugless, minimally invasive, and conservative care

A proactive approach that encourages patients to takes responsibility for their health

The patient and patient-centered practitioner act as partners in decision making, emphasizing clinically effective and economically appropriate care based on various levels of evidence.[6]

---

studies providing evidence and seed material for a patient-centered paradigm.[3-5] This patient-centered paradigm[6] was further refined and agreed to by both chiropractic and multidisciplinary nominal panels and a 60-member multidisciplinary Delphi panel that followed the same three-tiered consensus process used to develop chiropractic terminology.[7] (See Chapter 1.) The characteristics of this patient-centered paradigm are outlined in Box 2-1.

Patient-centered care is not unique to the chiropractic profession,[8] but those characteristics identified do distinguish chiropractic practice. As outlined, a chiropractic patient-centered paradigm encapsulates the uniqueness of the philosophical first principles of chiropractic that provide the basis for chiropractic practice.

Chiropractic Principles

Contemporary literature recognizes six doctrines that form the basis of the principles and philosophy of traditional chiropractic. These include vitalism, holism, naturalism, humanism, conservatism, and rationalism.[9-15]

Vitalism

The traditional philosophy of chiropractic has focused on the modulating function of the nervous system in the self-healing of the human organism.[16] This principle is exemplified in the following statement:

> The organism is a vital reactive entity, which is itself the first physician in disease.[17]

This philosophical first principle of chiropractic that each individual body has the innate capacity to fight disease is the answer to Palmer's query:

> One question was always uppermost in my mind in my search for the cause of disease. I desired to know why one person was ailing and his associate, eating at the same table, working in the same shop, at the same bench was not.[18]

Physical vitalism or that vital functioning of each individual was referred to by Palmer as the body's *innate intelligence*. Palmer saw this as a manifestation of the universal regularities and laws that govern nature that he referred to as *universal intelligence*.[18]

The belief that the true locus of health comes from within by modulation of the nervous system is embodied in the chiropractic first principle, physical vitalism. Recognition of the role of the nervous system in health and disease has increased since the mid-1980s. The focus on neuroimmunology provides evidence supporting a strong relationship between central nervous system function and immunology.[19] Short-term changes in immune function following manipulation have been demonstrated.[20] (See Chapter 15.) Palmer's concept that neural function enhances tissue resistance by modification of immune response and contributes to the body's innate ability to fight disease can no longer be ignored. Advances in neuroimmunology provide strong evidence that supports Palmer's 1890s convictions.[21]

Holism

The philosophy of holism states that the whole is greater than the sum of its parts.[22] Human beings are viewed as irreducible units with everything in them related to everything else. From its inception,

BOX 2-2 ■ Characteristics of Holism

The unity of body, mind, and spirit
Health as a positive state, not merely the absence
   of disease
Personal responsibility for health
Health education and self care, self healing
A relatively open, equal, and reciprocal relation-
   ship between patient and practitioner
Physical and/or emotional contact between
   patient and practitioner
A successful healing encounter that transforms
   both practitioner and patient
A preference for natural methods and an avoidance
   of highly technological health care procedures[23]

the chiropractic profession has embraced a holistic philosophy of health care, the object of which is to relate care to the total person. It is based on the view that the body is an integral unit, and that as long as integrity is maintained, the body is capable of maintaining it own health.[9] Chiropractic practice largely encompasses the conventional ideas of holism outlined in Box 2-2.

The chiropractic holistic approach views the patient as a whole person, not as a symptom-bearing organism. Rather than treating illness from the outside, doctors of chiropractic emphasize responsibility of patients for their own health and the importance of mobilizing their own health capacities. Recognition is given to personal, familial, social, and environmental factors that promote health.[24]

Naturalism

Doctors of chiropractic show a preference for natural therapies and avoid drugs and surgery. They incorporate the use of the hands for both diagnosis and therapeutics. Wellness and health promotion are encouraged through natural means (diet, exercise, and modification of risky behavior in both work and recreational activities). Patients are referred when more invasive methods, such as drugs and surgery, are required for infections, irreversible pathology, and life-threatening conditions.

Palmer conceived the body as built on Nature's order, thereby obeying Nature's laws. The body's ability to heal is supported by the use of natural remedies and recognition of the healing power of nature—Vis Medicatrix Naturae. Nature exerts pressure toward balance and this balance is the goal of doctors who employ natural remedies[9]:

Heal as Nature heals, in accordance with Nature's laws. Compelling the body to do its own healing with its own forces.[18]

It is as important today as in Palmer's time to avoid radical therapy when natural, noninvasive methods are safe and effective.

Humanism

Humanism implies a compassionate manner that requires empathy, nonjudgmental acceptance, congruence, and genuineness.[6] Humanism has been defined as follows:

Any system or mode of thought or action in which human interests, values, and dignity predominate.[25]

The primary importance of the patient's interests, values, and dignity is manifested in the patient-doctor interaction. By legitimizing a patient's complaints, the doctor of chiropractic appreciates that patients seek not just care but to be cared for.

The preferred relationship model of patient-practitioner interaction at the primary health care level is well demonstrated by the humanized approach used by chiropractors in clinical practice.[10]

Doctors of chiropractic legitimize their patients' health problems often after the patients have been rejected as "malingerers" or as "having psychosomatic illnesses."[4] Doctors of chiropractic use understandable language and effective aids to assist patients in visualizing health problems; each healing encounter is tailored to the individual.[3] The doctor of chiropractic is oriented to the patient, not the illness. Such a focus engenders positive feelings in patients and contributes an important social function to successful treatment. In addition, the patient is approached in a genuine and caring manner. The doctor of chiropractic fulfills the patient's needs by validating that some definable organic pathosis exists and empathizing with the patient with respect to how serious, painful, or disabling the condition is. It is impressed upon the patient that chiropractic intervention will help.[26] The patient-chiropractor interaction contributes greatly to patient healing because it is a process that promotes acceptance and validation, fulfills expectations, provides explanations, and engages the patient's commitment.[3]

Conservatism
Doctors of chiropractic are committed to a natural form of health care complemented by their conservative therapeutic ethic in the tradition of Hippocrates—*"Primum non nocere"* (first do no harm). The level of chiropractic treatment usually does not have radical side effects.[27] Minimal intervention on the part of the doctor promotes active participation of the patient in the healing process. With counseling to encourage positive lifestyle changes, the patient becomes a partner in health promotion and maintenance and reduces reliance on others for care. Health-related information is provided to the patient, enhancing the patient-doctor partnership.

The chiropractic physician's belief in the ability of the body to heal itself has a strong placebo effect, reassuring patients that their bodies will heal. A conservative approach to therapy serves the patient's best interests by eliminating unwanted side effects and complications caused by unwarranted invasive therapies. Economically, a conservative approach that employs the minimum amount of treatment necessary is the best path toward a sustainable health care system. This has significant implications for the good of society, as well as for individual patients.

Rationalism
Palmer intended his work to be a rational attempt to understand health and illness.[9] In the health sciences, clinical practice is based on scientific investigation wherein reason and logic are used to organize data collected by the senses. Rationalism thus invokes logic and evidence as a basis for clinical reasoning.[2] Utilizing logic and evidence, the doctor of chiropractic works with the patient

in a partnership that contributes to the success of care. Sackett[28] emphasizes that "Good doctors use both individual clinical expertise and the best available external evidence, and neither alone is enough." He notes that without clinical expertise, there is the risk that practice may become tyrannized by evidence for the reason that even excellent external evidence may be inapplicable or inappropriate for an individual patient. Without current best evidence, practice may become outdated, much to the detriment of the patient.

The ACC Chiropractic Paradigm
At the beginning of chiropractic's second century, a landmark event occurred. For the first time in the history of the profession, each president of every chiropractic program agreed upon a set of position papers that addressed the profession, practice, and the subluxation. These two position papers grew out of a series of retreats conducted by the Association of Chiropractic Colleges (ACC) in 1996 and 1997 (Figure 2-1, Box 2-3).

The achievement of this seminal piece of work did not come without great effort. It began with a debate between Drs. Gerard Clum and James Winterstein at the Centennial Grand Celebration in Davenport (September 1995) over issues that separated the profession, as well as areas where agreement existed. To everyone's surprise, the areas of agreement far outweighed the areas of difference.

In February 1996 the presidents held a retreat during which they developed a position statement focused on patient health and supported by the profession's purpose, principles, and practice. Realizing they had only made a dent in a major problem, the presidents decided to continue the dialogue. Additional retreats were held to discuss a more definitive statement of purpose, principles, and the practice of chiropractic. Several significant questions remained in need of clarification. What do we mean when we talk about optimizing health? What is the relationship of the body's recuperative powers to the nervous system? What do we mean when we say we perform a diagnosis, facilitate neurological and biomechanical integrity, and promote health?

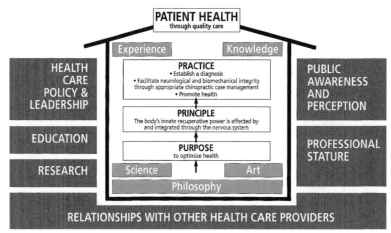

Figure 2-1   The ACC Chiropractic Paradigm (position paper 1). *(With permission, Association of Chiropractic Colleges, 1996.)*

BOX 2-3 ■ Chiropractic Paradigm (Position Paper 1)

1.0 Preamble

The Association of Chiropractic Colleges (ACC) is committed to affirming the profession by addressing issues facing chiropractic education. The ACC brings together a wide range of perspectives on chiropractic and is uniquely positioned to help define the chiropractic role within health care.

The ACC is committed to greater public service through reaching consensus on the following issues that are important to the chiropractic profession:

- continued enhancement of educational curricula;
- strengthening chiropractic research;
- participating and providing leadership in the development of health care policy;
- fostering relationships with other health care providers;
- affirming professional confidence and conduct; and
- increasing public awareness regarding the benefits of chiropractic care.

The member Colleges of the ACC represent a broad diversity of institutional missions. The presidents have drafted a consensus statement that includes the following:

- the ACC position on chiropractic;
- a representation of the chiropractic paradigm; and
- clarification regarding the definition and clinical management of the subluxation.

Additional statements will be forthcoming as the ACC continues to provide meaning and substance regarding what is taught in chiropractic colleges and how this information influences the present and future of the profession.

BOX 2-3 ■ Chiropractic Paradigm (Position Paper 1)—cont'd

2.0 ACC position on chiropractic

Chiropractic is a health care discipline that emphasizes the inherent recuperative power of the body to heal itself without the use of drugs or surgery.

The practice of chiropractic focuses on the relationship between structure (primarily the spine) and function (as coordinated by the nervous system) and how that relationship affects the preservation and restoration of health. In addition, Doctors of Chiropractic recognize the value and responsibility of working in cooperation with other health care practitioners when in the best interest of the patient.

The Association of Chiropractic Colleges continues to foster a unique, distinct chiropractic profession that serves as a health care discipline for all. The ACC advocates a profession that generates, develops, and utilizes the highest level of evidence possible in the provision of effective, prudent, and cost-conscious patient evaluation and care.

3.0 The chiropractic paradigm

Purpose
The purpose of chiropractic is to optimize health.
Principle
The body's innate recuperative power is affected by and integrated through the nervous system.
Practice
The practice of chiropractic includes:
• establishing a diagnosis;
• facilitating neurological and biomechanical integrity through appropriate chiropractic case management; and
• promoting health.
Foundation
The foundation of chiropractic includes philosophy, science, art, knowledge, and clinical experience.
Impacts
The chiropractic paradigm directly influences the following:
• education;
• research;
• health care policy and leadership;
• relationships with other health care providers;
• professional stature;
• public awareness and perceptions; and
• patient health through quality care.

4.0 The subluxation

Chiropractic is concerned with the preservation and restoration of health, and focuses particular attention on the subluxation.

A subluxation is a complex of functional and/or structural and/or pathological articular changes that compromise neural integrity and may influence organ system function and general health.

A subluxation is evaluated, diagnosed, and managed through the use of chiropractic procedures based on the best available rational and empirical evidence.

With permission, Association of Chiropractic Colleges, 1996.

The second position paper of the ACC provided answers to these questions. The participants realized that while there was agreement on general definitions and terms suitable for public usage, there were deeper issues that needed further dialogue and debate. In the *ACC Position on Chiropractic* (Figure 2-2, Box 2-4) the ACC advocated for a profession that generated, developed, and utilized the highest level of evidence possible in providing effective, prudent, and cost-conscious patient evaluation and care.

Both position papers resulted from consensus among the presidents of chiropractic educational institutions and programs. The papers were never intended to serve as testable hypotheses. Rather, they were written in a manner (it was hoped) that would be acceptable to the greater chiropractic community and provide a locus for future discussion from which testable hypotheses might be generated. Because of the generic nature of both position papers, widespread acceptance has been granted, including endorsements by the **American Chiropractic Association, International Chiropractic Association, Canadian Chiropractic Association, World Federation of Chiropractic, Congress of Chiropractic State Associations, World Chiropractic Alliance,** and the **Association of Chiropractic Colleges.**

Since the release of the position papers as the ACC Paradigm Statement, little has been done by the ACC to further address controversial issues within the profession. Only recently has the ACC reentered the arena in an attempt to address the meaning and usage of the term *diagnosis* within chiropractic education and practice. At this writing, no final statement has been released. (See Figure 2-1.)

This first position paper was actually titled *The ACC Chiropractic Paradigm.* In the preamble, the ACC stated its commitment to seek further consensus on issues of public interest. The group then rendered a definition as follows:

> Chiropractic is a health care discipline which emphasizes the inherent recuperative power of the body to heal itself without the use of drugs and surgery.

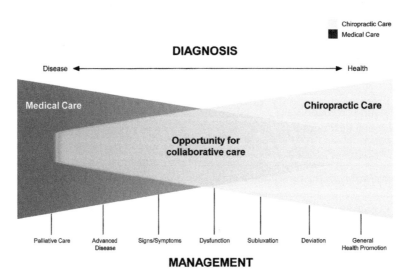

Figure 2-2   ACC Chiropractic Scope and Practice (position paper 2). *(With permission, Association of Chiropractic Colleges, 1996.)*

BOX 2-4 ■ Chiropractic Scope and Practice (Position Paper 2)

1.0 Introduction

The Association of Chiropractic Colleges (ACC) brings together a wide range of perspectives on chiropractic and is uniquely positioned to help define the chiropractic role within health care. In Position Paper 1 (July 1996), the ACC presidents described the practice of chiropractic within the chiropractic paradigm to include:

- establishing a diagnosis;
- facilitating neurological and biomechanical integrity through appropriate chiropractic case management; and
- promoting health.

As part of its ongoing commitment to affirming the profession by addressing issues facing chiropractic education, the ACC presidents have drafted a consensus statement on chiropractic scope and practice.

ACC member colleges educate students for the competent practice of chiropractic. These academic institutions have a direct interest in the definition of the chiropractic scope and practice. Clarity on chiropractic scope and practice will:

- enhance the consistency and excellence of educational outcomes;
- contribute to a better understanding of chiropractic education and practice, both within the profession and by the public; and
- provide direction to the profession for the advancement of chiropractic.

This second position paper includes:

- definition of the chiropractic scope; and
- a description of the practice of chiropractic with respect to diagnosis, case management, and health promotion.

2.0 Defining chiropractic scope

Since human function is neurologically integrated, Doctors of Chiropractic evaluate and facilitate biomechanical and neuro-biological function and integrity through the use of appropriate conservative, diagnostic and chiropractic care procedures.

Therefore direct access chiropractic care is integral to everyone's health care regimen.

3.0 Defining chiropractic practice

A. Diagnostic

Doctors of Chiropractic, as primary contact health care providers, employ the education, knowledge, diagnostic skill, and clinical judgment necessary to determine appropriate chiropractic care and management.

Doctors of Chiropractic have access to diagnostic procedures and /or referral resources as required.

B. Case Management

Doctors of Chiropractic establish a doctor/patient relationship and utilize adjustive and other clinical procedures unique to the chiropractic discipline. Doctors of Chiropractic may also use other conservative patient care procedures, and, when appropriate, collaborate with and/or refer to other health care providers.

C. Health Promotion

Doctors of Chiropractic advise and educate patients and communities in structural and spinal hygiene and healthful living practices.

With permission, Association of Chiropractic Colleges, 1996.

This statement is consistent with the concept of Naturalism discussed in the previous paradigm presented in this chapter.

The second effort at a definition was specific to the chiropractic profession:

> The practice of chiropractic focuses on the relationship between structure (primarily the spine) and function (as coordinated by the nervous system) and how that relationship affects the preservation and restoration of health.

The third definition was an attempt to find an acceptable way of describing an entity that has been fundamental to the core of chiropractic from its early beginnings—the subluxation:

> A subluxation is a complex of functional and/or structural and/or pathological articular changes that compromise neural integrity and may influence organ system function and general health.

While not offering specific definitions in the first paper, the practice of chiropractic was noted as follows:

> The practice of chiropractic includes:
> • establishing a diagnosis;
> • facilitating neurological and biomechanical integrity through appropriate chiropractic case management; and
> • promoting health.

The presidents of chiropractic educational institutions recognized it was beyond their purview to define or try to establish the scope of practice for the chiropractic profession. Nevertheless, the issue could not be easily swept from the table. (See Figure 2-2.)

This paper was titled *ACC Chiropractic Scope and Practice*. The health/disease continuum was used as a framework wherein the role of chiropractic care was positioned relative to the typical role of medical care. (See the diagram on position paper 2.) Note the overlap of the two triangles representing the area of care included in the scope of practice. This diagram supports the concept quite extensively for collaborative care with other health care practitioners.

Although the chiropractic profession continues to be confined by some to the care of back pain, the ACC statement is far more inclusive:

> Since human function is neurologically integrated, Doctors of Chiropractic evaluate and facilitate biomechanical and neuro-biological function and integrity through the use of appropriate conservative, diagnostic, and chiropractic care procedures.

This concept placed the role of the doctor of chiropractic solidly in the area of health promotion and more in the area of deviation from good health manifested by functional disorders. The area dealing with advanced disease management was relegated more to medicine. To recognize where a patient might fit in the health/disease spectrum, a diagnosis would be required. To this end, the following statement, although not a definition of "diagnosis," was an attempt to frame the concept:

> Doctors of Chiropractic, as primary contact healthcare providers, employ the education, knowledge, diagnostic skill, and clinical judgment necessary to determine appropriate chiropractic care and management.

In retrospect, everyone who participated in the development of these two position papers was surprised and amazed at the level of acceptance the work obtained. It was a bold step to make such statements, a badly needed one, on which some semblance of unity could be pursued for the future benefit and growth of the profession. Unfortunately, the consensus process developed something that everyone could not only agree to, but which was also subject to individual interpretation as well.

Since the release and widespread acceptance of the position papers, practitioners from both ends of the philosophical spectrum within chiropractic have excerpted statements that support their various points of view, claiming "evidence" of ACC support. Rather than fostering unity, the use of selected portions of the papers has only led to further debate and division within a profession that still struggles for identity, both within and outside of the profession.

This is not to infer the papers have failed. Quite the contrary. They have helped to frame the debate. The failure has been that the ACC (or other entities within chiropractic) has not continued the debate. At the time of this writing, the ACC is just now engaged in dialogue on the meaning of *diagnosis*—some eight years after the initial release of the position papers. While academic debate may be deliberate by intention and slow, eight years of lag time is unacceptable for a profession that struggles daily for existence.

Conclusion

Although both paradigms presented in this chapter have merit, I would hope they are not the end of the thought development process so vital to the continued existence and thriving of a profession. It is time for the next generation of intellectual, political, and practical leaders of the chiropractic profession to continue the debate, continue the dialogue, continue the development of a profession that is huddled around concepts in need of definition, practices in need of evaluation, and patients in need of quality care.

References

1. Kuhn TS. The structure of scientific revolutions. 2nd ed, enlarged. Chicago: University of Chicago; 1970.
2. Phillips RB, Mootz RD. Contemporary chiropractic philosophy. In: Haldeman S, editor. Principles and practice of chiropractic. 2nd ed. Norwalk, CT: Appleton and Lange; 1992. p. 45.
3. Coulehan JL. Chiropractic and the clinical art. Soc Sci Med 1985;21:383-90.
4. Kelner M, Hall O, Coulter I. Chiropractors: do they help? A study of their education and practice. Toronto: Fitzhenry and Whitehead; 1980.
5. Jamison JR. Clinical communication: the essence of chiropractic. J Chiro Human 1994;4:26-35.
6. Gatterman MI. A patient-centered paradigm: a model for chiropractic education and research. J Altern Complement Med 1995;4:371-86.
7. Gatterman MI, Hansen DT. Development of chiropractic nomenclature through consensus. J Manipulative Physiol Ther 1994;17:302-9.
8. Stewart M, Brown JB, Weston WW, McWhinney I, McWilliam CL, Freeman TR. Patient-centered medicine: transforming the clinical method. London: Sage; 1995.
9. Coulter ID. An institutional philosophy of chiropractic. Chiro J Aust 1991;21:136-42.
10. Jamison JR. Chiropractic philosophy versus a philosophy of chiropractic: the sociological implications of differing perspectives. Chiro J Aust 1991;21:153-9.
11. Kleynhans AM. An institutional perspective of philosophy in the chiropractic curriculum. Chiro J Aust 1991;21:144-8
12. Kleynhans AM. Developing philosophy in chiropractic. Chiro J Aust 1991;21:161-7.
13. Coulter ID. Alternative and investigatory paradigms for chiropractic. J Manipulative Physiol Ther 1993;16:319-26.
14. Jamison JR. The conundrum of contemporary chiropractic. Chiro J Aust 1993;23:136-40.
15. Phillips RB, Coulter ID, Adams A, Traina A, Beckman JA. Contemporary philosophy of chiropractic for Los Angeles College of Chiropractic. J Chiro Humanities 1994;4:20-5.
16. Gatterman MI. Principles of chiropractic. In: Gatterman MI, editor. Chiropractic management of spine related disorders. Baltimore: Lippincott, Williams & Wilkins; 2003. p. 49-68.
17. Coulter HL. Divided legacy: a history of the schism in medical thought. Washington, DC: Weehawken Books; 1988. p. x.
18. Palmer DD. The chiropractor's adjuster: the science, art, and philosophy of chiropractic. Portland, OR: Portland Printing House; 1910.
19. Blalock JE, Smith EM. A complete regulatory loop between the immune and neuroendocrine systems. Fed Proc 1985;44:108-11.
20. Brennan PC, Kokjohn K, Lohr GE. Enhanced phagocytic cell respiratory burst induce by spinal manipulation: potential role for substance P. J Manipulative Physiol Ther 1991;14:399-408.
21. Palmer DD. Chiropractic workshop. The Chiropractic 1897;17:4.
22. Phillips DC. Holistic thought in social science. Stanford, CA: Stanford University Press; 1976. p. 6.
23. McKee J. Holistic health and the critique of western medicine. Soc Sci Med 1998;26:775-84.
24. Jamison JR. Holistic health care in primary practice: chiropractic contributing to a sustainable health care system. J Manipulative Physiol Ther 1992;15:605-7.
25. Ullmann LP, Krasner L. A psychological approach to abnormal behavior. Toronto: Prentice-Hall; 1969. p. 599.
26. Firman GJ, Goldstein MS. The future of chiropractic: a psychological view. New Eng J Med 1975;293:639-42.
27. Coulter ID. The patient, the practitioner, and wellness: paradigm lost, paradigm gained. J Manipulative Physiol Ther 1990;13:107-11.
28. Sackett DL. Evidence-based medicine. Spine 1998;10:1085-6.

3

Anatomy Related to Spinal Subluxation

Gregory D. Cramer and

Susan A. Darby

Key Words   Zygapophyseal joint, intervertebral disc, intervertebral foramen, radicular pain

After reading this chapter you should be able to answer the following questions:

Question 1   What structures form the boundaries of the intervertebral foramen (IVF)?

Question 2   What is radicular pain?

Question 3   How might treatment of a subluxation decrease somatic referred pain?

The relationships between the anatomic components of the spinal motion segment are critical to understanding the spinal subluxation model. This three-joint complex consists of the two zygapophyseal (posterior) joints and the (anterior) intervertebral disc. These structures interact to form the functional unit of the spine. The position of the intervertebral foramen provides a significant boundary between the central nervous system and the peripheral nervous system, and in some cases it may be structurally important to nociception arising from the spinal motion segment (subluxation-generated pain). Pain of spinal origin is transmitted through peripheral and central neural structures and is modulated at various sites.

The Zygapophyseal Joints

General Description

The junctions between the superior and inferior articular facets of the articular processes (zygapophyses) on either side of two adjacent vertebrae are known as zygapophyseal joints (Z-joint). These joints are also referred to as facet joints or interlaminar joints.[1] There are left and right Z-joints between each pair of vertebrae and they are classified as synovial (diarthrodial) planar joints. These rather small joints allow motion to occur and, more importantly, determine the direction and limitations of movement that can occur between vertebrae. The Z-joint is of added interest to those who treat spinal conditions because loss of motion or aberrant motion may be a primary source of pain.[2]

Articular Capsules

Each Z-joint is surrounded by a capsule posterolaterally (Figure 3-1). The capsule consists of an outer layer of dense fibroelastic connective tissue, a vascular central layer made up of areolar tissue and loose connective tissue, and an inner layer consisting of a synovial membrane.[3] The anterior and medial aspects of the Z-joint are covered by the ligamentum flavum. The synovial membrane lines the articular capsule, the ligamentum flavum,[4] and the synovial joint folds (see following discussion), but not the articular cartilages of the joint surfaces.[1]

The Z-joint capsules throughout the vertebral column are thin and loose and are attached to the margins of opposing superior and inferior articular facets of adjacent vertebrae.[5] Superior and inferior protrusions of the joint capsules known as recesses bulge out from the top and bottom of the joint. These recesses are filled with adipose tissue and the inferior recess is larger than the superior recess.[6] The capsules are longer and looser in the cervical region than in the lumbar and thoracic regions to compensate for the greater amount of movement that occurs. As mentioned previously, the anteromedial aspect of the joint is formed by the ligamentum flavum,[4] and hyaline cartilage covers the surface of each facet.

The Zygapophyseal Joint Synovial Folds

Zygapophyseal joint synovial folds are synovium-lined extensions of the capsule that protrude into the joint space to cover part of the hyaline cartilage. The synovial folds vary in size and shape in the different regions of the spine. Engle and Bogduk in 1982[7] reported on a study of 82 lumbar Z-joints. (Cervical folds are discussed later.) They found at least one intraarticular fold (meniscus) within each joint. The intraarticular structures were categorized into three types. The first was described as a connective tissue rim found running along the most peripheral edge of the entire joint. This connective tissue rim was lined by a synovial membrane. The second type of meniscus was described as an adipose tissue pad, and the third type was identified as a distinct, well-defined fibroadipose meniscoid. This latter type was usually found entering the joint from the superior or inferior pole of the joint (or both).

Giles and Taylor[3] studied 30 zygapophyseal joints, all of which were found to have "menisci." The "menisci" were renamed zygapophyseal joint synovial folds because of their histologic makeup. Free nerve endings were found within the folds, and the nerve endings met the criteria for pain receptors (nociceptors). That is, they were distant from blood vessels and were of proper diameter

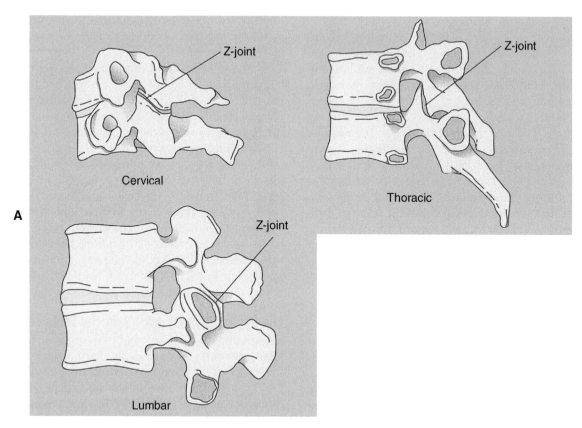

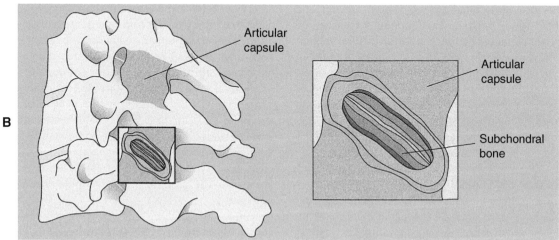

Figure 3-1   The zygapophyseal joint showing the layers of the articular capsule. **A,** Typical zygapophyseal joints of each vertebral region. **B,** Typical zygapophyseal joint. The layers of the Z-joint as seen in parasagittal section *(inset)* are color coded as follows: light blue, joint space; dark blue, articular cartilage; brown, subchondral bone; red, synovial lining of articular cartilage; pink, vascularized middle layer of the articular capsule; violet, fibrous outer layer of the articular capsule. *(From Cramer GD, Darby SA. Basic and clinical anatomy of the spine, spinal cord, and ANS. St. Louis: Mosby; 1995.)*

(6 to 12 μm). Therefore the synovial folds or menisci themselves were thought to be pain sensitive. This meant that if the Z-joint synovial fold became compressed by or trapped between the articular facets making up the Z-joint, back pain could result.

Unique Characteristics of the Cervical Zygapophyseal Joints

The cervical Z-joints are oriented approximately 45 degrees to the horizontal plane.[8] More specifically, the facet joints of the upper cervical spine lie at approximately a 35-degree angle to the horizontal plane, and the lower cervical Z-joints form a 65-degree angle to the horizontal plane.[9]

The superior articular processes and their hyaline cartilage–lined facets face posteriorly, superiorly, and slightly medially. The appearance of the cervical Z-joints changes significantly with age. Before the age of 20 years, articular cartilage is smooth and approximately 1 to 3 mm thick, and the subarticular bone is regular in thickness. The articular cartilage thins with age, and most adult cervical Z-joints possess an extremely thin layer of cartilage with irregularly thickened subarticular cortical bone. These changes in articular cartilage and the subchondral bone usually go undetected on magnetic resonance imaging and computed tomography scans. Osteophytes (bony spurs) projecting from the articular processes and sclerosis (thickening) of the bone within the articular processes are quite common in adult cervical Z-joints.

Cervical Zygapophyseal Joint Synovial Folds

Zygapophyseal joint synovial folds (menisci) project into the Z-joints at all levels of the cervical spine. Yu et al.[10] found four distinct types of cervical Z-joint menisci ranging from thin rims to thick protruding folds. They demonstrated several types of folds on magnetic resonance imaging scans.

Innervation of the Z-Joints

The Z-joint capsule receives a rich supply of sensory innervation. The sensory supply is derived from the medial branch of the posterior primary division (dorsal ramus) at the level of the joint, and each joint also receives a branch from the posterior primary division of the level above (Figure 3-2). In addition, Wyke[11] states that there

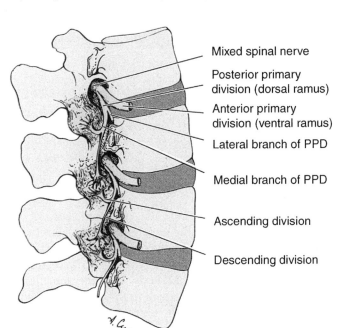

Mixed spinal nerve

Posterior primary division (dorsal ramus)

Anterior primary division (ventral ramus)

Lateral branch of PPD

Medial branch of PPD

Ascending division

Descending division

Figure 3-2   Innervation of the zygapophyseal joints. Notice each posterior primary division (dorsal ramus) divides into a medial and lateral branch. The medial branch has an ascending division which supplies the Z-joint at the same level and a descending division which supplies the Z-joint immediately below. *(From Cramer GD, Darby SA. Basic and clinical anatomy of the spine, spinal cord, and ANS. St. Louis: Mosby; 1995.)*

are three types of sensory receptors in the joint capsule of the Z-joints. These are as follows:

- Type I—very sensitive static and dynamic mechanoreceptors that fire continually to some extent even when the joint is not moving
- Type II—less sensitive and fire only during movement
- Type IV—slow conducting nociceptive mechanoreceptors

Type III sensory receptors are nociceptive fibers found in joints of the extremities, and Wyke[11] did not find these in the Z-joints.

The Intervertebral Disc

The intervertebral disc (IVD) is composed of water, cells (primarily chondrocyte-like cells and fibroblasts), proteoglycan aggregates, and collagen fibers. The proteoglycan aggregates are composed of many proteoglycan monomers attached to a hyaluronic acid core. However, the proteoglycans of the IVD are of a smaller size and are of a different composition than the proteoglycans of cartilage found in other regions of the body (articular, nasal, and growth plate cartilage).[12] The IVD is a dynamic structure that has been shown to repair itself and is capable of "considerable" regeneration.[13]

The IVD is composed of three regions known as the anulus fibrosus, the nucleus pulposus, and the vertebral (cartilage) end plate (Figure 3-3). Together they make up the anterior interbody joint or intervertebral symphysis. Each of these regions consists of different proportions of the primary materials that make up the disc. (See previous discussion.)

Anulus Fibrosus

The anulus fibrosus is made up of several fibro-cartilaginous lamellae, or rings, which are convex externally. The lamellae are formed by closely arranged collagen fibers and a smaller percentage (10% of the dry weight) of elastic fibers.[14] Most of the fibers of each lamella run parallel with one another at approximately a 65-degree angle from the vertical plane. Adjacent lamellae overlie one another, forming approximately a 130-degree angle between their fibers. The most superficial lamellae

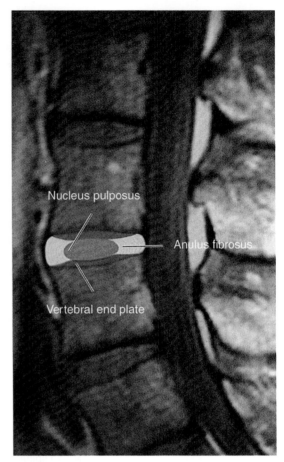

Figure 3-3   MRI of a sagittal section of the intervertebral disc with adjacent vertebral bodies. The parts of the intervertebral disc are labeled. *(From Cramer GD, Darby SA. Basic and clinical spinal anatomy of the spine, spinal cord, and ANS. St. Louis: Mosby; 1995. Photograph by Ron Mensching; illustration by Dino Juarez, The National College of Chiropractic.)*

send thick bundles of collagen into the bone of the vertebral rims in the region of the ring apophysis. These bundles are known as Sharpey's fibers. They form firm attachments between the intervertebral discs and the vertebral body. The inner lamellae of the anulus fibrosus attach to the cartilaginous vertebral end plate. The direction of the lamellae varies considerably from individual to individual and from one vertebra to the next.[15]

The lamellae of the anulus fibrosus are subject to tear. These tears occur in two directions, circumferentially and radially. Many investigators believe that circumferential tears are the most common. This type of tear represents a separation of adjacent lamellae of the anulus. The separation may cause the lamellae involved to tear away from their vertebral attachments. The second type of tear is radial in direction. These run from the deep lamellae to the superficial layers. Most authors[16] believe that this type of tear develops after circumferential tears. The presence of circumferential tears may make it easier for radial tears to occur because radial tears can then connect several adjacent circumferential tears. When this occurs, the inner nucleus pulposus may bulge or be extruded into the vertebral canal. This is known as intervertebral disc protrusion (bulging) or herniation (extrusion). However, this scenario probably occurs much less frequently than was once believed.

Nucleus Pulposus

The nucleus pulposus is a rounded structure located in the center of the IVD. It develops from the embryologic notochord. The nucleus pulposus is gelatinous and relatively large just after birth, and several multinucleated notochordal cells can still be found within its substance.[5]

Except for the most peripheral region of the anulus fibrosus, the disc is an avascular structure. The nucleus pulposus is responsible for absorbing most of the fluid received by the disc. The process by which a disc absorbs fluid from the superior and inferior vertebral bodies has been termed *imbibition*. When a load is applied to the spine, an IVD loses water but retains sodium and potassium. This increase in electrolyte concentration creates an osmotic gradient that results in rapid rehydration when the loading of the disc is stopped.[17]

The disc apparently benefits from activity during the day and rest during the hours of sleep. As a result, the disc is thicker (from superior to inferior) after rest than after a typical day of sitting, standing, and walking. Too much rest may not be beneficial, however. A decrease in the amount of fluid (hydration) of the intervertebral discs has

been noted on magnetic resonance imaging scans after five weeks of bed rest.[18] The disc reaches its peak hydration at approximately the age of 30 years, and the process of degeneration begins shortly thereafter.[19] As the disc ages, it becomes less gelatinous in consistency and its ability to absorb fluid diminishes. The changes in composition and structure caused by aging, common to all types of cartilage, occur earlier and to a greater extent in the IVD.[20] Breakdown of the proteoglycan aggregates and monomers is thought to contribute to the process of degeneration because this process results in a decreased ability of the disc to absorb fluid. In turn, there is a decrease in the ability of the disc to resist loads to which it is subjected. The degeneration associated with decreased ability to absorb fluid (water) has been identified with computed tomography[21] and magnetic resonance imaging and has been correlated with histologic structure and fluid content. As the disc degenerates, it becomes thinner (superior to inferior), and the adjacent vertebral bodies may become sclerotic (thickened and opaque on radiographs). Much of the disc thinning seen with age may also be the result of discs "sinking into" the adjacent vertebral bodies over the course of many years.[15]

Pathology of the intervertebral disc is seen frequently in clinical practice. As mentioned previously, the nucleus pulposus may cause bulging of the outer anular fibers or may protrude through the anulus. This was first described by Mixter and Barr.[22] Bulging or herniation of the disc may be a primary source of pain, or pain may result from pressure on the exiting nerve roots in the vertebral or intervertebral foramens. Such bulging is usually associated with trauma, although a history of trauma may be absent in as many as 28% of patients with confirmed disc protrusion.[23] Some investigators believe that proteoglycan leaks from tears in the anulus also may cause pain by creating chemical irritation of the exiting nerve roots. Pain caused by pressure on or irritation of a nerve root radiates in a dermatomal pattern. Such pain is termed *radicular pain* because of its origin from the dorsal root (radix) or dorsal root ganglion. Treatment for herniation of the nucleus ranges from conservative methods[24] to excision of the disc (discectomy) to chemical degradation of the disc (chymopapain chemonucleolysis).[25,26]

Vertebral End Plate

Vertebral end plates are cartilaginous plates that limit the disc (with the exception of the most peripheral rim) superiorly and inferiorly and are attached to the nucleus pulposus, anulus fibrosus, and the adjacent vertebral body. Although a few authors consider the vertebral end plate to be a part of the vertebral body, most authorities consider it to be an integral portion of the disc.[18,26] The end plates are approximately 1 mm thick peripherally and thicker centrally. They are composed of both hyaline cartilage and fibrocartilage. The hyaline cartilage is located against the vertebral body and the fibrocartilage is found adjacent to the remainder of the intervertebral disc. The end plates help to prevent the vertebral bodies from undergoing pressure atrophy and, at the same time, contain the anulus fibrosus and nucleus pulposus within their normal anatomic borders.[27]

Occasionally the nucleus pulposus ruptures through the vertebral end plate, causing a lesion known as a Schmorl's node. These nodes cause the vertebrae surrounding the lesion to move closer together. This movement is thought to increase pressure on the anterior intervertebral joints, speeding the degenerative process of the anterior interbody joint (by means of internal disc disruption). In addition, the disc thinning or narrowing resulting from such end plate herniations leads to more force being borne by the Z-joints. This shift in force application may result in more rapid degeneration of the Z-joints as well.

The vertebral end plates begin to calcify and thin with advancing years. This leaves them more brittle. The central region of the end plate in some vertebrae of certain individuals may be completely lost in the later years of life.

Innervation of Intervertebral Discs

The outer third of the anulus fibrosus receives both sensory and vasomotor innervation.[28] The sensory fibers are probably both nociceptive (pain sensitive) and proprioceptive in nature, and the vasomotor fibers are associated with the small vessels located along the superficial aspect of the anulus fibrosus. The posterior aspect of the disc receives its innervation from the recurrent meningeal nerve (sinuvertebral nerve). The posterolateral aspect of the anulus receives both direct branches from the anterior primary division and also branches from the gray communicating rami of the sympathetic chain. The lateral and anterior aspects of the disc primarily receive innervation from branches of the gray communicating rami and also from branches of the sympathetic chain (Figure 3-4).

The fact that the disc has direct nociceptive innervation is clinically relevant. The intervertebral disc itself is probably able to generate pain. Therefore, disorders affecting the intervertebral discs alone, including internal disc disruption and tears of the outer third of the anulus fibrosus, can be the sole cause of back pain. The disc also can generate pain by compressing (entrapping) an exiting dorsal root. Leakage of nerve-irritating (histamine-like) molecules from disrupted intervertebral discs has been found to be a cause of irritation to the exiting dorsal root. These latter conditions cause a sharp, stabbing pain that radiates along a dermatomal pattern. This type of pain is known as radicular pain because it results from irritation of a nerve root (radix).

Cervical Intervertebral Discs

The basic anatomy of the cervical intervertebral discs is similar to that of intervertebral discs throughout the spine. The discs of this region make up more than 25% of the superior-to-inferior length of the cervical spine and their substantial size facilitates much of the motion that occurs in this region. The intervertebral discs in the cervical region thin with age while at the same time the uncinate processes continue to enlarge. By the age of 40 years, the uncinate processes create a substantial barrier that prevents lateral and posterolateral herniation of the intervertebral disc. Bland[29] believes that the cervical discs dehydrate earlier in life than do the discs in the thoracic and lumbar regions. He states that there is no nucleus

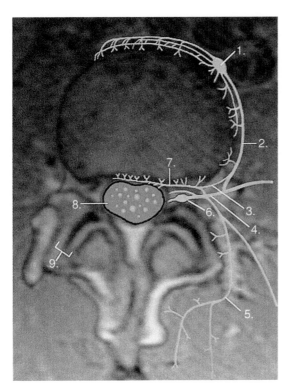

Figure 3-4   The innervation of the intervertebral disc in horizontal section. The neural elements have been drawn onto a horizontal magnetic resonance imaging scan. The top of the illustration is anterior and the bottom is posterior. Numbers indicate the following: *1*, sympathetic ganglion; *2*, gray ramus communicantes; *3*, branch of the gray ramus coursing toward the intervertebral foramen (IVF) to contribute to the recurrent meningeal (sinuvertebral) nerve; *4*, anterior primary division (ventral ramus); *5*, medial branch of posterior primary division (the lateral branch is seen coursing to the right of the medial branch in this illustration); *6*, dorsal root (spinal) ganglion and dural root sleeve (red) within the IVF; *7*, recurrent meningeal (sinuvertebral) nerve; *8*, cauda equina (yellow) within the cerebrospinal fluid (blue) of the lumbar cistern of the subarachnoid space; *9*, zygapophyseal joint. Notice the intervertebral disc is receiving innervation from branches of the sympathetic ganglion (anteriorly), gray communicating ramus (laterally and posterolaterally), and the recurrent meningeal nerve (posteriorly). Also notice that the zygapophyseal joint is receiving innervation from the medial branch of the posterior primary division. *(From Cramer GD, Darby SA. Basic and clinical anatomy of the spine, spinal cord, and ANS. St. Louis: Mosby; 1995. Photograph by Ron Mensching; illustration by Dino Juarez, The National College of Chiropractic.)*

pulposus in the cervical spine beyond the age of 45 years; therefore he believes that intervertebral disc protrusion in the cervical region has been over-diagnosed. Recall that there are no intervertebral discs between the occiput and the atlas or between the atlas and the axis. The C2-C3 interbody joint is the first joint to possess an intervertebral disc, making the C3 spinal nerve the most superior nerve that can be affected by disc protrusion.

Mendel et al.[13] studied the innervation of the cervical intervertebral discs and found sensory nerve fibers throughout the anulus fibrosus. These fibers were most numerous in the middle (from superior to inferior) third of the disc. The structure of many of the nerve fibers and their end receptors was consistent with those that transmit pain. In addition, pacinian corpuscles and Golgi tendon organs were found in the posterolateral aspect of the disc. These findings help to confirm

that the anulus fibrosus is a pain-sensitive structure and further indicate that the cervical discs are involved in proprioception, enabling the central nervous system to monitor the mechanical status of the intervertebral disc. Mendel et al.[13] hypothesized that the arrangement of the nerve fiber bundles may allow for the IVD to sense peripheral compression or deformation as well as alignment. No nerves were found in the nucleus pulposus.[13]

The Intervertebral Foramen

The intervertebral foramen (IVF) is a very important "hole" in the spine. The IVF is an area of great biomechanical, functional, and clinical significance.[5] Much of the importance stems from the fact that the IVF provides an osteoligamentous boundary between the central nervous system and the peripheral nervous system. Therefore knowledge of the specific anatomy of this clinically important area is needed in the differential diagnosis of back and extremity pain and can help with determining proper management for individuals with compromise to this region.

A pair (left and right) of intervertebral foramina are located between the adjacent vertebrae from C2 to the sacrum. There are no IVFs between C1 and C2. When present, the IVFs lie posterior to the vertebral bodies and between the superior and inferior vertebral notches of adjacent vertebrae. Therefore, the pedicles of adjacent vertebrae form the "roof" and "floor" of this region. The width of the pedicles gives depth to these openings, making them actually neural canals[30] rather than foramina, but the name remains.

Six structures form the boundaries of the IVF (Figure 3-5). Beginning from the most superior border ("roof") and continuing anteriorly in a circular fashion, the boundaries are as follows:
1. The pedicle of the vertebra above (more specifically, its periosteum)
2. The vertebral body of the vertebra above (again, its periosteum)
3. The intervertebral disc (posterolateral aspect of the anulus fibrosus)
4. The vertebral body of the vertebra below; in the cervical region is the uncinate process (periosteum)
5. The pedicle of the vertebra below forms the "floor" of the IVF (periosteum). A small part of the sacral base (between the superior articular process and the body of the S1 segment) forms the floor of the L5-S1 IVF.
6. The zygapophyseal joint (forms the "posterior wall"). Recall that the Z-joint is made up of (1) the inferior articular process (and facet) of the vertebra above, (2) the superior articular process (and facet) of the vertebra below, and (3) the anterior "articular capsule," which is composed of the ligamentum flavum.[1,4]

The IVFs are smallest in the cervical region and there is a gradual increase in IVF dimensions to the fourth lumbar vertebra. The IVFs between L5 and S1 are unique in size and shape. As mentioned previously, the IVFs are actually canals, varying in width from approximately 5 mm[31] in the cervical region to 18 mm[32] at the L5-S1 level. Many structures (surrounded by adipose tissue) traverse the IVF (Figure 3-5). They are as follows:
1. The mixed spinal nerve
2. The dural root sleeve
3. Lymphatic channel(s)
4. Three branches of the spinal ramus of a segmental artery—one to the posterior aspect of the vertebral body, one to the posterior arch, and one to the mixed spinal nerve (neural branch)
5. Communicating veins between the internal and external vertebral venous plexuses
6. Two to four recurrent meningeal (sinuvertebral) nerves

The dorsal and ventral roots unite to form the mixed spinal nerve in the region of the IVF. The

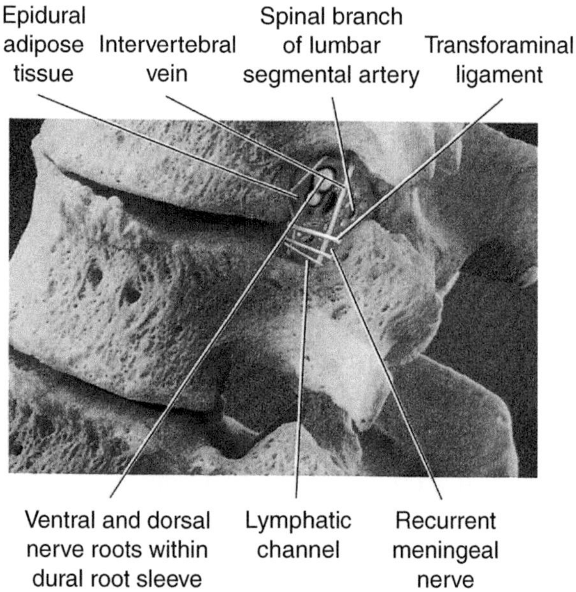

Epidural adipose tissue   Intervertebral vein   Spinal branch of lumbar segmental artery   Transforaminal ligament

Ventral and dorsal nerve roots within dural root sleeve   Lymphatic channel   Recurrent meningeal nerve

Figure 3-5   The intervertebral foramen (IVF). Notice the structures that normally traverse the IVF. The most common locations of the transforaminal ligaments are also shown on this illustration. *(From Cramer GD, Darby SA. Basic and clinical anatomy of the spine, spinal cord, and ANS. St. Louis: Mosby; 1995. Photograph by Ron Mensching; illustration by Dino Juarez, The National College of Chiropractic.)*

mixed spinal nerve is surrounded by the dural root sleeve, and the dural root sleeve is attached to the borders of the IVF by a series of fibrous bands. The dural root sleeve becomes continuous with the epineurium of the mixed spinal nerve at the lateral border of the IVF. The arachnoid blends with the connective tissue of the nerve root proximal to the dorsal root ganglion and at an equivalent region of the ventral root. Occasionally the arachnoid extends more distally; in such cases, the subarachnoid space extends to the lateral third of the IVF.

Each recurrent meningeal nerve (sinuvertebral nerve of Von Luschka) originates from the most proximal portion of the ventral ramus. It receives a branch from the nearest gray communicating ramus of the sympathetic chain before traversing the IVF. This nerve provides sensory innervation (including nociception) to the posterior aspect of the anulus fibrosus, the posterior longitudinal ligament, anterior epidural veins, periosteum of the posterior aspect of the vertebral bodies, and the anterior aspect of the spinal dura mater. Usually several recurrent meningeal nerves enter the same IVF.

Accessory Ligaments of the Intervertebral Foramen

Golub and Silverman[33] first used the term *transforaminal ligament* (TFL) when describing a ligamentous band seen to cross the IVF at any level of the spine. These ligaments vary considerably in size, shape, and location from one IVF to another. They found that the spinal arteries and veins ran above this structure and the anterior primary division ran underneath it. Bachop and Janse[34] reported that the higher the ligament is placed, the less space remains for the spinal vessels, which could conceivably lead to ischemia or venous congestion. The lower the ligament is placed, the greater the possibility of sensory and/or motor deficits.

Bachop and Hilgendorf[35] studied 15 spines and from these they dissected the lumbar IVFs on both the left and the right sides, making a total of 150 IVFs. From these dissections they found the following:

26 (17.3%) IVFs had TFLs
13 (50%) of TFLs were at L5-S1 and 11 (73.3%) of the 15 spines had 1 to 2 TFLs at L5-S1
2 (13%) had 1 to 2 TFLs at L5-S1

The term *corporotransverse ligament* is used when referring to a ligament that runs between the vertebral body and the transverse process at the L5-S1 junction.[34] Bachop and Hilgendorf[35] found that the corporotransverse ligaments were of two basic types; they were either broad and flat or they were rod-like. The rod-like ligaments were usually tougher (firmer) than the flat type. Golub and Silverman[33] reported that these could calcify and be seen on radiographs. Bachop and Ro[36] found the gray communicating sympathetic ramus running through the opening above the corporotransverse ligament.

Bachop and Janse[34] believed that the corporotransverse ligament could have a constricting effect on the anterior primary division (ventral ramus). For example, in patients with sciatica, raising the leg might cause the anterior primary division to stretch across the ligament, possibly mimicking the thigh and leg pain of a disc protrusion.

Amonoo-Kuoffi et al.[37] have recently discussed accessory ligaments of the IVF. They consistently found such ligaments throughout the lumbar region and mapped out the relationship of the spinal nerve, segmental veins and arteries, and the recurrent meningeal nerve through the openings between the ligaments. They concluded that the accessory ligaments tend to hold the above-mentioned structures in their proper places. Bakkum and Mestan[38] also found several ligaments at each level that decreased functional superior inferior diameter of the IVF by approximately one third.

Pain (Nociception) of Spinal Origin

The Perception of Pain

All pain should be considered as real and as having both physical and psychological components, one of which may predominate. All pain alters the personality of the individual.[39] This personality usually returns to the pre-pain state when the physical cause of the discomfort has sufficiently healed. In addition, pain is always subjective and is perceived by patients in relation to experiences they have had with pain in their early years.[40]

Pain of Somatic Origin

Once a nociceptor has depolarized, it changes its properties, frequently becoming more sensitive to subsequent noxious stimuli. This increased sensitivity to pain is known as hyperalgesia. The central nervous system also has several mechanisms by which it may create hyperalgesia in an area of injury. After tissue is damaged, it is usually more sensitive to pain until healing has occurred. After development of a pathologic condition or injury, hyperalgesia also may be present in the healthy tissues surrounding the site of the lesion. Pain of spinal origin is the result of damage to several structures, and the effects of hyperalgesia allow for pain to be felt in tissues that, if injured alone but to the same degree, may have gone unnoticed.[41]

Most pain of spinal origin has a physical cause. One way to organize possible pain generators is by listing them according to the four main sources of neural innervation to spinal structures. These sources are (1) the anterior primary division (ventral ramus), (2) the posterior primary division (dorsal ramus), (3) the recurrent meningeal nerve, and (4) sensory fibers that course with the sympathetic nervous system (including fibers that run with the sympathetic trunk and also the gray communicating rami). All of these afferent nerves have cell bodies in the dorsal root ganglia (DRG), which, with the exception of C1 and C2, are located within the intervertebral foramina of the spine. The sensory fibers that are associated with the recurrent meningeal nerve and the sympathetic nervous system provide a route for the transmission of pain arising from somatic structures of the anterior aspect of the vertebral column. Fibers arising from these sources pass through the anterior primary division for a short distance before reaching the mixed spinal nerve. The structures innervated by the ventral ramus, dorsal ramus, and recurrent meningeal nerve are listed in Box 3-1, Box 3-2, and Box 3-3.

BOX 3-1 ■ Spine-Related Structures Innervated by the Ventral Ramus
Possible Pain Generators

- Referred pain from structures innervated by plexuses
- Psoas muscle
- Quadratus lumborum muscle
- Intertransversarii muscles

BOX 3-2 ■ Structures Innervated by the Dorsal Ramus
Possible Pain Generators

Medial branch of the dorsal ramus innervates:

- Deep back muscles
- Zygapophyseal joints
- Periosteum of posterior vertebral arch
- Interspinous, supraspinous, and intertransverse ligaments, ligamentum flavum
- Skin (upper cervical, middle cervical, and thoracic)

Lateral branch of the dorsal ramus innervates:

- Erector spinae muscles
- Splenius capitis and cervicis muscles (cervical region)
- Skin

BOX 3-3 ■ Structures Innervated by the Recurrent Meningeal Nerve
Possible Pain Generators

- Periosteum of posterior vertebral bodies
- Internal vertebral (epidural) veins *and* basivertebral veins
- Epidural adipose tissue
- Posterior intervertebral disc
- Posterior longitudinal ligament
- Anterior spinal dura mater

Nerves Associated with the Sympathetic Nervous System

Several structures are innervated by nerves that arise from the sympathetic trunk and the gray communicating rami. The sensory fibers of these nerves follow the gray rami to the anterior primary division where they enter the mixed spinal nerve and then reach the spinal cord by coursing through the dorsal roots. Pathology of the periosteum of the anterior and lateral vertebral body, innervated by sensory fibers traveling with gray rami, may lead to pain. Some of the most common causes of this type of pathologic condition include fracture, neoplasm, and osteomyelitis.[42] Sprain of the anterior longitudinal ligament or the outer layers of the anterior or lateral anulus also may result in pain conducted by fibers that course with the gray communicating rami. The structures innervated by nerves associated with the sympathetic trunk and gray communicating rami are listed in Box 3-4.

Pain Generators Unique to the Cervical Region

Pain generators unique to the cervical region include irritation of the nerves surrounding the vertebral artery and also pain arising from uncovertebral "joints" (joints between the uncinate processes and the vertebral body immediately above). In addition, pain arising from pathology or dysfunction of the cervical Z-joints can refer to regions quite distant from the affected joint.[43] The

---

BOX 3-4 ■ Structures Innervated by Nerves Associated with the Sympathetic Trunk and the Gray Communicating Rami
Possible Pain Generators

- Periosteum of the anterior and lateral vertebral bodies
- Lateral intervertebral disc
- Anterior intervertebral disc
- Anterior longitudinal ligament

---

two most common types of pain referral are neck pain and head pain (headache) arising from the C2-C3 Z-joints, and neck pain and shoulder pain arising from the C5-C6 Z-joints.[44] However, pain arising from almost any structure innervated by the upper four cervical nerves may refer to the head, resulting in head pains and headaches.[43,45-47] Pain originating from the region of the basiocciput and occipital condyles frequently refers to the orbital and frontal regions. Sweating, pallor, nausea, alterations of pulse, and other autonomic disturbances have frequently been observed in association with disturbances of the suboccipital and upper cervical spine. The intensity of autonomic reactions seems to be proportional to the stimulus and its proximity to the suboccipital region. The autonomic responses range from mild subjective discomforts to measurable objective signs.[45]

Pain Generators Unique to the Thoracic Region

Pain generators unique to the thoracic region include pain arising from the costocorporeal and costotransverse articulations. Compression fracture of the vertebral bodies is also an important source of acute pain arising from the thoracic region.

The Dorsal Root Ganglia and Radicular Pain

The dorsal root ganglia serve as modulators of spinal pain. They contain many neuropeptides associated with the transmission of pain (substance P, calcitonin gene–related peptide, vasoactive intestinal peptide).[40] These substances may be released from the peripheral terminals of the sensory nerves that transmit pain, and the neuropeptides may reach these peripheral terminals (receptors) by axonal transport mechanisms. The presence of neuropeptides in and around the receptors may "prime" them by making them more susceptible to depolarization.[40] Direct pressure or irritation of the dorsal roots or dorsal root ganglia results in radicular pain. Radicular pain is sharp and stabbing in nature and radiates along a narrow band. It is accompanied by other sensory or motor deficits. Some of the causes of radicular pain include intervertebral disc protrusion, spinal (vertebral) canal stenosis, and other space-occupying lesions (Box 3-5).

Somatic Referred Pain

There are several possible mechanisms of pain referral from a somatic structure. Perhaps one of the most important is attributable to the internal organization of the spinal cord. The nociceptive information coming in from a pain generator is dispersed by ascending or descending within the tract of Lissauer for several cord segments before synapsing with tract neurons of several cord levels. Therefore nociceptive information entering from several vertebral levels may converge in the same interneuronal pool.

The dispersal of incoming afferents onto different tract neurons, in combination with the convergence of several different afferents onto single-tract neurons, may decrease the ability of the central nervous system to localize pain. This type of dispersal and convergence also may be found at the second synapse along the pain pathway, located in the ventral posterior lateral nucleus of the thalamus. Finally, the ventral posterior lateral thalamic nucleus projects to the postcentral gyrus of the cerebral cortex. The back and neck have very small regions allotted to them on the postcentral gyrus (sensory homunculus), and this also may contribute to the poor localization of spinal pain. In addition, the tract neurons for ascending pain pathways most frequently carry nociceptive information from cutaneous areas. Therefore when the tract neurons are stimulated to fire, the cerebral cortex (where conscious awareness of pain occurs) may interpret the impulse as coming from a cutaneous region or from another more recently injured region. Either of these areas may be distant to the structure that is currently damaged or inflamed. This phenomenon is sometimes referred to as "pain memory."[48,49]

Somatic referred pain is characterized as a dull aching pain that is difficult to localize and is constant in nature. Activity of the muscles and the Z-joints, as well as spinal manipulation of the Z-joints, tends to decrease pain through a "gate control" type of mechanism.[39] Therefore if pain is of somatic origin, the patient may benefit most by treatment that promotes activity and movement.[39] Of course, care must be taken not to compromise the damaged tissue in any way (Box 3-6).

Central Transmission of Pain

The afferent fibers that convey nociception are group A-delta and group C fibers. These fibers enter the dorsolateral tract of Lissauer located at the tip of the dorsal horn. Within this region, collateral branches of those fibers that continue directly into the gray matter ascend or descend numerous cord segment levels before they also enter the dorsal horn. The A-delta fibers, which convey pain quickly and rapidly, terminate in lamina I and laminas IV through VI. The group C fibers, which convey a dull sensation of pain at a slow rate, terminate in lamina II. The neurons that transmit the information to higher centers are located in various laminae of the gray matter. Surgical cordotomy procedures that relieve pain have shown that the major fibers that transmit nociception to higher centers decussate in the ventral white commissure and then ascend in the anterolateral quadrant of the white matter of the spinal cord.[50] Alternative pathways also may be involved, although their course and function in humans remain unclear.

The Neospinothalamic Tract

One of the tracts in the anterolateral quadrant is the neospinothalamic tract (Figure 3-6). This tract ascends through the brainstem to the ventral lateral nucleus (posterior part) and also to the posterior nucleus of the thalamus with little or no input to the brainstem. From the thalamus, axons course to the somesthetic region of the cortex; that is, the postcentral gyrus and the posterior part of the paracentral lobule of the parietal lobe. As the axons ascend, body parts are represented in specific regions of the tract, and in the cerebral cortex a pattern is retained such that a specific area of cortex corresponds to the region of the body from which the sensory fibers originate. This cortical representation is referred to as the sensory homunculus. The size of the body part represented on the homunculus reflects the amount of sensory innervation devoted to that body area. As previously mentioned, this unequal neuronal representation may explain why localization of sensations such as pain is more difficult in one region (the back, for example) than in another. The neospinothalamic tract synapses in the region of the sensory homunculus and provides the basis for the discriminatory qualities of pain sensation, including stimulus intensity and spatial localization.

The Paleospinothalamic and Spinoreticular Tracts

Two additional tracts that ascend in the anterolateral quadrant are the paleospinothalamic and spinoreticular tracts (Figure 3-7). The paleospinothalamic tract ascends through the brainstem and likely contributes collateral branches to the reticular

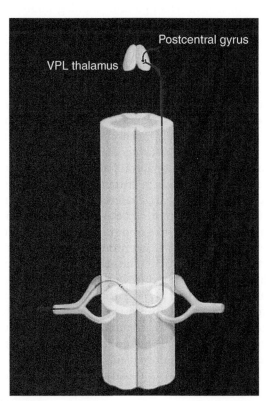

Figure 3-6   The primary pathway for transmittal of nociception—the neospinothalamic tract. *(Illustration by Dino Juarez, The National College of Chiropractic.)*

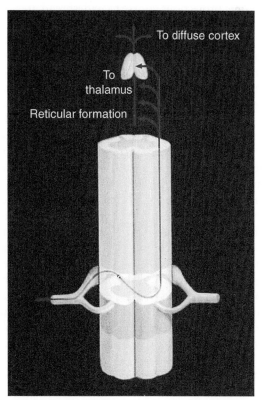

Figure 3-7   The paleospinothalamic tract and the spinoreticular tract. *(Illustration by Dino Juarez, The National College of Chiropractic.)*

formation. It terminates in the midline and intralaminar thalamic nuclei. From these nuclei, thalamic fibers travel to regions associated with the limbic system and to widespread areas of cerebral cortex, such as the orbitofrontal region. The spinoreticular tract ascends to the reticular formation of the brainstem. The reticular formation is a complex network of neurons located throughout the core of the brainstem. It has numerous functions and is a major component, along with the thalamus and the cerebral cortex, of the ascending reticular activating system. The ascending reticular activating system provides the circuitry through which arousal and attentiveness are maintained. The tract neurons that synapse in the reticular formation form complex connections within this region and subsequently project to brainstem nuclei, the hypothalamus, and the midline and intralaminar nucleus of the thalamus. Subsequent thalamic projections course to widespread areas of the cerebral cortex.

The paleospinothalamic and spinoreticular tracts possess similar characteristics. One of these is that they both terminate in the same region of the thalamus, which projects to nonspecific areas of cerebral cortex. Another similarity is that neither of them is somatotopically organized. Both the spinoreticular and paleospinothalamic tracts may be involved with the generation of chronic pain and the qualities associated with that sensation. The response of the brain to painful stimuli is quite involved. The perception of pain takes place in the thalamus, postcentral gyrus, frontal cortex (affective component), and temporal cortex (memory of previous pain component).[39] The unpleasant emotional response associated with pain, however, seems to be associated with the limbic system. The limbic system allows one to perceive a sensation as being uncomfortable, aching, or hurting.[41] The focus of one's attention on the painful area is likely a function of the ascending reticular activating system.

Supraspinal Control

Evidence from studies in which electrical stimulation of regions of the brainstem produced analgesia[51] indicates that there are descending pathways that can modulate nociceptive signals. One of the com-

ponents of this endogenous pain control system is the periaqueductal gray matter (PAG) of the midbrain. This region has a major projection to the nucleus raphe magnus, which is located in the midline of the rostroventral medulla. This nucleus is rich in the neurotransmitter serotonin. From this region, serotonergic fibers course into the dorsolateral funiculus of the spinal cord (raphe-spinal tract) and synapse heavily on neurons in the superficial dorsal horn (laminae I and II).

The superficial dorsal horn is the region that receives input from afferent fibers conveying nociception. In addition, it is the location of the origin of the spinothalamic tracts[51,52] and is the area involved with the segmental modulation of nociception. (See previous discussion.) Descending fibers synapse with neurons, which include enkephalin (an opioid peptide)-containing inhibitory interneurons, and also on the nociceptive projection neurons (tract neurons). The opioid-containing inhibitory interneurons are in close proximity to both primary nociceptive afferents and the tract neurons. In fact, the afferent endings and the dendrites of the tract neurons both contain opioid receptors.

Pharmacologic studies have shown that the release of opioid peptides from the inhibitory interneurons blocks transmission of nociception by two mechanisms. One mechanism is by binding to receptors and blocking the release of neurotransmitters, such as substance P from the primary afferent fibers. Although direct axoaxonic synapses between enkephalinergic neurons and the primary afferent fibers have not yet been found, enkephalins may possibly bind to receptors by diffusing from their site of release to the presynaptic membrane of the afferent fiber.[52-54] The second mechanism by which inhibitory interneurons can mediate spinal neurotransmission of nociception is by directly synapsing with the postsynaptic membrane of the tract neuron. This occurrence has been well documented.[52-54] Through these connections, nociceptive transmission is prevented.

As mentioned previously, analgesia can be produced by neural stimulation. Analgesia can also be produced by the administration of opiates into the central nervous system. The areas that are activated by the opiates are the same as those that produce analgesia when electrically stimulated, that is, the PAG and the rostroventral medulla. This lends credence to the theory that endogenous opioid peptides that have been found in the brain can activate the descending system.[52]

In addition to the serotonergic descending pathway, there are other fibers descending from the pons[50,53] that appear to be involved with control of the nociceptive system. These descending fibers contain norepinephrine and appear to inhibit nociception at the dorsal horn level. At the same time, however, collateral branches of these fibers synapse on the serotonergic neurons of the raphe nuclei. The subsequent release of norepinephrine at this level results in "tonic inhibition" of the raphe-spinal neurons.[53] Thus both systems provide a descending component to the mechanism for controlling pain. Feeding into these systems is the nociceptive information transmitted through ascending pathways,[41] possibly the spinomesencephalic tract and input from the reticular formation, and possibly stress induced input channeled through the limbic system and hypothalamus.[52]

Acknowledgments

The authors thank Mr. James McKay, Ms. Sheila Meadows, and Dr. Michael Kiely for invaluable assistance during the preparation of this chapter.

References

1. Giles LG. The surface lamina of the articular cartilage of human zygapophyseal joints. Anat Rec 1992;233:350-6.
2. Paris S. Anatomy as related to function and pain. Orthopedic Clinics of North America 1983;14:475-89.
3. Giles LG, Taylor JR. Human zygapophyseal joint capsule and synovial fold innervation. Br J Rheumatol 1987; 26:93-8.
4. Xu G, Haughton VM, Yu S, Carrera GF: Normal variations of the lumbar facet joint capsules. Clin Anat 1991;4:117-22.
5. Williams PL, Warwick R, Dyson M, Bannister LH: Gray's anatomy. 37th ed. New York: Churchill Livingstone; 1989.
6. Jeffries B. Facet joint injections. Spine: State of the Art Reviews 1988;2:409-17.
7. Engle R, Bogduk N. The menisci of the lumbar zygapophyseal joints. J Anat 1982;135:795-809.
8. Panjabi M, Oxland T, Parks E. Quantitative anatomy of cervical spine ligaments. Part II. Middle and lower cervical spine. J Spinal Dis 1991;4:277-85.
9. Oliver J, Middleditch A. Functional anatomy of the spine. Oxford: Butterworth Heinemann; 1991.
10. Yu S, Sether L, Haughton VM. Facet joint menisci of the cervical spine: correlative MR imaging and cryomicrotomy study. Radiology 1987;164:79-82.
11. Wyke B. The neurology of low back pain. In: Jayson M. The lumbar spine and back pain. 3rd ed. New York: Churchill Livingstone; 1987.
12. Buckwalter JA, Smith KC, Kazarien LE, Rosenberg LC, Ungar R. Articular cartilage and intervertebral disc proteoglycans differ in structure: An electron microscopic study. J Orthop Res 1989;7:146-51.
13. Mendel T, Wink CS, Zimny ML. Neural elements in human cervical intervertebral discs. Spine 1992;17:132-5.
14. Bogduk N, Twomey LT. Clinical anatomy of the lumbar spine. London: Churchill Livingstone; 1991.
15. Humzah MD, Soames RW. Human intervertebral disc: structure and function. Anat Rec 1988;220:337-56.
16. Ito S, Yamada Y, Tsuboi S, Yamada Y, Muro T. An observation of ruptured annulus fibrosus in lumbar discs. J Spinal Dis 1991;4:462-6.
17. Kraemer J, Kolditz D, Gowin R. Water and electrolyte content of human intervertebral discs under variable load. Spine 1985;10:69-71.
18. LeBlanc AD, Schonfeld E, Schneider VS, Evans HJ, Taber KH. The spine: Changes in T2 relaxation times from disuse. Radiology 1988;169:105-7.
19. Coventry MB. Anatomy of the intervertebral disc. Clin Orthop 1969;67:9-15.
20. Bayliss MT, Johnstone B, O'Brien JP. Proteoglycan synthesis in the human intervertebral disc: Variation with age, region, and pathology. Spine 1988;13:972-81.
21. Bahk YW, Lee JM. Measure-set computed tomographic analysis of internal architectures of lumbar disc: Clinical and histologic studies. Invest Radio11988;23:17-23.
22. Mixter WJ, Barr JS. Rupture of the intervertebral disc with involvement of the spinal canal. N Eng J Med 1934; 211:210-5.
23. Martin G. The role of trauma in disc protrusion, N Z Med J 1978;March:208-11.
24. Sanders M, Stein K. Conservative management of herniated nucleus pulposus: treatment approaches. J Manipulative Physiol Ther 1988;11:309-13.
25. Alcalay M, Bontoux D, Vincent MH, Valat JP, Fouquet B, Bregeon C et al. Traitement par nucleolyse a la chymopapaine des hernies discales a forme purement lombalgique. Rev Rhum Mal Osteoartic 1988;55:741-5.
26. Dabezies EJ, Langford K, Morris J, Shields CB, Wilkinson HA. Safety and efficacy of chymopapain (discase) in the treatment of sciatica due to a herniated nucleus pulposus: results of a randomized, double-blind study. Spine 1988;13:561-5.
27. Bogduk N. Clinical anatomy of the lumbar spine. London: Churchill Livingstone; 1991.
28. Bogduk N, Tynan W, Wilson A. The nerve supply to the human lumbar intervertebral discs. J Anat 1981;132:39-56.

29. Bland J. The cervical spine: from anatomy to clinical care. Medical Times 1989;117:15-33.
30. Czervionke LF, Daniels DL, Ho PS, Yu SW, Pech P, Strandt J et al. Cervical neural foramina: Correlative anatomic and MR imaging study. Radiology 1988;169:753-9.
31. Hewitt W. The intervertebral foramen. Physiotherapy 1970;56:332-6.
32. Pfaundler S. Pedicle origin and intervertebral compartment in the lumbar and upper sacral spine. Acta Neurochir 1989;97:158-65.
33. Golub B, Silverman B. Transforaminal ligaments of the lumbar spine. J Bone Joint Surg 1969;51:947-56.
34. Bachop W, Janse J. The corporotransverse ligament at the L5 intervertebral foramen [abstract]. Anat Rec 1983;205.
35. Bachop W, and Hilgendorf C. Transforaminal ligaments of the human lumbar spine [abstract]. Anat Rec 1981;199.
36. Bachop WE, Ro CS. A ligament separating the nerve from the blood vessels at the L5 intervertebral foramen. J Bone Joint Surg 1984;8:437.
37. Amonoo-Kuofi HS, el-Badawi MG, Fatani JA. Ligaments associated with lumbar intervertebral foramina. 1. L1 to L4. J Anat 1988;156:177-83.
38. Bakkum BW, Mestan M. The effects of transforaminal ligaments on the sizes of T11 to L5 human intervertebral foramina. J Manipulative Physiol Ther 1994;17:512-22.
39. Kirkaldy-Willis WH. The mediation of pain. In: Kirkaldy-Willis W, editor. Managing low back pain. 2nd ed. New York: Churchill Livingstone, 1988.
40. Weinstein WH. The perception of pain. In: Kirkaldy-Willis W, editor. Managing low back pain. 2nd ed. New York: Churchill Livingstone; 1988.
41. Haldeman S. The neurophysiology of spinal pain. In: Haldeman S, editor. Principles and practice of chiropractic. 2nd ed. East Norwalk, CT: Appleton and Lange; 1992.
42. Bogduk N. The innervation of the lumbar spine. Spine 1983;8:286-93.
43. Dwyer A, Aprill C, Bogduk N. Cervical zygapophyseal joint pain patterns. I. A study in normal volunteers. Spine 1990;15:453-7.
44. Bogduk N, Marsland A. The cervical zygapophyseal joints as a source of neck pain. Spine 1988;13:610-7.
45. Campbell D, Parsons C. Referred head pain and its concomitants. J Nerv Mental Dis 1944; 99:544-51.
46. Bogduk N, Engel R. The menisci of the lumbar zygapophyseal joints. Spine 1984;9:454-60.
47. Aprill C, Dwyer A, Bogduk N. Cervical zygapophyseal joint pain patterns. II. A clinical evaluation. Spine 1990; 15(6):458-61.
48. Carpenter MB, Sutin J. Human neuroanatomy. 8th ed. Baltimore: Williams & Wilkins; 1983.
49. Nolte J. The human brain. 2nd ed. St. Louis: Mosby; 1988.
50. Hoffert MJ. The neurophysiology of pain. Neurol Clin 1989;7(2):183-203.
51. Basbaum AI, Fields HL. Endogenous pain control mechanisms: review and hypothesis. Ann Neurol 1978;4:451-62.
52. Jessell TM, Kelly DD. Pain and analgesia. In: Kandel ER, Schwartz JH, Jessell TM, editors. Principles of neural science. 3rd ed. New York: Elsevier; 1991.
53. Basbaum AI. Cytochemical studies of the neural circuitry underlying pain and pain control. Acta Neurochir Suppl (Wien). 1987;38:5-15.
54. Besson JM. The physiological basis of pain pathways and the segmental controls of pain. Acta Anaesthesiol Belg 1988;39(3 Suppl 2):47-51.

4

Animal Models in the Study of Subluxation and Manipulation: 1964-2004

Charles N.R. Henderson

Key Words   Subluxation, animal model, basic science, neuroscience

After reading this chapter you should be able to answer the following questions:

Question 1   To what extent has chiropractic's subluxation theory been explored by basic science research?

Question 2   What issues arise from animal model research?

Question 3   What are eight reasons for using animal models in research?

Question 4   What are Haldeman's basic criteria for judging any proposed neurobiological mechanism for spinal manipulative therapy (SMT)?

"The lack of a relevant and reproducible animal model may be one important obstacle to clarification of these issues....Thus, subluxation remains a hypothesis yet to be evaluated experimentally."

Murray Goldstein, General Chairman, 1975

NINCDS Conference; The Research Status of Spinal Manipulative Therapy[1]

"The concept of chiropractic subluxation remains a hypothesis yet to be evaluated experimentally. We believe that this has been one of the most frustrating aspects of certain views of the pathology that is purported to be altered with spinal manipulative therapy. When one is correcting a 'subluxation' that cannot be perceived by independent scientific observers, it is difficult to convince those observers that the treatment is effective."

White & Panjabi, 1990

Biomechanics of the Spine[2]

"Studies to address these kinds of questions [autonomic effects of adjustment] are hampered by the absence of a reliable animal model." and "If the subluxation consists, at least in part, of fixation of the Z joints [zygapophyseal joints], then an animal model that mimics such fixation is clearly needed."

Basic Research Work Group Report, 1996

The National Workshop to Develop the Chiropractic Research Agenda[3]

The preceding quotes illustrate that scholars, both inside and outside the chiropractic community, see a need for an animal model of the subluxation. A useful model should allow researchers to evaluate effects predicted by chiropractic theory. In addition to clarifying theoretical mechanisms by which the subluxation may impact musculoskeletal and general health, important clinical questions may be addressed:

- Are different types of subluxation more serious in their biomechanical and systemic effects?
- Is there a "time window" when spinal manipulation is most effective in preventing or correcting the adverse consequences of subluxation?
- What are the effects of different therapeutic techniques for a given patient?
- What determines the optimal number or frequency of spinal manipulation treatments for a given patient?

Although studies conducted with animal models must be followed by human studies, the role of animal research is critical to human studies. Animal research provides essential data about biological mechanisms that are needed to identify and clarify questions for human research. In fact, the absence of relevant animal studies make clinical studies very difficult to justify to Institutional Review Boards that serve as the gatekeepers for human research.[4] Moreover, the absence of basic research evidence prompts the larger scientific and health care communities to treat lightly the results of such clinical studies. This is particularly true for studies examining chiropractic treatment of visceral complaints. In his review of animal models used in subluxation research, Vernon[5] noted the great need for basic science research if the chiropractic profession wants to persuade the larger health care community that chiropractic has a place in the treatment of nonmusculoskeletal conditions. He stated the following:

> It is my opinion that dozens of clinical trials can occur in such areas as the chiropractic treatment of asthma, dysmenorrhea, hypertension, etc., but they will all be relegated to insignificance and be dismissed as large-scale exercises in the placebo effect if a credible, valid biologic mechanism that links dysfunction in the spinal column with dysfunction in organ systems cannot be provided. This is the task that only the profession's basic scientists, in their pursuit of the scientific basis of subluxation, can accomplish.

Vernon presented eight reasons for using animal models in research:
1. Test theories derived from conceptual models
2. Provide data to support clinical experience
3. High level of experimental control
4. Prospective; therefore can explore cause and effect relationships
5. Explore "treatment" effects when lesion is reversed
6. Explore physiologic components of subluxation
7. Chronic experiments may allow for exploration of behavioral effects
8. Animal studies are the "Holy Grail" of clinical science

According to Vernon, there are essentially two ways to model the spinal subluxation. First, investigators may create the obligate precipitating elements of the subluxation, vertebral fixation, and misalignment and monitor the effects:

> ...this approach retains the highest fidelity to the natural circumstances and achieves the highest level of prospective validity, because...the disorder was created first and its putative effects were studied thereafter.

He also observed that this approach is by far the more difficult of the two, requiring a reproducible and biomechanically well-characterized model. He commented that one or more "first order" effects (e.g., nerve root pressure) must be demonstrated by an animal model before "second order" effects (e.g., changes in peripheral reflexes or nerve conduction velocities) can be studied and logically correlated with the theoretical subluxation model. Vernon considered this to be a difficult task and noted that it had never been achieved in total in any of the studies he reviewed.

The second approach suggested by Vernon is to accept the proposition that vertebral misalignment creates nerve interference as presented above and simply begin the experiment by modeling the effects of intervertebral foramen encroachment or altered somatic afferent input (for Vernon—spinal joint pain). He stated a preference for this second "alternative" approach because he considered it to be easier, both experimentally and logically: "When sufficient data have been gathered from studies like this, then investigators can return to the problem of whether the misalignment really produces the proximate [first order] effects."

In this chapter we present an overview of animal models that have been used to study subluxation, or in the case of osteopathy, the osteopathic lesion. Of course, not all basic research that investigates subluxation and manipulation must involve animals. A number of valuable basic science studies have been performed in humans.[6-8] However, as illustrated by Vernon's eight reasons for using animal models in research, animal research provides research opportunities that cannot be accomplished in human studies.

The issue of definition becomes preeminently necessary at this point. What do we mean by *subluxation* and why are studies of the *osteopathic lesion* relevant? For that matter, what do we mean by *manipulation* and why not use the term *adjustment*? In this chapter, key terms will be operationally defined and the essential features of a good animal model will be described. This will quite naturally lead to a general discussion of animal research issues. Animal research on subluxation (and the osteopathic lesion) that has been conducted in the last 40 years of the twentieth century will be reviewed. Lastly, the chapter will conclude with a few observations about where all of this appears to be going in the twenty-first century.

The definition and use of terms like *subluxation* and *adjustment* is a hotly contested issue, not simply because of differences in perspective, but because these terms are intertwined with the philosophical, legal, and political foundations of the chiropractic profession. They are central to the profession's collective sense of identity and autonomy. Simply stated, the chiropractic profession claims ownership of the *subluxation* and *adjustment*.

"Ownership" of the Subluxation

The profession that will be recognized as "owning" the subluxation and its correction will not simply be the first or loudest proclaimer. Rather, it will be the profession that is recognized for understanding the subluxation and converting that understanding into demonstrable clinical outcomes.

It is often a jolting surprise to those arguing chiropractic ownership due to "original discovery and development" that neither the term *subluxation* nor its chiropractic usage began with the Palmers. The first published use of the term in chiropractic was by Smith, Langworthy, and Paxson in their 1906 two-volume textbook, *Modernized Chiropractic*.[9] The earliest attribution of subluxation by the *Oxford English Dictionary* is to Holme in 1688; "Sublaxation [sic]—a dislocation, or putting out of joynt [sic]."[10] A more "chiropractic" definition of the term is found in the work of Joannes Heironymi in his 1746 thesis *De Luxationibus et Subluxationibus:*

> ...subluxation of joints is recognized by lessened motion of the joints, by slight change in position of the articulating bones and pain...most displacements of vertebrae are subluxations rather than luxations.[11]

Finally, Edward Harrison was an outspoken advocate for the manual correction of subluxations.[12-14] His words could have come right out of an early chiropractic text. Yet his description of the subluxation and its treatment was written at least 70 years before D.D. Palmer's historic discovery:

> A small irregularity in the height and disposition of some particular vertebrae is perceptible, on examination, in most delicate females. This disorderly arrangement and disposition of the component parts of the spinal column, though hitherto overlooked and wholly neglected, are I am persuaded, of great consequence to future health. The effects of this subluxation, not being distinguishable by the symptoms, have never been traced to their origin in the spine. A very slight and partial compression of the cord, or some of its nerves, will disturb the organs to which they run....When we take into account the number, the size and the distribution of the spinal nerves among the viscera and muscles, we are led to conclude that scarcely a complaint can arise in which they do not participate. In recent cases these subluxations are easily replaced: parents will therefore best consult the health and comfort of their children by frequently examining the spinal column, and taking the earliest opportunity of counteracting its defects.... Happily these vertebral dislocations from internal causes may be easily removed in every recent, and in many old cases, so as to leave no traces in the appearance of the back or in the health of the individual.

As noted at the beginning of this section, the chiropractic profession will be recognized as "owning" the subluxation and its successful treatment only if it is recognized as the most knowledgeable authority on this topic and can convert that knowledge into demonstrable clinical outcomes. Growing national and international recognition of the chiropractic profession is testimony to both the prevalence of spinal problems and the clinical success of chiropractic practitioners. The

inevitable consequence of this success is increased scrutiny by private and governmental agencies and an "ownership challenge" by other health care practitioners. Both of these consequences are likely to promote beneficial growth in the profession. With increased research, our understanding of the subluxation will grow and our ability to successfully treat subluxation and its clinical consequences will increase. The chiropractic profession will no longer need to assert ownership of the subluxation and proclaim its professional autonomy; the evidence will speak for itself. We can then define our terms for the appropriate purpose of clarity, not to buttress misguided claims based upon historical or philosophical ownership.

Definition of Subluxation

In the first edition of this text, Gatterman[15] stated the following:

> The conceptual definition of subluxation has been the foundation on which chiropractic science has stood. It is now time to operationally define subluxation by identifying the testable components of misalignment, aberrant motion, and dysfunction included in the definition. With these components delineated, we can examine current data and further study the topic of our discourse.

She presented a consensus definition of the chiropractic subluxation developed through nominal and Delphi methods using a cross-section of the political, academic, and clinical chiropractic community. The consensus definition of subluxation thus obtained was as follows:

> A motion segment in which alignment, movement integrity, and/or physiologic function are altered although contact between the joint surfaces remains intact.

Gatterman noted that it is important that the definition of a subluxation be broad enough to include the medical concept of subluxation, a lesion that is severe enough to be visible on radiographic examination. (See Chapter 8.) This led to further refinement of the term. It was acknowledged that some subluxations may be unstable, require surgical repair, or be aggravated by manipulation.

For this reason, the term *manipulable subluxation* has been defined. A manipulable subluxation is "a subluxation in which altered alignment, movement, or function can be improved by manual thrust procedures." (See Chapter 1.) Models that mimic subluxation in this chapter attempt to emulate the manipulable subluxation. They incorporate altered motion (fixation) with and without misalignment (malposition) while retaining contact between the joint surfaces. Gatterman noted that there are more than 100 synonyms for the subluxation. Why so many? Perhaps the reason can be found in two observations:

1. Most definitions of the *chiropractic subluxation, spinal manipulation,* or *adjustment* serve political or legal purposes. The originators of these definitions generally represent broad, sometimes conflicting, constituencies so their definitions are invariably broad and imprecise. By contrast, operational definitions used in scientific studies must be clearly defined, rather restrictive statements. These operational definitions permit scientists to write and subsequently test very focused research hypotheses.

2. The chiropractic subluxation remains an unvalidated theoretical construct because there is no widely accepted physical model of the subluxation. It remains an abstract concept, free to drift with the shifting winds of political/legal necessity and philosophical/entrepreneurial influence.

"Nothing is so firmly believed as what is least known."

Michel de Montaigne

Definition of Manipulation

As noted above, there has been a longstanding polemic in the chiropractic profession about the use of the term *manipulation* preferred by researchers and the term *adjustment* used historically by chiropractic field practitioners. In the research literature, *manipulation* is broadly used to refer to any manual or mechanical movement of a joint by an applied load. This may include the application of an impulse thrust, most characteristic of the "chiropractic adjustment" or the more slowly applied "mobilization" forces commonly used by physical therapists and osteopaths. In a widely referenced taxonomy for manipulation developed by the Technique Council of the American Chiropractic Association, a six-tiered system is used to categorize the various chiropractic treatment procedures.[16] (See Chapter 7.) This system distinguishes manually applied forces from mechanically applied forces, specific and nonspecific contacts, long and short lever applications, rate of application, and amplitude of joint motion. Authors using this taxonomy generally describe the doctor and the patient/subject setup, areas of contact (e.g., support and therapeutic load contacts), rate of load application, and the expected amplitude of joint motion. Therefore manual manipulations that are most common to chiropractic practice, impulse thrusts, are frequently described as high velocity, low amplitude (HVLA), while mobilization manipulations are often described as low velocity, high amplitude (LVHA). In clinical studies, descriptions of chiropractic manipulation are almost always based upon what the treating doctor "intended" to do. There are seldom kinetic (force) and kinematic (displacements, velocities, and accelerations) measurements of the applied loads and their outcomes. Therefore the actual application of the manipulation taxonomy relates more to the manipulator's intended mechanical outcome rather than the true nature of the procedure. By contrast, most basic science studies (examining mechanisms) report actual kinetic and kinematic data. In this chapter our report of the specific treatment(s) applied in a given study was limited by the quality of description given by the authors.

Characteristics of Animal Models

Models provide an essential component in our attempt to understand both normal and pathologic processes in human beings.[17,18] They are simplified representations of a system of interest that replicate or approximate critical features of that system. It follows that the validity of any given model lies in its ability to provide clarification or new understanding about the system of interest. Mechanical or computer models can provide useful information about simple physical or chemical interrelationships, but they are quickly overtaxed by complex interactions required to represent even the most primitive mammalian system. By contrast, direct examination of living tissues readily permit researchers to study complex biological interactions and even evaluate the effect of experimental intervention. Valuable work has been done with isolated tissue preparations, such as the study of cellular and synaptic pathologies in brain slices or the study of mechanical state encoding in isolated joint capsules.[19,20] However, only intact animal models allow investigators to examine complex global interactions between major body systems.[21,22] A good animal model for basic health care research should have at least five features. It should: (1) be appropriate for evaluating specific hypotheses relating to normal or pathologic mechanisms, (2) permit rapid and reproducible examination of numerous study subjects, (3) be economical, (4) not present serious ethical concerns, and (5) allow valid extrapolation to the human condition. One of the most powerful applications of a physical model is the emulation of a conceptual construct (conceptual model). In this chapter we introduce animal models that attempt to emulate the central foundational constructs of chiropractic—subluxation and spinal manipulation.

Issues in Animal Model Research

One of the five characteristics listed above for a good animal model was that it should "not present serious ethical concerns." For some this is an impenetrable boundary. They conclude that there are no "good" animal models because all animal research presents intractable ethical problems from their perspective.[23,24] However, researchers and the public generally recognize a continuum of animal research.[25-27] The ends of this continuum are defined by reasoned consideration of potential health benefits as well as threats to animal welfare. Unacceptable animal research has low potential benefit and/or involves a disproportionate loss of animal life, pain, or distress. By contrast, good animal research will have *both* a demonstrable

benefit to human and/or animal health and a proportionately low loss of animal life, pain, and distress. For this reason, animal research protocols must contain thorough explanations of why animals are required for the proposed work and include what steps were taken to find nonanimal alternatives. If it is established that there is no acceptable alternative to using animals, the animal species and the minimal number of animals required must then be explicitly justified. Potentially painful or stressful procedures must be explained and detailed strategies must be provided for limiting pain and distress (e.g., anesthetics, analgesics, and animal care). Critical review of proposed animal research projects and reasoned consideration of the potential benefits of each project, as well as its impact on animal welfare, are the responsibility of each institution's Institutional Animal Care and Use Committee (IACUC). The IACUC also establishes and monitors species-appropriate housing and care for all animals at the institution. The constituency of this important committee and its procedures are prescribed by federal statute and closely monitored by two federal agencies, the Office of Laboratory Animal Welfare (OLAW) at the National Institutes of Health (NIH), and the Animal and Plant Health inspection Service (APHIS) at the United States Department of Agriculture (USDA).[28] In addition, many state, county, and city statutes further govern animal research. The benefit of this work to human and animal health has been both essential and profound, demonstrated by the observation that 7 of the last 10 Nobel Prizes have relied, at least in part, on animal research.[25,26,29]

Frequently the question is asked: How can we learn anything meaningful about humans from animal studies when the differences between the species are so great? Most laboratory animals have organs and body systems that are quite similar to humans. From these similarities we have learned a great deal about human physiology. Also, many laboratory animals are susceptible to the same diseases that affect humans. Because of this, scientists have been able to apply information gained from animal studies not only to humans, but to pets, wildlife, and other animals. This information has led to a dramatic increase in life expectancy in the United States, from an average of 49 years in 1900 to 76 years at the turn of the twenty-first century. Americans are not only living longer—they are living healthier. Between 1994 and 1996, 72% of Americans 65 years of age and older reported their health was good or excellent.[30,31] In addition, disability among older Americans is declining dramatically and at an accelerating pace. According to analyses from the National Long Term Care Survey, the percentage of people age 65 and older with disabilities fell 1.6% per year from 1989 through 1994 and 2.6% annually from 1994 though 1999.[32] The improvements in recent years are also noteworthy for a newly observed decline in disability among black Americans as well as a decrease of at least 200,000 in the number of people estimated to live in nursing homes. These benefits are due in great part to improved health care that was advanced by animal research.

It is important to appreciate that many of the greatest scientific discoveries were achieved because researchers exploited important differences between humans and laboratory animals. Two animals used in neuroscience research nicely illustrate this point. The anatomy and physiology of the giant squid is dramatically different from that of a human (Figure 4-1). Giant squid axons can be up to 1 mm in diameter, 100 to 1000 times larger than mammalian axons! This tremendous size allowed researchers to obtain the first intracellular recordings of action potentials from nerve cells as well as the first experimental measurements of ionic currents, thereby allowing us to understand how the nervous system conveys information.[33,34] The great size of the axon also permitted researchers to extrude the cytoplasm by pressing it out with a small roller, much like toothpaste in a tube, and measure its ionic composition. They were subsequently able to replace the axoplasm with artificial solutions and observe resulting changes in membrane potential. Moreover, some giant squid nerve cells form very large synaptic contacts with other giant nerve cells, allowing extraordinary access to these important neurological structures.[35,36] Hodgkin and Huxley were

awarded the Nobel Prize in 1963 for their body of work, much of it done with the giant squid axon.

One final example suggests a possible *National Enquirer* headline decrying government waste: "US Government Spends Millions of Your Tax Dollars to Study Frog Eggs!" In reality, these studies combine molecular and physiological methods to make an exciting new research tool that takes advantage of unique features in the clawed African frog, *Xenopus laevis*.[37] The eggs of the female frog are huge (approximately 1 mm in diameter), are easily harvested, and have few endogenous membrane-bound ion channels (Figure 4-2). These attributes permit scientists to inject exogenous mRNA into the oocytes, causing them to synthesize proteins that then produce large quantities of membrane-bound ion channels.[38] The size of the eggs also permits the use of classical methods, such as the patch clamp technique, to study ionic currents generated by the newly formed channels.[39,40] With this powerful tool, scientists can now directly study the relationship between channel structure and function. Defined mutations common to neurological diseases (often affecting a single nucleotide) can also be produced to assess the functional consequences of a mutation. These and other extraordinarily valuable animal studies have formed the foundation of modern neuroscience and, subsequently, clinical practice.

Scientists interested in subluxation and spinal manipulation hope to make similarly important contributions, but we got off to a late start. It is generally agreed that modern chiropractic research began in earnest after the 1975 National Institutes of Neurological and Communicative Disorders and Stroke (NINCDS) conference, "The Research Status of Spinal Manipulative Therapy."[41] At the end of this conference, it was acknowledged that there was little or no direct evidence to support or deny the claims of manipulative therapists. The evidence presented was general and circumstantial. It was especially and painfully obvious that there were very few published clinical or basic science studies by members of the chiropractic community.

Two years later, a follow-up conference, "Research Workshop on Neurobiological Mechanisms in

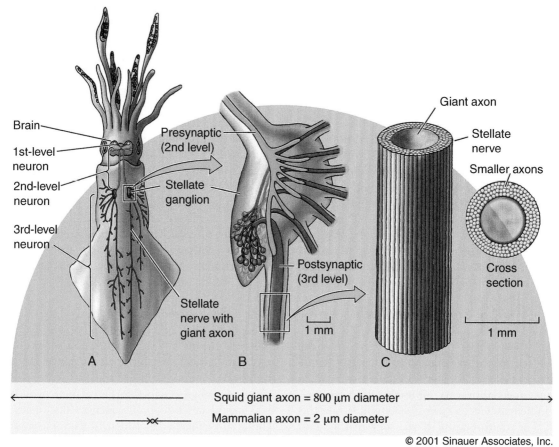

Figure 4-1   Giant squid axons can be up to 1 mm in diameter, 100 to 1000 times larger than mammalian axons! This tremendous size allowed researchers to attain the first intracellular recordings of action potentials from nerve cells as well as enabled the first experimental measurements of ionic currents, thereby allowing us to understand how the nervous system conveys information.[33,34] *(Reprinted with permission from Purves D, Augustine GJ, Fitzpatrick D, Katz LC, Lamantia A, McNamera JO et al. Neuroscience. 2nd ed. Sunderland, MA: Sinauer Associates, Inc.; 2001. p. 53.)*

Manipulative Therapy," was sponsored at Michigan State University by the National Institutes of Health (NIH). Scott Haldeman was asked to present a paper titled *The Clinical Basis for Discussions of Mechanisms in Manipulative Therapy.*[42] He was given a set of four basic criteria for judging any proposed neurobiological mechanism for spinal manipulative therapy (SMT):

1. SMT must produce consistent clinical results under controlled conditions in the treatment of a specific pathologic process, organ dysfunction, or symptom complex.
2. SMT must demonstrate a specific effect on the musculoskeletal system.
3. The musculoskeletal effect must have a specific influence on the nervous system.
4. The influence on the nervous system must demonstrate a beneficial influence on abnormal function of an organ, tissue pathology, or symptom complex.

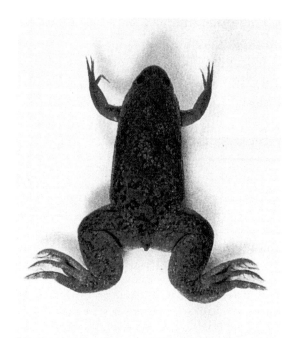

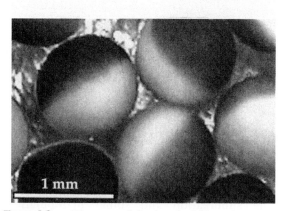

1 mm

Figure 4-2   The eggs of the female African frog, *Xenopus laevis,* are huge (approximately 1 mm in diameter), are easily harvested, and have few endogenous membrane-bound ion channels. These attributes permit scientist to inject exogenous mRNA into the oocytes, causing them to synthesize proteins, which then produce large quantities of membrane-bound ion channels.[38] With this powerful tool, scientists can now directly study the relationship between channel structure and function. *(Reprinted with permission from Purves D, Augustine GJ, Fitzpatrick D, Katz LC, Lamantia A, McNamera JO et al. Neuroscience. 2nd ed. Sunderland, MA: Sinauer Associates, Inc.; 2001. p. 85.)*

In a recent article, "Neurologic Effects of the Adjustment," Haldeman[43] noted that these criteria remain as valid today as they were in 1977. In agreement with this observation, each study synopsis in this review ends with an assessment of which of the four criteria are addressed by the study. Haldeman's criteria were specific to SMT research, but as discussed below, may also be applied to subluxation studies.

Review of Subluxation Research

With small modifications, a figure from Haldeman's article[43] provides an interesting overview of biomedical research (Figure 4-3). The original figure has been modified to encompass both SMT research and subluxation research. In Figure 4-3, criterion 1 highlights the outcome of SMT on organ dysfunction, tissue pathology, or symptom complex. This describes the focus of most clinical research studies. In these studies the patient is pretty much considered like the proverbial "black box." There is little attempt to examine mechanisms within the black box that underlie the clinical study observations. By contrast, it is precisely these mechanisms that are the focus of basic science research. Basic scientists are most interested in what goes on within the black box (criteria 2, 3, and 4). Sometimes this simple dichotomous distinction between clinical and basic science studies is blurred. Clinical studies may include the examination of mechanisms, and basic science studies may explore the outcome of a treatment or lesion upon clinically relevant outcomes, as can be seen in this review of animal models. Whether the focus of a study is SMT or subluxation, the Haldeman criteria may be applied. Figure 4-3 presents the original criteria as they relate to examining the purported therapeutic benefit of SMT as well as the putative consequence of subluxation. Figure 4-3 suggests the necessary integration of SMT-focused research and subluxation-focused research. To date, no published studies have combined an SMT model with a subluxation model. However, as will be described at the end of this chapter, research is currently under way that will accomplish just that. A successful subluxation mimic model is being

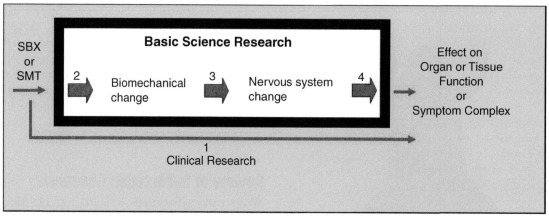

Figure 4-3   This diagram identifies four basic criteria for judging any proposed neurobiological mechanism for spinal manipulative therapy *(SMT)* or subluxation *(SBX)*. Criterion 1 highlights the focus of most clinical research studies. In these studies, the patient is pretty much considered like the proverbial "black box." There is little attempt to examine mechanisms within the black box that underlie the clinical study observations. By contrast, it is precisely these mechanisms that are the focus of basic science research. Basic scientists are most interested in what goes on within the black box (criteria 2, 3, and 4). *(Modified from Haldeman S. The clinical basis for discussion of mechanisms of manipulative therapy. In: Korr IM, editor. The neurobiologic mechanisms in manipulative therapy. New York: Plenum Press; 1978. p. 53-75.)*

used in conjunction with various SMT mimic models to study the effects of different spinal manipulative therapies on animals with established pathologic consequences of subluxation.

There have been relatively few attempts by scientists at chiropractic institutions to model the chiropractic subluxation. Rather than reflecting the difficulty of the task, as Vernon[5] suggested, this may actually reflect the small number of basic science researchers in chiropractic. Chiropractic colleges have a considerable number of basic science faculty, but the nearly fatal combination of heavy teaching loads, insufficient basic research facilities, and meager research funding makes this work a very rare occurrence at chiropractic institutions. The lack of follow-up on several proposed subluxation models that are reviewed here, despite positive initial studies, is symptomatic of this problem.

The four modified Haldeman criteria (see Figure 4-3) have been assigned to the reviewed studies as seemed appropriate. Some will assert that there

are many more studies addressing each of the criteria. Besides the 40-year time frame (1964 to 2004), this review is limited to animal studies of the spine by researchers examining the subluxation, osteopathic lesion, or spine manipulation. Of course, the greater body of published scientific research contains many additional articles that may be relevant to understanding, evaluating, or developing subluxation and spinal manipulation theory. The reader is encouraged to explore that body of literature as well as the works presented here. It is hoped that this review will serve as both an historical overview and a "state-of-the-art" introduction to field practitioners and students.

All studies (and reviews) have flaws and limitations. Some of the studies reported here, particularly the earliest ones, do not reflect the rigor of current day research standards. This issue will be addressed in the comments section for each study. Most of the synopses were made after reading full journal publications, but some studies were only available as conference abstracts.

The synopses are organized according to the primary construct they model (subluxation or spinal manipulation) and whether they represent a full mimic of the construct or just one of its components. To facilitate comparison and discussion, the reviewed subluxation studies are grouped as *Subluxation Mimic Models,* in which the study investigators attempted to mimic the subluxation, or *Subluxation Component Models,* wherein the investigators simply assume the subluxation produces a certain component effect and then examine the influence of that specific effect. *Spinal Manipulation Mimic Models* are dichotomized according to the method of manipulation, that is, manual or instrument.

Subluxation Mimic Models are further subdivided with regard to whether the subluxation was induced manually or surgically. Subluxation Component Models are subgrouped according to whether the effect of the component investigated was mechanical, chemical, or both.

Where studies address multiple elements of this taxonomy, the full synopsis is provided under the initial entry; a pointer to the location of the full description has been placed under the second entry within the list of studies. These studies have also been marked with an asterisk (*) after the large bold study number at both entries (e.g., both manual and surgical methods were used for inducing subluxation—studies 1 and 2).

Subluxation Mimic Models
Manual Subluxation Mimic Models

1*

DATE: 1964

AUTHORS: S.D. Miroyiannis, H.C. Hunter, J.W. Chatfield[44]

TITLE AND SOURCE: Effect of vertebral malalignment on Nissl granules in rabbit spinal cord

Journal of the American Osteopathic Association 1964;63:862-3

---

*This study is listed under both manually and surgically induced subluxation mimics.

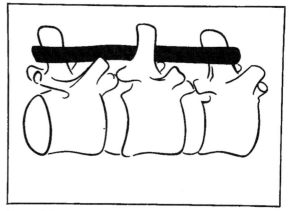

Figure 4-4   Surgically subluxated animals had a 1-cm, 20-gauge, aluminum wire implanted between the spinous processes of three lumbar vertebrae such that the middle vertebra was rotated relative to its two contiguous neighbors. The wire was secured by sutures. *(Reprinted with permission from Miroyiannis SD, Raines BA, Jurczenko VJ, Hunter HC. J Am Osteopath Assoc 1965;65:48-52.)*

ANIMAL: 21 Rabbits

METHODS: The rabbits were divided into three groups. Group 1 received a manually induced spine lesion. While under pentobarbital anesthesia, the upper lumbar spine was forcibly extended and rotated. Group 2 animals received a surgically implanted wire that was positioned to laterally malalign the spinous process of a lumbar vertebra relative to its contiguous neighbors (Figure 4-4). Group 3 animals served as nonmanipulated (normal) controls. The Nissl granule content of anterior horn cells was then compared between the control group and the two experimental groups at 2, 4, 6, 8, or 10 days following the experimental procedure.

FINDINGS: The Nissl content of cells in the manually manipulated group decreased progressively from the second to the tenth day. By contrast, the Nissl content of cells in the surgically malaligned group decreased in amount on the second day, but gradually increased such that by the tenth day following the surgery it was the same as the control group. The authors noted that these results were consistent with earlier work by Cole,[45] in which a similar manual spine trauma produced decreased Nissl granule content in anterior horn cells.

COMMENT: This study was one of the last of its kind in a long line of studies published in the osteopathic literature wherein the spine of an animal was manually traumatized to produce an "osteopathic lesion."[45-48] The study design did not permit the authors to discriminate between the consequences of acute trauma associated with the manual manipulation or surgical procedure and a possible chronic consequence of these interventions, an osteopathic lesion (or subluxation). In study 2, the authors did control for the surgical trauma.

Modified Haldeman Criteria: #3

2*

DATE: 1965

AUTHORS: S.D. Miroyiannis, B.A. Raines, V.J. Jurczenko, H.C. Hunter[49]

TITLE AND SOURCE: Effects of distortion of the spinal column of the rat with reference to the Nissl granules of the anterior horn cells: a pilot study

Journal of the American Osteopathic Association 1965;65:48-52

ANIMAL: 50 Rats

METHODS: The authors repeated the study previously conducted in rabbits (study 1), but with four groups of rats: (1) manual manipulation, (2) manual control, (3) surgical lesion, and (4) surgical control. The manual lumbar manipulation was as described above (under pentobarbital anesthesia) but was repeated until palpable paraspinal muscle spasticity was observed. The manual control group rats were anesthetized, but they received no procedure other than daily palpation. Rats in the surgical lesion group received the spinous displacing implant procedure described in study 1 (Figure 4-4), while animals in the surgical control group only had the wire placed next to but not displacing the T11-L1

---

*This study is listed under both manually and surgically induced subluxation mimics.

[sic] spinous processes. In each group, half of the animals were sacrificed at 8 days and the other half were sacrificed at 15 days. Rats in the manual manipulation group received regular, additional manipulations under anesthesia during the survival period to maintain paravertebral spasticity. At the end of the 8- and 15-day survival periods, spinal cord sections were examined for both the quality and quantity of Nissl granule changes.

FINDINGS: These investigators found that animals receiving traumatic manual manipulations had markedly diminished Nissl granule content at both 8 and 15 days. Manual control animals had normal Nissl granule presentation at both time intervals. The most interesting finding was the difference between the surgical lesion group and the surgical control group. At 8 days, the surgical control group experienced a similar loss in Nissl substance as that experienced by the traumatic manual manipulation group, but at 15 days the surgical control animals had recovered the Nissl content to a normal level (like the manual control group). By contrast, surgical lesion rats maintained a low Nissl granule appearance at both the 8- and 15-day exam periods. The authors concluded, "Apparently the experimentally produced malalignment [surgical lesion] was sufficient stress in itself to cause changes in the Nissl granules."

COMMENT: This study took an important step toward linking changes in spinal biomechanics with changes in the nervous system. However, they did not actually measure the biomechanical consequences of their experimental lesions and compare those changes against quantified changes in Nissl substance. This was a pilot study, but to my knowledge, a more definitive follow-up study was never published.

Modified Haldeman Criteria: #3

3

DATE: 1981

AUTHOR: K.F. DeBoer[50]

TITLE AND SOURCE: An attempt to induce vertebral lesions in rabbits by mechanical irritation

Journal of Manipulative and Physiological
Therapeutics 1981;4:119-27

ANIMAL: 8 Rabbits

METHODS: DeBoer evaluated the use of a Grostic
Adjusting Gun as a means of inducing
subluxation in rabbits using a single group pre-
post design. The C1 vertebra of each rabbit was
impacted with the gun in addition to one
thoracic vertebra (Figure 4-5). The Grostic gun
was set with a 4-mm tip displacement and
delivered 15 pulses at approximately 66.2
N/pulse (15 lb/pulse). The tip was placed against
the left or right C1 transverse process to drive
the vertebra laterally or at the base of a thoracic
spinous process (approximately 45-degree angle)
to produce rotary and anterior displacement.
These lesion inducements were performed two
times per day for four consecutive days for each
animal. Three blinded observers determined the
presence and location of subluxations before and
after subluxation inducement in the spine regions
C1, and T1 to T8. The observers were
chiropractic students with advanced standing,
who had all received training in palpation. They
were specifically trained to palpate normal and
"experimentally subluxated" rabbits for
approximately six weeks prior to the beginning
of the study. They recorded their palpation
findings as level (C1, T1, T2…T8) and severity
(0, no lesion, to 3, grossly obvious lesion). All
rabbits were also radiographed (lateral and
dorsal-ventral) before and after subluxation
inducement.

FINDINGS: DeBoer reported a statistically
significant higher "vertebral lesion score" from
palpatory findings after subluxation inducement
in the rabbits compared to the preinducement
score. However, he found that interexaminer
postinducement palpation scores were only
marginally significant. Also, radiographic
examination demonstrated no reliability. He
noted that inducing subluxations with the
Grostic gun produced considerable soft tissue
edema in some rabbits as well as muscle
splinting, which interfered with palpatory
assessment. Because of this and the benefit of

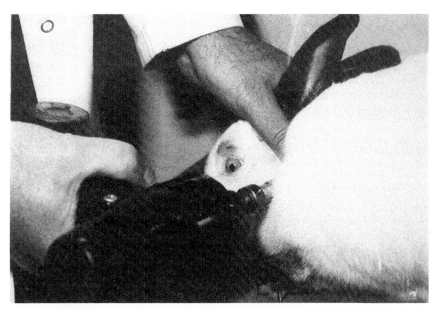

Figure 4-5   DeBoer evaluated the use of a Grostic Adjusting Gun as a means of inducing subluxation in rabbits using a single group pre-post design. The C1 vertebra of each rabbit was impacted with the gun in addition to one thoracic vertebra. *(Reprinted with permission from DeBoer KF. J Manipulative Physiol Ther 1981;4:119-27.)*

having tactile feedback, he suggested that future studies would probably use a manual method for producing subluxation lesions.

COMMENT: This study by DeBoer began a sequence of published work that, until recently, was the only sustained subluxation mimic investigation in chiropractic research (DeBoer studies 4, 5, 9, and 10). Recently, Henderson and Cramer have developed a reversible spine fixation model which has been characterized biomechanically (study 13) and has been shown to produced spine degeneration (study 14). In addition, Budgell (studies 23, 26, 27, and 28), Pickar (studies 19, 20, 21, 29, 30, 31, and 34), and Sato (studies 18, 23, 26, 27, and 28) have produced an impressive number of "subluxation component" and "spinal manipulation mimic" studies using animal models within the past decade. DeBoer's work also demonstrated the difficulty of developing reliable verification procedures, a situation that parallels the chiropractic clinical experience.

Modified Haldeman Criteria: #2

4*

DATE: 1984

AUTHOR: K.F. DeBoer[51]

TITLE AND SOURCE: Gastrointestinal myoelectric activity in rabbits with vertebral lesions: preliminary report

European Journal of Chiropractic 1984;32:131-42

ANIMAL: 9 Rabbits

METHODS: A subluxation mimic was attempted at T6 in these nine rabbits using one of two different methods. Six rabbits were "subluxated" using the Grostic gun technique described in study 3. Three rabbits were also "subluxated" using a surgically implanted 5 × 2 mm gold pin that was wedged between the pre- and post-zygapophyses of T6-T7. As in the earlier study

---

*DeBoer used both manually and surgically induced subluxation mimics in this study.

(study 3), three observers palpated the rabbits to determine the presence and degree of subluxation. In this investigation, the experimenter outlined strict palpation procedures requiring agreement between multiple examiners. Monopolar electrodes were implanted in the antrum and duodenum; both were located 5 cm from the sphincter. Gastrointestinal myoelectric activity was recorded in each fully conscious rabbit while restrained in a specially constructed frame for the 2- to 3-hour recording session. Three control recording sessions at least one week apart were performed prior to inducing subluxation lesions to obtain a stable baseline for each animal.

FINDINGS: DeBoer stated, "The EMG records from the stomach, and occasionally from the duodenum, were sometimes very noisy and difficult to interpret, even in the prelesioned (control) recordings. Visual analysis of the EMG recordings failed to reveal any obvious changes in pattern following induction of vertebral lesions, either by surgical or mechanical means." He also noted that demonstrating a "real" bony misalignment radiographically was problematic. The radiographs were inconclusive and at autopsy no visible spinal misalignment was observed in animals "subluxated" using the Grostic gun. In addition, the implanted pin had come completely out in two of the three surgically lesioned animals, and no residual spinal abnormality could be seen. In the one remaining surgically lesioned rabbit, the pin was still in place and radiographs revealed a small "very inconspicuous rotation of T6 and T7."

COMMENT: Once again, DeBoer's work demonstrated the twin problems of subluxation research—producing and verifying a successful subluxation lesion. As might be expected with problems obtaining a reliable vertebral lesion and the great variability in baseline EMG data, the results of this study were inconclusive. Despite this, he persisted in trying to develop an experimental subluxation lesion and studying the biological consequences of subluxation for an additional nine years. He succeeded in demonstrating gut EMG changes with a manual subluxation mimic in study 5.

Modified Haldeman Criteria: #2 and #3

5

DATE: 1988

AUTHORS: K.F. DeBoer, M. Schutz, M.E. McKnight[52]

TITLE AND SOURCE: Acute effects of spinal manipulation on gastrointestinal myoelectric activity in conscious rabbits

Manual Medicine 1988;3:85-94

ANIMAL: 22 Rabbits

METHODS: These investigators reported the acute effects of a manually induced vertebral lesion on gastrointestinal myoelectric activity in conscious rabbits. The subluxation mimic was produced by manually displacing the spinous processes of two contiguous vertebrae through the intact skin (Figure 4-6). They concurrently recorded EMG activity in the distal stomach and proximal duodenum in response to this vertebral displacement, and in additional control experiments. Control experiments consisted of a sham manipulation as well as noxious and nonnoxious stimulation of the skin overlying the vertebrae. The sham manipulation was accomplished by holding the same vertebral segments with slight ventral pressure, but no spinous rotation. The noxious stimulation was achieved by clamping a skin fold with a small forceps and nonnoxious stimulus consisted of light manual compression of the skin fold. The GI electrode placement and recording procedures are described in study 4. Manual vertebra displacement (the subluxation mimic) was applied to each rabbit at four different sites (T1-2, T5-6, T11-12, and L2-3) for about 2.5 minutes. The conscious rabbit remained calm during the subluxation lesion procedure after an initial startle response. No residual vertebral lesions were found upon subsequent palpation.

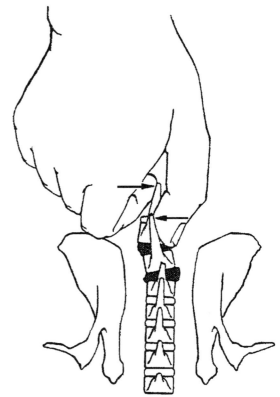

Figure 4-6   In a study of the acute effects of a manually induced vertebral lesion on gastrointestinal myoelectric activity in conscious rabbits, DeBoer et al. produced a subluxation mimic by manually displacing the spinous processes of two contiguous vertebrae through the intact skin. *(Reprinted with permission from DeBoer KF, Schutz M, McKnight ME. Manual Med 1988;3:85-94.)*

FINDINGS: DeBoer et al. reported a strong inhibition of gut EMG activity during the manually induced vertebral lesion, but not during the sham procedure or noxious and nonnoxious stimulation at the same vertebral sites. The response was also site specific, in that vertebral lesions at T1 and T6 produced complete inhibition of EMG activity in 19 of the 37 trials, while lesions at T12 and L3 produced complete inhibition in only 2 of 23 trials.

COMMENT: This interesting study provided support for the widely held view by chiropractic clinicians that visceral problems can be related to segmentally specific subluxations (the Meric System).[53-55] This work, along with that of Sato and Swenson (study 18), Budgell et al. (studies 23, 26, 27, and 28), and Kang et al. (study 31) demonstrate the existence of segmental and suprasegmental somatovisceral reflex pathways with afferent limbs in spinal and paraspinal tissues.

Modified Haldeman Criteria: #1 and #3

Surgical Subluxation Mimic Models
DATE: 1964*
AUTHORS: S.D. Miroyiannis, H.C. Hunter, J.W. Chatfield[44]
TITLE: Effect of vertebral malalignment on Nissl granules in rabbit spinal cord

DATE: 1965†
AUTHORS: S.D. Miroyiannis, B.A. Raines, V.J. Jurczenko, H.C. Hunter[49]
TITLE: Effects of distortion of the spinal column of the rat with reference to the Nissl granules of the anterior horn cells: a pilot study

6

DATE: 1965
AUTHOR: C.S. Cleveland[56]
TITLE AND SOURCE: Researching the subluxation on the domestic rabbit
International Review of Chiropractic: Scientific Edition 1965;1(8):1-23

---

*See study 1; these investigators used both manually and surgically induced subluxation mimics.

†See study 2; these investigators used both manually and surgically induced subluxation mimics.

ANIMAL: 2 Rabbits
METHODS: Cleveland applied a transcutaneous fixation system in which the spinous attachment device consisted of a compression clamp with a needle that pierced the spinous process of a single vertebra. Three contiguous spinous attachment devices were linked together by a superstructure that held the devices in various positions of fixation, with or without malposition (Figure 4-7). He reported two case studies in rabbits wherein a misalignment of T12 was produced—"the 12th dorsal vertebra was subluxated posterior and right."

FINDINGS: Cleveland reported that urinary system problems developed in both animals, but did not provide blood chemistries or histologic data. One rabbit developed proteinuria with blood casts and ascites within 1 month following the experimental subluxation. At the end of the month, the researchers corrected the vertebral malposition with the splinting device and the animal died 18 hours later. The second animal was similarly "subluxated" and observed for 3 months. This rabbit developed a transient proteinuria, but did not develop ascites. After 3 months with the experimental subluxation, the animal was euthanized and a necropsy was performed. A dense, white, fibrous mass was found in its right kidney. These investigators reported observing numerous pathologic and physiologic changes in "many, many other experiments," but no further detail was provided.

COMMENT: The introduction to this article explained that this was a report of their pilot studies to determine the feasibility of the model. Unfortunately, no follow-up work was ever published. This is the earliest recorded attempt to produce a small animal model of the chiropractic subluxation. Cleveland's approach is very similar to another subluxation mimic developed by Henderson and Cramer (studies 13 and 14).

Modified Haldeman Criteria: None. If control experiments had been performed, Haldeman criteria #1 would have applied.

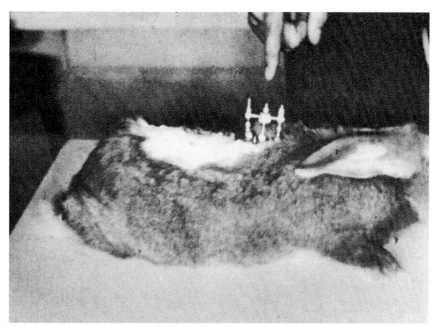

Figure 4-7   Cleveland produced a surgical subluxation mimic via a transcutaneous fixation system. Three spinous attachment devices were attached to contiguous vertebrae and subsequently linked together by a superstructure that held the devices in various positions of fixation, with or without malposition. *(Reprinted with permission from Cleveland CS. International Review of Chiropractic: Scientific Edition 1965;1(8):1-23.)*

7

DATE 1976

AUTHOR: M.Z. Awad[57]

TITLE AND SOURCE: Induction of intervertebral disrelationship in experimental animals and the preliminary effects of the dysarthrias

Proceedings of the 7th Annual Biomechanics Conference on the Spine. 1976;27-50

ANIMAL: 35 Rats

METHODS: Awad reported a surgical procedure to produce a reversible vertebral fixation rat model. He implanted small posts in the contiguous spinous processes (or anterior vertebral bodies) of rats which were then linked by a small rubber band, producing "an intervertebral disrelationship" (Figure 4-8). Vertebra linked via the spinous process posts could be released at a later date by making a small skin incision over the site and cutting the rubber band.

FINDINGS: Awad observed scoliosis in rats linked dorsally (in extension) or ventrally at the vertebral bodies (in flexion), but not in unlinked (control) rats. He commented that rats linked dorsally developed scoliosis more readily than ventrally linked animals (Figure 4-9). However, he did not provide data to support this observation.

COMMENT: This small study introduced a reversible animal model of spine fixation and suggested an interesting connection between fixation and scoliosis. However, no additional work with this model was ever published. A very similar subluxation mimic was suggested by Lin et al. two years later (study 8). Awad commented that previous animal models used methods that were

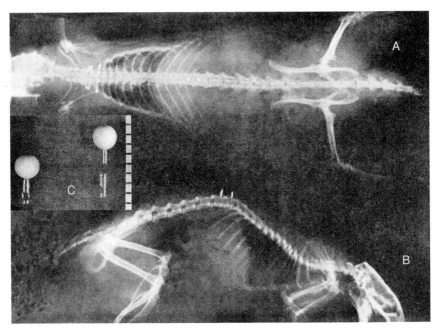

Figure 4-8   Awad reported a surgical procedure to produce a reversible vertebral fixation rat model. He implanted small posts in the contiguous spinous processes (or anterior vertebral bodies) of rats which were then linked by a small rubber band, producing "an intervertebral disrelationship." **A** and **C**, Radiographs of a rat three days after a successful spinous implant procedure. **B**, Stainless steel tube and post assemblies which were implanted and subsequently linked by a small rubber band. The scale on the extreme right side of this inset is 1 mm/division. *(Reprinted with permission Awad MZ. Induction of intervertebral disrelationship in experimental animals and the preliminary effects of the dysarthrias. In: Suh CH, editor. Proceedings of the 7th annual biomechanics conference on the spine. Boulder: University of Colorado; 1976. p. 27-50.)*

not reproducible. He was referring to previous studies in which an "osteopathic lesion" was created by manual manipulation of the spine.[44,58-60] This chapter reviews five studies that applied manual methods to produce a subluxation mimic (studies 1 to 5).

Modified Haldeman Criteria: #2

8

DATE: 1978

AUTHORS: H.L. Lin, A. Fujii, H. Rebechini-Zasadny, D.L. Hart[61]

TITLE AND SOURCE: Experimental induction of vertebral subluxation in laboratory animals

Journal of Manipulative and Physiological Therapeutics 1978;1:63-6

ANIMAL: Rats; number of animals not reported

METHODS: Lin et al. introduced a method for inducing an "experimental vertebral subluxation" in male rats. They fixed the T10 and T11 vertebrae in extension by attaching stainless steel screws to the spinous processes of these vertebrae which were then linked by a stainless steel spring. Sham operated, experimental, and normal animals were compared using line drawings on lateral radiographs.

FINDINGS: They reported a statistically significant intervertebral extension in the experimental group, but not the normal or sham groups.

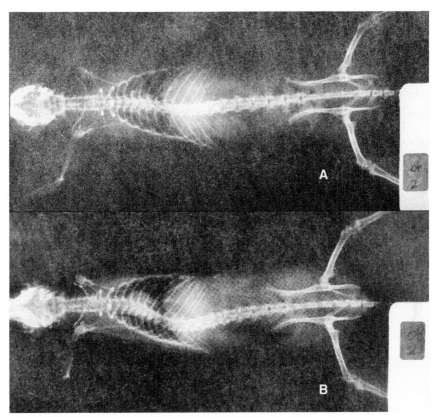

Figure 4-9   An experimentally induced scoliosis developed in the rat's lower thoracic region 15 weeks after the dorsal spine fixation procedure (**A**) and was significantly greater at 24 weeks following the fixation procedure (**B**). *(Reprinted with permission Awad MZ. Induction of intervertebral disrelationship in experimental animals and the preliminary effects of the dysarthrias. In: Suh CH, editor. Proceedings of the 7th Annual Biomechanics Conference on the Spine. Boulder: University of Colorado; 1976. p. 27-50.)*

COMMENT: The number of animals was not reported in this study and these investigators did not examine the putative pathophysiologic effects of the fixations they created. No further investigations were published with this model.
Modified Haldeman Criteria: #2

DATE: 1984[*]
AUTHOR: K.F. DeBoer[51]
TITLE: Gastrointestinal myoelectric activity in rabbits with vertebral lesions: preliminary report

---

*See study 4; DeBoer used both manually and surgically induced subluxation mimics in this study.

9

DATE: 1988
AUTHORS: K.F. DeBoer, M.E. McKnight[62]
TITLE AND SOURCE: Surgical model of a chronic subluxation in rabbits

Journal of Manipulative and Physiological Therapeutics 1988;11:366-72

ANIMAL: 16 Rabbits; actual number uncertain due to article discrepancies

METHODS: Ten adult rabbits were equally distributed between a control group and an experimental group. At least six additional animals originally planned for the experimental group were not used due to subsequent implant failure. In the experimental animals, a stainless steel bar was slid along the base of the spinous processes of three adjacent vertebrae within the T3-T7 region such that the bar moved the middle vertebra into rotatory misalignment with respect to the two end segments (Figure 4-10). The two ends of the bar were then sutured in place to the spinous processes of the end vertebrae. In the control animals, bars were initially placed similar to the experimental animals but then were immediately withdrawn and placed in a neutral force position (alongside, not between, the spinous processes). Successful "subluxations" were determined by static palpation and plain film radiographs. Successful bar implants were verified by visual inspection at the time of surgery and at autopsy.

FINDINGS: These investigators reported only a 50% success rate in producing a surgically induced vertebral lesion, determined by bar position at autopsy. Technical difficulties made palpation a poor outcome measure for evaluation of this model: "This palpation of the bar and surrounding fibrous or bony tissue was often judged by the palpators to, by itself, constitute a VL [vertebral lesion] of severity 1 even though no bony misalignment could be palpated." Radiographic data was equivocal, and the researchers commented that characterizing specific vertebral misalignments radiographically was confounded by difficulties obtaining standardized positioning of the rabbits.

COMMENT: This study has been credited with introducing the first surgical subluxation mimic. While DeBoer's work was certainly innovative and, until recently, has been the only continuous line of subluxation research in chiropractic, this was not the first surgical subluxation mimic. Four surgical models predate the DeBoer publication (studies 1, 2, 6, 7, and 8). Moreover, Miroyiannis introduced this very model in his 1964 and 1965 publications (studies 1 and 2).

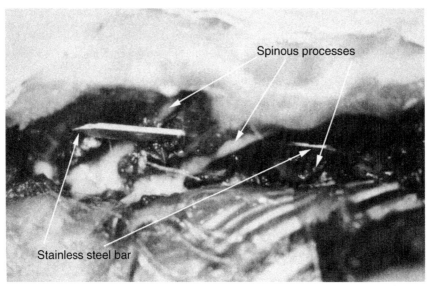

Figure 4-10   In DeBoer's surgical subluxation mimic, a 3.8-cm stainless steel bar was slid along the base of the spinous processes of three adjacent vertebrae such that the bar moved the middle vertebra into rotatory misalignment with respect to the two end segments. The two ends of the bar were then sutured to the spinous processes of the end vertebrae to hold the bar in position. In this figure, the wound has been enlarged for photography of the insert. *(Reprinted with permission from DeBoer KF, McKnight ME. J Manipulative Physiol Ther 1988;11:366-72.)*

Unfortunately, this productive researcher published only one further study before leaving Palmer college for nonresearch pursuits (study 10).

Modified Haldeman Criteria: #2

10

DATE 1993

AUTHORS: K.F. DeBoer, J. Hansen[63]

TITLE AND SOURCE: Biomechanical analysis of an induced joint dysfunction (subluxation-mimic) in the thoracic spine of rabbits

Journal of Manipulative and Physiological Therapeutics 1993;16:74-81

ANIMAL: 15 Rabbits

METHODS: Fifteen anesthetized rabbits received steel bar implants to produce the surgical subluxation-mimic described by DeBoer et al. in their 1988 publication (study 9). Twelve rabbits were equally divided into experimental and control groups. The fate of the additional three rabbits receiving implants was not clear in the paper. As in study 9, rotary vertebral displacements were produced in the experimental rabbits. These investigators commented that the control animals were not "true" controls in that they had originally been experimental group animals in which the bar implants had moved out of position shortly after surgery (demonstrated radiographically). They noted that there was a 50% failure rate in animals having the bars still in place after 3 to 12 months (determined at autopsy). The stated primary outcome measure for determining successful subluxation lesions in this study was a radiographic series (lateral views: neutral, flexed, and extended; and posteroanterior views: neutral and laterally flexed) that used 4-inch foam molds to standardize animal positioning. Films were taken before the surgical implant and at various times after the implant. Angular displacement measurements were obtained from lines drawn from specific reference points on the films. However, DeBoer and Hansen also examined the spine of each animal at autopsy to determine final bar position and visually discern misalignment

and fixation when the spine was moved through the same motions used in the radiographic exam.

FINDINGS: Visual and manual examination of animals at necropsy revealed that none of the controls were misaligned or fixated, but four of five experimental animals were relatively fixed in at least one motion. In addition, all but one experimental animal had a visually discernible spinous rotation. However, the researchers found no statistically significant decreases for radiographically determined intervertebral range of motion of experimentally lesioned areas.

COMMENT: Although these investigators reported vertebral lesion effects observed at necropsy examination, they did not find statistically significant decreases in their main outcome measure, radiographically determined intervertebral range of motion. Surprisingly, they did not examine range-of-motion differences within each animal (preimplant and postimplant). Rather, they compared postsurgical range-of-motion measurements between adjacent 3-segment regions for each experimental animal and between control and experimental animals. One is left to wonder why a prelesion versus postlesion ROM difference was not calculated for the lesioned and control procedure segments in each animal. Subsequent comparison across segmental levels within the experimental group and between the study groups appears to be the critical analysis for this study. DeBoer and Hansen concluded the study with this comment: "Of course, our model is inherently very tentative and crude, but nonetheless, we think it is a viable first generation model and one quite easy to produce."

Modified Haldeman Criteria: #3

11

DATE: 1991

AUTHORS: M. Papakyriakou, J.J. Triano, P.C. Brennan[64]

TITLE AND SOURCE: Spine stiffness measures in a dog model of restricted joint motion

Proceedings of The International Conference on Spinal Manipulation 1991:272-4

ANIMAL: 6 Dogs

METHODS: This data was drawn from a larger study (see study 12). The dogs were assigned to either an experimental group (n = 4) that received bilateral intraarticular zygapophyseal joint (Z-joint) injections of a nontoxic, nonimmunogenic fibrin adhesive or a control group (n = 2) that underwent the same surgical procedure without the adhesive injection. The experimental group animals were divided further into two subgroups, one group (n = 2) received the intraarticular injections into the L1/L2 and L2/L3 Z-joints bilaterally. The other group (n = 2) received the injections in the T11/T12, T12/T13, L1/L2, and L2/L3 Z-joints bilaterally. All animals were assessed for spine stiffness preinjection and at three months postinjection by stress radiographs and biomechanical stiffness tests (motion analysis system with reflective skin markers at T13, L2, and S1). Stress radiographs were taken of anesthetized animals held in extreme flexion and extreme extension. Angles were subsequently measured from posterior body lines drawn on the radiographs at L1, L2, L3, and L7. Motion analysis was performed with the anesthetized animals placed prone in a sling that left the lumbar spine unsupported. Dorsoventral loads (up to 20% body weight for 150 seconds) were placed at L2 during each test and the resulting marker translations were recorded.

FINDINGS: The radiographic stress analysis revealed increased spine stiffness in the experimental group as indicated by a range of motion loss at L1/L7 and L1/L2 in the experimental animals, but not in the controls. The L2/L3 radiographic data was equivocal. The motion analysis data failed to show any differences between the experimental and control groups. These investigators thought technical problems with regard to accurately repositioning markers between preinjection and postinjection tests may explain the motion analysis failure. In addition, they commented that the skin marker–dependent motion analysis system may be confounded by

hypermobile segments developing adjacent to fixed segments.

COMMENT: One of the investigators' explanations for the apparent failure of the motion analysis system (hypermobile segments developing adjacent to the fused segments) could probably have been evaluated by reexamining the radiographs. This is the only fixation model incorporating an intraarticular adhesive. An additional abstract using this model was published at the same conference (study 12).

Modified Haldeman Criteria: #2

12

DATE: 1991

AUTHORS: P.C. Brennan, K. Kokjohn, J.J. Triano, T.E. Friz, C.L. Wardrip, M.A. Hondras[65]

TITLE AND SOURCE: Immunologic correlates of reduced spinal mobility: preliminary observations in a dog model

Proceedings of the International Conference on Spinal Manipulation 1991:118-21

ANIMAL: 8 Dogs

METHODS: This study used the joint adhesion model reported by Papakyriakou et al. in study 11. The eight dogs were assigned in equal numbers to either a facet joint fusion group or a sham fusion group. The joint fusion animals received injections into the L1/L2 and L2/L3 facet joints (two of these dogs also received injections into the T11/T12 and T12/T13 joints). Dogs in the sham group had the same surgical injection procedure, but the adhesive was injected subcutaneously, adjacent to, but not in the target facet joints. In addition to the radiographic and motion analysis tests described in study 11 above, peripheral blood was collected in EDTA Vacutainer tubes at baseline and every two weeks after adhesive or sham injection. Isolated polymorphonuclear neutrophils were tested for respiratory burst activity using chemiluminescence and mitogen challenge according to methods previously published by these investigators.[66] Plasma substance P levels were also measured with a radioimmunoassay previously used by these investigators.[66] All dogs were euthanized and necropsied 12 weeks after the facet injection. The target facet joints and adjacent tissues were harvested for histopathologic examination.

FINDINGS: The respiratory burst activity of both the adhesion fused and sham groups were significantly impaired four weeks after the injection procedure. The sham group returned to baseline by the sixth post injection week, but the fusion animals remained depressed for the duration of the study. Plasma substance P levels were markedly elevated in both groups two weeks after surgery, but these levels returned to baseline values four weeks postinjection. Interestingly, the substance P plasma level for the fusion group rose again after the fourth week and remained elevated for the duration of the study. Physical examination of the spines at necropsy suggested that the joints of animals in the fused group were more restricted than animals in the sham group. No gross pathologic changes were observed in the tissues of animals in either group. These investigators concluded that animals in the fused group exhibited early functional impairment of immune function. They explained that it is unlikely that these changes were the result of facet joint pathology because the histologic examination of these structures was negative.

COMMENT: This preliminary work is the only study, to date, that has quantitatively assessed immune function in an animal model of spine fixation. This work appeared promising, but because of pressures associated with the use of dogs, it was abandoned (personal communication).

Modified Haldeman Criteria: #1 and #2

13

DATE: 2000

AUTHORS: C.N.R. Henderson, J.W. DeVocht, S.J. Kirstukas, G.D. Cramer[67]

TITLE AND SOURCE: In vivo biomechanical assessment of a small animal model of the vertebral subluxation

Proceedings of the International Conference on Spinal Manipulation 2000:193-195

ANIMAL: 90 Rats

METHODS: Stainless steel spinous attachment units (SAUs) were surgically attached to the L4, L5, and L6 spinous processes of experimental rats and time matched control rats (Figure 4-11). After a one-week recovery period, the SAUs on experimental rats were externally linked by interconnecting the SAUs with small steel bars, producing vertebral fixation in a neutral or flexed position. Control rats were never linked but were assigned to groups with survival times that matched the link periods of the experimental rats (1, 2, 4, 8, 12, or 16 weeks). Dorsoventral spine stiffness (D-V stiffness) was determined with a Mecmesin load frame that measured displacement while a dorsoventral loading force was progressively applied to the rat spine (up to 3 N). Immediate residual D-V stiffness was determined by calculating the proportional change from baseline stiffness (stiffness before the link period) to that measured immediately after link removal at the end of the link period. Long-term residual D-V stiffness was the proportional stiffness change from baseline to that stiffness measured at a variable time period (4, 8, or 12 weeks) after link removal.

FINDINGS: Due to the numerous combinations of study variables and the small number of animals with complete data for this preliminary report, only descriptive statistics were reported. Examining D-V spine stiffness over a wide range of age in control and prelinked experimental rats suggested no D-V stiffening with age. Stiffness during the link period was much greater than baseline stiffness and increased with the length of the link period (at least a 245% increase during a 1-week link period and at least a 323% increase during the 16-week link period). D-V stiffness measured immediately after removing the links (immediate residual stiffness) was also increased from baseline (greater than 22% increase after a

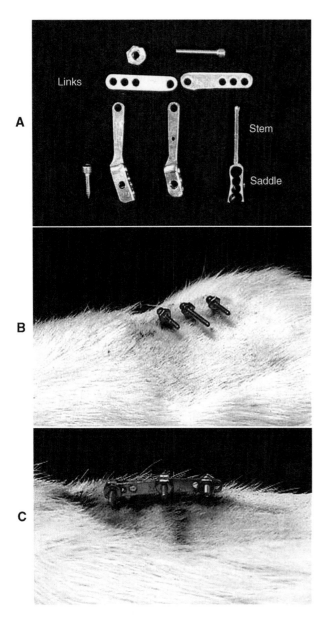

Figure 4-11   Henderson and Cramer produced a surgical subluxation mimic by implanting stainless steel spinous attachment units (SAUs) on the L4, L5, and L6 spinous processes of experimental rats and time-matched control rats. After a one-week recovery period, the SAUs on experimental rats were externally linked by interconnecting the SAUs with small steel bars, producing vertebral fixation in a neutral or flexed position. Control rats were never linked, but were assigned to groups with survival times that matched the link periods of the experimental rats (1, 2, 4, 8, 12, or 16 weeks). **A,** Three SAUs and two links. The far right SAU has been rotated to show the saddle region in profile. **B,** Either a control rat (never linked) or a rat before linking or after link removal. **C,** A rat linked in flexion. The black lines on the skin are residual marks from surgical guidelines.

1-week link period and greater than a 131% increase after a 16-week link period). Long-term residual stiffness was also increased above baseline, but there were insufficient animals in this presentation of preliminary data to suggest a trend. Lastly, no clear trend was noted with regard to the effect of link configuration (neutral versus flexed vertebral fixation).

COMMENT: This preliminary data demonstrated that the external link system used in this subluxation mimic could produce spine fixation and the links could be easily removed to allow measurement of residual stiffness effects. It was interesting that both D-V stiffness during the link period and immediately following, immediate residual stiffness appeared to increase with increased link time. It was surprising that the specific link configuration, neutral versus flexed, did not appear to have an effect. At the time of this conference abstract, the reported observations could not be statistically tested because of the relatively small amount of preliminary data and the large number of study hypotheses involved. However, those data are now available. A full journal article describing the surgical methods for the model as well as its biomechanical characteristics is expected to be published in 2005. A report of spine degeneration associated with this subluxation mimic was recently published (study 14). In addition, data relating neurological and behavioral changes observed with the model will be published soon. This model used a method for producing spine fixation that was very similar to the Cleveland subluxation mimic (study 6). However, these investigators incorporated a different spinous attachment unit (SAU) and they measured the changes in spine stiffness associated with linking the SAUs. The study reviewed below examined degenerative spine changes that developed as a biologically significant consequence of this subluxation mimic.

Modified Haldeman Criteria: #2

14

DATE: 2004

AUTHORS: G.D. Cramer, J.T. Fournier, C.N.R. Henderson, C.C. Wolcott[68]

TITLE AND SOURCE: Degenerative changes following spinal fixation in a small animal model

Journal of Manipulative and Physiological Therapeutics 2004;27:141-54

ANIMAL: 87 Rats

METHODS: Using the subluxation mimic described in study 13, three contiguous lumbar segments, L4, L5, and L6, were fixed with spinous attachment units in either a neutral, flexed, or rotated configuration (Figure 4-11). This study sought to answer three questions: (1) Will

experimentally induced lumbar spine fixation produce degenerative spine changes (hypertrophic spurs on the vertebral bodies and Z-joints, intervertebral disc thinning, or Z-joint articular cartilage and subchondral articular surface changes)? (2) Will the degenerative changes be greater with increased fixation time (1, 2, 4, 8, 12, or 16 weeks) or with a given experimental fixation position (neutral, flexed, or rotated)? (3) Is there a "time window" within which these degenerative changes will spontaneously remit if the experimental fixation is removed?

Rats were assigned to experimental and control subgroups such that spinal segments of control rats were compared with those of animals with 1, 4, or 8 weeks of fixation. Subgroups of the fixation animals subsequently had the fixation device removed for 1, 2, 4, 8, or 12 weeks to evaluate the effects of attempting to reestablish normal forces to the vertebral segments following hypomobility. Osseous and ligamentous spine structures were cleaned of all soft tissues by placing the carcasses of euthanized rats in a dermestid beetle colony. After the cleaned carcasses were removed from the colony, the spines (L3-S1) were harvested en bloc and then hydrated and fixed in a 5% formalin solution. The vertebral bodies, intervertebral disks, and zygapophyseal joints were subsequently examined for macroscopic degenerative changes using the 6X and 12X magnifications of a dissecting microscope. Both the occurrence (number of involved segments) and severity (scale of 0 to 3, least to most severe) of degenerative changes were recorded. No formal blinding procedures were used in the study.

FINDINGS: Significant differences were found between fixed segments and nonfixed segments within the same animal for all of the occurrence and severity Z-joint parameters in animals that had been linked, but not in comparable segments of control (never linked) animals (Figure 4-12). Both osteophytic and articular surface degeneration was greater on linked (fixated) vertebrae compared to adjacent, nonlinked

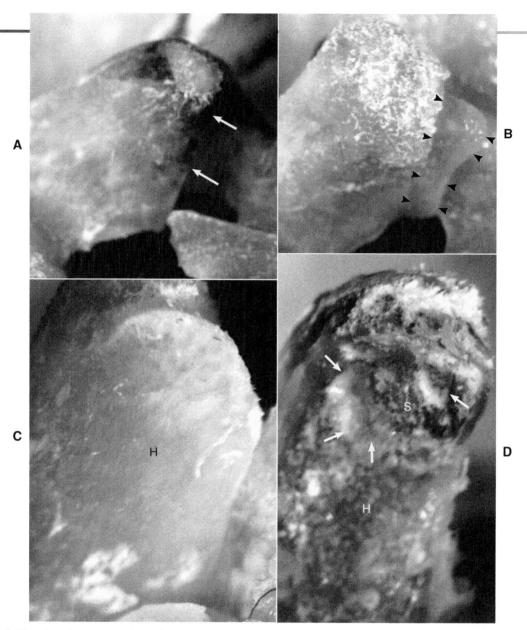

Figure 4-12   A and B, zygapophyseal joint (Z-joint) osteophyte formation on the external surfaces of two L5 cephalad articular processes for the degeneration severity parameter. **A** is from a control animal [Cnull, 8-week], and **B** is from an 8-week fixation animal. The large white arrows in **A** point to the smooth cephalad edge of the articular process, with no signs of osteophyte formation. The arrowheads in **B** outline a +3 osteophyte. C and D, Internal surfaces of two L5 cephalad articular processes demonstrating Z-joint articular cartilage degeneration for the degeneration severity parameter. **C** is from a control animal [Csau, 1-week], and **D** is from a 4-week fixation animal. Notice that the hyaline articular cartilage of the control animal (**C**) is quite smooth, while that of the 4-week fixation animal (**D**) has marked roughening, pitting, and remodeling. The remodeling is so marked in **D** that the ventral portion of the articular process (bottom) is out of the plane of maximum focus. In addition, subchondral bone is exposed on the dorsal portion of the articular process (hyaline articular cartilage has eroded). The arrows in **D** show deep pits within the Z-joint articular cartilage and subchondral bone. *H*, Hyaline cartilage on the Z-joint facet of a cephalad articular process. *S*, Subchondral bone. *(Reprinted with permission from Cramer GD, Fournier JT, Henderson CNR, Wolcott CC. J Manipulative Physiol Ther 2004;27:141-54.)*

(nonfixated) vertebrae. These differences were greater with longer link times. However, link configuration (fixation position) did not appear to influence the number of occurrences or the severity of the degenerative changes. In addition to these differences between adjacent vertebrae within animals, it was observed that the occurrence and severity of Z-joint osteophytes on rats with fixated vertebrae were significantly greater than similar degenerative changes on comparable segments in never-linked control rats. Moreover, longer link times were associated with greater osteophyte occurrence and severity. There was some evidence that osteophyte occurrence and severity improved when the links removed. However, this improvement appeared to have a link-time threshold. It was only observed in animals linked less than eight weeks. Degenerative changes to the articular surfaces paralleled the osteophytic changes with regard to both occurrence and severity. However, articular surface changes appeared earlier and the differences were more pronounced in animals linked for longer durations. Moreover, the link-time threshold above, which little or no improvement was obtained by removing the links, was lower than that observed for osteophytes, occurring somewhere between one and four weeks of link-time. Vertebral body changes were rare in this study, occurring in only three instances of 390 vertebral bodies examined (all three of these were from fixated animals). Similarly, only one intervertebral disc was found to have a degenerative severity score greater than 1.

COMMENT: This subluxation mimic study provided strong evidence that decreased vertebral motion (vertebral fixation) produced degenerative changes in the zygapophyseal joints that were greater for longer periods of fixation. Moreover, the data suggested that an "intervention time threshold" may exist, before which an active intervention may reduce or reverse the fixation-induced degenerative changes. This intervention time threshold appeared to be earlier for facet surface degeneration (occurring between one and four weeks of fixation time) and later for

osteophytic degeneration (occurring between four and eight weeks of fixation time). In addition, facet degeneration was observed to occur earlier than osteophyte formation. The existence of these time thresholds is intriguing and may have clinical significance. However, the authors warn that there is no known basis for projecting these time frames onto human subjects. This study was part of a larger project examining the physiologic consequences of spine fixation. Future publications with this model will examine neurological and behavioral changes as well as the putative benefits of spinal manipulation as a therapeutic intervention.

Modified Haldeman Criteria: #1 and #2

Subluxation Component Models

Mechanical Subluxation Component Models

15

DATE: 1967

AUTHORS: J.S. Denslow, T.F. Armour, E.A. Bruns, V.N. Kassicieh, R. Vomastek[69]

TITLE AND SOURCE: Evidence of osteopathic lesion in an experimental animal (dog): part I

Journal of the American Osteopathic Association 1967;66:94-5

ANIMAL: Dogs; number not reported

METHODS: These researchers describe the construction and application of a device that is very similar to a present-day pressure algometer. This device was used in conjunction with an electromyograph to record contractions of the musculus cutaneous trunci (MCT) in response to measured pressure applied to specific spinous processes.

FINDINGS: Denslow et al. reported that many older dogs demonstrated a region in the lower thoracic spine, particularly T10 and T11 that presented three elements common to the "osteopathic lesion": (1) palpable "abnormal" tissue tone overlying the spinous process, (2) hyperalgesic response to digital pressure on the spinous process (e.g., withdrawal, vocalization, and occasional snapping at the examiner), and (3) depressed "spinal reflex" threshold. The spinal reflex referred to was a contraction of the musculus cutaneous trunci in response to pressure over the tender spinous processes. These investigators drew a comparison between this observation and the "viscero-pannicular reflex" reported by Ashkenaz and Spiegal in 1935.[70] The viscero-pannicular reflex is a contraction of the musculus cutaneous trunci (MCT) in response to gallbladder distention with a rubber balloon. The old name for musculus cutaneous trunci is "panniculus carnosus."

COMMENT: This is a loosely written descriptive report. The number of animals used was not provided and specific experimental methods were not well described. Only brief qualitative observations were reported. However, the "spinal reflex" referred to in this animal study bears some similarities to the interesting observations of Lehman et al. (2001)[71] in a human study. Lehman et al. measured increased paraspinal muscle activity via surface electromyography (s-EMG) in response to dorsoventral pressure applied to tender spinous processes in the low back region of human subjects. The pressure was applied using a pressure algometer. Lehman et al. reported a reduction in pressure stimulated s-EMG activity following spinal manipulation of the involved segments.

Modified Haldeman Criteria: #2

16

DATE: 1967

AUTHORS: J.S. Denslow, T.F. Armour, E.A. Bruns, V.N. Kassicieh, R. Vomastek[72]

TITLE AND SOURCE: Evidence of osteopathic lesion in an experimental animal (dog): part II

Journal of the American Osteopathic Association 1967;66:95-7

ANIMAL: >20 Dogs. However, it is unclear that this number applies to this specific study.

METHODS: This study is a continuation of the work reported in study 15. Denslow et al. used a device that is very similar to a present-day pressure algometer in conjunction with an electromyograph to record contractions of the musculus cutaneous trunci (MCT) in response to measured dorsoventral pressure applied to thoracic and lumbar spinous processes. In this part of their study, they included radiographic examination of the spine and compared responses in young versus older dogs.

FINDINGS: They found that T10 was often the most sensitive spinous process in the dogs they examined, but this spinous was considerably shorter than that of adjacent segments and not readily contacted with their algometer-like device. They had no explanation for this anatomical feature. Denslow et al. reported three primary findings: (1) an apparent correlation between the presence of abnormal local paraspinous tissue tone, hyperalgesia, and a low "spine reflex" pressure threshold (contraction of the MCT with relatively low pressure on the involved spinous process), (2) animal-to-animal differences in spinal reflex pressure thresholds, and (3) spinal reflex thresholds varied between segments within the same animal (elevated at some and depressed at others). They noted that young, healthy dogs usually had no spinal reflex response to maximum spinous pressures applied with their algometer-like device, while older dogs frequently had tender spinous processes and demonstrated spinal reflexes to low dorsoventral pressures.

COMMENT: In this study (part II), the investigators reported the amount of pressure applied to spinous process at different segmental levels but made only qualitative comments about the associated spinous reflex response. They failed to adequately summarize their data and provided no study design information or statistical analysis. However, the observations reported are interesting and suggest hypotheses for examination in more rigorous studies. In addition, as mentioned in "comments" on part I of this study above, the "spinal reflex" referred to in this animal study bears similarities to the interesting observations of Lehman et al. (2001)[71] in a human study.

Modified Haldeman Criteria: #2

Unfortunately, this study was never presented in greater detail and no additional work was published by this investigator.

Modified Haldeman Criteria: #3

17

DATE: 1983
AUTHOR: V. Israel[73]
TITLE AND SOURCE: Changes in nerve physiology in the rat after induced subluxation
Articulations 1983;1(1):9-10
ANIMAL: 5 Rats
METHODS: This brief article summarizes a Master's Thesis conducted at California State University, Los Angeles. It appears to be a very small study with no controls. The rats were positioned in a stereotaxic frame while dorsoventral pressure was applied to the L6 vertebral process, driving that vertebra into "anterior [ventral] subluxation." Israel did not supply important information in this article about the applied load (e.g., magnitude, rate of application, duration). She monitored changes in the Hoffman reflex by stimulating the tibial nerve in the distal thigh and recording electromyographic activity in the ipsilateral foot with a bipolar needle electrode.
FINDINGS: She reported that following the experimental subluxation the H waves were delayed up to 15%. Israel noted that a comparable increase in H-wave latency in human clinical studies of the analogous nerve pathway would be considered conclusive evidence for spinal root lesions produced by chronic compression. She also noted that a significant number of blunted and fragmented H waves were observed in this study after experimental subluxation of L6 in the rat. According to Israel, blunted and fragmented action potentials are indicative of axonal degeneration.
COMMENT: Although this presentation of Israel's work was very brief and incomplete, the model and study findings were quite interesting.

18

DATE: 1984
AUTHORS: A. Sato, R.S. Swenson[74]
TITLE AND SOURCE: Sympathetic nervous system response to mechanical stress of the spinal column in rats
Journal of Manipulative and Physiological Therapeutics 1984;7(3):141-7
ANIMAL: 21 Rats
METHODS: Sato and Swenson monitored changes in heart rate, blood pressure, and the activity of renal and adrenal sympathetic nerves following lateral flexion stress (0.5 to 3.0 kg) applied to four mechanically isolated vertebrae segments in intact animals. The posterior and lateral muscular attachments had been carefully removed from the spine segments (T10-T13 or L2-L5), and the terminal vertebrae of each segment were then firmly held by spinal clamps, leaving two mobile vertebrae in between (Figure 4-13). Responses were compared to those obtained by noxious pinching (2 kg/cm^2) and nonnoxious cutaneous stimulation (brushing at 1 Hz) delivered to either the lower chest skin or hind limb/hindpaw skin.
FINDINGS: These investigators reported clear and consistent decreases in blood pressure but only a small and inconsistent decrease in heart rate with lateral stress stimulation of the spine. They observed decreased renal nerve activity during the mechanical spine stimulation (to 64% of control activity with thoracic stimulation and 50% of control activity with lumbar stimulation). Adrenal nerve activity also decreased, with the greatest change occurring within the first five seconds of mechanical stimulation (to 85% of control activity for thoracic stimulation and 89% of control activity for lumbar stimulation). The maximum drop in

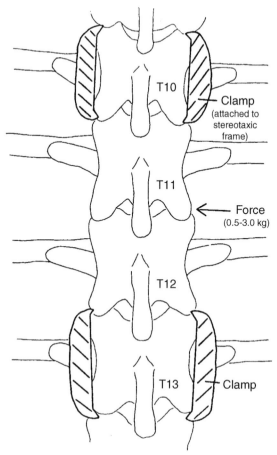

Figure 4-13 In this mechanical stimulation setup, the posterior and lateral muscular attachments had been carefully removed from the spine segments (T10-T13 or L2-L5). The terminal vertebrae of the segment were firmly held by spinal clamps in a stereotaxic frame, leaving two mobile vertebrae in between. A 0.5- to 3.0-kg force was applied to the right or left side of the mobile segment while Sato and Swenson monitored changes in heart rate, blood pressure, and the activity of renal and adrenal sympathetic nerves. *(Reprinted with permission from Sato A, Swenson RS. J Manipulative Physiol Ther 1984;7:141-7.)*

adrenal nerve activity within the first five seconds was followed by a gradual increase, reaching 121% and 116% of control levels (thoracic and lumbar, respectively) 25 seconds after the stimulation stopped. All of these effects were

greater with increased load (maximum of 3.0 kg). The direction of the lateral mechanical challenge (left or right) did not change the character of these responses. Baroreceptor denervation removed the adrenal nerve "overshoot" such that only activity decreases were observed with mechanical spine stimulation. Renal nerve activity had slightly greater stimulus-induced reductions after baroreceptor denervation. Spinalizing the animals (C1-C2 transection) reversed the effect of spinal stimulation. Lateral mechanical stimulation of the spine in spinalized rats caused slight increases in blood pressure, renal nerve activity, and adrenal nerve activity.

COMMENT: This elegant study was the first to demonstrate somatoautonomic spine reflexes using mechanical loads. The weights of the rats were not provided, but the common weight of Wistar rats used in laboratory studies is 250 g. Therefore it is probable that the applied mechanical force was 2 to 12 times each animal's body weight. Sato and Swenson did not determine whether their applied loads damaged articular structures. Consequently, it is not clear in this study whether the observed sympathetic nerve activities were in response to nociceptive signals. Subsequent studies reviewed here have clarified this matter. In addition, the force-time profiles associated with thrust manipulations, mobilization manipulations, or the static loads applied in this study may produce markedly different neurological responses. This issue is currently under investigation in J. Pickar's laboratory (personal communication). Sato and Swenson's study increased the level of scientific sophistication applied to basic subluxation research. Brian Budgell trained with Sato and continues the study of somatovisceral interactions arising from spine structures (studies 23, 26, 27, 28). Budgell's work, and work by Kang et al. performed in Pickar's laboratory (study 31) are clarifying the segmental and suprasegmental reflexes suggested in this early study by Sato and Swenson.

Modified Haldeman Criteria: #1, #3, and #4

19

DATE: 1999

AUTHOR: J.G. Pickar[75]

TITLE AND SOURCE: An in vivo preparation for investigating neural responses to controlled loading of a lumbar vertebra in the anesthetized cat

Journal of Neuroscience Methods 1999;89:87-96

ANIMAL: 2 Cats

METHODS: This article presents a modification of a unique surgical approach introduced by Pickar and McLain in 1995 (study 34). During spine loading, Pickar obtains single unit recordings in the L6 dorsal root from muscle spindle and Golgi tendon afferents supplying the local paraspinal muscles. The original preparation of Pickar and McLain allowed direct loading of an amputated L5-L6 articular pillar while preserving many of the associated muscles, ligaments, tendons, and the joint capsule. Although the paraspinal muscles were left largely intact in that procedure, some osseous attachments were removed to permit access to the caudal L5 articular pillar. In the procedure presented here, these limitations were largely overcome. The lumbar paraspinal tissues and their attachments from L5 to L7 were removed on the left side, but remained fully intact on the right side of the vertebral column. Access to the L6 dorsal root without damaging the L6 and L7 vertebrae was accomplished due to a unique anatomical feature of the lumbar spine. The L6 dorsal root (which innervates the L6-L7 facet joint) enters the spinal cord 2 to 2.5 vertebral segments rostral to the passage of the L6 spinal nerve through the L6-L7 intervertebral foramen. Therefore a full laminectomy at L5 and the inferior half of L4 was performed to permit access to the L6 dorsal root. During the laminectomy, care was taken to leave the multifidus muscles intact on the right side. This was accomplished by isolating the spinous processes and laminae from the intact paraspinal muscles on the right side using a subperiosteal approach. The periosteum was lifted from the bone surfaces using a Freer elevator, thereby allowing removal of bone without damaging the

multifidus muscles. With these paraspinal muscles intact, the L6-L7 facet joints were then physiologically loaded via attachment to the spinous process of the intact L6 vertebra using a 31-cm bridge connected to the lever arm of an electronic feedback motor (Figure 4-14). Loads were applied to the L6 vertebra at three angles (0 degrees, 45 degrees, and 90 degrees) relative to the long axis of each cat's vertebral column. This was thought to simulate decompression, bending, or rotation loads that might occur during segmental spine motion. Static loads (maintained for 15 seconds) were applied at 25%, 50%, 75%, and 100% of body weight such that the facet joints were either distracted (distractive loads) or compressed (compressive loads). The laminectomy procedure allowed single unit recordings from the right L6 dorsal root while the L6-L7 facet joints were loaded. The receptive area of each responding afferent was identified initially by stroking the paraspinal tissues through the overlying intact lumbar fascia with a cotton-tipped applicator. This large receptive area was subsequently narrowed to a relatively well-circumscribed area primarily over the longissimus or multifidus muscles by the use of nylon filaments (von Frey-like hairs). The mechanical threshold (von Frey) was also recorded for each afferent's receptive field. At the end of each experiment, the muscle proprioceptors were characterized by response to succinylcholine injection and by determining their conduction velocity.

FINDINGS: The responses of two paraspinal muscle proprioceptors to vertebral loading were reported. A proprioceptor located within the longissimus muscle was characterized as a muscle spindle because it had background-firing activity that increased with succinylcholine injection; its conduction velocity was 35 m/sec (consistent with Ia and II afferents). It was clearly a low threshold mechanoreceptor; the von Frey threshold was 20.9 g. By contrast, a receptor located in the multifidus muscle had no resting discharge and a minimal response to succinylcholine. The conduction velocity of this afferent was 54 m/s, consistent with group Ib

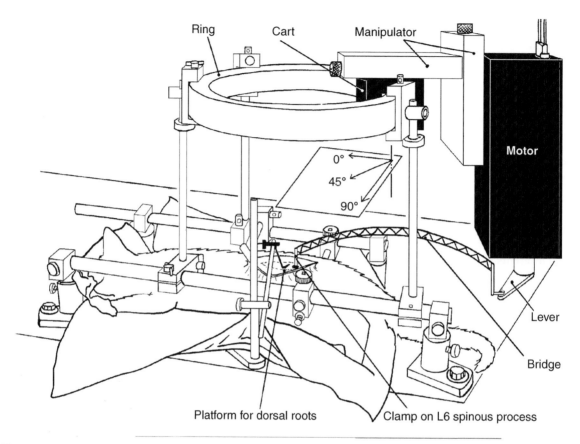

Figure 4-14   With the paraspinal muscles intact, the L6-L7 facet joints were physiologically loaded in anesthetized cats via attachment to the spinous process of the intact L6 vertebra using a 31-cm bridge connected to the lever arm of an electronic feedback motor. Loads were applied to the L6 vertebra at three angles (0 degrees, 45 degrees, and 90 degrees) relative to the long axis of each cat's vertebral column. During spine loading, Pickar obtained single unit recordings in the L6 dorsal root from muscle spindle and Golgi tendon afferents supplying the local paraspinal muscles. *(Reprinted with permission from Pickar JG. J Neurosci Meth 1999;89:87-96.)*

afferents in the cat cervical spine. Therefore it was considered to be a Golgi tendon organ. The von Frey threshold for this proprioceptor was high (164.3 g), but Pickar thought that this was probably due to the location of the tendon organ deep within the multifidus muscle mass. He noted that these characterizations must be considered tentative because he did not induce active muscle contraction, an action that would unload a muscle spindle (decreasing its activity) and load a Golgi tendon organ (increasing its activity). However, he observed that both of

these proprioceptors responded with unique activity patterns to changes in the magnitude and direction of lumbar loading. Pickar summarized his results with the observation that this preparation could be used to examine important questions with regard to central processing of paraspinal inputs, both somatic and autonomic. He specifically commented on the opportunity to use this preparation to investigate the combination of chemical mediators with mechanical loads, a combination thought to play a major role in low back pain.

COMMENT: In this article, Pickar makes a critical refinement to an important experimental preparation that he originally developed (study 34) and he demonstrates the value of this experimental setup in the study of sensory information arising from the lumbar paraspinal tissues during loading of the spine. In addition, he suggests possible applications of this experimental preparation in the study of somatic and autonomic reflexes as well as exploring possible low back pain mechanisms. In short, he identified a fruitful line of research that would occupy his laboratory for many years (studies 20, 21, 29, 30, and 31).

Modified Haldeman Criteria: #2 and #3

20

DATE: 2001

AUTHORS: J.G. Pickar, J.D. Wheeler[76]

TITLE AND SOURCE: Response of muscle proprioceptors to spinal manipulative-like loads in the anesthetized cat

Journal of Manipulative and Physiological Therapeutics 2001;24:2-11

ANIMAL: 10 Cats

METHODS: These investigators used the experimental preparation introduced in study 19 above. This preparation permitted physiologic loading of the L6-L7 facet joint while recording from the L6 dorsal root in each anaesthetized adult cat. As in the previous study, they obtained single fiber recordings and characterized the associated proprioceptors by examining afferent conduction velocities, mechanical threshold of receptive fields, the presence of resting discharge, and sensitivity to intraarterially administered succinylcholine. Vertebral loading was controlled using an electronically controlled feedback motor that moved the L6 spinous process via a rigid bridge with a specially fabricated "c"-clamp. (See Figure 4-14.) The motor was controlled to produce a force-time profile that mirrored a spinal manipulation, previously described by Hessel et al.[77] A specially constructed gantry

allowed the investigators to position the motor and its bridge such that the applied loads would distract or compress the L6-L7 facet joint.

FINDINGS: They obtained single unit recordings from 10 afferents with receptive fields in the multifidus or longissimus muscles of the lumbar spine. All but one of the afferents were classified as muscle proprioceptors (muscle spindles or Golgi tendon organs). Five afferents were classified as muscle spindles and four were classified as Golgi tendon organs (Figure 4-15, A and B). Due to its unique response characteristics, the nonmuscle proprioceptive afferent was thought to be a Pacinian corpuscle. Golgi tendon organ afferents generally had no resting discharge and increased more at the manipulation impulse than the preload. They usually became silent again immediately after the impulse. Muscle spindle afferents were characterized by a resting discharge, and they generally increased more at the impulse rather than the preload phase of the manipulation. Interestingly, spindle afferents often became silent immediately after the impulse (up to 4 seconds) and then resumed their background activity. In this study, both Golgi tendon and muscle spindle afferents responded more vigorously to loads that distracted rather than compressed the L6-L7 zygapophyseal joint.

COMMENT: This study was the first demonstration that muscle spindles and Golgi tendon organ afferents with receptive fields in the paraspinal muscles respond to vertebral loads with force-time profiles that are similar to spinal manipulation. Moreover, the unique response to the impulse (thrust) portion of the spinal manipulation–like load in this study suggests that paraspinal proprioceptors may contribute to the therapeutic effects of spinal manipulation. Pickar and Wheeler speculate that on the basis of their study findings, the combined activation of Golgi tendon organ and muscle spindle afferents during a spinal manipulation may decrease spontaneous EMG activity by reflex inhibition or disfacilitation of α-motor neurons. They also caution, "Clinical studies involving sham

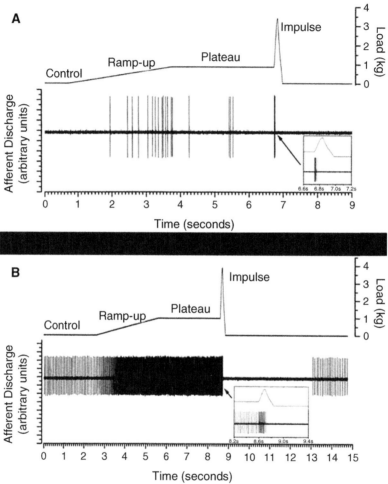

Figure 4-15   Pickar and Wheeler obtained single unit recordings were from afferents with receptive fields in the multifidus or longissimus muscles of the lumbar spine. Two afferents, classified as a Golgi tendon organ (**A**) and a muscle spindle (**B**), are shown here. Above each single unit recording, the force-time loading profile is shown. Each loading profile had four components (control, ramp-up, plateau, and impulse) replicating a typical spinal manipulation, as previously described by Hessel et al.[77] Golgi tendon organ afferents (**A**) generally had no resting discharge and increased more at the manipulation impulse than the preload. They usually became silent again immediately after the impulse. Muscle spindle afferents (**B**) were characterized by a resting discharge and they generally increased more at the impulse rather than the preload phase of the manipulation. Interestingly, spindle afferents often became silent immediately after the impulse (up to 4 seconds), and then resumed their background activity. *(Reprinted with permission from Pickar JG, Wheeler JD. J Manipulative Physiol Ther 2001;24:2-11.)*

manipulations should consider the types of sensory inputs they are trying to either mimic or exclude. Sham manipulations that provide a preload but not an impulse may still activate paraspinal muscle afferents." Perhaps this mechanism explains the recent observation by Dishman that both lumbar side posture manipulation and side posture set up alone (with a preload) inhibited the tibial H-reflex.[78]

Modified Haldeman Criteria: #3

21

DATE: 2001

AUTHORS: J.G. Pickar, Y.M. Kang[79]

TITLE AND SOURCE: Short-lasting stretch of lumbar paraspinal muscle decreases muscle spindle sensitivity to subsequent muscle stretch

Journal of the Neuromuscular System 2001; 9:88-96

ANIMAL: 5 Cats

METHODS: The work presented here used the approach developed by Pickar (see study 19). The great value of this approach is that it preserves the muscles, ligaments, tendons, and joint capsule of the facet joints, allowing physiologic loading and assessment of these intact joints. These investigators subsequently recorded single fiber afferent activity from the L6 dorsal root (which innervates the intact L6-L7 facet joint). The L6 spinous process was accessed with minimal trauma and controlled by an electronic feedback motor such that the vertebral column could be moved into flexion or extension (2 mm in either direction). Afferents and their receptive fields in the paraspinal muscles were identified. Mechanical thresholds were quantified with von Frey-like fibers, and conduction velocities were measured. Afferents with receptive fields in the multifidus or longissimus muscle were classified as muscle spindle afferents by the presence of resting discharge, increased discharge to succinylcholine, and decreased discharge to muscle contraction. Once identified as a muscle spindle afferent, the direction of spine motion (flexion or extension)

that loaded the spindle (stretched the muscle) was determined and a test sequence was initiated to evaluate the effect of previous muscle length history. Two previous histories were possible: "held short"—the muscle spindles had been unloaded (muscle shortened) for five seconds prior to a test movement that stretched the paraspinal muscle, or "held long"—the spindles had been loaded (muscle stretched) for five seconds prior to a test movement that stretched the muscle.

FINDINGS: Recordings were reported from five muscle spindle afferents. Four of these afferents had receptive fields in the longissimus muscle near the L6/L7 facet joint and one afferent had its receptive field in a multifidus muscle near the L7/S1 joint. All five spindles were loaded (stretched) by extension of the lumbar spine and unloaded by flexion. Hold short conditioning sensitized the paraspinal muscle spindles to subsequent muscle stretch.

COMMENT: This small but very interesting study found that holding the lumbar spine in two different static positions for as little as five seconds altered the sensitivity of paraspinal muscle spindles. This finding suggests that postural positions prior to spine motion will bias spindle-based information about joint motion and position. This "muscle history" effect could have serious clinical consequences. If sufficient proprioceptive error is introduced, the necessary synergy among and between muscle agonists and antagonists could be disrupted. This would certainly interfere with normal biomechanics and may predispose the joint to injury.

Modified Haldeman Criteria: #3 and #4

22

DATE: 1994

AUTHORS: B. Budgell, A. Sato[81]

TITLE AND SOURCE: Somatoautonomic reflex regulation of sciatic nerve blood flow

Journal of the Neuromuscular System 1994;2:170-7

ANIMAL: 24 Rats

METHODS: All rats in this study were anesthetized, artificially ventilated, and maintained normothermic at 80-mm systolic blood pressure for measuring autonomic nerve function. Mean arterial blood pressure (MAP) and heart rate (HR) were continuously monitored via an indwelling catheter in the right common carotid artery. Sciatic nerve blood flow (NBF) was assessed continuously via a Laser Doppler Flowmeter positioned over the left sciatic nerve. The animals were divided into three treatment groups. Group 1: Thirteen rats, 13 to 14 months old, received noxious mechanical stimulation (toe web pinch, 3 kgf for 10 seconds) before and after thoracolumbar spinalization; group 2: Six sympathectomized rats, 6 to 7 months old, received the same noxious mechanical stimulation before and after thoracolumbar spinalization; and group 3: Five rats, 13 to 14 months old, received the noxious mechanical stimulation after combined sympathectomy and spinalization. The age difference in group 2 was an attempt to obtain more stable sciatic nerve blood flow measurements associated with younger animals. This was abandoned after the group 2 data were gathered because the larger body size of older rats provided greater stability under prolonged anesthesia. Hence the age of group 3 animals was 13 to 14 months like group 1.

FINDINGS: Generally, for all rats with the spinal cord and lumbar sympathetic trunks intact, pinching either the forepaws or the hindpaws produced a brief increase in both MAP and NBF. In group 1 animals, spinalization produced a significant drop in MAP but an increase in NBF. Subsequent noxious mechanical stimulus to the forepaws increased both MAP and NBF. Interestingly, the increased NBF that followed noxious forepaw stimulation in these animals was greater after spinalization. Noxious hindpaw stimulation in these spinalized animals did not change MAP, but did produce a marked decrease in NBF. In group 2 animals there was a substantial drop in MAP following the sympathectomy procedure. Nevertheless, noxious forepaw or hindpaw stimulation in these

otherwise intact animals also produced an increase in both MAP and NBF. Due to technical problems, results from only three of the six group 2 animals were reported in the examination of noxious stimulus response after spinalization. After spinalization, noxious forepaw stimulation in these three sympathectomized animals increased NBF. However, the increased NBF following a hindpaw pinch that was seen previous to spinalization was abolished or decreased after spinalization in the sympathectomized animals. In the sympathectomized and spinalized group 3 rats, forepaw pinch continued to produce increased MAP and NBF. However, hindpaw pinch in these rats failed to materially change either MAP or NBF. It is known that sciatic nerve blood flow is relatively insensitive to changes in arterial CO_2 or pH levels. Further, although various naturally occurring chemical substances have been demonstrated in sciatic nerve tissue (e.g., substance P, serotonin, and vasoactive intestinal peptide), their role in the physiologic control of sciatic nerve blood flow is unknown. By contrast, both the presence and physiological role of noradrenergic fibers are well established. These experiments clarify that role (see Figure 4-17, study 26). They reveal that NBF is controlled by competing supraspinal and segmental influences. Lumbar sympathectomy removed segmental control (probably somatosympathetic constriction of the vasa nervorum) and thoracolumbar spinalization removed supraspinal control. Therefore noxious hindpaw stimulation failed to produce a change in either MAP or NBF in group 3 animals. Forepaw pinch increased MAP in these animals because neither afferent input from the forepaws nor supraspinal supply to the heart was blocked by the thoracolumbar spinalization. Consequently, the increased NBF seen with forepaw pinch in group 3 animals was probably just a passive response to increased MAP. By contrast, the increased MAP and NBF seen in intact group 1 rats following either forepaw or hindpaw pinch reflect the interplay between both a dominant supraspinal influence and a segmental influence. When supraspinal influences were removed by spinalization, a segmentally mediated decrease in NBF was unmasked with hindpaw pinch. This is most likely due to a somatosympathetic reflex constriction of the sciatic vasa nervorum.

COMMENT: These investigators point out that conclusions should not be drawn from this study about the possible effects of noxious stimulation at other sites (e.g., zygapophyseal joints or paraspinal tissues) or chronic noxious stimulation. In addition, they acknowledge that it is not known whether the magnitude of changes reported here could alter sciatic nerve function and thus have clinical consequences. However, their observations suggest a provocative question: Can noxious stimulation of somatic tissues at one site elicit reflex attenuation of blood flow in more distant nerves with resultant sensory and/or motor disturbance, producing aberrant end organ function? This question has great relevance to subluxation theory. In study 26, Budgell et al. further develop this interesting model of somatovisceral function. They examine the effect of noxious and innocuous stimulation of spinal and paraspinal tissues on sciatic nerve blood flow.

Modified Haldeman Criteria: #3

Chemical Subluxation Component Models

23

DATE: 1993
AUTHORS: J.W. Hu, X.M. Yu, H. Vernon, B.J. Sessle[80]
TITLE AND SOURCE: Excitatory effects on neck and jaw muscle activity of inflammatory irritant applied to cervical paraspinal tissues
Pain 1993;55:243-50
ANIMAL: 19 Rats

METHODS: All rats were anesthetized with halothane anesthesia and maintained in a stable experimental position by a stereotaxic apparatus. Electromyography (EMG) electrodes were inserted into the digastric, masseter, and trapezius muscles ipsilateral to the side of future algesic injection. Electrodes were also inserted bilaterally into the deep neck muscles (rectus capitis posterior). Electrode positions were evaluated by dissection after each experiment. EMG activity in all muscles was monitored before, during, and after injection of either mineral oil or mustard oil into the deep paraspinal tissues on the left side of the C1-C3 region. Changes in EMG activity after injection to either mineral oil or mustard oil were regarded as an increase if one or more EMG data points was elevated two standard deviations above the mean baseline level (mean of pooled preinjection levels). The "latency of response" was defined as the time from the beginning of an injection to an increase in EMG activity. The "duration of response" was the time interval between the beginning of an EMG response and the return of EMG activity to its preinjection baseline level. Mustard oil was also injected into the gastrocnemius-soleus muscle in three rats. Injection sites were visually examined for extravasation of Evans Blue dye, which was injected into the right external jugular vein at the end of each experiment. Neck tissues were also harvested and examined histologically for evidence of inflammation.

FINDINGS: Injection of mineral oil into the deep cervical tissues at C1-C3 produced only a small transient increase in EMG signal above baseline. By contrast, mustard oil injection produced a large increase in EMG activity that was observed in both the jaw and deep neck muscles. However, the response in the deep neck muscles was much more prominent than that seen in the jaw muscles. In addition, the response was generally biphasic (20 seconds after injection and 11 minutes after injection), with the second phase showing a larger EMG response with a longer response duration than that of the first phase (2 minutes versus 11 minutes). Mustard oil injected into distant noncervical muscles (gastrocnemius-soleus muscle) and noxious pressure to the hindpaw did not produce increased EMG activity in the jaw or neck muscles. Histologic examination revealed that mineral oil injections did not produce Evans Blue dye extravasation or an inflammatory reaction, while the mustard oil injections produced both in an area localized to the deep paraspinal tissues of the C1-C3 region. This was mostly ipsilateral to the injection site but did spread to the contralateral side in five of the nine animals receiving mustard oil injections.

COMMENT: This was the first study to demonstrate that irritation of deep cervical paraspinal tissues would result in a strong and moderately prolonged activation of both jaw and neck muscles. Moreover, this reaction was most pronounced in the deep cervical muscles. Mustard oil has been demonstrated to preferentially excite small-diameter nociceptive afferents and to act as an inflammatory irritant. The mechanisms involved in mustard oil-induced increases in EMG activity in the neck and jaw muscles are likely to be similar to those involved in paraspinal muscle hypertonicity resulting from subluxation as well as deep cervical injury and inflammation.

Modified Haldeman Criteria: #3

Mechanical and Chemical Subluxation Component Models

24

DATE: 1993

AUTHORS: R.G. Gillette, R.C. Kramis, W.J. Roberts[82]

TITLE AND SOURCE: Characterization of spinal somatosensory neurons having receptive fields in lumbar tissues of cats

Pain 1993;54:85-98

ANIMAL: 27 Cats

METHODS: All cats were anesthetized with sodium pentobarbital and maintained nonresponsive to toe pinch and without pressor response. Dura and dorsal horn access was accomplished by microlaminectomies 1 to 2 mm in diameter at the L4 vertebral level. Another laminectomy was

performed at T10 in 11 animals to permit transection of the right dorsolateral funiculus (to block conduction in most descending modulatory fibers) and implantation of microelectrodes in the left ventrolateral and right dorsolateral funiculus. Ethanol was injected bilaterally into paravertebral muscles at multiple sites (T9 to T11) to irreversibly block paraspinal muscle contractions in response to spinal stimulation. Extracellular single-unit recordings were made by advancing a recording electrode through the lateral dorsal horn in 6 μm steps. Electrode penetration depth was determined by recording the electrode tip relative to the cord surface (using a stepper drive) and by iontophoretic deposition of pontamine Sky Blue. Dye marks were located at the end of the study by histologic examination. While advancing the electrode, the lumbar region, hips and hind limbs were manually stimulated, first with nonnoxious and then with "just noxious" intensities (brief pinch and/or sustained pressure to skin and deep tissues). Nonnoxious cutaneous receptive fields were mapped prior to the application of noxious mechanical stimuli. Specific deep tissues were examined for low threshold and noxious mechanical response (dorsolateral dura and anterior longitudinal ligament/annulus fibrosis) while others were injected with saline, bradykinin, or capsaicin (multifidus muscles and facet joints).

FINDINGS: Most of the lateral dorsal horn neurons examined in this study (72% of 118 neurons) received converging excitatory input from skin and multiple deep tissues in the ipsilateral low back, hip, and thigh. These second order neurons were designated "sd," indicating convergence from skin and deep tissues. All sd neurons were nociceptive, responding to either noxious input alone (17 nociceptive specific neurons) or to both noxious and nonnoxious stimulation (68 wide dynamic range neurons). Some dorsal horn neurons (23% of 118 neurons) received only input from the skin and were designated "s" neurons. Very few (5% of 118 neurons) had input from only deep somatic tissues (designated "d" neurons). All "sd" and "d" neurons were activated by noxious stimulation of deep paraspinal tissues, including two or more of the following: facet joints, periosteum, ligaments, intervertebral disc, spinal dura, low back/hip/ proximal leg muscles, and tendons. The "sd" neurons also responded to skin stimulation. Although brush strokes, von Frey hair pressure, and pinching with forceps all produced a response, the most effective excitatory stimulus for "sd" neurons was injection of algesic substances (6% saline, bradykinin, or capsaicin) into deep paraspinal muscles and facet joints. In fact, some neurons that were unresponsive or only minimally responsive to brief or sustained noxious pressure on skin and deep paraspinal muscles responded vigorously to deep tissue algesic injections, suggesting input from mechanically insensitive nociceptors. Mechanical traction on the anulus of the intervertebral disc and the associated ventral longitudinal ligament produced a response in 9 of the 25 "sd" neurons (2 nociceptive specific and 7 wide dynamic range). In addition, 9 of 14 "sd" neurons (4 nociceptive specific and 5 wide dynamic range) tested by stimulating the spinal dura mater responded vigorously to noxious mechanical or chemical stimulation. The cutaneous receptive fields of most of the nociceptive dorsal horn cells were "very large." Most (75%) of the 28 neurons examined in detail showed expanded receptive fields after noxious stimulation that persisted more than a few seconds (e.g., injection of bradykinin into lumbar paravertebral tissues). Many (82%) of the 44 "sd" neurons examined had receptive fields that crossed the midline to involve a small additional area of skin on the contralateral back and hip. These same neurons responded to bilateral deep-tissue stimulation. Not all cells responded with increased activity. Ongoing background activity was attenuated by noxious and/or nonnoxious stimulation in 20% of the "sd" population (17 of 85). Most of these neurons had an inhibitory receptive field located within a larger excitatory receptive field of the low back or proximal leg. Twelve neurons were antidromically activated with stimuli localized to either the ipsilateral dorsal lateral funiculus or the contralateral ventral lateral funiculus. Eleven

of these dorsal horn neurons were "sd" neurons and one was a nociceptive specific "s" neuron.

COMMENT: This study is the first to examine dorsal horn neurons receiving noxious stimulation from deep lumbar paravertebral structures. The major finding was that most of the nocireceptive neurons (nociceptive specific and wide dynamic range) in the lateral border of the cat lumbar dorsal horn receive somatosensory input from many different deep somatic tissues and from skin in the low back, hip, and proximal leg. Gillette et al. refer to this observation as "hyperconvergence." The functional consequence of hyperconvergence is that these neurons are better suited to mediate diffuse, poorly localized pain than precisely localized pain. This is consistent with the observation that patients cannot readily localize the area of low back pain. Of course, this makes it very difficult for clinicians attempting to localize treatment on the basis of pain. Hyperconvergence also suggests a mechanistic explanation for the common referred pain pattern (hip and proximal thigh) associated with low back injury in humans. Gillette et al. demonstrated for the first time that noxious mechanical or chemical stimulation of the lumbar dura mater excite "sd" dorsal horn neurons (both nociceptive specific and wide dynamic range). This is consistent with recent studies in which the dura mater has become a focus for understanding neck and back pain and reexamining the interpretation of straight leg nerve tension tests.[83,84]

Modified Haldeman Criteria: #3

25

DATE: 1998

AUTHORS: R.G. Gillette, R.C. Kramis, W.J. Roberts[85]

TITLE AND SOURCE: Suppression of activity in spinal nocireceptive "low back" neurons by paravertebral somatic stimuli in the cat

Neuroscience Letters 1998;241:45-8

ANIMAL: 11 Cats

METHODS: The methods used here were the same as described in study 24. The primary focus of this investigation was to study the suppression of ongoing excitatory activity in a population of low back nocireceptive neurons. Receptive fields in the low back were identified using manual stimulation of lumbar paraspinal, hip, and hindquarter tissues at weak and intense levels (brushing, brief pinch, and/or sustained pressure onto deep tissues). Extracellular single-neuron recordings from mid to lateral L4-L5 dorsal horn neurons were obtained using micropipettes (3 M NaCl, 2-8 MΩ). After a nocireceptive neuron within the dorsal horn was located, its receptive fields were mapped and it was identified as responding to both skin and deep tissue stimulation (sd) or only to deep stimulation (d). It was then characterized as nociceptive specific (ns) or wide dynamic range (wdr), and its ongoing activity rate was recorded. Subsequently, local and distant mechanical stimuli (weak and intense) were applied to determine the location of inhibitory receptive fields. Five neurons were tested by antidromic stimulation above the T10 level (dorsolateral funiculus and ventrolateral funiculus).

FINDINGS: Fifteen neurons were identified that had stable ongoing activity throughout the recording periods (ranging from 40 to 280 minutes). Suppression was tested against this activity. Local mechanical stimuli (within the excitatory receptive fields) that were intense (pinch or 3.2 N von Frey) were effective in suppressing ongoing activity in 13 of the 15 low back nocireceptive neurons. Seven of 14 units tested with weak mechanical stimulation (brush or 0.09 N von Frey) also suppressed ongoing nocireceptive activity. The magnitude of suppression was similar in four units. Remote stimulus (pinna pinch) also produced suppression of similar magnitude in seven of seven units tested. This suppression was maintained throughout the period of stimulation for both weak and intense mechanical stimuli.

COMMENT: These investigators were the first to present data demonstrating suppression of activity in nocireceptive "low back" neurons by mechanical stimulation within their excitatory receptive fields. This suggested a mechanistic explanation for relief of low back pain following spine manipulation: a local, somatically induced suppression of low back nocireceptive neurons by mechanical stimulation of spinal and paraspinal structures. Interestingly, this was accomplished by both innocuous and intense local mechanical stimulation. These findings are consistent with the observation that the spinal cord is the initial site for pain modulation within the central nervous system. Interconnections between nociceptive and nonnociceptive afferent pathways can control the transmission of nociceptive information to higher centers within the brain. The concept that the pain experience results from a balance between nociceptive and nonnociceptive afferents, the Gate Control Theory, was first proposed by Melzack and Wall in 1965.[86] As in this study, the gate control mechanism is known to be topographically specific. The area of the body in which pain is regulated is linked anatomically to the segments of the spinal cord where the nociceptive afferents terminate.

Modified Haldeman Criteria: #3

26

DATE: 1995

AUTHORS: B. Budgell, H. Hotta, A. Sato[87]

TITLE AND SOURCE: Spinovisceral reflexes evoked by noxious and innocuous stimulation of the lumbar spine

Journal of the Neuromuscular System 1995;3:122-31

ANIMAL: 13 Rats

METHODS: The animals were prepared for measuring autonomic nerve function as described in study 23. Mean arterial blood pressure (MAP) and heart rate (HR) were continuously monitored via an indwelling catheter in the right common carotid artery. Sciatic nerve blood flow

(NBF) was assessed continuously via a Laser Doppler Flowmeter positioned over the left sciatic nerve. Experimental stimuli were *noxious mechanical* (pinched skin web between toes with a forceps, approximately 3 kg for 10 seconds), *injection of a nonnoxious agent* (20 µl of 0.9% saline), or *injection of a noxious agent* (20 µl of 10 mM capsaicin). These stimuli were applied to (1) the contralateral forepaw or hindpaw, (2) ipsilateral L4/L5 facet joint, or (3) L4/L5 interspinous ligament. The study consisted of two parts; Part 1 used nine intact rats, and Part 2 used four spinalized rats (cord transected at the thoracolumbar level).

FINDINGS: In intact animals, noxious mechanical *forepaw* stimulation produced a sharp

monophasic rise in both MAP and NBF followed by a slow fall toward normal values (NBF fell more rapidly than MAP). Saline injection into the contralateral *hindpaw* produced essentially no response (Figure 4-16, *A*). By contrast, similar to noxious mechanical stimulation, capsaicin injection into the contralateral hindpaw produced a sharp rise in both MAP and NBF and a slow return to baseline, with NBF falling more quickly (Figure 4-16, *B*). Saline injection into the ipsilateral L4/5 facet joint produced a small decline in both MAP and NBF (Figure 4-16, *C*). A slightly greater decline in both MAP and NBF was observed following capsaicin injection into the ipsilateral L4/L5 joint (Figure 4-16, *D*). Saline injection into the L4/L5 interspinous

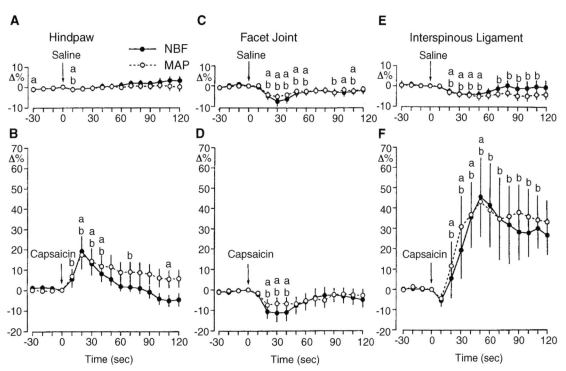

Figure 4-16   Budgell, Hotta, and Sato reported percentage change (mean ± SEM) in mean arterial blood pressure *(MAP)* and left sciatic nerve blood flow *(NBF)* in response to injection of the right (contralateral) hindpaw (**A, B**), left (ipsilateral) L4/5 facet joint (**C, D**), and the L4/L5 interspinous ligament (**E, F**) with 20 µl of isotonic saline (0.9% NaCl) or 20 µl of 10 mM capsaicin in 5% Triton X with saline carrier. Injection began at T = 0 and injection of the full bolus usually took 10 to 20 seconds, depending upon tissue resistance. a = p < 0.05 for NBF, b = p < 0.05 for MAP, per paired t-test, versus prestimulus levels of each parameter. n = 9 rats. *(Reprinted with permission from Budgell B, Hotta H, Sato A. J Neuromusculoskel Sys 1995;3:122-31.)*

ligament produced a small, but statistically significant drop in MAP and NBF (Figure 4-16, E). By contrast, capsaicin injection produced a very brief decrease followed by a very marked elevation and a long lasting return to baseline for both parameters (Figure 4-16, F). Interestingly, MAP remained elevated during this last phase while NBF dropped below the base level recorded prior to stimulation. The drop in NBF below baseline was seen in plots for individual animals, but due to averaging of overlapping second and third phases across animals, it is not reflected in Figure 4-16, F. In an effort to isolate

the different mechanisms acting upon MAP and NBF in this third phase of the capsaicin response, these investigators examined the various stimuli in four animals that were spinalized before stimulation (part 2). Saline injection into the L4/L5 facet joints of spinalized rats produced no changes in MAP and NBF. Surprisingly, the researchers observed that capsaicin injection into the L4/L5 facet joints or injection into the L4/L5 interspinous ligament produced dramatic changes in both MAP and NBF in some animals. In contrast to their expectations, the MAP and NBF were actually coupled more closely in the

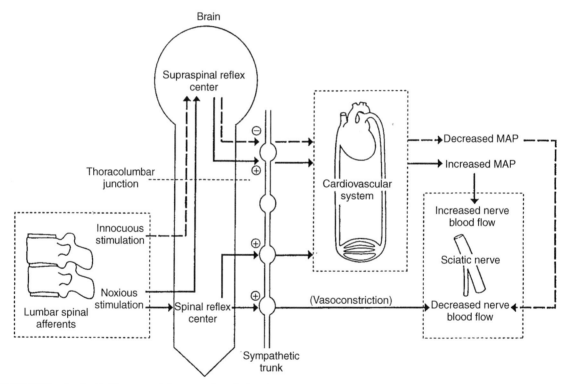

Figure 4-17   Budgell, Hotta, and Sato produced this diagrammatic summary of interactions between spinally mediated somatoautonomic reflexes and descending supraspinal influences elicited by noxious and innocuous stimulation of spinal afferents. Note that they sought, but did not find evidence of spinally mediated reflexes to innocuous spinal stimulation. However, noxious spinal stimulation elicited both supraspinal and spinal reflexes, which may compete for expression. For example, noxious stimulation elicits two competing somatoautonomic reflexes in the regulation of sciatic nerve blood flow: A suprasegmentally mediated cardiac pressor response causes an increase in MAP, and consequently, a passive increase in sciatic NBF; and a segmentally mediated reflex vasoconstriction of the vasa nervorum that attenuates NBF. *(Reprinted with permission from Budgell B, Hotta H, Sato A. J Neuromusculoskel Sys 1995;3:122-31.)*

spinalized rats. However, these changes were quite variable, and the four animals examined were too few to attain statistical significance. The explanation for these seemingly disparate results was attributed to the interplay of yet another reflex—a segmentally mediated shunting of blood from visceral to systemic beds in response to stimulation of somatic afferents. Figure 4-17 diagrammatically summarizes the spinally mediated somatoautonomic reflexes and descending supraspinal influences that appear to be operational in this study. Budgell et al. commented, "These results draw attention to the difficulty in predicting the integrated manifestation of somatoautonomic reflexes. A single stimulus may unleash a cacophony of responses which compete for expression in the end organ."

COMMENT: In this complex study, Budgell et al. continue a line of investigation that began with the pioneering work of Sato and Swenson (study 18). Although a considerable amount of work had been done examining the cutaneous and appendicular joint (and muscle) induction of somatovisceral reflexes, only Sato and Budgell had systematically examined how spinal articular and paraspinal afferents mediate these reflexes. This study and other work by Budgell et al. (studies 23, 27, and 28) and Kang et al. (study 31) are beginning to address mechanisms underlying the often-reported clinical observations of field practitioners that many visceral problems improve with spinal manipulation.

Modified Haldeman Criteria: #3

27

DATE: 1997

AUTHORS: B.S. Budgell, A. Sato, A. Suzuki, S. Uchida[88]

TITLE AND SOURCE: Responses of adrenal function to stimulation of lumbar and thoracic interspinous tissues in the rat

Neuroscience Research 1997;28:33-40

ANIMAL: 18 Rats

METHODS: All rats in this study were prepared for measuring autonomic nerve function as described in study 23. Mean arterial blood pressure (MAP) and heart rate (HR) were continuously monitored via an indwelling catheter in a common carotid artery. The study consisted of two series: In series 1, five CNS-intact and four spinalized (C1-C2) rats were used. Compound nerve activity was recorded in an adrenal sympathetic nerve while interspinous tissues (T8/9-T12/13 and L3/4-L6/S1) were stimulated by 20 μl injections of either 0.9% saline or 10 mM capsaicin. Catecholamine secretion was obtained via a catheterized adrenal vein and assayed by high performance liquid chromatography. Adrenal venous blood was collected at fixed intervals prior to and following interspinous tissue injections. In any animal, each site received only one injection to avoid the effects of altered sensitivity or dilution of subsequent injections. In series 2 experiments, five CNS-intact and four spinalized (C1-C2) rats received either graded single shocks or repetitive electrical stimulation of the L2 primary dorsal ramus. A-reflex and C-reflex potentials were concurrently recorded from the adrenal sympathetic nerve.

FINDINGS: Saline injection, either thoracic or lumbar interspinous tissues, did not produce a response in adrenal nerve activity. By contrast, capsaicin injection produced a clear and statistically significant response for all stimulation sites. CNS intact animals responded with similar increases in adrenal nerve activity for both thoracic and lumbar injections. Spinalized animals had greater increases in adrenal nerve activity with thoracic stimulation as compared to lumbar stimulation, but these differences were not statistically significant. The response of catecholamine levels, adrenaline (epinephrine) and noradrenaline (norepinephrine), to interspinous tissue stimulation was consistent with adrenal nerve response (Figure 4-18). This was observed in both CNS intact and spinalized animals,

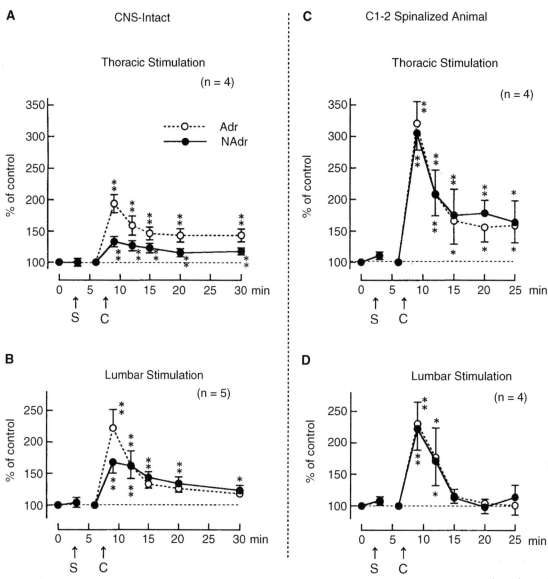

Figure 4-18 Budgell et al. recorded the response of catecholamine levels, adrenaline (epinephrine) and noradrenaline (norepinephrine), to injection of interspinous tissues with 20 µl or isotonic saline (S, 0.9% NaCl) or 20 µl of capsaicin (C, 10 mM capsaicin). The significance, per ANOVA, of any increase in secretion rate compared with the prestimulus rate is indicated by asterisks: *, p < 0.05, **, p < 0.01. Absolute secretion rates prior to saline (S) and successive capsaicin (C) injection were not identical. Therefore they have been normalized for presentation on these plots. The error bars represent ± SEM. (Reprinted with permission from Budgell B, Sato A, Suzuki A, Uchida S. Neurosci Res 1997;28:33-40.)

although the basal catecholamine levels fell markedly following spinalization. In addition, CNS intact animals had a statistically greater increase in adrenaline compared to noradrenaline, but this preferential increase was lost after spinalization. Repetitive electrical stimulation and single shock stimulation of the L2 dorsal primary ramus elicited similar A-reflex and C-reflex discharges in the adrenal sympathetic nerves for both CNS intact and spinalized animals.

COMMENT: These investigators stimulated interspinous tissues with the algesic agent capsaicin to model the intensity and chronicity of biomechanical back pain. Their previous work with this model (study 26) demonstrated that irritating lumbar interspinous tissue with capsaicin modified sciatic nerve blood flow, a somatovisceral effect, via both segmental and suprasegmental mechanisms. However, it was not clear whether this effect had clinical consequences. This study demonstrated that irritation of either thoracic or lumbar interspinous tissues would produce a strong somatovisceral reflex that modified adrenal function. Therefore evidence is mounting that irritation to paraspinal tissues produces somatovisceral effects. This is consistent with the Altered Somatic Afferent Input Theory for explaining the clinical effects of subluxation.[89] Moreover, support for this mechanism can be found in many of the studies reviewed in this chapter. Nonetheless, two major issues are constantly before us: (1) Are the observed biological effects reported in these animal studies relevant to humans? (2) Does a biomechanical lesion (the subluxation) exist outside of the laboratory which produces these effects? Research history strongly supports the general value of animal studies as a window into the biological mechanisms common to both animals and humans. However, the specific application of animal research to humans requires follow-up human studies. The reality of the subluxation, at least as an experimental phenomenon, is becoming clear with the use of subluxation

mimic models (studies 13 and 14). However, the existence of this entity in the "real world" outside the laboratory has not yet been established in either animals or humans.

Modified Haldeman Criteria: #3 and #4

28

DATE: 1998

AUTHORS: B.S. Budgell, H. Hotta, A. Sato[90]

TITLE AND SOURCE: Reflex responses of bladder motility after stimulation of interspinous tissues in the anesthetized rat

Journal of Manipulative and Physiological Therapeutics 1998;21:593-9

ANIMAL: 9 Rats

METHODS: The animals were prepared for measuring autonomic nerve function as described in study 23. In each animal, bladder pressure changes were monitored after the bladder was slowly inflated to 100 mm H_2O. This basal pressure was obtained by injecting saline into the bladder through a catheter that was sealed in the urethra with surgical glue. Following this procedure, basal bladder pressure changes were measured in all animals in response to a series of somatic stimuli (soft brushing, vapocoolant spray, or tissue pinch) that were applied to the forepaw or sacral skin. Subsequently, the skin over the spine was incised, and 20 µl solutions of either 0.9% saline or 10 mM capsaicin were injected into the interspinous tissues of the lower thoracic spine (T8/9-T10/11) or lower lumbar spine (L4/5-L6/S1). Bladder pressure changes were monitored in response to these interspinous injections. In five rats, capsaicin was injected both before and after bilateral transection of the pelvic nerves. Two rats had capsaicin injected before and after a mock transection surgery. Lastly, two rats with intact pelvic nerves were injected with capsaicin before and after spinalization at T9-T10. The five CNS intact rats were also assessed for bladder pressure changes in response to electrical stimulation of the lateral and medial branches of the lumbar spinal nerves. In two of these animals the L4 spinal nerve was electrically stimulated, while the other three rats were stimulated at the L2 spinal nerve. The L4 nerve provides afferent innervation to the L5/6 and L6/S1 interspinous tissues. The L2 nerve provides preganglionic sympathetic supply to the hypogastric nerve.

FINDINGS: In intact animals (Figure 4-19), forepaw or sacral brushing had no effect on bladder pressure, heart rate, or mean arterial blood pressure. Brief application of vapocoolant spray to the forepaws or sacrum produced a slight increase in bladder pressure, heart rate, and

mean arterial pressure. Only the forepaw stimulation produced a statistically significant response, and this was only in heart rate and blood pressure changes. Hindpaw pinching did not affect bladder pressure but consistently elevated heart rate and blood pressure (both statistically significant). Saline injection to interspinous tissues, thoracic or lumbar, produced no changes in bladder pressure, heart rate, or mean arterial pressure. By contrast, capsaicin injection to either thoracic or lumbar interspinous tissues produced a marked increase in bladder pressure and mean arterial pressure and a marked decrease in heart rate. The mock transection surgery made no difference in bladder

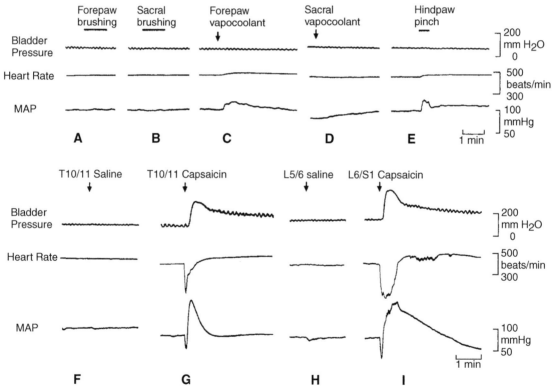

Figure 4-19   Budgell, Hotta, and Sato recorded bladder pressure, heart rate, and mean arterial blood pressure (MAP) in response to various forms of somatic stimulation (soft brushing, pinching, vapocoolant spray, 20 μl injection of isotonic saline, or 20 μl injection of 10 mM capsaicin). Duration of brushing (60 sec) and pinching (20 sec) is indicated by a horizontal bar above the recordings. Onset of cooling (5-second duration) and injection of interspinous tissues (approximately 20-second duration) is indicated by a vertical arrow above the recordings. *(Reprinted with permission from Budgell BS, Hotta H, Sato A. J Manipulative Physiol Ther 1998;21:593-9.)*

pressure response to capsaicin. However, bilateral transection of the pelvic (parasympathetic) nerves completely abolished the bladder response to capsaicin injection of both the thoracic and lumbar interspinous tissues. Spinalization also abolished the bladder response to capsaicin injection in lumbar interspinous tissues. Neither L2 nor L4 spinal nerve stimulation by graded electrical current produced a change in bladder pressure, although all of five animals tested had responded vigorously to thoracic interspinous capsaicin injection.

COMMENT: Consideration of the results observed in this interesting study requires an appreciation of the unique dependence of the urinary bladder on parasympathetic rather than sympathetic innervation. The rat bladder, like the human bladder, is richly innervated with parasympathetic fibers that, in the rat, originate primarily in the intermediolateral nucleus of the L6-S1 spinal cord. The rat hindpaw is innervated by the L4/5 spinal nerves. Pinching the hindpaw produces a clear cardiovascular response that is mediated through the sympathetic nervous system but does not provide nociceptive input to the L6/S1 intermediolateral nucleus and therefore does not activate bladder motility. Noxious but not nonnoxious stimulation of the L6-S1 interspinous tissues produced profound increases in bladder pressure that were abolished by spinalization. This observation suggests that this reflex response to noxious chemical stimulation was mediated at the supraspinal level with little local segmental participation. Since the L6-S1 interspinous tissue is innervated by afferents from spinal nerves two or more levels rostral, there is little opportunity for a segmentally mediated parasympathetic reflex. The sympathetic driven, cardiovascular responses reported in this study are consistent with the previously discussed studies above (studies 18, 23, and 26). This work underscores critical differences between somatovisceral reflex mechanisms originating in spinal and paraspinal tissues and those commonly seen in appendicular structures. As noted previously, these

observations are provocative, but it remains to be seen if these unique features have clinical relevance. Modified Haldeman Criteria: #3 and #4

29

DATE: 2001

AUTHORS: Y.M. Kang, J.D. Wheeler, J.G. Pickar[91]

TITLE AND SOURCE: Stimulation of chemosensitive afferents from multifidus muscle does not sensitize multifidus muscle spindles to vertebral loads in the lumbar spine of the cat

Spine 2001;26:1528-36

ANIMAL: 25 Cats

METHODS: This study used the unique subperiosteal laminectomy approach developed by Pickar (study 19). Single unit recordings from muscle spindle afferents in the lumbar multifidus muscle were recorded from the L6 dorsal root. Receptive fields within the multifidus were located by probing the muscle with a cotton-tipped applicator. Muscle spindle afferents were identified by their increased discharges to succinylcholine injection and decreased discharges to muscle contraction. Chemosensitive afferents in the L5 and L7 multifidus muscles were stimulated with bradykinin (5-100 µg), capsaicin (100 µg-100 mg), or isotonic saline (volume control) administered under the fascial covering of the muscles (n = 10) or via intramuscular injection (n = 15). Testing protocols began within 2 minutes of injections and were separated by at least 15 minutes. After muscle injection, an electronic feedback controlled motor was used to apply mechanical loads (25%, 50%, 75%, and 100% body weight) to the L6 spinous process sufficient to produce a robust activation of the multifidus spindles.

FINDINGS: Neither the intact anesthetized cat nor the nonanesthetized decerebrate cat showed any effect on L6 muscle spindle activity when bradykinin, capsaicin, or saline were injected (subfascial or intramuscular) into the multifidus muscles and the L6 vertebra was mechanically loaded.

COMMENT: These results suggest that the stimulation of small-caliber afferents in the deep lumbar muscles by noxious chemicals (e.g., bradykinin and capsaicin) does not sensitize the associated muscle spindles to mechanical loading of the spine. Therefore these data do not support the widely accepted theory known as the "pain-spasm-pain cycle" which holds that pain elicits muscle spasm, causing noxious metabolites to accumulate and stimulate Aδ and C fibers, thereby increasing pain and sensitizing muscle spindles via a gamma reflex. The sensitized spindles then maintain the muscle spasm, closing the loop in this putative cycle. Since muscle pain and spasm are common findings in neck and back pain, the pain-spasm-pain mechanism has been suggested as one possible cause, or at least a perpetuator of vertebral subluxation. As these investigators note, other studies in the cat have demonstrated that intramuscular injection of bradykinin increases the sensitivity of muscle spindles in neck muscles.[92,93] The reason for these contrasting findings is unclear. It will be interesting to see if the current findings are duplicated or supported by the future work of other investigators. It is also possible that differences in the specific muscles examined may explain the apparent conflict between this study and the two studies demonstrating algesic sensitization of neck muscles.[92,93] This study examined the effect in lumbar multifidus muscles, small, deep muscles, which act on individual low back vertebrae. The other two studies in the cat examined the splenius and trapezius muscles (superficial neck muscles), which act upon large spinal segments.

Modified Haldeman Criteria: #2, #3, and #4

30*

DATE: 2002

AUTHORS: Y.M. Kang, W.S. Choi, J.G. Pickar[94]

TITLE AND SOURCE: Electrophysiologic evidence for an intersegmental reflex pathway between lumbar paraspinal tissues

---

*This study examines a neurological pathway critical to both subluxation and spinal manipulation.

Spine 2002;27:E56-E63

ANIMAL: 23 Cats

METHODS: Two series of experiments were performed in α-chloralose anesthetized cats. (1) The investigators directly stimulated the medial branch of a dorsal primary ramus at L3, L4, or L5 and recorded any resulting compound action potentials in the medial branch of a dorsal primary ramus of a vertebra one or two segments away (L3, L4, or L5). This was done to determine the presence of intersegmental reflexes between adjacent lumbar paraspinal tissues. At the end of each nerve stimulation protocol, the nerve was cut just proximal to the electrode to confirm that the recorded action potential was reflexive and not simply due to volume conduction (spread of the stimulating current through the intervening tissue volume to the multifidus muscle). (2) They also electrically stimulated the lumbar facet capsule of one vertebra while recording any evoked multifidus EMG activity in adjacent vertebrae. This was done to evaluate the claim that electrically stimulating a facet capsule reflexively activates multifidus muscles one or two segments away. Three experimental procedures were performed to determine that any recorded EMG activity produced by electrically stimulating the facet capsule was indeed a reflex and not due to volume conduction: (1) They anesthetized the facet joint capsule receptors by injecting 0.05 to 0.2 ml 2% lidocaine into the joint; (2) The dorsal roots of the spinal cord were anesthetized via intrathecal lidocaine injections; and (3) The putative afferent reflex pathway was interrupted by cutting the medial branch of the dorsal primary ramus innervating the stimulated joint capsule. Surgically exposed facet joint capsules were stimulated with bipolar electrodes positioned on the capsule surface. A range of square wave pulses were used (4-80 V, 50-200 μsec at 0.2 Hz for 25 sec). Multifidus EMG activity was recorded with subdermal needle electrodes inserted 3 mm lateral to the interspinous space immediately cranial to the more caudal spinous process.

FINDINGS: Stimulating the medial branch of a lumbar dorsal primary ramus evoked a compound action potential in a lumbar medial nerve branch one to two segments away. In all cases the action potential was abolished by cutting the medial branch of the dorsal ramus just proximal to the stimulating electrode. Intracapsular lidocaine injection significantly decreased the magnitude of the multifidus EMG evoked by electrical stimulation of the facet joint capsule in all groups. Intrathecal injection had no effect on multifidus EMG activity due to electrical stimulation of the facet capsule but did decrease activity when subsequently injected into the joint capsule. In addition, cutting the medial branch of the dorsal primary ramus supplying the joint did not significantly decrease the multifidus EMG activity.

COMMENT: This study suggests the presence of intersegmental paraspinal reflexes that span at least one to two vertebrae. In addition, these investigators provide evidence that the medial branch of the dorsal primary ramus may be a critical part of the pathway for these reflexes. Their study supported previous reports that electrical stimulation of a facet joint capsule increases multifidus muscle activity but suggests that this observation is due to volume conduction rather than a reflex response. These mechanisms may mediate critical intersegmental coordination during spine motion and prove to be a neural substrate for biomechanical spine failure and the beneficial effects of spinal manipulation. Once again, these findings are consistent with the Altered Somatic Afferent Input Theory for explaining the clinical effects of subluxation.[89]

Modified Haldeman Criteria: #4

31

DATE: 2003

AUTHORS: Y.M. Kang, M.J. Kenny, K.F. Spratt, J.G. Pickar[95]

TITLE AND SOURCE: Somatosympathetic reflexes from the low back in the anesthetized cat

Journal of Neurophysiology 2003;90:2548-59

ANIMAL: 27 Cats

METHODS: Heart rate (HR), blood pressure (BP), and splenic and renal sympathetic nerve discharge activity (splenic SND and renal SND) were evaluated in response to dorsoventral loading of the L3 vertebra with and without multifidus muscle inflammation. The splenic and renal sympathetic nerves were isolated via a retroperitoneal approach and their electrical activity was monitored under five experimental conditions: (1) intramultifidus mustard oil injection, (2) intramultifidus mustard oil injection in conjunction with dorsoventral mechanical loading at the L3 vertebra, (3) intramultifidus mineral oil (vehicle) injection, (4) transection of peripheral nerves innervating multifidus and intramultifidus mustard oil injection in conjunction with dorsoventral mechanical loading at the L3 vertebra, and (5) spinal cord transection at C2-3 and intramultifidus mustard oil injection in conjunction with dorsoventral mechanical loading at the L3 vertebra. The mustard oil (or mineral oil vehicle) was injected at two sites in each left multifidus muscle at L2, L3, and L4 (two 10 µl injections per each of three muscles, 20% vol/vol allyisothiocyanate). The static dorsoventral mechanical force (100% of body weight) simulated a lumbar extension load. It was delivered to L3 and held for 20 minutes using the electronic feedback motor system described in study 19. Measurements were compared across three intervals: (1) baseline, the first 5 minutes of each experimental protocol, (2) intervention, the 20-minute period beginning 3 minutes after the start of injection, and (3) a 5-minute mechanical load recovery period following the 20-minute intervention interval. Nerve activity was digitized and integrated with heart rate and blood pressure data over 25-second intervals, and the mean value of each interval was placed in 25-second bins. At the end of each experimental protocol, the ganglionic blocker hexamethonium was injected to differentiate sympathetic activity from electrical noise. Integrated postganglionic sympathetic nerve discharge was obtained in each animal by subtracting the residual electrical activity following hexamethonium injection from the mean in each of the 25-second bins.

FINDINGS: These investigators reported significantly increased HR (52 bpm), splenic SND (60%), and renal SND (31%) following mustard oil injections into the multifidus muscles (experiment 1). Dorsoventral mechanical loading alone did not affect these outcome measures (control protocols in experiments 2 and 3), but combined mustard oil and loading (experiment 2) produced smaller increases in HR (27 bpm), splenic SND (55%), and renal SND (16%). Following both the nonloaded and the loaded mustard oil injections, BP rose early in the intervention period and fell below baseline later during that same period; therefore there was little mean change for the overall period. While this pattern was maintained with loading, the total change from baseline in both the early and late portions of the interval was reduced. By contrast, the pattern of mustard oil–induced HR and SND increases over time were different with and without vertebral loading. With loading (experiment 2), the observed HR and SND increases were prolonged compared to the nonloaded mustard oil increases. These changes were clearly due to the effect of mustard oil, since vehicle alone (mineral oil) did not produce them (experiment 3). Cutting the medial branches of the T11-L5 dorsal primary rami abolished the mustard oil–induced changes. Therefore the investigators concluded that these responses were mediated by neural reflexes with afferent limbs that traveled through the peripheral nerves. Lastly, transecting the spinal cord at C2-3 also abolished the increases, suggesting a supraspinal contribution to these reflexes.

COMMENT: The findings of this interesting study suggest that sensory feedback from paraspinal tissues may have a role in adaptive and homeostatic mechanisms that influence autonomic regulation via reflex pathways. Moreover, the prolonging effect of a static mechanical spine load on the autonomic responses to mustard oil highlights the significant interaction between joint biomechanics and tissue inflammation on neural function. While

underscoring the likely role of Altered Somatic Afferent Input[89] in autonomic regulation, it remains to be determined if the autonomic changes reported here can be expressed as clinically significant effects.

Modified Haldeman Criteria: #3 and #4

Spinal Manipulation Mimic Models
Manual Manipulation Mimic Models

32

DATE: 1966
AUTHORS: J. Greenspan, J. Melchior[96]
TITLE AND SOURCE: The effect of osteopathic manipulative treatment on the resistance of rats to stressful situations
Journal of the American Osteopathic Association 1966;65:1205-7
ANIMAL: 200 Rats approximately; number not clearly identified
METHODS: Litter mates were divided into pairs of equal weight (within 3 g). In a series of stress experiments, one rat in each pair served as a control while the other received an experimental stress. The stresses were of two types, (1) cold stress (3°, for 20 hours each of 3 days) or (2) translocation stress, psychic stress experienced by rats when simply moved from the cage room to the basement by elevator and remained in the basement for 2 to 3 hours; this was repeated each day for 3 days. In a series of therapeutic assessment experiments, both rats in littermate pairs were stressed (with either cold or translocation). One rat in each pair was also given osteopathic treatment (spine mobilization and soft tissue massage) while the other rat in each pair was handled ("gentled") for 4 minutes each day. The effects of stress and the potentially ameliorating effects of the osteopathic treatment were assessed by comparing differences in body weight and adrenal and pituitary weights between the rats in each pair.

FINDINGS: Statistically significant decreases in body weight were reported in animals receiving the cold stress and in animals receiving the translocation stress. In addition, cold stress was shown to increase adrenal and pituitary weights. No data was provided for the effect of translocation on adrenal and pituitary weights. Decreased body weight induced by either cold stress or by translocation stress was ameliorated by osteopathic manipulation therapy compared to rats receiving control treatment (handling). The study authors did not report the effect of osteopathic therapy on adrenal and pituitary weights.

COMMENT: These authors present an interesting study of the effects of osteopathic therapy as an ameliorating treatment for two nonspecific stress agents (the Selye[97] method). However, their presentation of data was incomplete and not well explained.

Modified Haldeman Criteria: #1

Instrument Manipulation Mimic Models

33

DATE: 1990

AUTHORS: R.J. Thomas, T. Salem, J. Nance, D. McGee, A.S. Bonci[98]

TITLE AND SOURCE: Ligamentous changes in the rat spine following repeated adjustments: a pilot study

Proceedings of the International Conference on Spinal Manipulation 1990;122-3

ANIMAL: 23 Rats, number unclear

METHODS: Eighteen adult male rats were divided equally into two treatment groups, each receiving a regimen of spinal manipulation to the L3-L5 spine region. Treatment group 1 was "adjusted left-to-right" and treatment group 2 was "adjusted right-to-left." Five (additional?) rats were assigned to a control group that received no treatments. The spinal manipulations were delivered five times weekly for six weeks to identical segments using

an Activator Adjusting Instrument with a mean force of 16.7 lbs/in². At the conclusion of this treatment period, all rats were euthanized and the L3-L5 region was harvested for histological examination. In this brief abstract these investigators did not describe their methods but referenced the study of Chazal et al., 1985.[99]

FINDINGS: The authors reported no statistically significant histological differences between the control rats and the rats in either of the two treatment groups, but they did note some cellular evidence of inflammation. They did not identify the group(s) in which this inflammation was present or provide quantified data.

COMMENT: This small pilot study was published only in a loosely written abstract, and no further studies were reported by these investigators.

Modified Haldeman Criteria: #2

34

DATE: 1995

AUTHORS: J.G. Pickar, R.F. McLain[100]

TITLE AND SOURCE: Responses of mechanosensitive afferents to manipulation of the lumbar facet in the cat

Spine 1995;20:2379-85

ANIMAL: 9 Cats

METHODS: These researchers used a unique subperiosteal laminectomy to permit single fiber recording of type III and IV afferents in the L5[†] dorsal root during loading of the ipsilateral L5-L6 facet joint in anaesthetized adult cats. Their subperiosteal laminectomy method allowed access to the L5 dorsal root while preserving the muscles, ligaments, tendons, and joint capsule of the L5-L6 vertebral segment. The L5 dorsal root innervates the L5-L6 facet joint. The paraspinal receptive field of each afferent was determined by probing the tissues with a blunt instrument.

[†]The original paper erroneously indicated that recordings were obtained from the L6 dorsal root (personal communication).

Following this, the mechanical threshold of the field was approximated with a calibrated set of nylon filaments (von Frey-like hairs). The L5-L6 facet joint was manipulated by applying directionally varied loads to the amputated caudal articular pillar of L5 using fine tissue forceps.

FINDINGS: Single unit recordings were obtained from 16 afferent fibers in the lumbar spine (7 with receptive fields at or near the facet joint and 9 with fields some distance from the joint). Nine of these afferents were group III and three were group IV; most responded in a graded fashion to the direction of the applied load.

COMMENT: This study demonstrated for the first time that group III and IV afferents located in tissues throughout the low back region respond in a directionally sensitive fashion to movement of a lumbar facet joint. These afferents were found in all tissues of the lumbar spine examined by these investigators (facet joint, connective tissue immediately surrounding the facet joint, and paraspinous muscles and fascia distant from the facet joint). This suggests a complex neural network of small diameter fibers in the low back that respond to specific movements of the lumbar spine. Pickar and McLain comment that surgical disruption of this system may contribute to dysfunction in some individuals and its stimulation or modulation may explain the beneficial effects many patients receive through physical therapy, bracing, and spinal manipulation. This is consistent with the Altered Somatic Afferent Input Theory for explaining the clinical effects of subluxation.[89]

Modified Haldeman Criteria: #3

DATE: 2002*

AUTHORS: Y.M. Kang, W.S. Choi, J.G. Pickar[94]

TITLE AND SOURCE: Electrophysiologic evidence for an intersegmental reflex pathway between lumbar paraspinal tissues (see study 30)

---

*This study examines a neurological pathway critical to both subluxation and spinal manipulation.

Where Do We Go from Here?

Most chiropractic research seeks to clarify the unique subject of our therapeutic focus, the subluxation, or examine our primary therapeutic tool, spinal manipulation. This is done with the ultimate goal of refining the clinician's ability to render optimal care to patients. The field is wide open. Despite strong advances since the 1975 NINCDS conference,[1] we have only established a small toehold in understanding the chiropractic clinical experience. The most researched area to date, the spinal musculoskeletal system, is still relatively unexplored. When we consider the extremities, only a few published studies are available.[101] Similarly, subluxation-associated visceral problems are frequently mentioned by field practitioners, but despite the recent contributions of Budgell, Sato, and Pickar, we know very little about this important area of study. The small animal subluxation model described in studies 13 and 14 is currently the only research model that fulfills Vernon's description[5] of the preferred approach for studying subluxation:

> ...create the obligate precipitating elements of the subluxation, vertebral fixation and misalignment, and monitor the effects.... [T]his approach retains the highest fidelity to the natural circumstances and achieves the highest level of prospective validity, because...the disorder was created first and its putative effects were studied thereafter.

The model needs further refinement, but it promises to be an important tool for evaluating and developing chiropractic theory.

Evaluation and development of foundational theories is a critical activity for all professions. Studies can be cobbled together to make a case for virtually any theory, but this is not definitive evidence. The popular practice of building an evidence base solely from studies that support a pet theory constitutes "mosaic evidence" (Figure 4-20, *A*) and should be discouraged by the profession.

Theories integrate and expand observations, providing an essential framework for a profession. But they may be transformed into lethal dogma. Louis Pasteur's remarks on "preconceived ideas" may also apply to a profession's foundational theories:

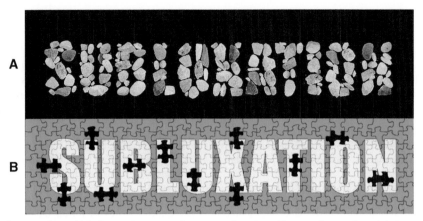

Figure 4-20   Studies can be cobbled together to make a case for virtually any theory, but this is not definitive evidence. The popular practice of building an evidence base solely from studies that support a pet theory constitutes "mosaic evidence" (**A**) and should be discouraged by the profession. By contrast, the integration of all pertinent studies, with an attempt to understand and reconcile points of disagreement, provides the proper basis for theory validation. This is comparable to fitting the pieces of a puzzle together (**B**). To successfully complete the puzzle, one must carefully examine each new piece (study) and fit it into the developing picture (body of evidence), taking care not to jam "near fits" into place. As the puzzle takes shape, the form of specifics pieces needed to complete the picture become clear.

Preconceived ideas are like searchlights which illumine the path of the experimenter and serve him as a guide to interrogate nature. They become a danger only if he transforms them into fixed ideas. This is why I should like to see these profound words inscribed on the threshold of all the temples of science: "The greatest derangement of the mind is to believe in something because one wishes it to be so."[102]

The integration of all pertinent studies with an attempt to understand and reconcile points of disagreement provides the proper basis for theory validation. This practice is implicit in the peer-reviewed publication process. Moreover, the most compelling evidence is provided by studies that were specifically designed to examine a given theory. This is very much like an a priori analysis of data as contrasted with a post hoc analysis. To continue the mosaic evidence analogy, this form of theory validation is comparable to fitting the pieces of a puzzle together (Figure 4-20, *B*). To successfully complete the puzzle, one must carefully examine each new piece (study) and fit it into the developing picture (body of evidence), taking care not to jam "near fits" into place. As the puzzle takes shape, the form of specific pieces needed to complete the picture become clear. Fortunately, this too occurs in the research experience. We presently have few pieces of the subluxation puzzle, but we have a good start and the work is exciting.

"If we begin with certainties, we shall end in doubts; but if we begin with doubts, and are patient, we shall end in certainties."

Sir Francis Bacon

References

1. Aspects of Manipulative Therapy. 2nd ed. Melbourne: Churchill Livingstone; 1985. p. 1-194.
2. White A, Panjabi MM. Clinical biomechanics of the spine. 2nd ed. Philadelphia: J.B. Lippincott Company; 1990. p. 21.
3. Brennan PC, Cramer GD, Kirstukas SJ, Cullum ME. Basic science research in chiropractic: the state of the art and recommendations for a research agenda. J Manipulative Physiol Ther 1997;20:150-68.

4. Fifty-second World Medical Association General Assembly. World Medical Association declaration of Helsinki: Ethical principles for medical research involving human subjects (5th revision). Edinburgh, Scotland: World Medical Association; 2000.

5. Vernon H. Basic scientific evidence for chiropractic subluxation. In: Gatterman MI, editor. Foundations of chiropractic: subluxation. St. Louis: Mosby; 1995. p. 35-55.

6. Dishman J, Cunningham B, Burke J. Comparison of tibial nerve H-reflex excitability after cervical and lumbar spine manipulation. J Manipulative Physiol Ther 2002;25:318-25.

7. Cramer GD, Gregerson DM, Knudsen JT, Hubbard BB, Ustas LM, Cantu JA. The effects of side-posture positioning and spinal adjusting on the lumbar Z joints: a randomized controlled trial with 64 subjects. Spine 2002;27:2459-66.

8. Little JS, Ianuzzi A, Chiu JB, Baitner A, Khalsa PS. Human lumbar facet joint capsule strains II: alteration of strains subsequent to anterior interbody fixation. Spine 2004;4:153-62.

9. Smith OG, Langworthy SM, Paxson MC. Subluxations in modernized chiropractic. 1st ed. Cedar Rapids, IA: Laurance Press; 1906. p. 23-9.

10. The Oxford English Dictionary. New York: Oxford University Press; 2000. p. 33.

11. Hieronymi JH. Dissertatio inauguralis medico-chirurgica de luxationibus et subluxationibus [dissertation]. Jena: Litteris Ritterianis; 1746. p. 1-30.

12. Harrison E. Observations respecting the nature and origin of the common species of disorder of the spine: with critical remarks on the opinions of former writers on this disease. London Med & Phys J 1821;45:103-22.

13. Harrison E. Observations on the pathology and treatment of spinal diseases. London Med & Phys J 1824; 51:350-64.

14. Harrison E. Pathological and practical observations on spinal diseases. Illustrated with cases and engravings. Also, an inquiry into the origin and cure of distorted limbs. London: Thomas & George Underwood; 1827.

15. Gatterman MI. What's in a word? In: Gatterman MI, editor. Foundations of chiropractic: subluxation. St. Louis: Mosby; 1995. p. 4-17.

16. Bartol KM. A model for the categorization of chiropractic treatment procedures. Chiro Tech 1991;3:78-80.

17. Henderson CNR. Three neurophysiologic theories on the chiropractic subluxation. In: Gatterman MI, editor. Foundations of chiropractic: subluxation. St. Louis: Mosby; 1995. p. 225-33.

18. Schimandle JH, Boden SD. Spine update: animal use in spinal research. Spine 1994;19:2474-7.

19. Knowles WD. In vitro electrophysiology of human brain slices from surgery for epilepsy. In: Lüders H, editor. Epilepsy surgery. New York: Raven Press; 1991. p. 729-36.

20. Khalsa P, Hoffman A, Grigg P. Mechanical states encoded by stretch-sensitive neurons in feline joint capsule. J Neurophysiol 1996;76:1-13.

21. Kawakami M, Tamaki T, Hashizume H, Weinstein J, Meller S. The role of phospholipase A2 and nitric oxide in pain related behavior produced by an allograft of intervertebral disc material to the sciatic nerve of the rat. Spine 1997;22:1074-9.

22. Nakano M, Matsui H, Miaki K, Yamagami T, Tsuji H. Postlaminectomy adhesion of the cauda equina. Spine 1997;22:1105-14.

23. Regan T. The case for animal rights. In: Singer P, editor. In defense of animals. Oxford: Basil Blackwell; 1985. p. 13-26.

24. Singer P. Tools for research: your taxes at work. Animal liberation. 2nd ed. New York: Avon Books; 1990. p. 25-94.

25. Cohen C. The case for the use of animals in biomedical research. N Engl J Med 1986;315:865-70.

26. Paton W. Man and mouse: animals in medical research. 2nd ed. New York: Oxford University Press; 1993. p. 1-288.

27. Macrina FL. Scientific integrity: an introductory text with cases. 2nd ed. Washington, D.C.: ASM Press; 2000. p. 1-338.

28. National Research Council. Guide for the care and use of laboratory animals. 7th ed. Washington, D.C.: National Academy Press; 1996. p. 1-125.

29. Foundation for Biomedical Research. Nobel Prizes: the payoff from animal research; 2002. www.fbresearch.org/education/nobels.htm. Accessed October 4, 2004.

30. Department of Health and Human Services. Method for constructing complete annual U.S. life tables: data evaluation and methods research. Series 1999;2(129):1-28. Hyattsville Maryland, DHHS. Publication No. (PHS) 2000-1329.

31. National Institute on Aging. Health disparities strategic plan; 2000. www.rcmar.ucla.edu/documents/nia-sphd.pdf. Accessed October 4, 2004.

32. Manton KJ, Gu.X-L. Changes in the prevalence of chronic disability in the United States black and non-black population above age 65 from 1982 to 1999. PNAS 2001;98:6354-9.

33. Hodgkin AL. The conduction of the nervous impulse. Liverpool, England: Liverpool University Press; 1964.

34. Llinás RR. Calcium in synaptic transmission. Sci Am 1982;247:56-65.

35. Markovich SE. Pain in the head: a neurological appraisal. In: Gelb H, editor. Clinical management of head, neck, and TMJ pain and dysfunction; a multidisciplinary approach to diagnosis and treatment. Philadelphia: WB Saunders Company; 1977:125-39.

36. Evans PJ. Simple rating system for assessing treatment outcome in chronic pain patients. Adv Pain Res Ther 1985;9:377-85.

37. Gordon JB, Lane CD, Woodland HR, Marbaix G. Use of frog eggs and oocytes for the study of messenger RNA and its translation in living cells. Nature 1971;233:177-82.

38. Gundersen CB, Miledi R, Parker I. Slowly inactivating potassium channels induced in Xenopus oocytes by messenger ribonucleic acid from Torpedo brain. J Physiol 1984;353:231-48.

39. Stühmer W. Electrophysiolgical recordings from Xenopus oocytes. Meth Enzym 1998;293:280-300.

40. Sumikawa K, Houghton M, Emtage JS, Richards BM, Barnard EA. Active multi-subunit ACh receptor assembled by translation of heterologous mRNA in Xenopus oocytes. Nature 1981;292:862-4.

41. Goldstein M. The research status of spinal manipulative therapy: NINCDS monograph 15. Bethesda: U.S. Department of Health, Education, and Welfare; 1975.

42. Haldeman S. The clinical basis for discussion of mechanisms of manipulative therapy. In: Korr IM, editor. The neurobiologic mechanisms in manipulative therapy. New York: Plenum Press; 1978. p. 53-75.

43. Haldeman S. Neurologic effects of the adjustment. J Manipulative Physiol Ther 2000;23:112-4.

44. Miroyiannis SD, Hunter HC, Chatfield JW. Effect of vertebral malalignment on Nissl granules in rabbit spinal cord. J Am Osteopath Assoc 1964;63:862-3.

45. Cole WV. Osteopathic lesion syndrome. Academy of applied osteopathy yearbook of selected osteopathic papers. Carmel, CA: Academy of Applied Osteopathy; 1951:149-78.

46. McConnell C P. The osteopathic lesion. J Am Osteop Assoc 1910;9(8):315-34.

47. Hoskins ER. A preliminary study of the motility of the gastro-intestinal tract in lesioned animals. Still Research Institution Bulletin 5 1917:16-37.

48. Burns L, Vollbrecht WJ, Steunenberg G. Methods of lesioning. In: A study of certain growth changes due to vertebral lesions in rabbits and other mammals. Chicago: The A. T. Still Research Institute; 1926. p. 9-11.

49. Miroyiannis SD, Raines BA, Jurczenko VJ, Hunter HC. Effects of distortion of the spinal column of the rat with reference to the Nissl granules of the anterior horn cells: a pilot study. J Am Osteopath Assoc 1965;65:48-52.

50. DeBoer KF. An attempt to induce vertebral lesions in rabbits by mechanical irritation. J Manipulative Physiol Ther 1981;4:119-27.

51. DeBoer KF. Gastrointestinal myoelectric activity in rabbits with vertebral lesions: preliminary report. Eur J Chiropr 1984;32:131-42.

52. DeBoer KF, Schutz M, McKnight ME. Acute effects of spinal manipulation on gastrointestinal myoelectric activity in conscious rabbits. Manual Med 1988;3:85-94.

53. Craven JH. The Meric system. A textbook on chiropractic orthopedy. 2nd ed. Davenport, IA: J.H. Craven; 1922. p. 220-32.

54. Beal MC. Viscerosomatic reflexes: a review. J Am Osteopath Assoc 1985;85:786-801.

55. Christensen MG, Kerhoff D, Kollasch MW. Job analysis of chiropractic: a project report, survey analysis, and summary of the practice of chiropractic within the United States. Greeley, Colorado: National Board of Chiropractic Examiners; 2000. p. 129.

56. Cleveland CS. Researching the subluxation on the domestic rabbit: a pilot research program conducted at the Cleveland Chiropractic College, Kansas City, Missouri. International Review of Chiropractic Scientific Edition 1965;1(8):1-23.

57. Awad MZ. Induction of intervertebral disrelationship in experimental animals and the preliminary effects of the dysarthrias. In: Suh CH, editor. Proceedings of the 7th Annual Biomechanics Conference on the Spine. Boulder: University of Colorado; 1976. p. 27-50.

58. McConnell CP. The osteopathic lesion. J Am Osteopath Assoc 1910;9:315-34.

59. Burns L, Gibbon H. Changes in the circulation of the brain of the white rat due to upper cervical lesions. J Am Osteopath Assoc 1931;30:201-8.

60. Cole WV. The osteopathic lesion syndrome: VIII. The effects of an experimental vertebral lesion on the gross structure of the atlanto-occipital region. J Am Osteopath Assoc 1950;49:447-50.

61. Lin HL, Fujii A, Rebechini-Zasadny H, Hartz DL. Experimental induction of vertebral subluxation in laboratory animals. J Manipulative Physiol Ther 1978;1:63-6.

62. DeBoer KF, McKnight ME. Surgical model of a chronic subluxation in rabbits. J Manipulative Physiol Ther 1988;11:366-72.

63. DeBoer KF, Hansen JM. Biomechanical analysis of an induced joint dysfunction (subluxation-mimic) in the thoracic spine of rabbits. J Manipulative Physiol Ther 1993;16:74-81.

64. Papakyriakou M, Triano JJ, Brennan PC. Spine stiffness measures in a dog model of restricted joint motion. Proceedings of the International Conference on Spinal Manipulation. Des Moines: Foundation for Chiropractic Education and Research; 1991. p. 272-4.

65. Brennan PC, Kokjohn K, Triano JJ, Fritz TE, Wardrip CL, Hondras MA. Immunologic correlates of reduced spinal mobility: preliminary observations in a dog model. Proceedings of the International Conference on Spinal Manipulation. Des Moines: Foundation for Chiropractic Education and Research; 1991. p. 118-21.

66. Brennan PC, Kokjohn K, Kaltinger CJ, Lohr GE, Glendening C, Hondras MA et al. Enhanced phagocytic cell respiratory burst induced by spinal manipulation: potential role of Substance P. J Manipulative Physiol Ther 1991;14:399-408.

67. Henderson CNR, DeVocht JW, Kirstukas SJ, Cramer GD. In vivo biomechanical assessment of a small animal model of the vertebral subluxation. Proceedings of the International Conference on Spinal Manipulation 2000:193-5.

68. Cramer GD, Fournier JT, Henderson CNR, Wolcott CC. Degenerative changes following spinal fixation in a small animal model. J Manipulative Physiol Ther 2004; 27:141-54.

69. Denslow JS, Armour TF, Bruns EA, Kassicieh VN, Vomastek R. Evidence of osteopathic lesion in an experimental animal (dog). Part I. J Am Osteopath Assoc 1967;66:94-5.

70. Ashkenaz DM, Spiegel EA. The viscero-pannicular reflex. Amer J Physiol 1935;112:573-6.

71. Lehman GJ, Vernon H, McGill SM. Effects of a mechanical pain stimulus on erector spinae activity before and after a spinal manipulation in patients with back pain: a preliminary investigation. J Manipulative Physiol Ther 2001;24:402-6.

72. Denslow JS, Armour TF, Bruns EA, Kassicieh VN, Vomastek R. Evidence of osteopathic lesion in an experimental animal (dog). Part II. J Am Osteopath Assoc 1967;66:95-7.

73. Israel V. Changes in nerve physiology in the rat after induced subluxation. Articulations 1983;1(1):9-10.

74. Sato A, Swenson RS. Sympathetic nervous system response to mechanical stress of the spinal column in rats. J Manipulative Physiol Ther 1984;7:141-7.

75. Pickar JG. An in vivo preparation for investigating neural responses to controlled loading of a lumbar vertebra in the anesthetized cat. J Neurosci Meth 1999; 89:87-96.

76. Pickar JG Wheeler JD. Response of muscle proprioceptors to spinal manipulative-like loads in the anesthetized cat. J Manipulative Physiol Ther 2001;24:2-11.

77. Hessel BW, Herzog W, Conway PJW, McEwen MC. Experimental measurement of the force exerted during spinal manipulation using the Thompson Technique. J Manipulative Physiol Ther 1990;13:448-53.

78. Dishman JD, Bulbulian R. Spinal reflex attenuation associated with spinal manipulation. Spine 2000;25: 2519-25.

79. Pickar JG, Kang YM. Short-lasting stretch of lumbar paraspinal muscle decreases muscle spindle sensitivity to subsequent muscle stretch. J Neuromusculoskel Sys 2001;9:88-96.

80. Hu JW, Yu XM, Vernon H, Sessle BJ. Excitatory effects on neck and jaw muscle activity of inflammatory irritant applied to cervical paraspinal tissues. Pain 1993;55: 243-50.

81. Budgell B, Sato A. Somatoautonomic reflex regulation of sciatic nerve blood flow. J Neuromusculoskel Sys 1994;2:170-7.

82. Gillette RG, Kramis RC, Roberts WJ. Characterization of spinal somatosensory neurons having receptive fields in lumbar tissues of cats. Pain 1993;54:85-98.

83. Kallakuri S, Cavanaugh JM, Blagoev DC. An immunohistochemical study of innervation of lumbar spinal dura and longitudinal ligaments. Spine 1998;23:403-11.

84. Konnai Y, Honda T, Sekiguchi Y, Kikuchi S, Sugiura Y. Sensory innervation of the lumbar dura mater passing through the sympathetic trunk in rats. Spine 2000; 25:776-82.

85. Gillette RG, Kramis RC, Roberts WJ. Suppression of activity in spinal nocireceptive "low back" neurons by paravertebral somatic stimuli in the cat. Neurosci Lett 1998;241:45-8.

86. Melzack R, Wall P D. Pain mechanisms: a new theory. Science 1965;150:971-9.

87. Budgell B, Hotta H, Sato A. Spinovisceral reflexes evoked by noxious and innocuous stimulation of the lumbar spine. J Neuromusculoskel Sys 1995;3:122-31.

88. Budgell B, Sato A, Suzuki A, Uchida S. Responses of adrenal function to stimulation of lumbar and thoracic interspinous tissues in the rat. Neurosci Res 1997; 28:33-40.

89. Henderson CNR. Three neurophysiologic theories on the chiropractic subluxation. In: Gatterman MI, editor. Foundations of chiropractic: subluxation. St. Louis: Mosby; 1995. p. 225-33.

90. Budgell BS, Hotta H, Sato A. Reflex responses of bladder motility after stimulation of interspinous tissues in the anesthetized rat. J Manipulative Physiol Ther 1998; 21:593-9.

91. Kang YM, Wheeler JD, Pickar JG. Stimulation of chemosensitive afferents from multifidus muscle does not sensitize multifidus muscle spindles to vertebral loads in the lumbar spine of the cat. Spine 2001;26:1528-36.

92. Pedersen J, Sjolander P, Wenngren BI, Johansson H. Increased intramuscular concentration of bradykinin increases the static fusimotor drive to muscle spindles in neck muscles of the cat. Pain 1997;70:83-91.

93. Wenngren BI, Pedersen J, Sjolander P, Bergenheim M, Johansson H. Bradykinin and muscle stretch alter contralateral cat neck muscle spindle output. Neurosci Res 1998;32:119-29.

94. Kang YM, Choi WS, Pickar JG. Electrophysiologic evidence for an intersegmental reflex pathway between lumbar paraspinal tissues. Spine 2002;27:E56-E63.

95. Kang YM, Kenney MJ, Spratt KF, Pickar JG. Somatosympathetic reflexes from the low back in the anesthetized cat. J Neurophysiol 2003;90:2548-59.

96. Greenspan J, Melchior J. The effect of osteopathic manipulative treatment on the resistance of rats to stressful situations. J Am Osteopath Assoc 1966; 65:1205-7.

97. Selye H. The stress of life. New York: McGraw-Hill Book Company; 1956. p. 1-475.

98. Thomas RJ, Salem T, Nance J, McGee D, Bonci AS. Ligamentous changes in the rat spine following repeated adjustments: a pilot study. Proceedings of the International Conference on Spinal Manipulation. Des Moines: Foundation for Chiropractic Education and Research; 1990:122-3.

99. Chazal J, Tanguy A, Bourges M, Gaurel G, Escande G, Guillot M, Vanneuville G. Biomechanical properties of spinal ligaments and a histological study of the supraspinal ligament in traction. J Biomech 1985;18:167-76.

100. Pickar JG, McLain RF. Responses of mechanosensitive afferents to manipulation of the lumbar facet in the cat. Spine 1995;20:2379-85.

101. Meeker W, Mootz R, Haldeman S. The state of chiropractic research. Top Clin Chiro 2002;9:1-13.

102. Dubos RJ. Louis Pasteur: free lance of science. Boston: Little, Brown & Co.; 1950. p. 376.

5

Palpatory Diagnosis of Subluxation

**Mitchell Haas and
David M. Panzer**

Key Words   Palpation, motion palpation, joint play, end feel, reliability

After reading this chapter you should be able to answer the following questions:

Question 1   What are the three most frequently cited adjustive indicators evaluated by palpation?

Question 2   What is the reliability of spinal palpation?

Question 3   What strategies can be used to improve the reliability of palpatory procedures?

The hands are the primary tool of the chiropractor and are of utmost importance in identifying subluxation. The origin of the term *chiropractic* is the Greek *cheiroprattien* (done by hand), and current texts used in chiropractic education are replete with comprehensive palpatory techniques.[1-4] Manual therapies are, however, not unique to chiropractic.

Historically, manual therapies can be traced to Eastern and Western cultures thousands of years before the advent of chiropractic.[5] Hippocrates was a notable proponent of manual treatment, particularly for spinal conditions such as scoliosis and subluxation.[5,6]

In light of modern advances in diagnostic imaging and other procedures, it may seem that the tedious process of palpation to evaluate the neuromusculoskeletal system is outdated. However, palpation remains recognized as an essential skill by disciplines such as osteopathy[7] and physical therapy,[8,9] which employ many techniques quite similar to those used by chiropractors. Beal,[7] an osteopath, notes that "palpation is of prime importance in diagnosis, manipulative treatment, and prognosis" of musculoskeletal conditions. Magee[9] describes numerous static and dynamic palpatory procedures for spinal and extremity articulations.

In quite another realm, Goble[10] offers practical advice for purchasing a horse. He states that

> with recent advances in diagnostic techniques...there is a tendency to reduce our reliance on the most important part of purchase evaluation of the horse, the hands-on physical examination.

Human parallels are obvious in our age of cost-conscious health care, in which a thorough physical examination may render more useful information than expensive diagnostic tests.

History of Palpation in Chiropractic

Because the use of diagnostic palpation has stood the test of time, a brief review of its history in the chiropractic profession is of interest. In 1912 Gregory[11] defined palpation as "the gentle application of the hand or fingers to the surface of the body for the purpose of determining the condition of the surface and adjacent parts of a certain locality or organ of the body." He described palpable characteristics of the "spinal lesion" as follows:
1. Pain
2. Tender nerves
3. Thermic alterations
4. Congested neural cords
5. Contractured or contracted muscle
6. Spinous process malposition
7. Transverse process malposition

A contemporary study by Keating et al.[12] to evaluate interexaminer reliability of currently used palpation procedures showed remarkable similarity to indicators listed in 1912, with the addition of a dynamic component:
1. Osseous pain
2. Soft tissue pain
3. Temperature difference
4. Visual observation
5. Passive motion palpation
6. Muscle tension palpation
7. Active motion palpation
8. Misalignment palpation

Among the earliest chiropractic palpation techniques was nerve tracing, defined as

> the art of following, by palpation, a tender nerve from its spinal origin to some inflammatory or pathological lesion or zone, or the act of tracing a tender spinal nerve from an inflammatory zone back to its spinal exit.[11]

D.D. Palmer[13] identifies himself as the originator of nerve tracing, but B.J. Palmer[14] also wrote extensively on the subject. According to B.J. Palmer, methodologic consistency and reliability appear to have been recognized as a problem even in his day (early twentieth century) shown by his observation that

> so far all of the nerve tracing in chiropractic, while it has been excellent, has produced excellent results—has been used by many chiropractors with a large degree of success—has still shown a remarkable divergence of method and accuracy.[14]

It is interesting that early nerve tracing was not unique to the chiropractic profession. Cyriax, a medical doctor, published a paper on "nerve palpation" in 1914.[15] Nerve tracing is no longer emphasized in chiropractic education.

In addition to the aforementioned static palpation techniques, various dynamic forms of palpation have developed within the chiropractic profession. Gillet[16-18] developed and systematized motion palpation techniques that have been expanded and disseminated by Faye[2,19,20] and Schafer.[20] Palpation is currently defined as the application of manual pressures through the surface of the body to determine the shape, size, consistency, position, and inherent motility of the tissues beneath.[21]

Palpatory Indicators for Manipulation

Contemporary palpation techniques can be divided into static and motion procedures used in the adjustment decision-making process[1,4]:
A. Static Palpation
  1. Soft tissue
    a. Tenderness
    b. Edema
    c. Temperature
    d. Moisture
    e. Muscle tone
    f. Hyperemia response
    g. Motility
    h. Trophic changes
  2. Bony
    a. Tenderness
    b. Malposition
    c. Anomalies
B. Motion Palpation
  1. Active/passive segmental range of motion
    a. Tenderness
    b. Quantity
    c. Quality
  2. Accessory motions
    a. Joint play
    b. End play or end feel
    c. Joint challenge/tenderness
Of the aforementioned palpatory techniques, some seem to be emphasized more than others. Bryner[22] surveyed 27 manuals and texts from chiropractic, osteopathic, physical therapy, and medical sources. He reported the frequency of citation of 15 different indicators for knee manipulation. He found the three most frequently cited indicators to be: (1) joint play abnormality, fixation, adhesion, tissue tension; (2) misalignment, displacement, prominence; and (3) tenderness, swelling.

He concluded that "more consensus between professional groups exists than is suggested in most professional forums." A survey of chiropractic colleges[23] found that all of the respondents (9 of 18 colleges surveyed) reported using joint play assessment and motion palpation as important indicators for joint manipulation. It was further concluded that improved standardization of procedures is needed, a concern also noted by others.[8,24-27]

Previous mention was made of selection of palpatory techniques that identify manipulable subluxation or manipulable lesion. Jull, Bogduk, and Marsland[28] looked at this issue, as well as the accuracy of manual diagnostic techniques for specific localization of cervical zygapophyseal pain and dysfunction. The three palpatory criteria selected were: (1) abnormal end feel, (2) abnormal quality of resistance to movement, and (3) local pain on palpation.

This study was unique in many respects. First, its subjects were 20 patients with chronic (more than one year) neck pain. Second, they were evaluated with diagnostic nerve blocks to establish with certainty the vertebral level of their symptoms and that the zygapophyseal (facet) joints were indeed the source of pain. Third, the examiner blindly examined the subjects either before or after the diagnostic nerve block (1) to establish if the pain was the result of facet joint dysfunction; (2) if so, to identify the precise level of pain; and (3) to identify patients with nonfacet pain. The results were as follows:
1. The examiner correctly identified 15 of 20 patients with confirmed facet pain or dysfunction.
2. The correct segmental level was identified in all 15 patients.
3. Five patients with confirmed nonfacet pain were correctly identified.
4. It was concluded that "manual diagnosis by a trained manipulative therapist can be as accurate

as can radiologically-controlled diagnostic nerve blocks in the diagnosis of cervical zygapophyseal syndrome."[28]

5. The three diagnostic indicators chosen were "highly specific for symptomatic zygapophyseal joints."[28]

These results are quite impressive, and although they have been replicated in the cervical spine (see Chapter 17), they cannot be generalized to other areas of the spine. Still they invite a closer look at the issue of reliability as it relates to palpation procedures.

Test Reliability

Background

Reliability is the reproducibility or consistency of measurement or diagnosis.[29-31] It is the extent to which a test can produce the same result on repeated evaluation of an unchanged characteristic. When a test result is categorical in nature, such as the decision of whether to perform an adjustment, reliability is also called chance-corrected agreement or concordance.

Reliability evaluation is only one step in the determination of the clinical usefulness of a diagnostic or evaluative procedure.[32,33] The accuracy or validity of a procedure—to what degree the test is on the mark and to what degree it actually evaluates what is intended—is of paramount importance. Direct assessment of the validity of adjustive indicators has remained elusive because of the absence of a "gold standard" for identifying manipulable subluxation. Reliability assessment thus continues to be the primary research being conducted on the clinical usefulness of palpation. Although strong consistency of measures does not ensure validity, reliability assessment is extremely important because it estimates the contribution of a test itself to the clinical decision-making process beyond what would be expected by examiner guessing or random measurement error.[34]

Assessment

Reliability is evaluated by multiple blinded measurements performed on a sample of subjects.

Table 5-1

Types of Reliability

Type	Evaluation
Interexaminer	≥ 2 raters
Intraexaminer	≥ 2 times
Interinstrument	≥ 2 instruments
Test-retest	≥ occasions

There are several types of reliability relevant to palpation (Table 5-1). Interexaminer reliability evaluates the consistency of different examiners and is determined through repeated assessment by two or more raters. Intraexaminer reliability is a measure of self-consistency; each rater must perform at least two measurements. Intraexaminer reliability is susceptible to overestimation because of difficulty of blinding the rater[35] and a tendency toward consistency of measurement error.[36]

Interinstrument reliability evaluates the agreement between two diagnostic techniques or two instruments (same type or different kinds). For example, the reproducibility of pain thresholds by two different types of pressure algometer can be evaluated. Intertechnique reliability can be assessed only if both instruments use the same units of measurement.

Test-retest reliability seeks to determine if examiners or instruments are consistent over time. Measurement of this type of reliability is problematic because the stability of manipulable subluxation and other palpatory entities is largely unknown. Biomechanical changes may be responsible for any apparent lack of consistency over time.

Reliability Indices

The choice of the most appropriate reliability statistic depends on the type of measurement being made (Table 5-2). Although other statistical measurements have been used, they tend to give ambiguous results; in-depth discussions of reliability statistics may be found elsewhere.[29-31]

The most common data collected on patients through palpation are nominal. A prime example

Table 5-2

Reliability Statistics

Scales and Indices

Nominal	Kappa
Ordinal	Weighted kappa
Interval	Intraclass correlation

Strength of Agreement

0.0	Chance
0.00-0.39	Poor-fair
0.40-0.59	Moderate
0.60-1.00	Good-excellent
1.00	Perfect

is the yes-or-no decision on the site of a manipulable subluxation. Another, with a four-category outcome, is the determination of whether motion restriction is observed on the left, on the right, both, or neither. The reliability statistic of choice in the case of a clinical decision based on such categorical data is kappa. Kappa is often described as a chance-corrected measure of examiner agreement.[6,30,31,33]

When the measurement categories are ordered in some way, the data are called ordinal. A clinical decision of degree, such as mild, moderate, or severe joint play restriction, is a common example. The reliability of ordinal data is evaluated with the weighted kappa statistic. When the data are continuous (interval or ratio), for example, the force required to cross the patient's pain threshold, the statistic of choice is the intraclass correlation coefficient (ICC). When applied appropriately, the ICC also can be used to evaluate concordance for ordinal and two-category nominal data.[37,38]

Strength of Concordance

The indices of reliability, for all practical purposes, are measured on a zero to one scale. Zero implies no relationship between ratings and that agreement between examiners can be attributed to chance alone; one represents perfect consistency. Negative values, which are possible, are taken to mean that the procedure itself contributes nothing to the measuring process beyond guessing and measurement error. Although interpretation of values between zero and one are somewhat arbitrary,

there appears to be consensus that values less than 0.4 represent inadequate reliability.[39-41] Just what represents good reliability depends on the nature of the test performed; clearly a test for acute myocardial infarction would require a greater level of consistency than a test for manipulable subluxation. Table 5-2 provides a rule of thumb for the interpretation of reliability for palpatory procedures.

Reliability of Chiropractic Spinal Palpatory Procedures

There have been close to 90 articles published in the peer-reviewed chiropractic literature on the subject of reliability; 28 address palpation. Because it is beyond the scope of this text to do an exhaustive review of the literature, average study findings are reported here in summary form for those studies reporting the statistics just discussed. However, there are in-depth review articles (Table 5-3) available that explore the original research on the reliability of palpatory procedures and several articles that carefully examine reliability study design, analysis, and interpretation in general.[30,35,42,43] Further studies may be found in the physical therapy and medical literature. These have not been included here because of their questionable generalization to chiropractors; other professionals may have different training in these procedures and may apply and interpret outcomes in a different manner.

Table 5-3

Review Articles

Author	Year	Subject
Alley[57]	1983	MP
Russel[58]	1983	MP, SP
Dishman[59]	1988	MP, SP
Keating[60]	1989	MP
Haas[35]	1991	MP, SP
Breen[24]	1992	MP, SP
Panzer[27]	1992	MP

MP, Motion palpation; *SP*, static palpation.

Specificity Assumption

The assessment of the reliability of palpatory procedures in the chiropractic literature has been guided by a fundamental chiropractic precept, the assumption that spinal manipulation must be and can be performed at specific spinal segments or motion segments to engender the appropriate therapeutic effect.[44] It then follows that palpatory procedures must be equally specific and it would seem reasonable that investigators have focused on the examiner consistency of identifying individual segments with manipulable subluxation. What must be kept in mind in reviewing study findings is that the specificity assumption has compelled the profession to accept a stringent standard for determining reliability; this precept still awaits clinical verification.

Motion Palpation

Fifteen studies report original data on the reliability of motion palpation in various regions of the spine and pelvis (five cervical, two thoracic, eight lumbar, and six sacroiliac) (Table 5-4). The interexaminer reliability of identifying motion or

Table 5-4

Motion Palpation Reliability Studies

Author	Year	Region
Wiles[61]	1980	SI
DeBoer et al.[56]	1985	C
Mior et al.[47]	1985	C
Bergstrom and Courtis[62]	1986	L
Love and Brodeur[25]	1987	L
Carmichael[46]	1987	SI
Boline et al.[45]	1988	L
Rhudy et al.[63]	1988	C, T, L
Nansel and Jansen[64]	1988	C, T, L, SI
Herzog et al.[65]	1989	SI
Leboeuf et al.[66]	1989	L, SI
Nansel et al.[49]	1989	C
Mootz et al.[26]	1989	L
Mior et al.[48]	1990	SI
Keating et al.[12]	1990	L

SI, Sacroiliac; *C*, cervical; *L*, lumbar; *T*, thoracic.

Table 5-5

Average Reliability of Palpatory Procedures

Motion Palpation		
Interrater	0.00-0.15	Poor
Intrarater	0.45-0.53	Moderate
Static Palpation		
Interrater		
Malposition	0.00	Poor
Muscle tension	0.07-0.20	Poor
Pain provocation	0.20-0.69	Fair-good
Intrarater	—	—

end-feel restriction at specific segmental levels was poor, averaging 0.00 to 0.15 (Table 5-5).[12,26,45-49] Raters agree little more than would be expected by chance. Intraexaminer reliability was considerably better, averaging 0.45 to 0.53.[26,46-48] However, the latter findings must be viewed with caution. Within the context of the specificity assumption, two examiners who are self-consistent but do not agree with one another requires the assumption that at least one rater must be consistently in error. Further, any clinical findings that cannot be replicated by others are always considered suspect.

Static Palpation

Ten studies on the various areas of the spine (three on the cervical region, one on the thoracic spine, seven on the lumbar region, and four on the sacroiliac joints) appear in the literature addressing static palpatory procedures (Table 5-6). Interexaminer concordance of vertebral malposition (0.00) and muscle tension (0.07 to 0.20) have been found to be little more than happenstance (see Table 5-5).[12,45,50] However, some results for provocative pain over the spinous processes and paravertebral soft tissue have been encouraging (0.20 to 0.69).[12,45,50] There have been no intraexaminer reliability studies on static palpation.

Conclusion

Although the reliability of palpation appears discouraging, all is far from lost as will be seen in the next section. Many interesting and provocative

Table 5-6

Static Palpation Reliability Studies

Author	Year	Region
DeBoer et al.[56]	1985	C
Boline et al.[45]	1988	L
Nansel and Jansen[64]	1988	C, T, L, SI
Owens[67]	1988	C
Leboeuf et al.[66]	1989	L
Jansen et al.[42]	1990	L, SI
Keating et al.[12]	1990	L
Byfield et al.[68]	1992	L, SI
Byfield et al.[69]	1992	SI
Boline et al.[50]	1993	L

C, Cervical; L, lumbar; T, thoracic; SI, sacroiliac.

Table 5-7

Clinical Judgment and Reliability Literature

Author	Year
Department[52]*	1980
Department[53]*	1980
Feinstein[70]	1964
Feinstein and Kramer[71]	1980
Feinstein[72]	1987
Sackett et al.[33]	1991
Wright and Feinstein[51]	1992

*Department of Clinical Epidemiology and Biostatistics, McMaster University, Hamilton, Ontario, Canada.

questions have arisen from more than a decade of research. For example, to what degree does the clinical decision-making process actually depend on individual palpatory procedures? How do chiropractors weigh the evidence from a variety of adjustive indicators? Are palpatory tests more valuable in certain patient populations than in others? Do chiropractors effect successful adjustments and patients show clinical improvement in spite of the diagnostic tests performed? Finally, we must ask ourselves if the specificity assumption led us astray from investigating the reliability of palpation in a context relevant to the actual biomechanical and clinical effects of manipulation on the body.

Improving the Reliability of Palpation

There is a rich supply of literature on the need for enhancing the reliability of diagnostic tests, sources of inconsistency, and recommendations for reliability improvement (Table 5-7). This literature is as valuable to the practicing clinician as it is to clinical researchers.

Why Bother?

We must first ask ourselves why improving consistency is so important. After all, experience tells us that we can successfully identify manipulable subluxations and make our patients better. Unfortunately, even accurate recollection of our experience can lead us to wrong conclusions about the effect of diagnostic tests on patient outcome,[33] and there are several good reasons why it is imperative that reliability of palpatory procedures be improved.[51]

Our first motivation is the justification of using palpatory procedures in the first place. A test in which the findings cannot be replicated will always be called into question. How can we be sure that we can identify a manipulable subluxation; how can we be sure that a patient really has a motion restriction or malposition and that it responded to treatment? Furthermore, poor reliability implies that a test performs little better than guesswork and as such contributes only marginally to the decision-making process[34]; why bother wasting the time and effort? An unreliable test can hardly be justified as cost-effective.

Improving reliability can also enhance the accuracy of a test; an unreliable test can never be accurate.[51] Improving accuracy can lead to increased efficiency of care because false-negative findings can lead to underadjusting, and false-positive findings can lead to excessive intervention. Finally, better consistency increases our confidence in finding manipulable subluxations and monitoring changes in clinical status.

Sources of Inconsistency

Three sources of test inconsistency are discussed in the literature: the examined, the examination, and the examiner.[51,52] Different clinical findings may be attributable to variability in the procedure. For example, intersegmental orientation and motion characteristics may vary greatly in the various patient positions—sitting, supine, prone, or side posture—used to perform the examination. Chiropractic physicians also use different landmarks to locate malposition and sites of provocative pain, as well as different methods for evaluating quality of motion, joint play, and end feel.

Even when the same procedure is used, there is variability in its performance. Chiropractic physicians hold patients in slightly different positions or palpate with varying degrees of force. Procedure and performance being equal, inconsistency still arises from variability in interpretation, including differences in principle and perception. Where do individual clinicians draw the line in identifying manipulable subluxations from hard end feel or joint play restriction? What constitutes a malposition? Perception also can vary with physician expectation, alertness, and mood. After an adjustment, what chiropractor is not confident that a manipulable subluxation has been rectified?

What We Can Do

Standardization

There are several important strategies for improving the reliability of palpatory procedures (Box 5-1).[53] Most difficult to implement is probably standardization of test procedure, performance, and interpretation. Chiropractic colleges

BOX 5-1 ■ Steps to Be Taken to Improve Reliability

- Standardization of test procedures
- Repetition of test findings
- Corroboration of test findings
- Identification of suitable patient subpopulations
- Reevaluation of specificity assumption

need to make a concerted effort to research and develop instructional methodologies that foster consistent terminology and palpation outcomes. It has been suggested that improved standardization of techniques and enhanced ability to evaluate psychomotor skills may be facilitated by the use of mechanical devices to assist in quantitative feedback by the quantification of manual forces.[8,54,55] Examples include bathroom scales,[8] pressure plate with oscilloscope,[55] and a mechanical spinal model with simulated fixations.[54] Instructors also must emphasize to their students the potential influences of perception and expectation on clinical findings. Ambiguity not only affects measurement consistency but also undermines the ability of chiropractors with diverse ideologies and treatment strategies to communicate with each other.

Repeated Tests

It is well known that for a test with nonzero reliability, the reliability of the average finding of test repetitions is greater than the reliability of a single evaluation.[29-31] For example, when repeated tests are conducted independently (examiner blinded to previous results), if the intraclass correlation coefficient (ICC) = 0.50 for a single measurement, the reliability of two evaluations would be ICC = 0.67, and for three assessments ICC = 0.75. Although repeated palpations are not blinded in clinical practice, they should reduce diagnostic error. However, because of the likelihood of some consistent error, the physician should regard high self-consistency with caution.[36]

Corroboration

Another strategy for strengthening the reliability of manipulable subluxation detection is the use of diagnostic test regimens.[42] Reliability might be increased by using multiple tests for the evaluation of a single palpatory dimension of the subluxation (e.g., motion, alignment, or palpatory pain). The evaluation of multiple palpatory dimensions as well as the inclusion of other clinical information is also strongly recommended to avoid false-negative results. Research into the value of multitest regimens is in its early stages.[12,45,50] Further investigation is required to clearly identify individual dimensions of the subluxation and to establish regiments of related tests for evaluation of these dimensions.

Identification of Suitable Patients

It is possible that various palpation techniques are more suitable for certain subpopulations of patients than for others. These subpopulations could be identified through studies of carefully defined homogeneous groups of patients, probably patients with more severe and extensive problems. It also must be pointed out that, in general, concordance depends on the prevalence of the entity being assessed.[30,34] For patient populations with a dearth of manipulable subluxation, it is difficult for any test to perform better than guessing that the patient is normal at any particular segmental level. Reliability will inevitably be low in this case, and the contribution of palpation to the clinical evaluation of the patient will be minimal.

Challenging the Specificity Assumption

With two exceptions,[26,56] reliability has been exclusively evaluated within the context of the specificity assumption. What we must ask ourselves is whether this precept is clinically valid. Are we really investigating the reliability of detecting what we actually treat? If not, are we underestimating the reliability of our adjustive indicators?[44] The specificity of the vertebral contact may not be necessary for correction of the "true" underlying manipulable subluxation. Alternatively, the specific adjustment of different manipulable subluxations may have the same clinical effects; two chiropractors may rightfully treat different segments.

If contact specificity is not valid, examiners would not have to agree on specific segments but only on a specific region to have the same clinical outcome. In this case, "regional" rather than "segmental" concordance in the site of an adjustment might be a sufficient condition to establish acceptable interexaminer reliability of palpatory procedures. If adjustment specificity is not required to treat a clinical condition, however, self-consistency may be paramount and intraexaminer concordance the key to the reliability of palpation (the concerns listed previously notwithstanding).

Clearly it is easier to find agreement over a wider range of vertebral segments and with oneself than it is to find interexaminer agreement segment by segment. However, enhancing reliability is no justification for abandoning the specificity assumption a priori. There is no biomechanical model or clinical evidence to suggest how big the zone of agreement might be or how it might vary for different regions of the spine or different clinical conditions.

Future Research

The goal of investigators must be to represent the adjustive decision-making process as realistically as possible in measurement evaluation research. Clinically relevant reliability assessment must include the study of de facto test regimens as well as the evaluation of individual procedures. The viability of the specificity assumption will be investigated in part through studies of the biomechanical relationship of the spinal contact with the motion segments being affected.

Further research must be conducted to establish the clinical usefulness of palpatory procedures.[32,33] The validity of palpation to detect manipulable subluxations will be measured indirectly in the short term through the assessment of its theoretical properties (construct validity); these include the correlation of palpatory findings with patient symptomatology, other diagnostic findings, adjustive intervention, and treatment outcomes. Ultimately, the utility of palpation must be evaluated: Is the patient better off for having had the procedures performed?

References

1. Peterson DH, Bergman TF. Chiropractic technique. 2nd ed. St. Louis: Churchill Livingstone; 2002.
2. Faye LJ, Wiles MR. Manual examination of the spine. In: Haldeman S, editor. Principles and practice of chiropractic. 2nd ed. San Mateo, CA: Appleton and Lange; 1992. p. 301-18.
3. Gatterman MI. Chiropractic management of spine related disorders. 2nd ed. Baltimore: Lippincott, Williams & Wilkins; 2003.
4. Plaugher G, Lopes MA, editors. Textbook of clinical chiropractic. Baltimore: Williams & Wilkins; 1993. p. 86-93.
5. Schiotz EH, Cyriax I. Manipulation past and present. London: William Heinemann Medical Books; 1975. p. 5-27.

6. Anderson R. Spinal manipulation before chiropractic. In: Haldeman S, editor. Principles and practice of chiropractic. 2nd ed. San Mateo, CA: Appleton and Lange; 1992.

7. Beal MC. Perception through palpation. J Am Osteopath Assoc 1989;89(10):1334-52.

8. Keating I, Matyas TA, Bach TM. The effect of training on physical therapists' ability to apply specified forces of palpation. Phys Ther 1993;73(1):45-53.

9. Magee DJ: Orthopedic physical assessment. 4th ed. Philadelphia: WB Saunders; 2002.

10. Goble DO. Medical evaluation of the musculoskeletal system and common integument relevant to purchase. Vet Clin North Am Equine Pract 1992;8:285-302.

11. Gregory AA. Spinal treatment science and technique. Oklahoma City: The Palmer-Gregory College; 1912. p. 345-6.

12. Keating JC Jr, Bergmann TF, Jacobs GE, Finer BA, Larson K. Interexaminer reliability of eight evaluative dimensions of lumbar segmental abnormality. J Manipulative Physiol Ther 1990;13:463-70.

13. Palmer DD. The science art and philosophy of chiropractic. Portland, OR: Portland Printing House; 1910. p. 20.

14. Palmer BJ. The philosophy, science, and art of nerve tracing. In: The science of chiropractic. Vol. 6. Davenport, IA: Palmer School of Chiropractic; 1911. p. 11-18.

15. Cyriax E. On the technique of nerve palpation by nerve "friction." Review of Neurology & Psychiatry (GB) 1914;12:148-51.

16. Gillet H. Vertebral fixations: an introduction to movement palpation. Ann Swiss Chiro Assoc 1960;1:30.

17. Gillet H, Liekens M. A further study of spinal fixations. Ann Swiss Chiro Assoc 1969;4:41.

18. Gillet H, Liekens M. Belgian chiropractic research notes. Huntington Beach, CA: Motion Palpation Institute; 1981.

19. Faye LJ. Motion palpation of the spine [MPI notes and review of literature]. Huntington Beach, CA: Motion Palpation Institute; 1981.

20. Schafer RC, Faye LJ. Motion palpation and chiropractic technique: principles of dynamic chiropractic. Huntington Beach, CA: Motion Palpation Institute; 1989.

21. ACA Council on Technique. Chiropractic terminology: a report. J Am Chiro Assoc 1988;25(10):46.

22. Bryner P. A survey of indications: knee manipulation. Chiro Tech 1989;1(4):140-5.

23. Bryner P, Bruin J. Extremity joint technique: survey of the status of technique teaching in chiropractic colleges. Chiro Tech 1991;3(1):30-2.

24. Breen A. The reliability of palpation and other diagnostic methods. J Manipulative Physiol Ther 1992;15:54-56.

25. Love RM, Brodeur RR. Inter- and intra-examiner reliability of motion palpation for the thoracolumbar spine. J Manipulative Physiol Ther 1987;10:1-4.

26. Mootz RD, Keating JC, Kontz HP. Intra- and inter-examiner reliability of passive motion palpation of the lumbar spine. J Manipulative Physiol Ther 1989;12:440-5.

27. Panzer D. The reliability of lumbar motion palpation. J Manipulative Physiol Ther 1992;15:518-24.

28. Jull G, Bogduk N, Marsland A. The accuracy of manual diagnosis for cervical zygapophyseal joint pain syndromes. Med J Aust 1988;148:233-6.

29. Bartko JJ, Carpenter WT. On the methods and theory of reliability. J Nerv Ment Dis 1976;163:307-17.

30. Haas M. Statistical methodology for reliability studies. J Manipulative Physiol Ther 1991;14:119-32.

31. Kramer MS, Feinstein AR. Clinical biostatistics. LIV. The biostatistics of concordance. Clin Pharmacol Ther 1981; 29:111-23.

32. McMaster University Department of Clinical Epidemiology and Biostatistics. How to read clinical journals. II. To learn about a diagnostic test. Can Med Assoc J 1981;124:703-9.

33. Sackett DL, Haynes RB, Guyatt GH, Tugwell P. Clinical epidemiology: a basic science for clinical medicine. 2nd ed. Boston: Little Brown; 1991.

34. Feinstein AR, Cicchetti DV. High agreement but low kappa. I. The problem of two paradoxes. J Clin Epidemiol 1990;41(6):543-9.

35. Haas M. The reliability of reliability. J Manipulative Physiol Ther 1991;14:199-208.

36. Rosner B, Willett WC, Spiegelman D. Correlation of logistic regression relative risk estimates and confidence intervals for systematic within-person measurement error. Am J Epidemiol 1989;8:1051-69.

37. Fleiss JL. Estimating the accuracy of dichotomous judgments. Psychometrika 1965;30(4):469-79.

38. Fleiss JL, Cohen J. The equivalence of weighted kappa and the intraclass correlation coefficient as measures of reliability. Ed Psychol Meas 1973;33:613-9.

39. Fleiss JL. Statistical methods for rates and proportions. New York: John Wiley & Sons; 1981. p. 212-36.

40. Landis JR, Koch GG. The measurement of observer agreement for categorical data. Biometrics 1977;33:159-74.

41. Rosner B. Fundamentals of biostatistics. 2nd ed. Boston: Duxbury Press; 1986.

42. Jansen RD, Nansel DD, Slosberg M. Normal paraspinal tissue compliance: the reliability of a new clinical and experimental instrument. J Manipulative Physiol Ther 1990;13:243-6.

43. Haas M. Interexaminer reliability for multiple diagnostic test regimens. J Manipulative Physiol Ther 1991;14:95-103.

44. Haas M, Peterson D, Hoyer D, Ross G. The reliability of muscle testing response to a provocative vertebral challenge. Chiro Tech 1993;5(3):95-100.

45. Boline PD, Keating JC, Brist J, Denver G. Interexaminer reliability of palpatory evaluation of the lumbar spine. Am J Chiro Med 1988;1:5-11.

46. Carmichael JP. Inter- and intra-examiner reliability of palpation for sacroiliac joint dysfunction. J Manipulative Physiol Ther 1987;10:164-71.

47. Mior SA, King RS, McGregor M, Bernard M. Intra- and interexaminer reliability of motion palpation in the cervical spine. J Can Chiro Assoc 1985;29:195-8.

48. Mior SA, McGregor M, Schut AB. The role of experience in clinical accuracy. J Manipulative Physiol Ther 1990; 13:68-71.

49. Nansel DD, Peneff AL, Jansen RD, Cooperstein R. Interexaminer concordance in detecting joint-play asymmetries in the cervical spines of otherwise asymptomatic subjects. J Manipulative Physiol Ther 1989;12:428-33.

50. Boline PD, Haas M, Meyers LL, Kassak K, Nelson C, Keating J. Interexaminer reliability of a multi-dimensional index of lumbar segmental abnormality. Part II. J Manipulative Physiol Ther 1993;16(6):363-74.

51. Wright JG, Feinstein AR. Improving the reliability of orthopaedic measurements. J Bone Joint Surg 1992; 74B:287-91.

52. McMaster University Department of Clinical Epidemiology and Biostatistics. Clinical disagreement. I. How often it occurs and why. Can Med Assoc J 1980;123:499-504.

53. McMaster University Department of Clinical Epidemiology and Biostatistics. Clinical disagreement. II. How to avoid it and how to learn from one's mistakes. Can Med Assoc J 1980;123:613-17.

54. Harvey D, Byfield D. Preliminary studies with a mechanical model for the evaluation of spinal motion palpation. Clin Biomech 1991;6(2):79-82.

55. Lee M, Moseley A, Refshauge K. Effect of feedback on learning a vertebral joint mobilization skill. Phys Ther 1990;70(2):97-104.

56. DeBoer KF, Harmon R, Tuttle CD, Wallace H. Reliability study of detection of somatic dysfunctions in the cervical spine. J Manipulative Physiol Ther 1985;8:9-16.

57. Alley JR. The clinical value of motion palpation as a diagnostic tool: a review. J Can Chiro Assoc 1983;27:97-100.

58. Russell R. Diagnostic palpation of the spine: a review of procedures and assessment of their reliability. J Manipulative Physiol Ther 1983;6:181-3.

59. Dishman RW: Static and dynamic components of the chiropractic subluxation complex: a literature review. J Manipulative Physiol Ther 1988;11:98-107.

60. Keating JC. Interexaminer reliability of motion palpation of the lumbar spine: a review of the chiropractic literature. Am J Chiro Med 1989;2:107-110.

61. Wiles MR. Reproducibility and interexaminer correlation of motion palpation findings of the sacroiliac joints. J Can Chiro Assoc 1980;24:59-69.

62. Bergstrom E, Courtis G. An inter- and intra-examiner reliability study of motion palpation of the lumbar spine in lateral flexion in the seated position. Eur J Chiro 1986;34:121-41.

63. Rhudy TR, Sandefur MR, Burk JM. Interexaminer/ intertechnique reliability in spinal subluxation assessment: a multifactorial approach. Am J Chiro Med 1988;1:111-4.

64. Nansel DD, Jansen RD. Concordance between galvanic skin response and spinal palpation findings in pain-free males. J Manipulative Physiol Ther 1988;11:267-72.

65. Herzog W, Read LJ, Conway PJ, Shaw LD, McEwen MC. Reliability of motion palpation to detect sacroiliac joint fixations. J Manipulative Physiol Ther 1989;12:86-92.

66. Leboeuf C, Gardner V, Carter AL, Scott TA. Chiropractic examination procedures: a reliability and consistency study. J Aust Chiro Assoc 1989;19:101-4.

67. Owens E An objective measurement of muscle tone. Chiro Res J 1988;1:34-42.

68. Byfield D, Humphreys K. Intra- and inter-examiner reliability of bony landmark identification in the lumbar spine. Eur J Chiro 1992;40:13-7.

69. Byfield DC, Mathiasen J, Sangren C. The reliability of osseous landmark palpation in the lumbar spine and pelvis. Eur J Chiro 1992;40:83-8.

70. Feinstein AR. Scientific methodology in clinical medicine. N. Acquisition of clinical data. Ann Intern Med 1964; 61(6):1162-93.

71. Feinstein AR, Kramer MS. Clinical biostatistics. LIII. The architecture of observer/method variability and other types of process research. Clin Pharmacol Ther 1980; 28(4):551-63.

72. Feinstein AR. Clinimetrics. New Haven, CT: Yale University Press; 1987.

73. Jansen RD, Nansel DD. Diagnostic illusions: the reliability of random chance. J Manipulative Physiol Ther 1988; 11:355-65.

6

The Role of Radiography in Evaluating Subluxation

John A.M. Taylor

Key Words   Static radiography, spinographic analysis, functional radiographs

After reading this chapter you should be able to answer the following questions:

Question 1   What are the common clinical indications for obtaining radiographs?

Question 2   What are the clinical findings that indicate functional radiography may be useful?

Question 3   What are the clinical indications for full-spine radiography?

The role of radiography in the evaluation of the chiropractic spinal vertebral subluxation has evolved considerably over the years.[1,2] Both static and functional radiographs are used in chiropractic to evaluate posture and biomechanics. In clinical practice, emphasis on one method or the other appears to depend largely on the individual practitioner's concept of a subluxation. Although some chiropractors view subluxation as a purely static phenomenon of vertebral misalignment, more recently an increasing number of chiropractors have begun to view the subluxation as a more dynamic, functional concept encompassing abnormalities of articular motion.[3-5]

Chiropractors use radiography for several reasons. Sherman[6] identifies the following clinical reasons for taking radiographs:
1. To establish a clinical (pathologic) diagnosis
2. To evaluate biomechanics and posture
3. To identify anomalies
4. To screen for contraindications
5. To monitor degenerative processes

Nonclinical reasons for taking radiographs are inappropriate and include the following[6,7]:
1. Financial gain for the practitioner
2. Force of habit
3. Medicolegal advantage
4. Patient education

Current epidemiologic studies examining the role of lumbar spine radiography question the value of taking radiographs for many clinical situations. Howard and Rowe[8] and Deyo and Diehl[9] recommend several criteria for selecting low-back pain patients for radiography (Box 6-1).

Some chiropractors argue that these recommendations ignore factors unique to the chiropractic approach to patient care.[6,10] For instance, Gatterman[11] identifies 31 conditions that contraindicate or require modification of spinal manipulation and suggests that in at least 20 of those conditions radiographic examination is part of the standard of practice for establishing the diagnosis. The fact remains that radiography should never be used as a general screening procedure without specific clinical indication.[9,12] Howe[13] stresses that routine or stereotyped methods of

BOX 6-1 ■ Spine Radiography: Clinical Indications for Patient Selection

Patient history

- Patients older than 50 years
- Significant trauma
- Neuromotor deficits
- Unexplained weight loss
- Suspicion of ankylosing spondylitis
- Drug or alcohol abuse
- History of cancer
- Corticosteroid use
- Increased temperature, above 100° F
- Diabetes or hypertension
- Recent visit for same problem and not improved
- Patients seeking compensation for back pain

Physical findings

- Dermopathy (psoriasis, melanoma)
- Cachexia
- Deformity and immobility
- Scars (surgical, accidental)
- Lymphadenopathy
- Localized pain, tenderness, spasm
- Motor or sensory deficit
- Elevated erythrocyte sedimentation rate
- Elevated acid or alkaline phosphatase
- Positive rheumatoid factor
- Positive HLA B27
- Serum gammopathy

Adapted from Deyo RA, Diehl AK. J Gen Intern Med 1986;1:20-5; and Howard BA, Rowe LJ. Spinal x-rays. In: Haldeman S, editor. Principles and practice of chiropractic. 2nd ed. East Norwalk, CT: Appleton and Lange; 1992. p. 361-4.

radiographic examination do not serve the best interests of the patient.

The following discussion focuses on the indications and limitations of some of the more commonly employed static and functional radiographic procedures employed in the evaluation of posture, biomechanics, and misalignment.

Static Radiography and Spinographic Analysis

Spinography, the procedure of analyzing spine radiographs for postural and structural abnormalities, dates from 1910 when it was first introduced at Palmer School of Chiropractic by Dr. B.J. Palmer.[1] Marking radiographs to identify misalignments was a natural extension of the popular static concept of subluxation in the early 1900s. From 1918 until 1936, full-spine radiographic techniques were developed.[1,2,14] Texts on chiropractic spinography have been published by Thompson,[15] Hildebrandt,[16] and Winterstein.[17] In addition, technique systems using spinographic analysis have been developed by several chiropractors, including Clarence C. Gonstead[10,18] and Hugh B. Logan.[14,19]

The utility of many spinographic methods requires more study. One fundamental criticism of measuring misalignments on radiographs is the problem of anatomic asymmetry. Asymmetric developmental anomalies are common and can simulate true misalignments.[20] The role of full-spine radiographs in chiropractic analysis remains controversial.[2] Opinions held by chiropractors vary widely and include those who consider full-spine radiography a routine procedure and those who consider it an overused procedure that never should be used. The literature suggests, however, that with proper patient selection, careful attention to technical detail, and use of several technologic advancements, full-spine radiography is a diagnostic and analytic procedure with an acceptable risk/benefit ratio.[2] The circumstances in which full-spine radiographs might be preferred over sectional radiographs are as follows: (1) cases in which clinical examination discloses the need for radiography of several spinal sections; (2) cases in which severe postural distortion is evident; (3) for scoliosis evaluation after clinical assessment; (4) cases in which a mechanical problem in one spinal area adversely affects other spinal regions; (5) to specifically evaluate complex biomechanical or postural disorders of the spine and pelvis under weight-bearing conditions.[2,16,21,22]

Many chiropractors agree that full-spine radiography should be reserved for evaluating scoliosis after a thorough clinical evaluation. Scoliosis measurement using the Cobb method is well established (Figure 6-1). This measurement is reported to be accurate to within 2.8 to 11 degrees.[23-25] Mehta concluded that rotation of up to 15 degrees is necessary for clear-cut identification of vertebral rotation on scoliosis radiographs.[26] This observation calls into question many of the methods used to measure millimetric changes in vertebral rotation. A high correlation has been

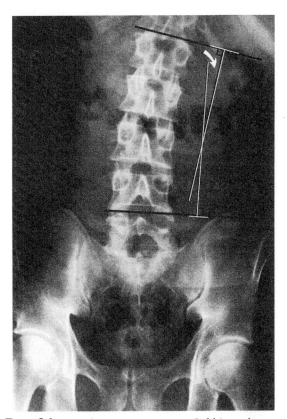

Figure 6-1   Scoliosis measurement: Cobb's angle. Cobb's angle is obtained from frontal (AP or PA) spine radiographs by constructing lines along the end plates of the end vertebra located at the superior and inferior extremes of the scoliosis. Perpendicular lines are then constructed and the intersecting angle is measured. This angle is used to assist in management decisions and as a comparison to previous and future studies to monitor scoliosis progress. This measurement is accurate within 2.8 to 11 degrees.

demonstrated between Cobb's angles measured on posteroanterior (PA) and anteroposterior (AP) radiographs.[27]

Conflicting evidence regarding the reliability of pelvic spinographic analysis has been reported. Plaugher and Hendricks[28] found excellent interobserver and intraobserver reliability, and Phillips[29] found very little consistency between the various methods used. Many errors arise from faulty patient positioning.[30]

Leg length inequality (LLI) can be measured reliably from spine radiographs,[31] but most authors agree that specialized orthoradiography or clinical examination is more accurate in the assessment of LLI (Figure 6-2).[31-34]

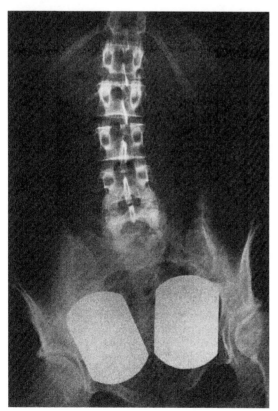

Figure 6-2   Scoliosis secondary to leg length inequality. This 35-year-old woman sustained a severe femur fracture when she was 12 years old, resulting in significant growth retardation of one lower extremity. This has resulted in obvious disparity in the heights of the femoral heads and iliac crests as well as scoliosis.

Some chiropractic analytical procedures are based on the premise that static misalignments can be confirmed by radiography and that these misalignments can be corrected by chiropractic adjustments. In one large study,[35] the only demonstrable postmanipulation change was a 34% reduction in retrolisthesis. No posttreatment change was observed in cervical lordosis, sacral base angle, lumbar lordosis, scapular angle, or Cobb's angle.

This study[35] raises the question of the clinical validity of spinographic analysis. Phillips et al.[36] concluded that spine radiographs, analyzed by measurements, have minimal value in predicting the presence or absence of low-back pain complaints. Mootz and Meeker[37] and Phillips agree that the use of radiography for biomechanical (postural) evaluation requires further clarification and research. Evidence is lacking that these parameters demonstrate any clinical significance.

Owens's review of the literature and summary of the role of line drawing analyses of static cervical radiographs used in chiropractic[38] is consistent with those of Phillips et al.[36] and Mootz and Meeker.[37] Owens concludes that, although some studies demonstrate reliability of some of these procedures, the accuracy and clinic significance remain in question:

> The major question should no longer be if x-ray analysis can be used as a tool in the scientific investigation of chiropractic subluxation. Rather, studies should be designed, using x-ray analysis, to test the fundamental hypothesis of the analysis techniques, that static structural misalignment in the neck and occiput can be a causative factor in the chiropractic subluxation.[38]

In his review, Owens lists 15 named chiropractic radiographic analysis techniques that are "systems" taught primarily through entrepreneurial postgraduate weekend seminars. Of the 15 techniques, only two (Gonstead and upper cervical specific-hole in one [HIO]) are taught as part of the curriculum at more than one accredited chiropractic college.[38]

In addition to the many "systems approaches" to marking radiographs, several lines and angles of measurement have been developed in the fields of radiology and chiropractic for assessing static and functional radiographs.[39,40] Table 6-1 outlines some of the more common procedures and their clinical significance, and Box 6-2 lists the classification for intersegmental subluxations that sometimes can be seen on static and functional radiographs (Figure 6-3).[41] Figures 6-4 to 6-10 illustrate some of the more commonly used lines, angles, and measurements. It should be emphasized, however, that the clinical significance of static misalignment subluxations has never been clearly established. Many of the patterns listed in

Box 6-2 actually only occur as a result of articular derangements, such as severe inflammatory or degenerative disc and apophyseal joint disease, or long-standing developmental articular changes.

One area of radiographic analysis that has received considerable attention is the cervical curve and its degree of lordotic configuration (Figure 6-11). Over the years, chiropractors have attributed various degrees of significance to the presence of hyperlordosis, hypolordosis, flattened lordosis, and kyphosis. After his review of the literature on the curve of the cervical spine, Gay[42] concluded that there is a wide range of normal,

Table 6-1

Commonly Used Radiographic Lines, Angles, and Measurements

Line, angle, measurement	Figure	Proposed clinical significance
Lumbar Spine		
Lumbar gravitational line	6-5	Anterior or posterior weight-bearing on lumbosacral disc
Lumbar lordosis angle		Hyperlordosis or hypolordosis determines stress on discs or facets
Lumbosacral base angle	6-7	Determines shearing or compressive forces on discs and facets
Lumbosacral disc angle		Can be increased in facet syndrome
Lumbar intervertebral disc angles	6-7	Can be increased in hyperlordosis
McNab's line		Unreliable method of assessing facet impingement or imbrication
Flexion-extension analysis	6-12	Measure of instability on lumbar flexion-extension views
Hadley's "S" curve		Method of assessing facet impingement or imbrication
Ullman's line		For assessing presence of L5-S1 anterolisthesis
Meyerding's grading	6-4	Method of grading spondylolisthesis (Grades 1-5)
Eisenstein's method		Lumbar sagittal canal diameter: stenosis or widening
Interpediculate distance		Lumbar coronal canal diameter: stenosis or widening
Canal/body ratio		Combined sagittal and coronal canal diameter
George's line	6-6	Disrupted in anterolisthesis or retrolisthesis
Cervical Spine and Skull Base		
Chamberlain's line		Basilar invagination, cranial settling, basilar impression
McGregor's line		Basilar invagination, cranial settling, basilar impression
George's line		Cervical or lumbar, anterolisthesis or retrolisthesis
Posterior cervical line		Anterolisthesis or retrolisthesis or neural arch fracture
Jackson's lines		Alterations in physiologic stress lines on flexion-extension views
Angle of cervical lordosis	6-11	Hypolordosis or hyperlordosis measurement
Cervical gravity line	6-10	Anterior or posterior weight-bearing
Cervical range of motion		Measurement performed on flexion-extension views
Atlantodental interval (ADI)		Indicates atlantoaxial instability from transverse ligament damage
Sagittal canal diameter	6-8	Stenosis or widening from intraspinal mass
Prevertebral soft tissue spaces	6-9	Inflammation, hemorrhage, or mass in soft tissues

that many traumatic and nontraumatic factors influence the curve, and that there is little evidence-based support of the contention that altered cervical curvature has any prognostic significance.[43] He found, based on the literature, that lordotic straightening or reversal could result from muscle spasm, but that more specific interpretation is speculative. He emphasized that, although acute angular kyphosis could represent an unstable ligamentous injury such as is seen in hyperflexion sprains, it could represent a normal variant in the absence of clinical and further radiographic corroboration.[43]

Text continued on p. 125.

BOX 6-2 ■ Radiographic Classification of Subluxation

Static intersegmental misalignments

- Flexion malposition
- Extension malposition
- Lateral flexion malposition
- Rotational malposition
- Anterolisthesis
- Spondylolisthesis
- Retrolisthesis
- Laterolisthesis
- Decreased interosseous spacing
- Foraminal encroachments

Kinetic intersegmental dysfunctions

- Hypomobility
- Hypermobility
- Aberrant motion

Sectional subluxations

- Scoliosis secondary to muscle imbalance
- Scoliosis secondary to structural asymmetry
- Decompensation of adaptational curvatures
- Abnormalities of global motion

Paravertebral subluxations

- Costovertebral
- Costotransverse
- Sacroiliac

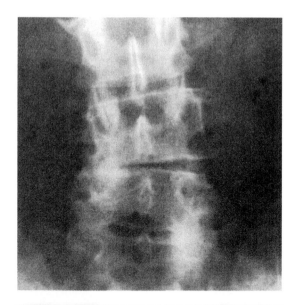

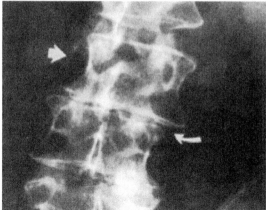

Figure 6-3   Static intersegmental misalignments. *Top,* lateral flexion malposition. *Bottom,* lateral listhesis. Although an extensive classification of static intersegmental misalignments exists (see Table 6-3), it is unusual to observe genuine malpositions on radiographs in the absence of severe degenerative or inflammatory joint changes. Note in both top and bottom the advanced discovertebral and apophyseal degenerative changes allowing these nonphysiologic malpositions to occur. Most nondegenerative or noninflammatory misalignments seen on radiographs actually represent asymmetry of vertebral structures.

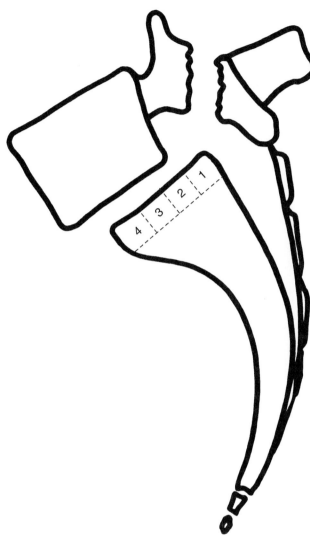

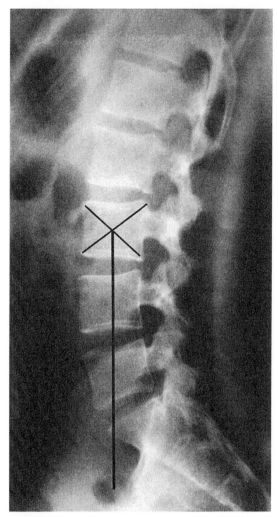

Figure 6-4 Lumbosacral spondylolisthesis. Myerding's method of measuring slippage in spondylolisthesis involves dividing the sacrum into four equal quadrants on the lateral lumbosacral radiograph. The degree of slippage is graded based on the alignment of the posterior aspect of the L5 vertebral body with one of the quadrants. The illustration above demonstrates a grade 2 spondylolisthesis.

Figure 6-5 Lumbar gravitational line. This line is constructed by identifying the central portion of the L3 vertebral body on a weight-bearing lateral lumbar radiograph. A vertical line is constructed inferiorly from this center point. In the "ideal" weight-bearing posture, this line should intersect the anterior portion of the sacrum. In anterior weight bearing, the line falls anterior to the sacrum; in posterior weight bearing, frequently associated with hyperlordosis, the line falls posterior to the anterior portion of the sacrum.

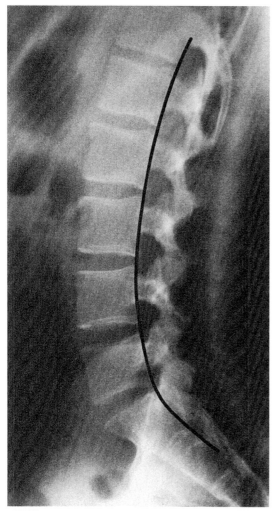

Figure 6-6   George's line. George's line is drawn to detect evidence of anterolisthesis or retrolisthesis. On a lateral radiograph of either the lumbar or cervical spine, a continuous vertical line is drawn along the posterior margins of the vertebral bodies. In the normal situation, this line should be smooth, curvilinear, and uninterrupted.

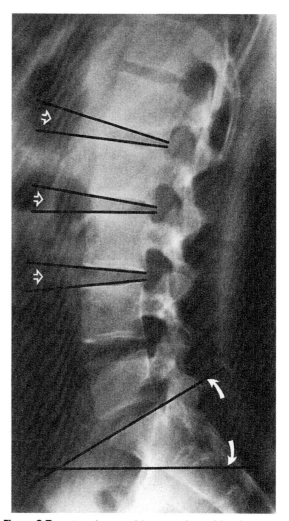

Figure 6-7   Lumbosacral base angle and lumbar intervertebral disc angles. Ferguson's angle or the lumbosacral base angle is obtained on the lateral lumbar radiograph by constructing a line along the superior aspect of the sacral base. The angle formed between this line and an intersecting horizontal line is then measured *(curved arrows)*. On upright radiographs, this measurement ranges from 26 to 57 degrees. An increase in this angle has been associated with an increased incidence of spondylolytic spondylolisthesis. In measuring the lumbar intervertebral disc angles, lines are constructed along the vertebral end plates of the lumbar vertebrae. The intersecting angles indicate the configuration of the intervertebral disc *(open arrows)*. The normal range is 10 to 15 degrees. Excessive angulation is seen in hyperextension or hyperlordosis, and diminished angulation is seen in patients with hypolordosis or acute flexion antalgia.

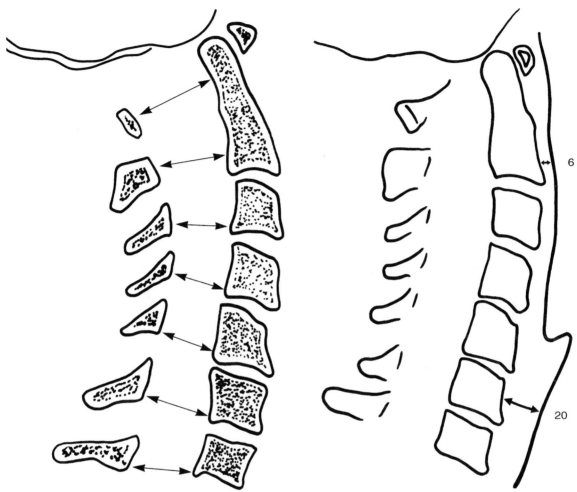

Figure 6-8   Sagittal canal diameter: cervical spine. The sagittal canal diameter is measured on a neutral lateral cervical radiograph taken at 72-inch-target film distance. Measurements less than 12 mm suggest canal stenosis and excessive measurements (more than 22 to 31 mm) suggest a space-occupying lesion expanding the spinal canal.

Figure 6-9   Prevertebral soft tissue measurements. The prevertebral soft tissues can be measured on a neutral lateral cervical radiograph taken at 72-inch-target film distance. The measurement at C2 should not exceed 5 to 6 mm and at C6 should not exceed 20 mm. These measurements are wider in cases of retrotracheal, retropharyngeal, or retrolaryngeal abscess, neoplasm, or posttraumatic hematoma.

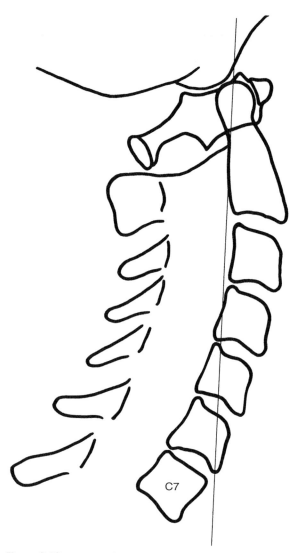

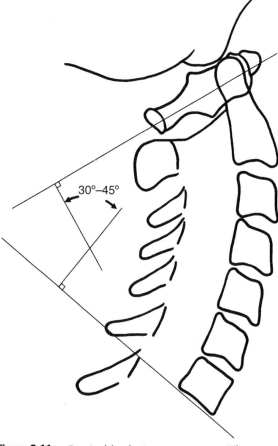

Figure 6-10   Cervical spine center of gravity. The cervical gravity line is measured by constructing a vertical line from the superior tip of the odontoid process. This line should intersect the C7 vertebral body. When the line passes anterior to the C7 body, such as in the schematic diagram above, the patient is said to have anterior head carriage or anterior weight bearing.

Figure 6-11   Cervical lordosis measurement. The cervical lordosis is measured by constructing lines along the atlas plane line and the inferior end plate of C7 on a neutral lateral radiograph. Perpendicular lines then are constructed and the intersecting angle is measured. Although 30 to 45 degrees is generally considered "normal," a wider range of normal exists. Several factors, including muscle spasm, influence the degree of curve, but there appears to be no prognostic significance of altered curvature.

Functional Radiography and Spinal Dysfunction

Gillet and Leikens[4] and Schafer and Faye[5] are responsible for raising chiropractic awareness of the importance of spine function and placing more emphasis on dynamic concepts, such as fixation analysis and movement palpation. This paradigm shift, from a static to a dynamic approach to spine analysis, initiated an increase in the use of functional radiography in chiropractic. Many authors, both chiropractic and nonchiropractic, have addressed the issue of functional radiography of the lumbar[43-51] and cervical[52-63] spine.

Functional radiography typically is used to establish the presence of the following:
1. Segmental or global hypomobility or fixation
2. Segmental or global hypermobility
3. Segmental instability
4. Aberrant segmental or global motion
5. Paradoxical motion
6. Postsurgical arthrodesis evaluation

Considerable disagreement persists regarding the indication for functional radiography. The chief concern revolves around the issue of radiation exposure.[64-68] In all cases the anticipated benefit of the study must outweigh the potential risk of ionizing radiation. Although some practitioners use functional radiography routinely, most authorities agree that it should be reserved as a supplementary procedure.

The following guidelines are suggested for the use of functional radiography based on clinical findings:
1. Persistent signs and symptoms or unsatisfactory response to a conservative trial of chiropractic care
2. Suggested persistent segmental dysfunction
3. Suggested segmental instability
4. When other appropriate imaging studies are inconclusive in establishing joint dysfunction

Meticulous attention to patient positioning is essential in functional radiography. Because of the difficulty of precise, standardized positioning in each patient, quantitative measurements derived from these films are subject to inaccuracies.[55] Therefore functional radiographs should be used more as qualitative indicators of spine motion rather than as a precise quantitative assessment. Another significant limitation of functional radiography is that the range of "normal" segmental motion in the general population has never been established. Wide variations of spinal motion exist in the normal population, and there is no evidence to confirm that too much or too little motion correlates with pain or disability, except in some cases of obvious instability.[59]

Lumbar Spine

Functional radiographs of the lumbar spine include flexion-extension and lateral bending studies.

Flexion-extension radiographs are used most often to evaluate translational movements between segments. Excessive translational movements indicate the possibility of instability and must be correlated with the clinical examination. Most authors agree that more than 3 to 5 mm translation from flexion to extension must raise the possibility of ligamentous instability[47,50] (Figure 6-12).

Tanz[49] has identified the average ranges of segmental lumbar flexion at various ages as indicated in Table 6-2. Tanz's study showed that segmental flexion increases at each successive level descending from L2-L3 through L5-S1 in the young healthy spine. With increasing age, motion decreases throughout the spine such that only

Table 6-2

Range of Lumbar Flexion at Various Ages

	Age (years)			
	2-13	35-49	50-64	65-77
Level				
L1-L2	—	5 degrees	4 degrees	2 degrees
L2-L3	10 degrees	8 degrees	5 degrees	5 degrees
L3-L4	13 degrees	9 degrees	8 degrees	3 degrees
L4-L5	17 degrees	12 degrees	8 degrees	7 degrees
L5-S1	24 degrees	8 degrees	8 degrees	7 degrees

Adapted from Tanz SS. AJR 1953;69:399.

Flexion   Extension

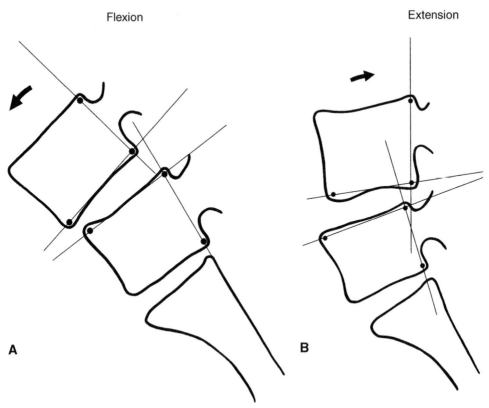

A   **B**

Figure 6-12   Flexion-extension analysis of the lumbar spine. Several methods have been developed to analyze functional radiographs of the lumbar spine for evidence of instability. The schematic diagrams above illustrate tracings of the L4-5 and L5-S1 levels from flexion (**A**) and extension (**B**) radiographs. Many authors contend that excessive translational movements measuring above 3 to 5 mm suggest ligamentous instability.

minimal differences in segmental motion are observed at successive levels.

Lateral bending radiographs have attracted significant interest within the chiropractic profession since the articles by Cassidy[43] and Grice[44] appeared in the 1970s. They recommended using lateral bending radiographs for several assessments, including the following:

1. Global range of motion
2. Segmental body rotation
3. Segmental disc wedging
4. Aberrant lateral flexion analysis

They developed a method for studying lateral bending radiographs to evaluate the coupled lumbar motions of rotation and lateral flexion. They identified four types of segmental coupling

motions and have attempted to correlate these aberrant patterns to various muscular imbalances and joint dysfunctions.[43,44] A more recent study by Haas, Cassidy, and others[69] questions the use of lateral bending radiographs for categorization of the lumbar spine in clinical practice. It should be emphasized that all radiographic findings must be correlated with clinical findings to be considered significant (Figure 6-13).

Table 6-3 lists the average ranges of segmental lumbar lateral flexion at various ages.[49] The values indicate maximum lateral flexion occurring at the L3-L4 and L4-L5 levels with very minimal motion occurring at L5-S1. Significant reduction in lateral flexion occurs at all levels with increasing age.

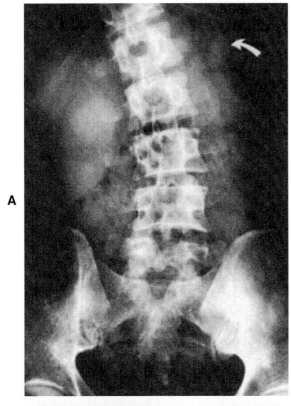

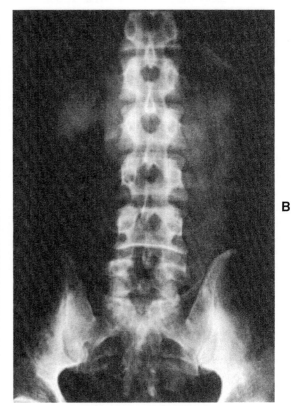

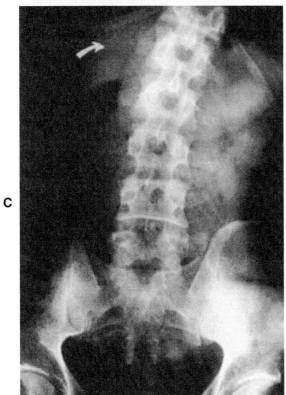

Figure 6-13 Lateral flexion analysis of the lumbar spine. Left lateral flexion (**A**), neutral AP (**B**), and right lateral flexion (**C**) radiographs of the lumbar spine in a 30-year-old man with acute low back pain. The analysis of coupled motion on lateral flexion radiographs was advocated in the 1970s and 1980s. Recent studies, however, suggest that these analyses are of little value in categorization of the lumbar spine in clinical practice. Information from all radiographs must be correlated with clinical findings.

Table 6-3

Range of Lumbar Lateral Flexion at Various Ages

Level	Age (years)			
	2-13	35-49	50-64	65-77
L1-L2	12 degrees	5 degrees	5 degrees	4 degrees
L2-L3	12 degrees	8 degrees	7 degrees	7 degrees
L3-L4	16 degrees	8 degrees	8 degrees	6 degrees
L4-L5	15 degrees	8 degrees	7 degrees	5 degrees
L5-S1	7 degrees	2 degrees	1 degrees	0 degrees

Adapted from Tanz SS. AJR 1953;69:399.

Cervical Spine

Flexion and extension views of the cervical spine form an integral part of the cervical Davis series. Coupled with routine views of the cervical spine, flexion-extension views can provide important information about the osseous and soft tissues of the cervical spine.[52,53,58] Coupled motions of rotation and lateral flexion are difficult to analyze in the lower cervical spine because of the complexity of motions involved, and radiographic evaluation in these planes is not recommended.

The flexion-extension examination is used extensively in assessing the effects of trauma on the cervical spine (Figure 6-14, A, B, C). Excessive (more than 3 mm) translational segmental movements can signify instability. Atlantoaxial instability is recognized radiographically as an increase in the atlantodental interval measuring more than 3 mm in adults and 5 mm in children on the neutral lateral or flexion views.[39] Similarly, hypermobility, hypomobility, and aberrant and paradoxical motion can be identified, according to some authors.[52-54]

Cervical overlay studies are useful in identifying flexion-extension motion abnormalities.[51-53]

In this procedure, outlines of the vertebral bodies from the radiographs are traced on acetate transparencies with colored fine-tip pens. In this way, a depiction of segmental motion can be compared between flexion, neutral, and extension positions (Figure 6-14, D, E).

Another method of evaluating motion on cervical flexion-extension radiographs is to identify the instantaneous axis of rotation (IAR) at each vertebral level. The IARs are then compared with well-established normal values.[55-57] Although this method appears reliable and valid, it has yet to gain widespread clinical use.

Open-mouth views taken in lateral flexion can demonstrate excessive lateral translation of the atlas lateral masses in relation to axis in atlantoaxial instability and abnormal motion in rotary atlantoaxial subluxation.[61]

Conclusion

The role of radiography in chiropractic is well established. Several clinical indications for radiography based on patient history and physical findings have been identified. In addition to using radiographs for identifying pathologic processes, chiropractors often use both static and dynamic radiographs to derive postural and biomechanical information. Many radiographic lines, angles, and measurements have been demonstrated as reliable indicators of postural and biomechanical abnormalities. These indicators help identify static and dynamic subluxation, dysfunction, and abnormal or excessive motion. Further research is necessary, however, to determine the precise clinical significance of many of these procedures. Although many studies have established the reliability of certain spinal displacement analysis procedures,[70] the validity and clinical relevance for many of these procedures remain in question.[71]

Acknowledgments

Special thanks to Drs. R. Sherman and T. Bergmann for reviewing the manuscript for this chapter and offering many helpful suggestions.

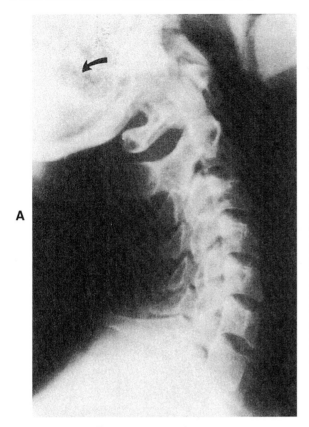

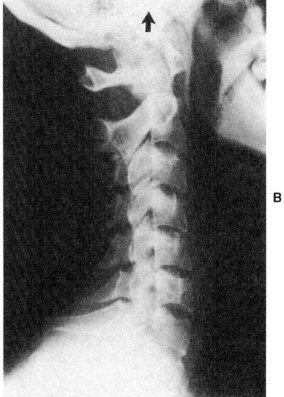

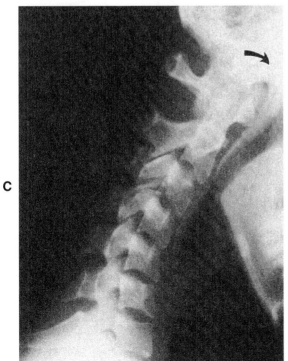

Figure 6-14 Cervical flexion-extension overlay study. Extension (**A**), neutral (**B**), and flexion (**C**) radiographs can be analyzed for intersegmental motion by tracing the anatomic outlines from the neutral radiograph (solid line in **D** and **E**) and comparing these with the extension (**D**) and flexion (**E**) tracings (dotted line in **D** and **E**), which are superimposed on the neutral tracings. This procedure is performed most frequently in patients after spine trauma and is used to detect excessive or abnormal motion.

Continued.

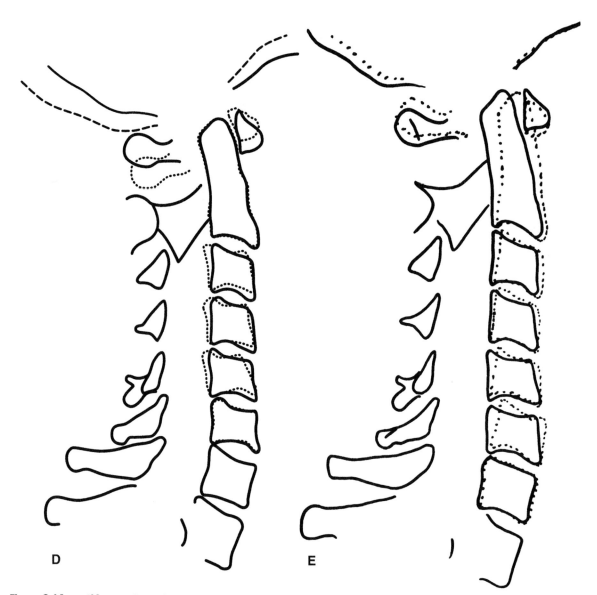

Figure 6-14, cont'd For legend, see previous page.

References

1. Hildebrandt RW. Chiropractic spinography and postural roentgenology. Part I. History of development. J Manipulative Physiol Ther 1980;3:87-92.
2. Taylor JAM. Full-spine radiography: a review. J Manipulative Physiol Ther 1993;16:460-74.
3. Sandoz R. Some reflections on subluxations and adjustments. Ann Swiss Chir Assoc 1989;7-29.
4. Gillet H, Leikens M. Belgian chiropractic research notes. 7th ed. Brussels: Authors; 1967.
5. Schafer RC, Faye LC. Motion palpation and chiropractic technic: principles of dynamic chiropractic. Huntington Beach, CA: ACAP and MPI; 1989.
6. Sherman R. Chiropractic x-ray rationale. J Can Chiro Assoc 1986;30:33-5.
7. Phillips R. Plain film radiology in chiropractic. J Manipulative Physiol Ther 1992;15:47-50.
8. Howard BA, Rowe LJ. Spinal x-rays. In: Haldeman S, editor. Principles and practice of chiropractic. 2nd ed. East Norwalk, CT: Appleton and Lange; 1992. p. 361-4.
9. Deyo RA, Diehl AK. Lumbar spine films in primary care: current use and effects of selective ordering criteria. J Gen Intern Med 1986;1:20-5.
10. Herbst RW. Full spine radiography. In: Gonstead chiropractic science and healing art. Mt. Horeb, WI: Sci-Chi Publications; 1977. p. 145-56.
11. Gatterman MI. Standards of practice relative to complications of and contraindications to spinal manipulative therapy. J Can Chir Assoc 1991;35:232-6.
12. Wyatt LH, Schultz GD. The diagnostic efficacy of lumbar spine radiography: a review of the literature. In: Hodgson M, editor. Current topics in chiropractic. Sunnyvale, CA: Palmer College of Chiropractic-West; 1987.
13. Howe JW. The role of x-ray findings in structural diagnosis. In: The research status of spinal manipulative therapy, NINCDS Monograph No. 15, DHEW Publication No. (NIH) 76-998. Washington, D.C.: U.S. Government Printing Office; 1975. p. 239-47.
14. Sausser WL. New spinographic technique: the full-length x-ray plate is a success. The Chiropractic Journal 1933;18-9.
15. Thompson EA. Chiropractic spinography. 2nd ed. Davenport, IA: Palmer School of Chiropractic; 1919. p. 15-27.
16. Hildebrandt RW. Chiropractic spinography. 2nd ed. Baltimore: Williams & Wilkins; 1985. p. 1-259.
17. Winterstein JF. Chiropractic spinographology. Lombard: National College of Chiropractic; 1970.
18. Plaugher G, Hendricks AH. The inter- and intra-examiner reliability of the Gonstead pelvic marking system. J Manipulative Physiol Ther 1991;14:503-8.
19. Logan HB. In: Logan VF, editor. Textbook of Logan basic methods. St. Louis: Logan Chiropractic College; 1950.
20. Van Schaik JPJ, Verbiest H, Van Schaik FDJ. Isolated spinous process deviation: a pitfall in the interpretation of the lumbar spine. Spine 1989;14:970.
21. Howe JW. Facts and fallacies, myths and misconceptions in spinography. J Clin Chiro Archives Edition 1972;II:1-7.
22. Hildebrandt RW. Chiropractic spinography and postural roentgenology. II. Clinical basis. J Manipulative Physiol Ther 1981;4:191-201.
23. Beekman CE, Hall V. Variability of scoliosis measurement from spinal roentgenograms. Phys Ther 1979;59:764-5.
24. Ylikoski M, Tallroth K. Measurement variations in scoliotic angle, vertebral rotation, vertebral body height, and intervertebral disc space height. Spinal Dis 1990;3:387-91.
25. Carman DL, Browne RH, Birch JG. Measurement of scoliosis and kyphosis radiographs: intraobserver and interobserver variation. J Bone Joint Surg 1990;72A:328-33.
26. Mehta MH. Radiographic estimation of vertebral rotation in scoliosis. J Bone Joint Surg 1973;55B:513-20.
27. DeSmet AA, Goin JE, Asher MK, Scheuch HG. A clinical study of the differences between the scoliotic angles measured on posteroanterior and anteroposterior radiographs. J Bone Joint Surg 1982;64A:489-93.
28. Plaugher G, Hendricks AH. The interexaminer reliability of the Gonstead pelvic marking system. J Manipulative Physiol Ther 1991;14:503-8.
29. Phillips RB. An evaluation of the graphic analysis of the pelvis on the A-P full spine radiograph. J Am Chiro Assoc 1975;9:139-45.
30. Schram SB, Hosek RS, Silverman HL. Spinographic positioning errors in Gonstead pelvic x-ray analysis. J Manipulative Physiol Ther 1981;4:179-81.
31. Mannello DM. Leg length inequality: a review. In: Proceedings of the sixth annual conference on research and education (CORE) for the Consortium for Chiropractic Research. Washington, D.C.: 1991.
32. Friberg O. The statics of postural pelvic tilt scoliosis: a radiographic study on 288 consecutive chronic LBP patients. Clin Biomech 1987;2:211-9.
33. Danbert RJ. Clinical assessment and treatment of leg length inequalities. J Manipulative Physiol Ther 1988;11:290-5.
34. Aspergren DD, Cox JM, Trier KK. Short leg correction: a clinical trial of radiographic vs. non-radiographic procedures. J Manipulative Physiol Ther 1987;10:232-8.
35. Plaugher G, Cremata EE, Phillips RB. A retrospective consecutive case analysis of pretreatment and comparative static radiological parameters following chiropractic adjustments. J Manipulative Physiol Ther 1990;13:498-506.
36. Phillips RB, Frymoyer JW, MacPherson BV, Newburg AH. Low back pain: a radiographic enigma. J Manipulative Physiol Ther 1986;9:183-7.
37. Mootz RD, Meeker WC. Minimizing radiation exposure to patients in chiropractic practice. ACA J Chir 1989;26:65-70.
38. Owens EF. Line drawing analyses of static cervical x-ray used in chiropractic. J Manipulative Physiol Ther 1992;15:442-9.

39. Yochum TR, Rowe LJ. Radiographic positioning and normal anatomy. In: Essentials of skeletal radiology. Baltimore: Williams & Wilkins; 1987. p. 1-94.

40. McRae J. Roentgenometrics in chiropractic. Toronto: CMCC; 1974. p. 1-160.

41. Bergmann T, Albers V. Stress x-rays and spinal dysfunction [lecture notes]. In: The chiropractic subluxation complex. Minneapolis: UCERF; November 1991.

42. Gay RE. The curve of the cervical spine: variations and significance. J Manipulative Physiol Ther 1993;16:591-4.

43. Cassidy JD. Roentgenological examination of the functional mechanics of the lumbar spine in lateral flexion. J Can Chiro Assoc 1976;13-6.

44. Grice A. Radiographic, biomechanical and clinical factors in lumbar lateral flexion. Part 1. J Manipulative Physiol Ther 1979;2:26-34.

45. Bronfort G, Jochumsen OH. The functional radiographic examination of patients with low back pain: a study of different forms of variations. J Manipulative Physiol Ther 1984;7:89-97.

46. Dupuis PR, Yong-Hing K, Cassidy JD, Kirkaldy-Willis WH. Radiologic diagnosis of degenerative lumbar spinal instability. Spine 1985;10:262-76.

47. Dvorak J, Panjabi MM, Chang DG, Theiler R, Grob D. Functional radiographic diagnosis of the lumbar spine. Flexion-extension and lateral bending. Spine 1991; 16:562-71.

48. Phillips RB, Howe JW, Bustin G, Mick TJ, Rosenfeld I, Mills T. Stress x-rays and the low back pain patient. J Manipulative Physiol Ther 1990;13:127-33.

49. Tanz SS. Motion of the lumbar spine. AJR 1953; 69:399-412.

50. Van Akerveeken PF, O'Brien JP, Park WM. Experimentally induced hypermobility in the lumbar spine. Spine 1979;4:236-40.

51. Vernon H. Static and dynamic roentgenography in the diagnosis of degenerative disc disease: a review and comparative assessment. J Manipulative Physiol Ther 1982;5:163-9.

52. Grice AS. Preliminary evaluation of 50 sagittal cervical motion radiographic examinations. J Can Chiro Assoc 1977;21:33-4.

53. Henderson DJ, Dormon TM. Functional roentgenometric evaluation of the cervical spine in the sagittal plane. J Manipulative Physiol Ther 1985;8:219-27.

54. Mannen EM. The use of cervical radiographic overlays to assess response to manipulation: a case report. J Can Chiro Assoc 1980;24:108-9.

55. Amevo B, Macintosh JE, Worth D, Bogduk N. Instantaneous axes of the typical cervical motion segments. I. An empirical study of technical errors. Clin Biomech 1991;6:31-7.

56. Amevo B, Worth D, Bogduk N. Instantaneous axes of the typical cervical motion segments. II. Optimization of technical errors. Clin Biomech 1991;6:38-46.

57. Amevo B, Worth D, Bogduk N. Instantaneous axes of the typical cervical motion segments. III. A study in normal volunteers. Clin Biomech 1991;6:111-7.

58. Dvorak J. Soft tissue injury to the cervical spine. Manual Med 1989;4:17-21.

59. Lind B, Sihlbom H, Nodwall A, Malchau H. Normal range of motion of the cervical spine. Arch Phys Med Rehabil 1989;70:692-5.

60. Monu J, Bohrer SP, Howard G. Some upper cervical spine norms. Spine 1987;12:515-9.

61. Reich C, Dvorak J. The functional evaluation of craniocervical ligaments in sidebending using x-rays. Manual Med 1986;2:108-13.

62. Sigler DC, Howe JW. Inter- and intra-examiner reliability of the upper cervical x-ray marking system. J Manipulative Physiol Ther 1985;8:75-80.

63. Vorro J, Johnston WL, Hubbard RP. Clinical biomechanic correlates for cervical function. Dl. Intermittent secondary movements. JAOA 1991;2:145-55.

64. Sherman R. Optimal kilovoltage technique for spinography. ACA J Chir 1990;(Dec):41-4.

65. Andersen PE, Andersen Poule E, Van der Kooy P. Dose reduction in radiography of the spine in scoliosis. Acta Radiol Diag 1982;23:251-3.

66. Hardman LA, Henderson DJ. Comparative dosimetric evaluation of current techniques in chiropractic full-spine and sectional radiography. J Can Chiro Assoc 1981; 25:141-5.

67. Field T, Buehler MT. Improvements in chiropractic full spine radiography. J Manipulative Physiol Ther 1981; 4:21-5.

68. Buehler MT, Hrejsa AF. Application of lead-acrylic compensating filters in chiropractic full spine radiography: a technical report. J Manipulative Physiol Ther 1985; 8:175-80.

69. Haas M, Nyiendo J, Peterson C, Thiel H, Sellers T, Cassidy D et al. Interrater reliability of roentgenological evaluation of the lumbar spine in lateral bending. J Manipulative Physiol Ther 1990;13:179-89.

70. Harrison DE, Harrison DD, Troyanovich SJ. Reliability of spinal displacement analysis on plain X-rays: a review of commonly accepted facts and fallacies with implication for chiropractic education and technique. J Manipulative Physiol Ther 1998;21:252-6.

71. Haas M, Taylor JA, Gillette RG. The routine use of radiographic displacement analysis: a dissent. J Manipulative Physiol Ther 1999;22:254-9.

7

Chiropractic Technique

Thomas F. Bergmann

Key Words   Subluxation, mobilization, manipulation, adjustment, long lever arm, short lever arm, force, thrust, facilitation, nociceptors, somatic dysfunction, trigger points, spondylotherapy

After reading this chapter you should be able to answer the following questions:

Question 1   What has led to the multiplicity of chiropractic techniques?

Question 2   What causes cavitation? Is it a necessary outcome of manipulation?

Question 3   What distinguishes manipulation from mobilization?

Question 4   How can the amount of force be minimized in manipulative procedures?

Question 5   What are the common mechanical, soft tissue, neurologic, and psychologic effects of manual therapy?

Question 6   What is the proposed effect of chronic segmental facilitation?

Question 7   What is the rationale for the use of manual therapy to ameliorate negative somatoautonomic reflexes?

Chiropractic has maintained that the most specialized and significant therapy employed involves the adjustment of the articulations of the human body especially the spinal column. This may be done manually or mechanically, actively or passively, with the purpose of restoring normal articular relationships and function, as well as reestablishing neurologic integrity and thereby influencing physiologic processes. Although most chiropractic techniques impart a thrust, many techniques are designed to affect physiologic processes without involving the use of a thrust procedure. This chapter discusses the theory and evidence supporting these procedures.

Historical Perspective

Osseous manual thrust techniques have been used to treat various conditions since early recorded history. Records of 4000-year-old artwork from Thailand depict the use of manual therapy, as do artifacts from early Egyptian, Polynesian, Japanese, Chinese, and Native American cultures. It appears that many ancient civilizations developed various forms of manipulation for the treatment of various disease processes.[1,2]

In the Corpus Hippocratum, Hippocrates (The Father of Medicine, 460-370 BC) described a form of spinal manipulation assisted by long axis distraction. The patient lay prone and was stretched by applying long axis distraction. When sufficient long axis distraction was applied, the physician would make palmar contact, reinforced by the opposite hand, over the "hump." The doctor could then deliver a straight thrust in a posterior to anterior direction or, if indicated, change the line of correction superiorly or inferiorly (Figure 7-1). Hippocrates also described variations of this manipulative technique; instead of contacting the hump with a palmar contact, the physician could sit on the hump or even place a foot over the hump. When even more force was indicated, a board was used. With one end anchored to the wall and the middle of the board resting over the hump, the physician could push down on the free end of the board, using it as a lever to induce a posterior to anterior force onto the hump.[3] Galen, Celisies, and Orbsius all used spinal manipulation techniques for various spinal deformities, neurologic deficiencies, and disease processes.

During the Middle Ages, there exists a void in writings describing manual procedures. By the

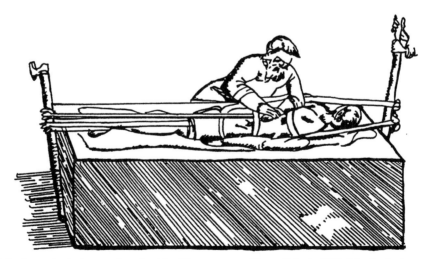

Figure 7-1   Spinal manipulation as described by Hippocrates. *(From Schoitz EH. Manipulation treatment of the spinal column from the medical-historical standpoint. Part I. Journal of the Norwegian Medical Association 1958; 78:359-72. Norske Laegeforening.)*

nineteenth century, a renewed interest in manual therapy was seen. In the early 1800s, Doctor Edward Harrison was renowned in London for his expertise in manual procedures. Like many others in the nineteenth century, he was shunned by his colleagues, who were more interested in practicing pharmacology and surgery.

"Bonesetters" became popular in both Europe and the United States in the nineteenth century. English bonesetters, including Hutton, Paget, Hood, Sweet, Mapp, and Barker, became famous. Herbert Barker developed such eminence as a bonesetter that in 1922 he was knighted by the Crown.

The nineteenth century was a time of turmoil and controversy in the health care world. It was this dissatisfaction with current medical practice that produced Daniel David Palmer and Andrew Taylor Still, the founders of chiropractic and osteopathy. Palmer and Still organized the knowledge of bonesetting and manual medicine into health care systems. Palmer believed in the "innate intelligence" of the brain and the central nervous system and thought that alterations in the spinal column (subluxations) interfered with neural function, thereby causing disease. Removal of the subluxation by a chiropractic adjustment was viewed as the treatment of choice. Still endorsed the osteopathic lesion and emphasized motion segment hypomobility and its effect on the vascular and lymphatic systems. Unlike Palmer's model, Still's model was more inclusive, taking into consideration the soft tissues as well as the primary role of the circulatory system. A major difference between Still's early osteopathy and Palmer's early chiropractic is that Still employed long lever arm techniques with nonspecific contacts; Palmer's system of chiropractic consisted of short lever arm adjustments to vertebrae using specific contacts on spinous and transverse processes.

In the days of the bonesetters, knowledge and techniques were passed down from generation to generation without formal training. After Palmer organized chiropractic into a system, he opened the first chiropractic college in 1896.[4] Many of his early students went on to establish schools of chiropractic that in turn produced students who opened other schools.

In the next century, more than 100 "named techniques" were developed.[5] It is necessary to understand that because a wide variety of methods exists, the assumption that all forms of manual therapy are equivalent must be avoided.[6] Many of the developed technique systems do not use high velocity low amplitude thrusts. One can only speculate about the reasons why technique systems not using thrust procedures developed. One such reason may be that certain patient presentations would either contraindicate or at least not indicate the use of a thrust technique. Examples are patients who are elderly or osteoporotic, in extremely acute pain, in later stages of pregnancy, or who have specific pathologies. Another reason might be the doctor's inability to produce a thrusting force that is capable of making a joint change. If the doctor's size, strength, or ability to develop the needed speed is inadequate to produce the appropriate force, some other type of technique application is necessary. Most of these "named techniques" had their origins in devoted and inquiring practitioners. These practitioners may have modified a particular technique to fit their own physical needs or to fit the needs of their subluxation conceptual model. Some observed a phenomenon of patients' improvements and developed a technique around this phenomenon. Regardless, many of the named techniques were developed out of the desire to improve the practitioner's ability to deliver health care.

As these named techniques sprang up, it was evident that many practitioners were creating their own language, redefining terms, and creating new words. This lack of a common language fanned the flames of miscommunication.

Terminology

As the chiropractic profession developed into the second largest health care delivery system outside of medicine, it also developed in many directions. With the lack of communication between the practitioners of different chiropractic techniques, each school of thought evolved as an independent entity. Schools expanded philosophies, refined techniques, and redefined terms. Although communication was a necessity for survival, there existed a severe communication gap. After the 1975 National Institute of Neurological Communicative Disorders and Stroke (NINCDS) Conference that evaluated the research status of spinal manipulative therapy, manual procedures were no longer considered invalid and became the object of study for a number of professions besides chiropractic. Practitioners of medicine, naturopathy, and physical therapy, in addition to osteopathy, began to study and employ manipulation and other manual techniques. The chiropractic profession was being forced to communicate with other branches of medicine, but a common language no longer existed to allow successful dialogue. Out of this dilemma, a subcommittee of the Standards of Care Committee from the Consortium for Chiropractic Research began to develop nomenclature through consensus. (See Chapter 1.) Through this consensus process, Gatterman and Hansen[7] defined the terms *manual therapy, manipulation, mobilization, adjustment, subluxation, subluxation complex,* and *subluxation syndrome* (Box 7-1).

The term *technique* should not be confused with the terms *therapy* or *treatment. Technique* should be reserved for describing a specific manual procedure, whereas *therapy* and *treatment* include the application of the primary and ancillary procedures indicated in the management of a patient with a given health disorder. These procedures are limited by individual statutory practice acts, but they may include such procedures as joint mobilization, therapeutic muscle stretching, soft tissue manipulation, sustained and intermittent traction, meridian therapy, physiological therapeutic modalities, application of heat or cold, dietary and nutritional counseling, therapeutic and rehabilitative exercises, and biofeedback and stress management.[2]

Manual therapy is therefore applied in many forms, including massage, mobilization, traction, muscle energy techniques, adjustment, and manipulation. The common characteristic in all of these methods is the application of external forces to the body for the purpose of affecting the flexibility and pain-free function of the spine and its contiguous tissues.[8] Moreover, all of these methods

---

BOX 7-1 ■ Manual Therapy Terminology

Manual therapy:

Procedures by which the hands directly contact the body to treat the articulations and/or soft tissues.

Mobilization:

Movement applied singularly or repetitively within or at the physiological range of joint motion, without imparting a thrust or impulse, with the goal of restoring joint mobility.

Manipulation:

A manual procedure that involves a directed thrust to move a joint past the physiological range of motion, without exceeding the anatomical limit.

Adjustment:

Any chiropractic therapeutic procedure that utilizes controlled force, leverage, direction, amplitude, and velocity that is directed at specific joints or anatomical regions. Chiropractors commonly use such procedures to influence joint and neurophysiological function.

Subluxation:

A motion segment in which alignment, movement integrity, and/or physiologic function are altered although the contact between the joint surfaces remains intact.

Subluxation complex:

A theoretical model of motion segment dysfunction (subluxation) that incorporates the complex interaction of pathologic changes in nerve, muscle, ligamentous, vascular, and connective tissues.

Subluxation syndrome:

An aggregate of signs and symptoms that relate to pathophysiology or dysfunction of spinal and pelvic motion segments or to peripheral joints.

From Gatterman MI, Hansen D. J Manipulative Physiol Ther 1994;17:302-9.

act on sensory receptors, usually in the region where the pain is felt or where it originates to produce a reflex response.[9] Pain warns us mainly against harmful functioning, and it is disturbance of function that is the most common cause of pain originating in the locomotor system. Movement restriction (blockage) at the segmental level and disturbed motor patterns at the central level may serve as examples.[10] The form of therapy used must vary according to the structures upon which it is to act. The optimal treatment for joint or spinal segment movement restriction is some form of manual therapy (Box 7-2).[9]

Sandoz[11,12] defines the chiropractic adjustment as a passive manual maneuver during which the

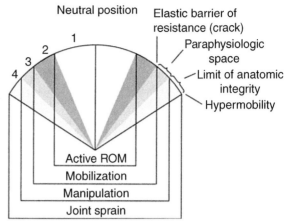

Figure 7-2   Sandoz chart: Four stages of range of movement in diarthrodial joints: *1*, Active range of movement (motion produced by muscular action). *2*, Passive range of movement (motion produced by traction or springing the joint-joint play, up to the elastic barrier of resistance); characterizes mobilization. *3*, Paraphysiologic range of movement (motion beyond the elastic barrier of resistance up to the limit of anatomic integrity produced by manipulation and accompanied by an audible release). *4*, Pathologic movement (motion beyond the limit of normal anatomic integrity, which damages ligaments and capsule, resulting in joint hypermobility). Manipulation that is too forceful may move the joint beyond the limit of anatomic integrity, creating or perpetuating joint instability.

BOX 7-2 ■ Goals of Manual Therapy

Mechanical effects

Manual therapy is thought to produce changes in the following:
- Joint alignment
- Dysfunction of motion
- Spinal curvature dynamics
- Entrapment or extrapment of a synovial fold[71]

Soft tissue effects

- Changes in the tone and strength of supporting musculature
- Influencing the dynamics of supportive capsuloligamentous connective tissue (viscoelastic properties of collagen)

Neurologic effects

- Reduction in pain
- Altering motor and sensory function
- Influencing autonomic nervous system regulation

Psychologic effects

- Laying on of hands
- Placebo factor
- Patient satisfaction

---

three-joint complex is suddenly carried beyond the normal physiological range of movement without exceeding the boundaries of anatomical integrity (Figure 7-2). However, various forms of manual therapy exist affecting different aspects of joint function and without the use of a thrust. (See Figure 7-2.) Regardless of the procedure used, the therapeutic emphasis is not on forcing a particular anatomical movement of a joint, but on restoring normal joint mechanics. Most forms of manual therapy result in movement of joint surfaces either actively or passively with the purpose of restoring normal articular relationships and function as well as restoring neurologic integrity and influencing physiologic processes.

Regardless of the specific form, the goals of manual therapy include a combination of mechanical effects, soft tissue effects, neurologic effects, and psychological effects. Although these effects are usually considered or discussed separately, the division is purely academic because the effects of manual therapy cannot be specifically directed or limited. In other words, one cannot apply a manual procedure and consistently achieve a single or specified effect. For example, when using a thrust technique to create a motion or alignment change (mechanical effect), input to the joint receptors (neurologic effect) occurs, muscles and ligaments (soft tissue effect) are compressed, stretched, or lengthened, and the patient is aware that something was done (psychologic effect). Therefore these categories are developed and designed only for an easier understanding of the principles for applying the various forms of manual therapy.

Mechanical Effects

The mechanical effects of manual therapy include changes in joint alignment, dysfunctional joint motion, and spinal curvature dynamics. Generally, the mechanical effects of an adjustment will be on derangements of the somatic structures of the body that have altered joint function. Causes of altered joint function are acute injury, repetitive use injury, faulty posture or coordination, aging, congenital or developmental defects, or primary disease states. There are several causes of acute and chronic mechanical joint dysfunction (Box 7-3).

Gatterman[13] and Rahlmann[14] have reviewed the causes of joint dysfunction (subluxation) and concluded that more than one mechanism is likely to be involved in the development of joint dysfunction, although immobilization due to adhesions had the strongest literature support. Therefore all mechanisms will be considered here. (See Chapter 11.)

Intraarticular meniscoids are leaflike fibroadipose folds of synovium that are attached to the inner surfaces of the joint capsules and project into the joint cavities (Figure 7-3). These meniscoids have been found to be present in all of the posterior joints of the spine. Bogduk and Jull[15] have suggested that extrapment of these meniscoids may be the cause of restricted joint motion. Upon flexion, the inferior articular process of a zygapophyseal joint moves upward, taking the meniscoid with it. Upon extension, the inferior articular process returns towards its neutral position. Instead of reentering the joint cavity, the meniscoid impacts the edge of the articular cartilage and buckles, creating a space-occupying lesion under the capsule. Pain occurs because of capsular tension and extension motion is restricted. The application of a procedure that will separate the articular surfaces may release the extrapped meniscoid.[15]

Cyriax[16] espouses the belief that displaced nuclear material along an incomplete radial fissure is the source of joint fixation. Postmortem dissection studies of degenerated discs have indeed identified radial fissures in the annulus fibrosis. Nuclear migration along these radial fissures has also been demonstrated by CT discography and correlated with the patient's pain.[17] A couple of questions remain unanswered regarding the disc's ability to restrict motion. First, annular fissures are apparently irreversible and do not mend with manipulation, yet manipulation can have an immediate and, often, lasting effect on joint dysfunction. Moreover, joint dysfunction and fixation can occur at segments where there are no intervertebral discs, such as the atlanto-occipital articulation and the sacroiliac articulations, to say nothing of the extremity joints. Finally, disc pathology can lead to spinal fixation through reflex muscle spasm. A painful and inflamed annular tear or disc herniation will cause reflex muscle spasm that restricts motion.

BOX 7-3 ■ Causes of Acute and Chronic Joint Dysfunction

Meniscoid entrapment or extrapment
Muscle spasm
Displaced disc fragments
Periarticular connective tissue adhesions

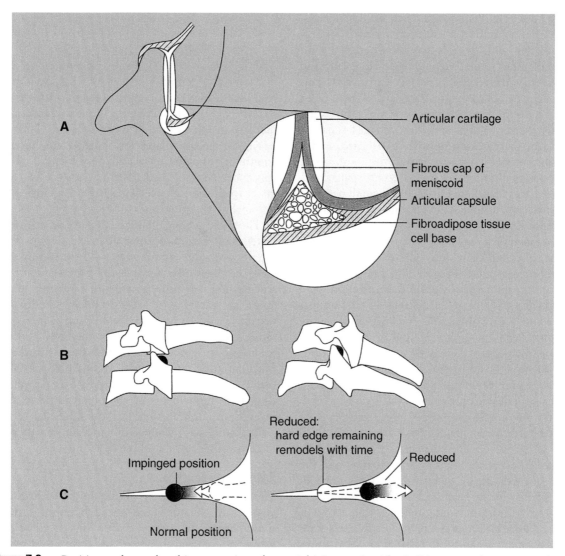

Figure 7-3   Position and postulated incarceration of synovial joint meniscoids. **A,** Diagrammatic representation of the structural components of a meniscoid in a lumbar facet. **B,** Meniscoids entrapment in cervical facet joints restricting extension and flexion movements. **C,** Entrapment of meniscoids in postulated to produce deformation of the articular cartilage surface; after reduction and over time the articular cartilage will remodel. *(Modified from Bergmann T, Peterson D, Lawrence D. Chiropractic technique. New York: Churchill Livingstone; 1993.)*

Specific joint derangements are thought to create a mechanical blockage of movement and an unleveling of the motion segment, resulting in tension on the joint capsule and posterolateral annulus. Because the joint capsule and posterior annulus are pain-sensitive structures, tension on these elements may reflexively induce muscle splinting with further joint restriction. Mechanical joint dysfunction is therefore considered a significant and frequent cause of spinal pain and a potential source of spinal degeneration.

A mechanical effect of manipulation that is intriguing, but not necessarily clinically important, is the process of joint cavitation. Studies performed by Roston et al.[18] and Unsworth et al.[19] demonstrate that as tension is applied causing a separation of the joint, there is a point where the joint surfaces jump apart, coinciding with a cracking noise. Once the tension is removed from the joint, the surfaces approximate themselves once again but at a distance slightly more apart. As the elastic barrier is passed, the articular surfaces separate suddenly, the cracking noise can be heard, and a radiolucent space appears within the joint space. The explanation of the radiolucent space rests with the fact that there is normally a small negative pressure present in a synovial joint. Its purpose is to maintain the cartilage surfaces in apposition and augment joint stability. Separation of the joint surfaces beyond the elastic barrier creates a drop in the interarticular pressure and gas is suddenly liberated from the synovial fluid to form a bubble in the joint space. The bubble bursts almost immediately with an audible crack. Analysis of the gas produced by synovial fluid cavitation was shown to consist of over 80% carbon dioxide.[19]

Brodeur[20] has presented a slightly different model of joint cavitation and cracking based on a mechanism described by Chen and Israelachvili.[21] Within this model, the capsular ligament plays a primary role in the production of joint cavitation and cracking. During the first phase of joint manipulation as the joint is being loaded and the joint surfaces are being distracted, the joint and the capsular ligament invaginate (draw inward) to maintain a constant fluid volume within the joint space. As distractive pressure is increased, the capsular ligament reaches its elastic limits and snaps away from the synovial fluid, producing cavitation at the capsular-synovial interface. A rapid increase in joint volume follows and the gas bubbles formed at the periphery rush to form a single coalesced bubble in the center of the joint space. Brodeur[20] speculates that the "snap-back" of the capsular ligament is the event responsible for the audible crack. He also proposes that this mechanism explains why some individuals with very tight or loose joint capsules do not crack:

> For loose joints, the volume of the articular capsule is larger and traction of the joint does not cause a sufficient tension across the ligament to initiate the

snap-back of the joint capsule. Similarly, an overly tight joint reaches the limits of its anatomic integrity before the joint capsule can begin to invaginate.

The only definitive effect of this cavitation response is the temporary increase in resting joint space. There is, however, an implication that an increase in joint range of motion occurs, but this has not been adequately established nor has the length of time for increased movement or joint space been established. There is also a placebo effect from the patient hearing the cracking noise and feeling the joint release.

There are other potential causes of noises associated with various forms of manual therapy that are not a product of cavitation. In the instance of cross linkages that have formed in traumatized soft tissues, a manual procedure can break them apart, thereby theoretically producing an audible tearing sound. With some mobilizing or manipulating procedures, the necessary movements of the parts can cause muscle tendons to move over bony protuberances, producing an audible snapping sound. Bony outgrowths can produce impingement that, with movements of the involved parts, can produce an audible clunking sound. Degenerative joint disease can produce crepitus on joint movement, producing an audible crackling sound.

Soft Tissue Effects
The soft tissue effects of manipulation include changes in the tone and strength of supporting musculature and influences on the dynamics of supportive capsuloligamentous connective tissue (viscoelastic properties of collagen). Connective tissue elements lose their extensibility with immobilization.[22] With immobilization, water is released from the proteoglycan molecule, allowing connective tissue fibers to contact one another, which encourages abnormal cross-linking that causes loss of extensibility.[23] It is hypothesized that certain manual therapies can break the cross-linkages and any intraarticular capsular fibroadipose adhesions, thereby providing free motion and allowing water imbibition to occur. Furthermore, action of these manual therapies can stretch segmental muscles, causing spindle reflexes that may decrease the

BOX 7-4 ■ Effects of Immobilization

Microscopic effects:

Loss of parallelism of collagen fibers
Distorted cellular alignment
Increased randomness of matrix organization
Increased collagen cross-link formation

Periarticular effects:

Thickening of joint capsule
Raised capsular tension
Connective tissue shrinking
Muscle atrophy
Bone demineralization

Intraarticular effects:

Proliferation of fatty tissue
Obliteration of joint space
Pressure necrosis of the articular cartilage
Extension of marrow space into the subchondral
  plate
Cartilage erosion and ulceration in noncontact
  areas
Adhesions to articular cartilage
Articular cartilage tears at the site of adhesions

Biochemical effects:

Decreased ligament strength
Decreased lineal stiffness
Decreased energy absorbing capacity

Adapted from Akeson WH, Amel D, Woo SLY. Cartilage and ligament: physiology and repair processes. In: Nicholas JA, Hershman EB, editors. The lower extremity and spine in sports medicine. St. Louis: Mosby; 1986. p. 3-41.

state of hypertonicity.[24] The effects of immobilization are summarized in Box 7-4.[25]

After immobilization, joints become stiff. Although some stiffness results from intraarticular adhesions to surfaces that normally glide past one another,[26] there is also evidence that ligamentous structures can shorten (contract) and limit joint motion.[27] It is likely that joint stiffness results from a combination of adhesion formation between normally gliding surfaces and active

changes in ligament length. Manual therapy applied to restricted joints will presumably tear the collagen cross-links and fibrous adhesions formed during joint immobilization. However, when articular or nonarticular soft tissue contractures are encountered, incorporation of procedures that minimize inflammation and maintain mobility should be considered. Viscoelastic structures are more amenable to elongation and deformation if they are first warmed and then stretched for sustained periods.[28] Therefore the application of moist heat, ultrasound, and other warming therapies might be considered before applying sustained manual traction or home-care stretching exercises.[2]

Neurologic Effects

The neurologic effects of manipulation include reducing pain, influencing spinal and peripheral nerve conduction, thereby altering motor and sensory function, and influencing autonomic nervous system regulation. Wyke[29] reported that manipulative procedures can stimulate the mechanoreceptors associated with synovial joints and thereby affect joint pain. He has identified four types of joint receptors. Types I, II, and III are corpuscular mechanoreceptors that detect static position of the joint, acceleration and deceleration of the joint, direction of movement and over-displacement of the joint. The Type IV receptor is a network of free nerve endings that have nociceptive capabilities. Type IV receptors are inactive under normal conditions. However, if noxious mechanical or chemical stimulation or if Types I-III receptors are not able to function, Type IV receptors become active and the sensation of pain is perceived. If manipulative therapy can restore normal function to the joint, allowing Types I-III receptors to function, the Type IV pain receptors should be inhibited, thereby decreasing the patient's pain. The structures most sensitive to noxious stimulation are the periosteum and joint capsule.

There is also evidence to support the concept that the spinal adjustment increases pain tolerance in the skin and deeper muscle structures, raises beta-endorphin levels in the blood plasma, and has an impact on the nerve pathways between the body wall and viscera that regulate general health.[30-35] Furthermore, a significant factor in musculoskeletal function is the musculature and its nerve control. Each individual will have a "postural personality" that is an expression of the individual's muscular patterns and posture. A frequent cause of joint dysfunction may therefore be faulty neuro-motor patterns due to muscular imbalance and postural strain[9] or an inability on the part of the patient to consciously control musculoskeletal function.

There are many controversies in the application of manual therapy. Of significance is the role of pain in deciding on the appropriateness of manual procedures. Mitchell[36] states that if one treats the part where the patient experiences the pain, one will be treating the wrong part of the body most of the time. He goes on to quote Osler, stating "pain is a liar." Mitchell bases this idea on the concept that in the musculoskeletal system, pain almost always develops and persists in the structures which are stressed the most by the adaptation to the dysfunction. The opposite idea is extolled by Lewit,[9] who states that if a manual therapy treatment is successful, it will usually produce immediate relief of pain. He adds that by far the most frequent cause of pain is disturbed function. This may involve passive joint mobility or active movement patterns. Manual therapy is directed to movement restriction of joints or motion segments of the spinal column. Pain in the locomotor system is therefore looked upon as a warning sign of harmful functioning that should be corrected in time before it causes permanent damage. Lewit also emphasizes that undiagnosed impairment of motor function is the most frequent cause of pain without a specific diagnosis, and that treatment of the pain without a thorough understanding of the functioning of the locomotor system is courting failure.[9]

Psychologic Effects

The psychologic effects of the laying on of the hands cannot be denied nor overlooked. Paris[37] states that with the addition of a skilled evaluation involving palpation for soft tissue changes and altered joint mechanics, the patient becomes convinced of the interest, concern, and manual skills of the clinician. If at the conclusion of the exami-

nation, a manual procedure is performed that results in an audible "pop" or "snap," the placebo factor will be undeniably high. Paris[37] states that some patients report total relief within a second or two following such a procedure which he considers far too short a time for any genuine benefit to be appreciated. The astute clinician accepts and reinforces this phenomenon, recognizing that the patient is in need of all possible assistance. It should be noted, however, that the response rate to manipulative treatment cannot be totally accounted for by the placebo effect.

Moreover, the body and mind are not separate, but really one system coordinated by the neuropeptides.[38] The tendency in the health care delivery system is to deal primarily with the physical aspects of health and ignore the emotional dimension—thoughts, feelings, the spirit, the soul. Today's health care provider should recognize the interconnectedness of all aspects of human emotion and physiology. The skin, the spinal cord, and the organs are all nodal points of entry into the psychosomatic network.

Joint Assessment Procedures

Primary health care providers, with whom patients can consult, must as portal-of-entry physicians use findings derived from the case history, physical examination, clinical laboratory, and indicated special testing procedures to assess the patient's state of health and determine the nature and cause of any ailments. The steps leading to a decision about how and what to treat are the most important part of any interaction between a doctor and a patient.[1] The differentiation of many conditions responsible for joint pain, including distinguishing an intervertebral disc lesion from facet or articular involvement, is sometimes based upon clinical intuition rather than true objective procedures. This is especially the case when the back pain is not typical for either. However, the chiropractic spinal examination and joint assessment set chiropractic apart from other areas of the healing arts. Knowing how complex the human body is, specifically the neuromusculoskeletal system, it would seem inappropriate to use a single evaluative procedure to decide on the presence of a manipulable lesion. No one evaluative tool should be used or relied on to make clinical decisions.

Structured evaluation of the integrity of the joint systems of the body should be viewed in terms of a multidimensional index of abnormality. The examination of the musculoskeletal system should never be done in isolation, but should be done within the confines of the rest of the clinical evaluation. The methods used in identifying the presence of joint dysfunction (subluxation) include the usual physical examination processes of observation, palpation, percussion, and auscultation. Because of the complexity of the human body and, more specifically, the neuromusculoskeletal system, it is appropriate to employ an evaluative system that combines clinical indicators to decide on those joints in greatest need of intervention. No one evaluative procedure should be used or relied upon to make clinical decisions. The structural evaluation of the spinal column should be viewed in terms of a multidimensional index of segmental abnormality. The mnemonic PARTS (Box 7-5) is used to identify

---

BOX 7-5 ■ PARTS Mnemonic for Identifying Characteristics of Joint Dysfunction

P—Pain/Tenderness
A—Asymmetry/Alignment
R—Range of Motion Abnormality
T—Tone/Texture/Temperature of Soft Tissues
S—Special Tests

P—Pain/Tenderness. The perception of pain and tenderness may be evaluated in terms of location, quality, and intensity. Most primary musculoskeletal disorders manifest as a painful response. The patient's description and location of pain is obtained with the location and intensity of tenderness produced by palpation of osseous and soft tissues noted. Pain and tenderness findings are identified through the procedures of observation, percussion, and palpation. Furthermore, changes in pain intensity can be objectified using Visual Analog Scales, algometers, pain questionnaires, and so forth.

A—Asymmetry. Asymmetrical qualities on a sectional or segmental level are noted. The homeostatic processes in the body seek a balance in structure and function. While the complex structure of the human body and especially its frame is never completely or perfectly symmetrical, focal changes in symmetry may be clinically significant. Body symmetry is evaluated using postural examination, static palpation, and static x-ray interpretation. This would include observation of posture and gait, palpation for misalignment of vertebral segments, and evaluation of static plain film radiographs for malposition of vertebral segments.

R—Range of Motion Abnormality. Changes in active, passive, and accessory joint motions are noted. These changes may be identified as an increase or a decrease in mobility. It is thought that a decrease in motion is a common component of joint dysfunction. Global range of motion changes are measured with inclinometers or goniometers. Segmental range-of-motion abnormalities are identified through the procedures of motion palpation and stress x-ray. The mechanical assistance of a moving table section can be used to assess passive joint movement as well. The advantage of this procedure is adding the assessment of long axis distraction movement in the spine joints.

T—Tissue Tone, Texture, Temperature Abnormality. Changes in the characteristics of contiguous and associated soft tissues including skin, fascia, muscle, and ligament are noted. These changes are identified through the procedures of observation, palpation, instrumentation, and tests for length and strength.

S—Special Tests. Those testing procedures that are specific to a technique system are performed (e.g., leg check, arm fossa test, therapy localization). Additionally, visceral relationships are considered as well as other testing procedures deemed necessary from data previously obtained.

the five diagnostic criteria for identification of joint dysfunction.[2,39]

The findings derived from the PARTS evaluation can be used to decide which areas are in need of an adjustment. The clinical decision as to whether an adjustment will be made, how it is done, where and when it is applied can be determined by which area has the most findings from each category. Minimum findings can be established, that is, one from each of the first four categories. Furthermore, the examination of the musculoskeletal system should never be performed in isolation, but should be done within the context of the history and physical examination of the patient.

If the examination is inadequate, failing to reveal the source or the extent of the problem, treatment cannot be maximally effective. Moreover, the use of joint assessment procedures should comprise part of a critical continual assessment of the patient so that the effects of care can be monitored. Perceiving when to stop is as important as knowing how to start and recognizing whether to continue. Even if a complete and thorough examination can be completed during the first visit, signs and certainly symptoms must be rechecked during the course of treatment to determine the extent of patient progress. This ongoing evaluation and assessment forms the basis for treatment modification and is a key factor in total patient management. The initial examination, no matter how thorough, cannot be expected to provide all the answers. A treatment trial should be instituted with effects assessed to determine whether it should be continued or a different plan devised. It is the examination that forms the foundation for treatment, guiding the doctor in selecting appropriate treatment techniques, frequency, and course. If practitioners were to standardize their evaluations, comparisons of treatment effectiveness and efficiency could be done.

Characteristics of the Adjustive Thrust

Whereas *manual therapy* is a term broadly used to define the therapeutic application of a manual force (see Chapter 1), chiropractors emphasize the application of specific adjustive techniques.[40] Chiropractic manipulation is a unique form of manipulation characterized by a specific high-velocity, short-amplitude thrust.[41]

It is necessary to understand that a wide variety of methods exist so that the assumption that all forms of manipulations are equivalent can be avoided.[41] Factors that influence the selection of manipulative procedures include age of the patient, acuteness or chronicity of the problem, general physical condition of the patient, clinician's size and ability, and effectiveness of previous therapy, present therapy, or both. Other factors to consider are knowledge of the local anatomy, including the geometric planes of the articulations, the nature of the condition and presence of comorbidities, and the mechanical characteristics of the manual procedure. These factors determine whether to use a long or short lever procedure, the positioning of the patient, specific contact points, the magnitude and vector of the force, and the type of thrust. Box 7-6 lists the factors governing the selection of adjustment methods.[42]

The adjustive thrust is further characterized by a transmission force that uses a combination of muscle power and the body weight of the practitioner. The force is delivered with controlled speed, depth, and magnitude through a specific contact on a particular structure such as the transverse or spinous process of a vertebra.[43] The adjustive thrust can be defined as the application of a controlled directional force. The adjustive vector describes the direction of applied force; the adjustive thrust refers to the production and implementation of that force. The adjustive force is typically generated through a combination of practitioner muscular effort and body weight transfer. The chiropractic adjustive thrust is a high-velocity, low amplitude force designed to induce joint distraction and cavitation without exceeding the limits of anatomic joint motion.[44]

The specific high-velocity, low amplitude manipulation is performed in one of two ways. Both require a sudden impulse delivered to the joint. In the first instance, the joint is maintained in a neutral position while specific contacts are made over indicated bony elements and a thrust

BOX 7-6 ■ Factors Governing the Selection of the Specific Application of Manual Therapy

Anatomic location of joint disorder or dysfunction

- Morphology of tissues: size, strength, and mobility of structures
- Some areas necessitate more power (mass and leverage)

Patient's age and physical condition

- Ability to assume specific positions
- Degree of pretension (force, mass, leverage, and depth of thrust) the patient can withstand
- Stress to adjacent spinal or extremity joints and soft tissues

Patient's size and flexibility

- Large or inflexible patient: need increased mechanical advantage in the development of pretension and thrust
- Table selection: height, articulating vs. nonarticulating, release or drop pieces, mechanized
- Method: leverage and type of thrust (e.g., push vs. pull)
- Flexible patient
- Focus force preloading of joint: removal of articular slack, use of nonneutral patient positions
- Selection of method: shorter lever methods

Presence of mitigating disorders or defects

- Preexisting congenital or developmental defects
- Preexisting degenerative defects
- Coexisting disease states
- Adjacent motion segment instability (focused force minimizes stress to adjacent joints)

Doctor's technical abilities and preferences
Patient treatment preferences

- Cannot compromise safety and effectiveness

Specific mechanical and physical attributes of adjustive methods

- Adjustive localization and pretension
  - Patient position
  - Doctor position
  - Contact points
  - Leverage
- Adjustive thrust
  - Leverage
  - Velocity
  - Amplitude (depth)
  - Mass
  - Point of delivery
  - Pause-nonpause
- Short lever preferred to long lever
  - Issue of specificity
  - Patient of manageable size
  - Flexible patient
  - Patients with clinical motion segment instability
- Long lever preferred to short lever
  - Spinal regions where additional leverage is desired
  - Patient size and flexibility demand additional leverage and power

From Hofkosh JM. Classical massage. In: Basmajian JV, editor. Manipulation, traction, and massage. 3rd ed. Baltimore: Williams & Wilkins; 1985. p. 263.

applied in a specific direction. Neutral joint slack and tissue elasticity are taken out before delivering the thrust. A typical example of this type of procedure is correction of thoracic spine dysfunction by use of a posterior-to-anterior force vector on the transverse processes with the patient lying in the prone position. The second approach moves the joint through its active and passive ranges of motion in the specific direction of the adjustment. The thrust is given at the end point of movement beyond the elastic barrier and into the paraphysiologic space.

The typical method of impulse thrust delivery is executed with controlled extension of the clinician's elbows by sustained isolated contractions of the triceps and anconeus muscle groups in combination with a shoulder-stabilizing contraction from the pectoralis major muscle. However, a body-drop thrust or a recoil thrust may also be used. The clinician locks the elbows and shoulders while using body weight to deliver the impulse thrust. The recoil thrust uses controlled extension of the elbow followed by a quick release and elbow flexion. It is quite commonly associated with a mechanical drop-section of the adjusting table. Impulse thrusts can be developed using pulling maneuvers as well.

In manipulative therapy it is accepted that although technique applications may be highly variable, the underlying principles are fairly constant. The lever is used to produce motion at an articulation or group of articulations. The longer the lever is, the greater the mechanical advantage and applied force will be. The levers and generated forces are used in such a way that the applied force will cause motion between the affected segments and will not be dissipated by the elasticity or mobility of other spinal or appendicular structures.[45] White and Panjabi[28] state that, regardless of external forces or manipulation, the movement of a vertebra is limited to the combinations possible within six degrees of freedom. They describe the manual application of forces directly to the spinous process and posterior elements of a given vertebra, thereby loading and displacing it along the X, Y, and Z axes. The issue of leverage becomes more complex when vectors of force are considered in connection with muscle attachments and the effect of soft tissues on the intervertebral joint.

Application of forces to spinous or lateral processes (articular, transverse, or mammillary) in the spine would be short lever procedures. Short lever techniques are also used in the extremities when a direct contact is taken on the involved segment. Greenman[46] defines the short lever as one in which a portion of one vertebra (spinous process) is held firmly while a force is applied to a bony prominence of the adjacent vertebra. A force is then applied with sufficient velocity to move one segment on the other. Velocity relates to the speed in which the impulse is given. Furthermore, Nwuga[47] believes that short lever thrust techniques require less amplitude (the distance over which the thrusting force is applied) than long lever technique to achieve the same movement at the joint being treated. The implied significance or rationale for the use of short lever procedures is increased specificity, which is thought to be important for influencing a specific joint complex for a specific joint dysfunction. However, there are only opinions and reasoned conclusions to support this idea.

A long lever technique may use a specific or general primary contact on the body part but the second contact is remote from the segment, forming a broad or long lever system of forces.[48] Maigne[49] uses the term *indirect manipulation* for a long lever procedure, stating that the body is used as a lever to move the vertebral column. All side posture lumbar and pelvic techniques employ a long lever, the femur of the flexed knee, as a means to apply preadjustive tension or the thrust itself. Citing side-posture low back techniques as examples, Nwuga[47] also uses the term *indirect manipulation* to describe techniques that use the limbs as natural levers to influence the spinal column.

Long and short lever combinations are apparently frequently used procedures. The long lever provides the necessary leverage for general distraction and articular prestress to the spine while the short lever contact focuses the force to a smaller section. The general or nonspecific technique thereby becomes more efficient and more specific.[48]

The term *specific contact* has two meanings in the literature. First, it can refer to the point on the clinician's hand or body that makes contact with the patient. Secondly, this term is used to describe the actual anatomical part of the patient that is being contacted. Virtually all texts written on manipulative therapy procedures that use thrust techniques describe specific hand contacts to be used by the clinician. Although some different terms are used, with few exceptions the descriptions are the same. Similarly, the part of the patient's body that is being contacted is described in common terms among authors. Specific contact in reference to a patient's spine means a contact is made on a spinous process or lateral process (articular process or lamina in the cervical spine, transverse process in the thoracic spine, or mammillary process in the lumbar spine) via the overlying soft tissues. These points of contact constitute a short lever when an external force is applied to them. Specificity in either case is thought to be important to influence a definite intervertebral joint complex for identified joint dysfunction; however, there is nothing but opinions or reasoned conclusions to support this idea.[50]

A specific manipulation attempts to focus the force of the thrust to one articulation or joint complex as much as possible. In comparison, a nonspecific manipulation is used to affect a region or group of articulations. Nwuga[47] used the term *nonspecific* in this manner and stated that most of the techniques described by Cyriax[16] would fall into this category. Grieve[51] used the terms *localized* and *regional* to distinguish between procedures that affect a single joint or a sectional area. In addition, the term *general* has been used to denote the nonspecific, regional, or sectional forms of manipulation.[52] Therefore techniques that are considered nonspecific would use broad contacts taken over multiple sites with the purpose of improving motion and/or alignment in an area that is generally stiff or distorted.

In an attempt to study the intent of osseous manual thrust procedures and to be more precise in the distinction, classification, and validation of chiropractic procedures, Bartol,[53,54] with the Panel of Advisors to the ACA Council on Technic, developed a generic classification system of treatment procedures based on a mechanistic approach (Figures 7-4 and 7-5). The theory behind this model is that the physical characteristics of the treatment procedure are directly related and consequently should be driven by the therapeutic intention of the procedure. This six-tiered flow chart attempts to classify treatment procedures based on the following physical characteristics:

1. Manual and nonmanual procedures: Manual procedures are those procedures in which direct physical contact is necessary between the doctor and the patient.
2. Area primarily being affected: anatomic joint, physiologic joint, or viscera
3. Type of contact employed: specific, nonspecific, or mechanical
4. Type of lever arm used: short lever arm, long lever arm, or a combination
5. Type of force used

This model is a first step; many other physical characteristics of osseous manual thrust procedures can affect the intent of applying the procedure.

Adjustive Mechanics

Each grouping of adjustments has its own mechanical characteristics based on adjustive contacts, patient positioning, doctor positioning, and adjustive vectors. Efficient and effective selections cannot be made without an understanding of each adjustment's unique physical attributes.[42] For example, side posture lumbar adjustments may be used to develop rotational tension and perpendicular facet distraction. In contrast, prone lumbar adjustments maintain a more neutral position of the lumbar spine and minimize the amount of rotational tension. Side posture positions also provide additional leverage and more latitude in the development and use of the doctor's body weight, providing a possible mechanical advantage. Therefore if rotational lumbar distraction is desired, a side posture method of adjustment should be considered over a prone method. If lumbar distraction without rotational tension is desired, then a prone lumbar position might be more appropriate. If these mechanical principles are not clear

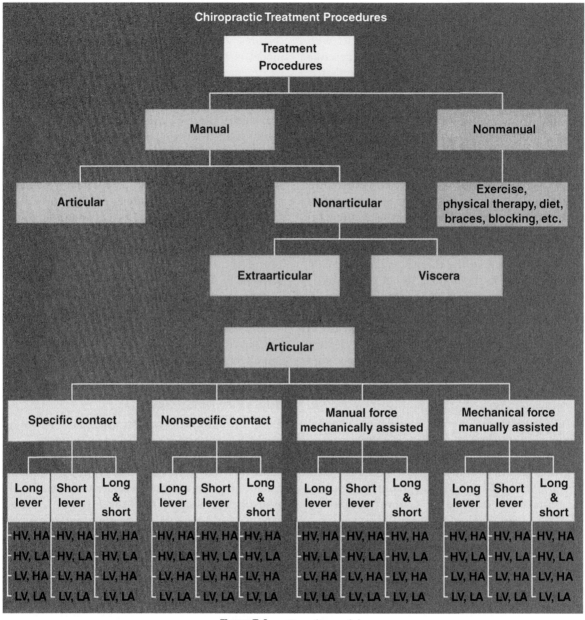

Figure 7-4   Bartol's model.

to the practitioner, the adjustive selections may be made by habit or chance instead of reason.

Adjustive localization refers to the preadjustive procedures that are designed to localize adjustive forces and joint distraction. They involve the application of physiologic and nonphysiologic positions, the removal of articular "slack," and the development of appropriate patient positions, contact points, and adjustive vectors. These factors are critical to the development of necessary preadjustive tension and adjustive efficiency. Attention to these components is intended to

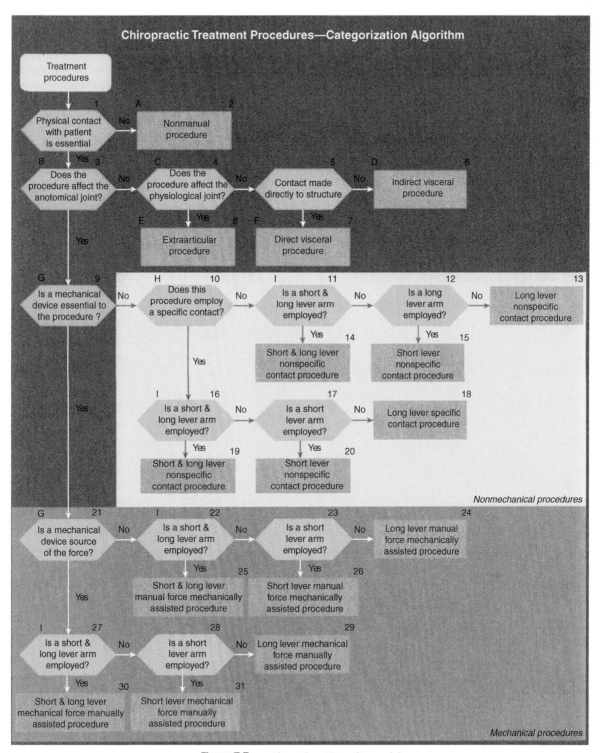

Figure 7-5 Algorithm: Bartol's model.

improve adjustive specificity and to minimize the distractive tension on adjacent joints.

Preadjustive joint tension and localization are dependent on patient placement and leverage. Localization of adjustive forces may be enhanced by using patient placement to position a joint at a point of distractive vulnerability. Locking adjacent joints and positioning the joint to be adjusted at the apex of curves during patient positioning enhances this process and adjustive specificity. Joint localization and joint distraction may be further enhanced if forces are used to either assist or oppose the adjustive thrust. Assisting or opposing forces may be generated either during the adjustive setup and/or during the adjustive thrust.

The notion of applying assisted and opposing forces during the performance of manipulation was first described relative to thoracic manipulation by the French orthopedist Robert Maigne.[55] In the chiropractic profession, Sandoz[11] was the first to describe similar terms. Sandoz[11] proposed using the terms *assisted* and *resisted* to describe patient positions that either assist or resist adjustive thrusts. Good[56] has presented examples of these concepts in relation to Diversified technique. As originally described, assisted and resisted methods were only applied to side posture lumbar adjustments and those procedures involving a single primary thrust.[11] Both methods are employed to improve the localization of preadjustive tension. Their application is based on the mechanical principle that the point of maximal tension will be developed at the point of opposing counter-rotation. Assisted and resisted methods are distinguished from each other by the positioning of vertebral segments relative to the adjustive thrust. In both circumstances the trunk and vertebral segments superior to the adjustive contact are prestressed in the direction of desired joint movement. In the assisted method, the contact is established on the superior vertebral segments and movement of the trunk and the thrust are directed together. Assisted procedures are designed to induce preadjustive tension and positions that assist the adjustive thrust. Resisted procedures employ patient positions in which the segments superior to the adjustive contact are stabilized or moved in a direction opposing the adjustive thrust. In the resisted method, the contact is established on the lower vertebral segment and the direction of trunk movement and adjustive thrust are in opposing directions. Sandoz[11] has suggested that resisted positions bring maximal tension to the articulation superior to the established contact and assisted positions bring maximal tension to the articulation inferior to the established contact. In the assisted method, the point of counter-tension is inferior to the point of contact because the segments below are stabilized or rotated in a direction opposite the adjustive thrust. In the resisted approach, the site of counter-tension is superior to the point of contact because the segments above are stabilized or rotated in a direction opposite the adjustive thrust. Therefore either method can theoretically be used to induce cavitation and motion within the same articulation. Although the movement generated is the same, the points of contact and the line of drive are different.

Assisted methods incorporate segmental contacts established on the superior vertebrae of the dysfunctional motion segment. They are applied to focus the adjustive force in the joint inferior to the level of segmental contact. The adjustive vectors are directed to produce movement of the superior vertebra relative to the inferior vertebra in the direction of joint restriction.[42]

Resisted methods incorporate segmental contacts established on the inferior vertebrae of the dysfunctional motion segment. They are applied to focus the adjustive effect in the joint superior to the level of segmental contact. The adjustive vectors are directed to produce movement of the joint in the direction of restriction (direction opposite malposition), but this is accomplished by moving the inferior vertebra of the dysfunctional joint in the direction opposite the joint restriction.[42]

Counter-resisted methods incorporate segmental contacts established on both sides of the joint to be adjusted.[42] Pretension and the adjustive thrusts are directed in opposing directions to maximize distraction across a given joint. The adjustive thrust may be focused through segmental contacts or incorporate additional contacts and reinforcing thrusts applied at levels superior to and inferior to the segmental contacts. In the spine, this procedure is most commonly applied in the treatment of rotational dysfunction.

Other Forms of Manual Therapy

Another form of manual therapy is termed *mobilization,* which is applied within the physiologic passive range of joint motion and is characterized by a nonthrust passive joint movement. (See Figure 7-2.) By taking the joint to its barrier and repetitively moving along or beside it, the barrier may be encouraged to recede.[57] Characteristics of a mobilization include a general contact on a number of bony structures with a single movement, a specific contact on a single bony structure with a multiple, repetitive movement action, or a general contact on a number of bony structures with a multiple repetitive movement action. Mobilization procedures help to loosen and break adhesions and fixations, allowing the adjustment to be more effective.

Manual traction is yet another form of manual therapy in which joint surfaces are held in sustained separation for a period of time. Traction may be solely through contacts made by the clinician or may be aided by a mechanized table or other devices. These forces may be applied manually or mechanically.[58] Traction techniques serve to aid adjustments by accomplishing the following:
1. Allowing physiologic rest to the area
2. Relieving compressive pressure due to weight bearing
3. Applying an imbibing action to the synovial joints and discs
4. Opening the intervertebral foramen to allow a break in reflex neurologic cycles

Mechanical assistance for manual therapy procedures is produced by an adjusting table that has a movable pelvic section. Cox developed this type of table in the early 1970s, blending osteopathic and chiropractic principles based on the early McManis table.[59-62] The mobile pelvic piece uses a long lever action to place the lumbar spine through the normal individual ranges of motion of flexion, extension, lateral bending, and rotation, as well as the combined movement of circumduc-

tion. Cox has developed a protocol for the use of flexion/distraction in the treatment of lumbar disc protrusion, spondylolisthesis, facet syndrome, subluxation, and scoliotic curves of a nonsurgical nature. His contention is that the axial traction of the vertebral motion segment while in flexion creates a force that tends to reduce extrusion of disc material.[59]

Eckard has also developed a mechanized distraction table that differs from the Cox table in that the axial traction of the motion segment is done in slight extension. The drop-away abdominal piece maintains the neutral or lordotic posture and is thought to mechanically separate the facet joints during traction, thereby requiring much less force than a conventional manipulative procedure.[63] Eckard further contends that the extended position, which is actually the normal lordotic position, reduces pressure in the motion segment and venous engorgement in the spinal veins. Both of these characteristics would be desirable in cases of low back pain of mechanical origin. Data supporting these claims have not been published and the theory remains unsubstantiated. Markey[64] has also described a distraction technique using flexion/distraction. His use of the Lloyd distraction table allows the possibility of both flexion and extension positions.

An apparent contradiction exists between the theories of Cox and Markey and those of Eckard. Cox and Markey advocate flexion/distraction, while Eckard prefers extension/distraction. However, the procedures are used for the same conditions but are based on different hypotheses about the mechanisms involving traction forces on the three-joint complex of the spinal motion segment. In each procedure the doctor places a specific contact on a spinous process (short lever) and applies headward pressure, while the distal end of the pelvic section is moved toward the floor (long lever). Therefore each technique uses a specific short-lever contact that is mechanically assisted by a long lever.[65] Schneider[66] notes that even with an acute disc herniation, mechanical compression of nerve roots by extruded disc material is not the only source of low back pain, nor its reduction the sole relief of such pain. He identifies other mechanisms such as chemical irritation of the nerve roots, facet synovitis, and intrinsic lumbar muscles (especially the multifidus) as sources of low back pain that may or may not accompany disc herniation. Schneider discusses the different effects of the two traction methods on the possible mechanisms.[66]

Soft Tissue and Reflex Techniques

Manual procedures can be specifically directed to the soft tissues. Even though all manual techniques have some effect on the soft tissues, the justification for a separate classification is to draw attention to the prime importance of including techniques that have the specific purpose of improving the vascularity and extensibility of the soft tissues,[51] as well as to reflexively influence neurologic elements and physiologic processes. Furthermore, soft tissue manipulation tends to relax hypertonic muscles so that when other forms of manual therapy are applied equal tensions are exerted across the joint.

Soft tissue manipulation includes massage (stroking or effleurage, kneading or pétrissage, vibration or tapotement, transverse friction massage), trigger point therapy, connective tissue massage, body wall reflex techniques (Chapman lymphatic reflexes, Bennett vascular reflexes, acupressure point stimulation), and muscle energy techniques. In addition, some methods of chiropractic adjustment apparently have a greater direct effect on the soft tissues or have a greater effect on the homeostasis of the body through reflex mechanisms.

Meeker[67] identifies chiropractic soft tissue techniques as those physical methods applied to muscles, ligaments, tendons, fascia, and other connective tissues with the goal of therapeutically affecting the body. He also defines nonforce techniques as very light force methods sometimes applied to the soft tissues, but most often to the bony parts of the spine and pelvis with the goal of improving the health of the patient.

Mechanical devices have been used with manual therapy to provide light force contacts and to produce purportedly controlled, repeatable percussion forces. Although some evidence exists to

support that these procedures move joints, there is seldom an audible release or cavitation response.[68]

A factor that seems to be common to body-wall reflex technique procedures is that the irritable "lesion" resides in fascial tissue. Therefore it is necessary to explore the structure and function of connective tissue, because it is a significant component of the fascia and all the soft tissues. Connective tissue contributes to kinetic joint stability and integrity by resisting the rotatory moments developed by forces acting at each joint. When these rotatory moments of force are large, considerable connective tissue power is required to produce the needed joint stability and integrity.

Within the past several decades, a great deal of scientific investigation has been directed at defining the physical properties of connective tissue. Connective tissue is made up of various densities and arrangements of collagen fibers embedded in a protein-polysaccharide matrix commonly called *ground substance*. Collagen is a fibrous protein that has a very high tensile strength. Collagenous tissue is organized into many different higher-order structures, including tendons, ligaments, joint capsules, aponeuroses, and fascial sheaths. Under normal and pathologic conditions, the range of motion in most body joints is predominately limited by one or more connective tissue structures. The relative contribution of each to the total resistance varies with the specific area of the body.

After trauma or surgery, the connective tissue involved in the body's reparative process frequently impedes function because it may abnormally limit the joint range of motion. Scar tissue, adhesions, and fibrotic contractures are common types of pathologic connective tissue that must be dealt with during chiropractic manipulative procedures. Understanding the physical factors influencing mechanical behavior of connective tissue under tensile stress is therefore essential for determining the optimal means through manipulation to restore normal function.

All connective tissue has a combination of two qualities, elastic stretch and plastic (viscous) stretch. The term *stretch* refers to linear deformation that increases length (elongation). Stretching, then, is the process of elongation. Elastic stretch represents springlike behavior. Elongation produced by tensile loading is reversible after the load is removed. It is also described as temporary or recoverable elongation. Plastic (viscous) stretch refers to puttylike behavior, in which the linear deformation produced by tensile stress remains even after the stress is removed. This is described as nonrecoverable or as a permanent elongation. The term *viscoelastic* is used to describe tissue that has both viscous and elastic properties.[2]

There are different factors that influence whether the plastic or elastic component of connective tissue is predominately affected. These include the amount of applied force and the duration of the applied force. Therefore the major factors affecting connective tissue deformation are force and time. A high force over a short period generally results in elastic deformation. A lower amount of force sustained over a longer period tends to produce plastic deformation.

When connective tissue is stretched, the relative proportion of elastic and plastic deformation can vary widely depending on how and under what conditions the stretching is performed. When tensile forces are continuously applied to connective tissue, the time required to stretch the tissue a specific amount varies inversely with the forced used. Therefore a low force stretching method requires more time to produce the same amount of elongation than that produced by a higher force method. However, the proportion of tissue lengthening that remains after the tensile stress is removed is greater for the low force, long-duration method. Of course, high force and long duration also cause stretch and possibly rupture of the connective tissue.

Trauma generally occurs because of a high force of short duration that influences the elastic deformation of the connective tissue. If the force is beyond the elastic range of the connective tissue, it enters the plastic range. If the force is beyond the plastic range, tissue rupture occurs. Commonly encountered is the microtrauma seen in postural distortions, muscle imbalance, and joint dysfunction because of low gravitational forces occurring over a long period, thus creating plastic deformation.

Connective tissue elements lose extensibility when their related joints are immobilized.[25] With immobilization, water is released from the proteoglycan molecule, allowing connective tissue fibers to contact one another, thereby permitting abnormal cross-linking and resulting in a loss of extensibility.[23] It is hypothesized that manual therapy can break the cross-links and any intraarticular capsular fiber fatty adhesions, allowing resumption of free motion and water imbibition. Furthermore, it is theorized that procedures can stretch segmental muscles, stimulating spindle reflexes that may decrease the state of hypertonicity.[24]

Muscle tightness or shortness develops after periods of immobilization as well. Length changes in muscle are associated with changes in sarcomere number and reorganization of the connective tissue elements within the muscle.[69] Muscle immobilized in a shortened position develops less force and tears at a shorter length than nonimmobilized muscle with normal resting length.[70] For this reason, vigorous muscle stretching has been recommended for muscle tightness.[71] For the stretch to be effective, however, the underlying joints should be freely mobile. Patients often require manipulation before muscle stretching.

Cantu and Grodin[72] reviewed the literature on the effects of manual therapy on fascia; such effects include circulatory changes, blood flow changes, capillary dilation, cutaneous temperature changes, metabolic changes, and reflexive autonomic changes. However, most of the citations were quite old.

Effects on Blood Flow and Temperature

Deep stroking and kneading of the soft tissues in the extremities of normal subjects, patients with rheumatoid arthritis, and subjects with spasmodic paralysis create a consistent and clinically significant increase in total blood flow and cutaneous temperature.[73] These findings are supported by other studies.[74-76] However, it must be emphasized that the clinical procedure being tested in all of these reports was deep or heavy massage application. Therefore conclusions on the effects of light force stimulation of the body wall cannot be drawn from these data.

Effects on Metabolism

Cuthbertson[77] conducted a literature review on the effects of massage on metabolic processes, including vital signs and waste products of the body. He reported that in normal subjects there was no increase in basal consumption of oxygen, pulse rate, or blood pressure, although an increase in urine output was observed. To effect a change in the vital signs, however, a systemic effect must be achieved. Localized changes in basal oxygen consumption may occur, but this has yet to be studied. Schneider and Havens[78] did find an increase in red blood cells needed to bring oxygen to the tissues being massaged. This provides some support that soft tissue procedures are able to increase circulation and nutrition to desired areas. Again, these were vigorous massage procedures that were described; caution is necessary when trying to apply these principles to other procedures.

Reflexive (Autonomic) Effects

Reflexive or autonomic effects relate to evidence of change in tissues or structures distal to or distant from the site of therapeutic application. Lesions in the soft tissue can initiate sensory irritation, which produces referred pain and tenderness. Moreover, autonomic nervous involvement may be activated through connections with the lateral horn cells in the cord to produce vasomotor, trophic, visceral, or metabolic changes. The impulse-based paradigm of neurodysfunction that has been developed from the work of Homewood[79] and Korr[80] suggests that somatic dysfunction or joint dysfunction induces persistent nociceptive and altered proprioceptive input. This persistent afferent input triggers a segmental cord response, which induces the development of pathologic somatosomatic or somatovisceral reflexes.[81-83] If these reflexes persist, they are hypothesized to induce altered function in segmentally supplied somatic or visceral structures. Manual therapy, including soft tissue techniques and other forms of adjustive therapy, would have the hypothetical potential for arresting both the local and distant somatic and visceral effects by terminating the altered neurogenic reflexes that are associated with somatic joint dysfunction.

BOX 7-7 ■ Stimuli for Evoking a Somatosomatic Reflex Response

Variation in temperature
Mechanical stress
Chemical irritation
Environmental stress
Structural stress

Reflex pathways exist such that when a stimulus (Box 7-7) is applied to a somatic structure of the body, the response occurs in another somatic structure of the body. This is referred to as a somatosomatic reflex. Although they are considered the most primitive reflexes in the human body, somatosomatic reflexes are essential to the control of normal physiologic activities and may become involved in abnormal reactions.

The somatosomatic reflex has direct application to the problem of muscle alterations in the paravertebral region. When conditions are such that the stimulus elicits and abnormally prolongs a muscle contraction in this area, the tissues become a secondary source of irritation with the potential of disturbing homeostatic balance. If the individual's inherent resistance cannot compensate for the imbalance, clinically recognizable symptoms may result.[45]

One of the signs of somatic dysfunction is the presence of muscle hypertonicity. Localized increased paraspinal muscle tone can be detected with palpation and in some cases with electromyography. Janda[71] recognizes five different types of increased muscle tone: limbic dysfunction, segmental spasm, reflex spasm, trigger points, and muscle tightness. Liebenson[84] has discussed the treatment of these five types using active muscle contraction and relaxation procedures.

Reflex Muscle Spasm from Spinal Injury

Reflex muscle spasm or splinting follows trauma or injury to any of the pain-sensitive structures of the spine. The pain-sensitive spinal tissues include the zygapophyseal joints, posterior ligaments, paravertebral muscles, dura mater, anterior and posterior longitudinal ligaments, and intervertebral discs.[85] Mechanical deformation or chemical irritation of any of these tissues causes restricted motion by way of muscle spasm. Treatment directed at the tissue source of pain reduces the reflex muscle spasm and increases the range of motion; however, if the muscle spasm has been present for some time it requires direct treatment as well.

Reflex Muscle Spasm from Visceral Disease

Visceral disease also can cause reflex muscle splinting. The diagnosis of a viscerosomatic reflex is based on a history of visceral disease, or current visceral disease symptomatology, and objective palpation findings.[86] Objective palpation findings include two or more adjacent spinal segments that show evidence of fixation located within a specific autonomic reflex area, a deep paraspinal muscle splinting reaction, resistance to segmental joint motion, and skin and subcutaneous tissue changes that are consistent with the acuteness or chronicity of the reflex.[86]

Somatoautonomic Reflex Theory

Korr[80] proposed that spinal muscles when under strain or tension caused the firing of proprioceptive nerve receptors embedded in the muscles. Korr believed that this proprioceptive information, which is conveyed to second-order neurons located in the spinal cord, facilitated or lowered the firing threshold of the second-order neurons. When second-order neurons are facilitated, they act as a "neurologic lens" and are hyperresponsive to impulses arriving from any source in the body. He termed this hyperirritability *chronic segmental facilitation*.[80]

Second-order neurons synapse with a variety of cells in the nervous system. Korr focused primarily on the local segmental connections in the spinal cord. In the spinal cord, second-order neurons synapse with anterior horn cells (involved in muscle innervation) and with lateral horn cells (part of the sympathetic nervous system). Korr proposed that continuous irritation of the lateral horn cells caused these (sympathetic) neurons to become facilitated. A facilitated or hyperirritable

sympathetic nervous system is considered by Korr to be a major contributing factor in perpetuation of musculoskeletal dysfunction and visceral organ exhaustion and disease.[80] Numerous conditions have been linked to hyperactivity of the sympathetic nervous system, including various types of cardiovascular, gastrointestinal, and genitourinary disorders, and certain musculoskeletal disorders such as reflex sympathetic dystrophy.

Evidence of Chronic Segmental Facilitation

Korr and his osteopathic colleagues performed several elaborate studies that supported his theory of chronic segmental facilitation.[87] The presence of segmental muscle spasm at the site of spinal dysfunction supported the reflex connection to the anterior horn cells. The presence of vasomotor changes (vasoconstriction or dilation), sudomotor changes (sweating or dryness), and pilomotor changes (hair follicle elevation) at the site of spinal dysfunction supported the reflex connection to the sympathetic nervous system. Korr proposed that, because hyperactivity was demonstrated in the sympathetic fibers innervating the skin, the sympathetic fibers innervating the viscera would also be hyperactive and possibly contribute to visceral disease.

The clinical evidence supporting this theory is primarily indirect and is based on the correlation of physical symptoms with spinal lesions. Because the spinal soft tissues are loaded with receptors, it seems plausible that any acute injury would result in increased sensory input to the spinal cord, which might then result in segmental facilitation.

The segmental facilitation theory is also called the *impulse-based theory* because it depends on impulses from the proprioceptive nerve receptors located in the spinal muscles. Nerve compression is not a factor in this theory; in fact, facilitated nerves are functioning as they are designed—to carry information. Facilitated nerves become sensitized by the vast amount of stimulation they receive from strained muscles.

Korr also postulated that when facilitated nerves become overburdened with activity, their axoplasmic flow rate can become reduced. However, the primary lesion stressed in the segmental facilitation theory is sympathetic nervous system hyperactivity.[80]

Nociceptors Reflexively Activate Sympathetic Neurons

Recent advances in the understanding of muscle spindle physiology raise questions as to the ability of muscle spindles to activate sympathetic fibers.[87] In response to this discrepancy in Korr's theory, Van Buskirk[87] has proposed that nociceptors are the primary receptors causing chronic segmental facilitation and sustained sympatheticotonia.

Sato[88] has recently reviewed the experimental studies of somatovisceral reflexes. He and his colleagues have been able to alter the heart rate, blood pressure, and renal and adrenal sympathetic nerve activity by applying mechanical pressure to the rat spine.[34] In addition, it has been discovered that stimulation of periarticular nociceptors causes a significant reflex activation of sympathetic neurons; in contrast, stimulation of nonnociceptive receptors has a minimal influence on sympathetic activity.[89]

Unfortunately, the stimulation threshold required to cause nociceptor activity and subsequent sympathetic facilitation in the living human is unknown. In addition, the extent to which spinal dysfunction in patients mimics experimental animal lesions is unknown. Korr[90] has recently discussed some of the limitations of the segmental facilitation theory and points out the need for clinical outcome research that tests manipulative therapy as it is practiced.

Musculoskeletal Dysfunction and Visceral Disease

Whether musculoskeletal dysfunction causes visceral disease appears to depend on many factors, such as the amount of nociceptive input from the musculoskeletal tissues, the previous threshold of the sympathetic neurons determined in part by the central nervous system's ability to reduce (or enhance) sympathetic activity, and the previous condition of the viscera. For this reason, musculoskeletal dysfunction is considered to be one of many potentiating factors that can lead to visceral dysfunction and disease.

It is thought that altered or impaired function of the musculoskeletal system components may either cause or be presymptomatic signs of disease. There is, however, little more than anecdote or personal opinion to support these ideas. Basic scientific information does exist to support the occurrence of somatovisceral and viscerosomatic reflexes.[80-83,86]

This information does not, however, support a clinical utility for intervention. Although theory and clinical practice suggest that events affecting the musculoskeletal structures may influence visceral function and that disturbances of visceral function may be reflected as altered musculoskeletal function, the chiropractic profession has done next to nothing to adequately show the relationship between manipulative therapy and visceral disease. The hypothesis is, of course, that the musculoskeletal component may be treated with chiropractic procedures (adjustments and other modalities), thereby altering the course of both the musculoskeletal and visceral disturbances, and allowing the physiologic process to return to optimal function.

Musculoskeletal Manifestations of Visceral Disease

It has been suggested that the body wall manifestations of visceral disease are an integral part of the disease process rather than just physical signs and symptoms.[91] However, the definitive causative factors and the characteristic response of the individual are still unknown.

Early signs of most disease states are manifested as symptoms and signs that are part of a common reaction pattern to injury or stress. Pain in the somatic tissues is a frequent presenting symptom in acute conditions related to visceral dysfunction. Palpatory cues of transient muscle hypertonicity and irritation or subcutaneous edema may be accompaniments of ill-defined subclinical states.[86] Subtle changes in tissue texture, joint position, and joint mobility identified by

From Meeker WC. Soft tissue and nonforce techniques. In: Haldeman S, editor. Principles and practice of chiropractic. East Norwalk, CT: Appleton and Lange; 1992. p. 520.

discerning palpatory skills appear to be latent manifestations of the somatic component of visceral disease (Box 7-8).

In a study[92] performed on cardiac patients in an intensive care unit, the following was noted in the autonomic spinal reference site for the involved viscus:

Vasomotor reaction: increase in skin temperature
Sudomotor reaction: increase in skin moisture
Increase in muscle tone/contraction
Skin texture changes: thickening
Increased subcutaneous fluid

In studies by Kelso[93] and Beal,[94] it was noted that as the visceral condition progresses, the somatic stress pattern subsides and the typical visceral reflex pattern is seen. Therefore the chronic phase of reflex activity is characterized by trophic changes in the skin and subcutaneous tissues, as well as by local muscle contraction. This typically results in joint misalignment and decreased segmental mobility. It is not known whether the continuation of reflex somatic dysfunction is related to the initial impact of the visceral disease or whether it is a result of long-term segmental facilitation.

In a blind study of 25 patients, Beal[94] was able to differentiate patients with cardiac disease from those with gastrointestinal disease with a reported accuracy of 76% by using a compression test to examine for soft tissue texture changes and resist-

ance to segmental motion. Similarly, Beal and Dvorak[95] examined 50 patients in a physician-blind format and were able to identify characteristics specific to patients with cardiovascular, pulmonary, gastrointestinal, or musculoskeletal diseases.

The use of spinal manual therapy in the treatment of visceral conditions has been advocated on the hypothetical basis that it is designed to reduce somatic dysfunction, to interrupt the viscerosomatic reflex arc, and to influence the viscus through stimulation of the somatovisceral reflex. However, the effectiveness of manipulative procedures for the musculoskeletal manifestations of organic disease has not been clearly established. There is a definite need for further data on the incidence of viscerosomatic reflexes and the relationship to manipulative therapy.

Manual Therapy and Somatoautonomic Reflexes

Manual therapies, and specifically chiropractic adjustments, are thought to disrupt harmful somatoautonomic reflexes by reducing the noxious input into the spinal cord. For example, a patient with a strained posterior joint capsule that is accompanied by reflex muscle spasm may have nociceptive bombardment of the spinal cord. If the nociceptive bombardment is of sufficient strength and duration, it can cause segmental facilitation.

If a manipulative procedure can reduce the strain on the joint capsule or reduce muscle spasm, nociception from these tissues into the spinal cord may be ameliorated or reduced. Because manual techniques stimulate many different types of neuroreceptors, the result is a degradation of a negative somatoautonomic reflex.

Specific Soft Tissue and Reflex Technique Procedures

What follows is a brief description of some manual therapies used by chiropractic physicians and other health care providers. Although this is not meant to be a comprehensive treatise on soft tissue and reflex techniques, it is designed to present the concepts or foundations applicable to many of the forms of technique that have been modified or adapted from them. Moreover, inclusion does not presume efficacy, nor does exclusion signify ineffectiveness but rather oversight.

Massage

Classical or traditional massage procedures form the basis for many other procedures. Simply defined, massage consists of hand motions practiced on the body surface with a therapeutic goal.[96] A more clinical or practical definition is that *massage* is a term used to describe certain manipulations of the soft tissues of the body; these manipulations are most effectively performed by the hands and are administered for the purpose of producing effects on the nervous system and the muscular system as well as on the local and general circulation of the blood and lymph.[97] The variations of massage movements include effleurage, pétrissage, roulemont, tapotement, and friction. Effleurage, or stroking, is applied over a large area, using broad contacts. It may be deep or superficial, creating general relaxation and superficial warming caused by mild erythema. Pétrissage involves grasping the skin and lifting it while applying a pinching action to the held tissue and a stroking or stretching action to the tissue beneath. Roulemont, or skin rolling, lifts the skin away from fascial surfaces beneath; when adhesive areas are encountered, a pull is applied to the skin to allow freer movement. Tapotemont is described as a tapping or vibratory action applied to the soft tissue in a rapid fashion, creating a stimulatory effect. Friction is done with slow, deep, circular stroking with the ball of the thumb to move the underlying tissue.

Nimmo Technique (Ischemic Compression)

Raymond Nimmo was one of the first chiropractics to incorporate the trigger point work of individuals such as Travell and Simon into chiropractic practice. He termed the procedure the Receptor Tonus Technique to emphasize his theory that this is a reflex technique and not a form of massage therapy. Emphasis is placed on posture and muscular involvement, as well as on the neurologic involvements that then may occur. The soft tissues are palpated for tenderness, spasm, and trigger points, with each muscle exhibiting a unique and characteristic pattern of referred pain (Figures 7-6 to 7-8). Nimmo technique uses deep pressure applied directly over the irritable lesion to produce an ischemic compression effect[98-100] (Figure 7-9). Travell advocates stretching the irritable tissue, as well as the injection of an antiinflammatory medication (procaine) into the trigger point.[101]

Connective Tissue Massage

Ebner[102] defined connective tissue massage as a form of manipulation carried out in the layers of connective tissue on the body surface. The patient is usually treated in the sitting position with a long or short stroking action carried out using the second and third fingertips of the relaxed hand to draw the skin slack (Figure 7-10). The effects include marked hyperemia and sweat gland stimulation. Bruising sometimes occurs after treatment depending on the degree of capillary fragility. This procedure is purported to cause a release of a histamine-like substance that acts on the autonomic nervous system.

Chapman's (Neuro) Lymphatic Reflexes

Frank Chapman, an osteopath, was of the opinion that body wall reflexes are clinically useful for diagnosis, for influencing the motion of fluids (mostly lymph), and for influencing visceral function via the nervous system. The surface changes of Chapman's reflex are palpable and are thought to arise from changes in the deep fascia such as gangliform contractions located at specific points and consistently associated with the same viscera. The amount of tenderness is an important consideration in differentiating the gangliform contraction from subcutaneous fat globules. After the surface locus has been contacted by the pad of the middle finger, a firm, gentle contact is maintained and a rotary motion imparted to the finger through the arm and hand so as to express the fluid content of the locus into the surrounding tissues. The actual application of attention to a given reflex is expressed in terms of seconds, but in practice it is actually determined by a response to

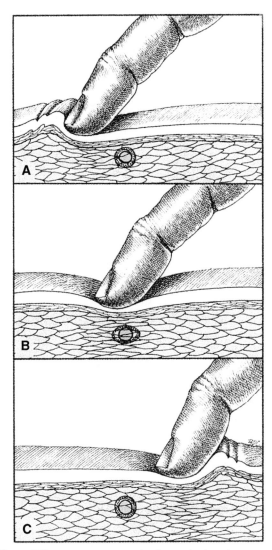

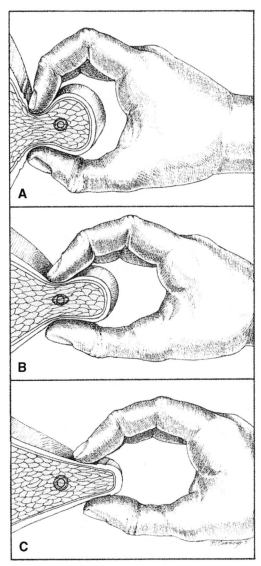

Figure 7-6   Cross-sectional schematic drawing showing flat palpation of a taut band *(black ring)* and its trigger point. Flat palpation is used for muscles that are accessible only from one direction, such as the infraspinatus. **A,** Skin pushed to one side to begin palpation. **B,** Fingertip slid across muscle fibers to feel the cordlike texture of the taut band rolling beneath it. **C,** Skin pushed to other side at completion of snapping palpation. *(From Travell JG, Simons DG. Myofacial pain and dysfunction: the trigger point manual. Baltimore: Williams & Wilkins; 1983.)*

Figure 7-7   Cross-sectional schematic drawing showing pincer palpation of a taut band *(black ring)* at a trigger point. Pincer palpation is used for muscles that can be picked up between the digits, such as the sternocleidomastoid, pectoralis major, and latissimus dorsi. **A,** Muscle fibers surrounded by the thumb and fingers in a pincer grips. **B,** Hardness of the taut band felt clearly as it is rolled between the digits. The change in the angle of the distal phalanges produces a rocking motion that improves discrimination of fine detail. **C,** Edge of the taut band sharply defined, as it escapes from between the fingertips, often with a local twitch response.

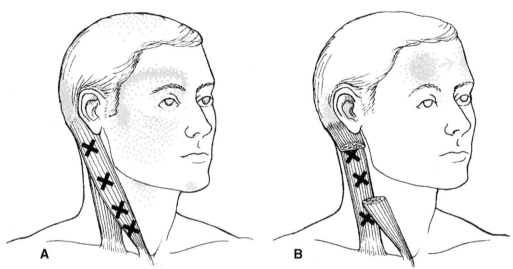

Figure 7-8   Referred pain patterns (shows essential zones and stippling shows the spillover areas) with location of corresponding trigger points *(X's)* in the right sternocleidomastoid muscle. A, The sternal (superficial) division. B, The clavicular (deep) division. *(From Travell JG, Simons DG. Myofascial pain and dysfunction: the trigger point manual. Baltimore: Williams & Wilkins; 1983.)*

palpation. The actual time of treatment may vary from 20 seconds to two minutes or more.[103]

Bennett's (Neuro) Vascular Reflexes

Terrence Bennett, a chiropractor, described reflex points mainly on the skull but also on other body parts. He believed that an irritable reflex reflected the vascular condition of organs and other structures. Bennett developed the Neurovascular Dynamics Technique, which he proposed alters and restores autonomic homeostasis. Treatment involves the stretch of a long muscle to initiate a palpable arteriole pulse at a specific location. A light but steady pressure is applied for at least one minute.[104,105]

Acupressure Point Stimulation

Acupressure is a method of massage to acupuncture points for the usual purpose of analgesia. Much has been written on the clinical aspects of acupuncture, acupressure, and meridian therapy. Acupuncture points are organized along meridians that have no known neurologic or vascular pattern. There appears to be a measurable change in electrical potential in irritable points, and they can

be treated by electrical stimulation, needle application, or manual pressure. Theoretically, blockage or other dysfunction in the meridian causes a departure from health.[67] Acupressure can be applied with the fingertip with a magnitude sufficient to cause pain. A possible explanation for the mechanism of pain relief is, therefore, in the modulation of endorphin levels.[106]

Muscle Energy Techniques

Described by Fred Mitchell, this technique uses specific muscle activity to restore physiologic joint function. Active muscle contractions are used at varying intensities from a precisely controlled position in a specific direction against a distinctly executed counterforce. The patient is therefore active in the corrective process, which encourages responsibility for self-care.[106]

Logan Basic

Basic technique was developed by Hugh B. Logan, who noted that the body must have normal structure to have normal function. In part, this system takes into account the effects of gravity on the spine and its related structures. Logan hypothesized that

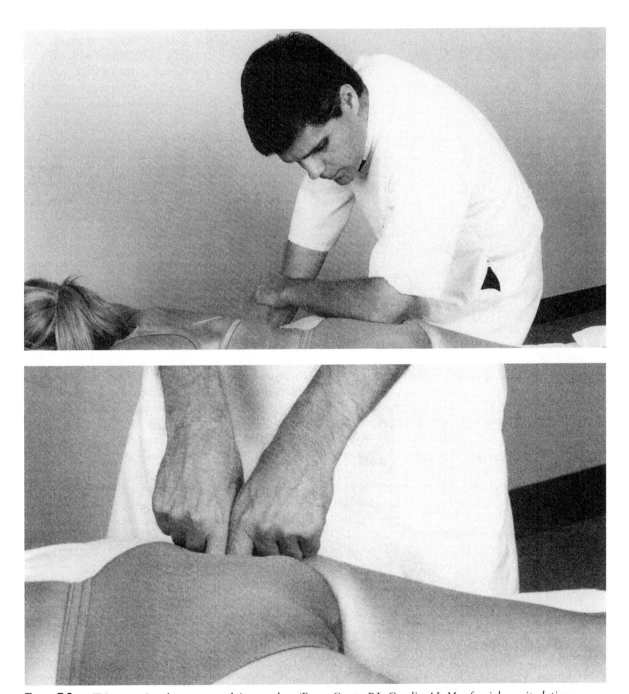

Figure 7-9   Trigger point therapy to pelvic muscles. *(From Cantu RI, Grodin AJ. Myofascial manipulation: theory and clinical application. Gaithersburg, MD: Aspen; 1992.)*

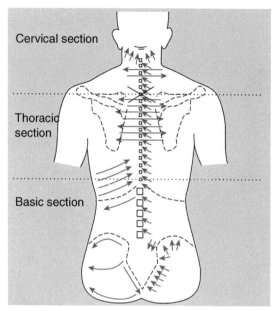

Cervical section

Thoracic section

Basic section

Figure 7-10   The approximate direction and position of connective tissue massage strokes applied to basic, thoracic, and cervical sections. *(Modified from Grieve GP, editor. Modern manual therapy of the vertebral column. New York: Churchill Livingstone; 1986.)*

the body of the lowest freely movable vertebra will rotate toward the low side of the sacrum (or the vertebra on which it rests); that is, the body of that vertebra rotates toward the side of least support. This is usually the low side of the sacrum. Logan believed that the sacrum was the biomechanical keystone of the body because it supported the spine and also allowed for locomotion; he also believed that the spine would respond to changes in the sacrum. Returning the sacrum to normal relations with its articulating bones was essential in reducing spinal involvements. He thought this required little force to accomplish with specific types of contacts on and around the sacrum. Pressure is applied steadily to these contacts with no true thrust delivered. One of the most common contacts involves approximately 2 to 10 ounces of pressure applied to the junction of the sacrotuberous and sacrospinalis ligaments. Somatic changes in muscle tone, skin and core body temperature, respiration, and perspiration are not uncommon.[107,108]

Spondylotherapy

Spondylotherapy was defined by Janse[109] as a method of treating visceral disease through the stimulation of involved sluggish reflexes by application of mechanical or electrical force in properly judged fashion on the vertebra overlying the reflex center. The principle of interrupted percussion or vibration is usually employed. A light, continuous contact held beyond the initial stimulation time is thought to produce relaxation through sedation, whereas a heavy continuous contact eventually produces inhibition because of actual nerve blockage. Continuous percussion, concussion, or vibration eventually inhibits reflexes because they become fatigued. Interrupted moderate percussion, concussion, vibration, or sinusoidalization prolongs the initial stimulation of the reflexes involved.

Activator Methods

Activator technique was developed by chiropractors W.C. Lee and A.W. Fuhr. Their emphasis from the start was on body mechanics and how light-force contact could be used to effect changes. The roots for the principles of activator methods can be traced to Logan. The analysis is centered on isolation testing, which involves specific patient positioning, causing changes in leg length. Therefore the prone leg check is the main evaluative tool used to identify specific segmental levels of joint dysfunction. The Activator method is known for its use of a handheld mechanical adjusting device called the Activator Adjusting Instrument (AAI), or Activator for short. The device is purported to produce a controlled and repeatable percussion force when it is triggered, so it induces a known force into the human body. It was developed to simulate a light-force thumb thrust (Logan Basic). This device has now begun to be examined with more rigorous research. In addition, there have been efforts to place it into a basic science model. Evidence exists to support the idea that the Activator thrust moves a spinal joint; however, there is seldom an audible release or cavitation response. Mechanoreceptor coactivation is theorized to be the mechanism for the observed effects.[68]

Sacro-Occipital Technique (SOT)

Major Bertrand DeJarnette was the developer of the sacro-occipital technique (SOT) system,[110] which is purported to restore normal functioning to the central and peripheral nervous systems through the effects on the meninges by the mechanical relationship between the cranium and pelvis. Padded wedges called *blocks* are placed between the patient's pelvis and the table, with the patient in either the prone or supine position, and gravity is allowed to affect the relationship of the innominata to the sacrum. Occipital fibers that apparently represent texture changes in the upper trapezius muscles are evaluated and treated. Cranial manipulative procedures based on the work of osteopaths Sutherland and Upledger[111] are also used. Evaluation is based on postural assessment, as well as on some reflex phenomena (the arm fossa test, dollar sign, and heel tensions). The evaluative process places the patient in one of three categories, and blocks then are placed under the pelvis in a specific manner, with the patient in either the prone or supine position. Category 1 involves slipping of the synovial part of the sacroiliac joint, placing a stress into the dura and primary respiratory cycle. Category 2 is the most common distortion pattern and involves a slip in the weight-bearing hyaline portion of the sacroiliac joint caused by trauma. Category 3 usually involves a lumbar disc or vertebral subluxation and is characterized by sciatica, antalgia, and possible neurologic signs.

Manual Cranial Therapy

Manual cranial therapy directed to the intrinsic joints of the skull has been described by Cottam[112] in chiropractic and Vredevoogd and Upledger[111] in osteopathic literature. It is reasoned that the sutures of the skull are intricately fashioned for maintenance of motion. The sutures are present throughout life, have consistent areas of bevel edge, and consistently separate when the skull is "exploded" (filled with beans and immersed in water).[46] It is further hypothesized that the skull has normal mobility during health and will show restrictions in response to trauma or disease. The perception of relatively low amplitude widening and narrowing of the skull can be made in association with respiration. This response is theorized to be the mechanism of cerebrospinal fluid flow. Evaluation consists of observation and palpation of the skull for symmetry, followed by sutural palpation for widening, narrowing, and tenderness. Sacral movements are also evaluated. Treatment involves various direct and indirect manual procedures as well as molding and disengagement procedures. All involve a relatively light force or sustained pressure applied in conjunction with the primary respiratory mechanism.

Conclusions

The science of chiropractic is beginning to investigate the art of chiropractic. The profession has a body of credible research to document some of its claims. Because of this, chiropractic is rapidly gaining increased acceptance. This acceptance of spinal manipulation by other health care professions, industry, and the general population continues to grow despite controversies that still exist in clinical practice, as well as lack of adequate validation. Advocates of manipulative therapy in the healing arts of chiropractic, medicine, osteopathy, and physical therapy have independently concluded that the high-velocity, low-amplitude thrust is an important clinical intervention for the treatment of dysfunctional conditions associated with the neuromusculoskeletal system.

Evidence also supports the existence of irritable lesions in soft tissues, including muscles, ligaments, and fascia. These lesions can produce noxious effects in various parts of the body remote from themselves and can cause pain or dysfunction. Specific techniques have been theorized and designed to affect and eliminate the irritable lesion using soft tissue and reflex mechanisms. Various forms of soft tissue and reflex therapy have been described.

Although many of these procedures have some overlap with the location of treated areas, there has been no acceptance or indication that they could be treated in the same fashion. The one thing that all of these pathologic reflexes seem to have in common is that they are all organismic responses to various types and degrees of tissue injury; that is, physical trauma, infection, degeneration, and chemical irritation.[103] Rational use of manual stimulation of the skin and soft tissues places the physiologic status of the skin at an optimum, invigorates circulation of the blood and lymph, and alerts the central and peripheral nervous systems.[113] Little evidence exists to validate the greater efficacy of any one therapy for a specific dysfunction. Although a few case reports have been published, no comparative studies have been conducted. Is it necessary to have validity or even an understanding of something before it is used clinically? If a procedure is observed to have a clinical effect, should it not be used? Full understanding and absolute validation may not be attainable with the technology and knowledge of today. Clinical success may carry weight for a time, but not as a general rule. The notion of clinical success is relative and fragile. It is necessary that practitioners further substantiate the principles and procedures of clinical practice.[114]

References

1. Gatterman M. Chiropractic management of spine related disorders. 2nd ed. Baltimore: Williams & Wilkins; 2003.
2. Bergmann T, Peterson D, Lawrence D. Chiropractic technique. New York: Churchill Livingstone; 1993.
3. Hippocrates. Hippocrates (with an English translation by Withington ET). 3rd ed. Cambridge: Howard University Press; 1959.
4. Gibbons RW. The evolution of chiropractic: medical and social protest in America. In: Haldeman S, editor. Modern developments in the principles and practice of chiropractic. East Norwalk, CT: Appleton Century Crofts; 1980.
5. Bergmann TF. Various forms of chiropractic technique. Chiro Tech 1993;5(2):53-5.
6. Haldeman S. Spinal manipulative therapy and sports medicine. Clin Sports Med 1986;5:277-93.
7. Gatterman MI, Hansen D. Development of chiropractic nomenclature through consensus. J Manipulative Physiol Ther 1994;17:302-9.
8. Triano JJ. Studies on the biomechanical effect of a spinal adjustment. J Manipulative Physiol Ther 1992;15:71-5.
9. Lewit K. Manipulative therapy in rehabilitation of the motor system. London: Butterworths; 1985. p. 1-256.
10. Nachemson A. A critical look at the treatment for low back pain. Scand J Rehab Med 1979;11:143-7.
11. Sandoz, R. Some physical mechanisms and effects of spinal adjustments. Ann Swiss Chiro Assoc 1976;6:91.
12. Sandoz, R. Some reflex phenomena associated with spinal derangements and adjustments. Ann Swiss Chiro Assoc 1981;7:45.
13. Gatterman MI. Indications for spinal manipulation in the treatment of back pain. ACA J Chiro 1982; 19(10):51-66.
14. Rahlmann JF. Mechanisms of intervertebral joint fixation: a literature review. J Manipulative Physiol Ther 1987:10:177-87.
15. Bogduk N, Jull G. The theoretical pathology of acute locked back: a basis for manipulative therapy. J Manual Medicine 1985;1:78-82.
16. Cyriax J. Textbook of orthopedic medicine. 9th ed., Vol. 2. London: Ballier Tindall; 1974. p. 57-66.
17. Vanharanta H, Sachs BL, Spivey MA, Guyer RD, Hochschuler SH, Rashbaum RF et al. The relationship of pain provocation to lumbar disc deterioration as seen by CT discography. Spine 1987;12:295-8.
18. Roston JB, Wheeler-Haines RW. Cracking in the metacarpophalangeal joint. J Anat 1947;81:165.
19. Unsworth A, Dowson D, Wright V. Cracking joints, a bioengineering study of cavitation in the metacarpophalangeal joint. Ann Rheum Dis 1971;30:348.
20. Brodeur R. The audible release associated with joint manipulation. J Manipulative Physiol Ther 1995;18:155.
21. Chen YL, Israelachvili J. New mechanism of cavitation damage. Science 1991;252:1157.
22. Akeson WH, Amiel D, Woo S. Immobility effects of synovial joints: the biomechanics of joint contracture. Biorheology 1980;17:95.
23. Akeson WH, Amiel D, Mechanic GL, Woos SLY, Harwood FL, Hamer ML. Collagen cross-linking alterations in joint contractures: changes in reducible cross-links in periarticular connective tissue collagen after nine weeks of immobilization. Connect Tissue Res 1977;5:5.
24. Burger AA. Experimental neuromuscular models of spinal manual techniques. Manual Med 1983;1:10.
25. Akeson WH, Amiel D, Woo SLY. Cartilage and ligament: physiology and repair processes. In: Nicholas JA, Hershman EB, editors. The lower extremity and spine in sports medicine. St. Louis: Mosby; 1986. p. 3-41.
26. Evans EB, Eggers GWN, Butler JK, Blumel J. Experimental immobilization and remobilization of rat knee joints. J Bone Joint Surg 1960;42A:737-58.
27. Dahners LE. Ligament contraction: a correlation with cellularity and actin staining. Trans Orthop Res Soc 1986;11:56.
28. White AA, Panjabi MM. Clinical biomechanics of the spine. 2nd ed. Philadelphia: JB Lippincott; 1990. p. 692-4.
29. Wyke BD. Articular neurology and manipulative therapy. In: Glasgow EF, Twomey LT, Schull ER, Kleynhans AM, editors. Aspects of manipulative therapy. New York: Churchill Livingstone; 1985. p. 72-80.
30. Terrett ACJ, Vernon H. Manipulation and pain tolerance. Am J Phys Med 1984;63(5):217-25.

31. Vernon HT, Dhami MSI. Spinal manipulation and Beta-endorphin: a controlled study of the effect of a spinal manipulation on plasma Beta-endorphin levels in normal males. J Manipulative Physio Ther 1986;9:115-23.
32. Vernon HT. Pressure pain threshold evaluation of the effect of spinal manipulation on chronic neck pain: a single case study. JCCA 1988;32:191-4.
33. Tran TA, Kirby JD. The effectiveness of upper cervical adjustment upon the normal physiology of the heart. ACA J Chiropractic 1977;11:58-62.
34. Sato A, Swenson RS. Sympathetic nervous system response to mechanical stress of the spinal column in rats. J Manipulative Physiol Ther 1984;7:141-7.
35. Briggs L, Boone WR. Effects of a chiropractic adjustment on changes in pupillary diameter: a model for evaluating somatovisceral response. J Manipulative Physiol Ther 1988;11:181-9.
36. Mitchell FL. Elements of muscle energy technique, In: Basmajian JV, Nyberg R, editors. Rational manual therapies. Baltimore: Williams & Wilkins; 1993. p. 318-9.
37. Paris SV. Spinal manipulative therapy. Clin Orthop 1983;179:55-61.
38. Pert C. Molecules of emotion. New York: Schribner; 1997.
39. Bergmann TF. Chiropractic spinal examination. In: Ferezy JS, editor. The chiropractic neurological examination. Gaithersburg, MD: Aspen Publications; 1992.
40. Peterson DR. Western States Chiropractic College adjustive technique manual. Portland, OR: Western States Chiropractic College; 1988.
41. Bergmann TF. Short lever, specific contact articular chiropractic technique. J Manipulative Physiol Ther 1992;15:591-5.
42. Peterson DR, Bergmann TF. Chiropractic technique. 2nd ed. St. Louis: Mosby; 2002.
43. Grice AS. Biomechanical approach to cervical and dorsal adjusting. In: Haldeman S, editor. Modern developments in the principles and practice of chiropractic. New York: Appleton-Century-Croft; 1980.
44. Bergmann TF. Low amplitude high velocity thrust techniques. In: Haldeman S, editor. Principles and practice of chiropractic. 3rd ed. Norwalk, CT: Appleton and Lange; 2004.
45. Hoag, JM, Cole, WV, Bradford, SG. Osteopathic medicine. New York: McGraw-Hill; 1969.
46. Greenman PE. Principles of manual medicine. 2nd ed. Baltimore: Williams & Wilkins; 2000.
47. Nwuga VC. Manipulation of the spine. Baltimore: Williams & Wilkins; 1976.
48. Grice A, Vernon H. Basic principles in the performance of chiropractic adjusting: historical review, classification, and objectives. In: Haldeman S, editor. Principles and practice of chiropractic. 2nd ed. San Mateo, CA: Appleton and Lange; 1992. p. 443-58.
49. Maigne R. Manipulation of the spine. In: Basmajian JV, editor. Manipulation, traction, and massage. 3rd ed. Baltimore: Williams & Wilkins; 1985.
50. Bergmann TF. Short/long lever, non-specific contact, articular chiropractic technique: a review of the literature. Chiro Tech 1993;5(3):107-110.
51. Grieve GP. Common vertebral joint problems. 2nd ed. New York: Churchill Livingstone; 1988.
52. Nyberg, R. Role of physical therapists in spinal manipulation. In: Basmajian JV, editor. Manipulation, traction, and massage. 3rd ed. Baltimore: Williams & Wilkins; 1985.
53. Bartol KM. A model for the categorization of chiropractic treatment procedures. J Chiro Tech 1991;3:78.
54. Bartol KM. Algorithm for the categorization of chiropractic technic procedures. J Chiro Tech 1992;4:8.
55. Maigne R. Localization of manipulation of the spine. In: Orthopedic medicine. 3rd ed. Springfield, IL: Charles C Thomas; 1979.
56. Good C. An analysis of diversified (lege artis) type adjustments upon the assisted-resisted model of intervertebral motion unit prestress. Chiro Tech 1992;4(4):117-23.
57. Bourdillon JF, Day EA. Spinal manipulation. 4th ed. London: William Heinemann Medical Books; 1987.
58. Bergmann TF, Davis PT. Mechanically assisted manual techniques: Distraction procedures. St. Louis: Mosby; 1997.
59. Cox JM. Mechanism, diagnosis, and treatment of low back pain. 5th ed. Baltimore: Williams & Wilkins; 1990.
60. Cox JM. Chiropractic manipulation in sciatica: statistical data on the diagnosis, treatment, and response of 576 consecutive cases. J Manipulative Physiol Ther 1984;7:1-11.
61. Lawrence I, Mattioni S. A fluoroscopic study of lumbar spine biomechanics during passive motion in the prone position [doctoral thesis]. Bournemouth, England: Anglo-European College of Chiropractic; 1987.
62. Deutro CL, Meeker WC, Menke JM, Keene K. The efficacy of flexion-traction manipulation and inverted gravity traction for treatment of idiopathic low back pain. Transactions of the Pacific Consortium for Chiropractic Research, First Annual Conference on Research and Education. Sunnyvale, CA: Palmer College of Chiropractic West; June 1986.
63. Eckard L. Literature packet and training manual for use with the Leander table. Port Orchard, WA: Leander Research, 12300 Sidney Road; no date available.
64. Markey LP. Markey distraction technique: new protocol for doctor and patient's safety. A pragmatic approach, part 1. Dig Chiro Econ 1985;Jul/Aug:66-9.
65. Bergmann TF. Manual force: mechanically assisted articular chiropractic technique using long and/or short level contacts: a literature review. J Manipulative Physiol Ther 1993;16:33-6.
66. Schneider MJ. The traction methods of Cox and Leander: the neglected role of the multifidus muscle in low back pain. J Chiro Tech 1991;3:109-15.
67. Meeker WC. Soft tissue and nonforce techniques. In: Haldeman S, editor. Principles and practice of chiropractic. East Norwalk, CT: Appleton and Lange; 1992. p. 520.

68. Osterbauer PJ, Fuhr AW. The current status of activator methods, chiropractic technique, theory, and training. Chiro Tech 1991;3(1):19-25.

69. Osterbauer PJ, Fuhr AW. The current status of activator methods chiropractic technique, theory, and training. Chiro Tech 1991;3(1):19-25.

70. Jones VT, Garrett WE, Seaber AV. Biomechanical changes in muscle after immobilization at different lengths. Trans Orthop Res Soc 1985;10:6.

71. Janda V. Muscle spasm: a proposed procedure for differential diagnosis. Manual Med 1991;6:136-9.

72. Cantu RI, Grodin AJ. Myofascial manipulation theory and clinical application. Gaithersburg, MD: Aspen; 1992. p. 53-7.

73. Wakim KG. The effects of massage on the circulation in normal and paralyzed extremities. Arch Phys Med 1949;30:135.

74. Wolfson H. Studies on effect physical therapeutic procedures on function and structure. JAMA 1931;96:2020.

75. Carrier EB. Studies on physiology of capillaries: Reaction of human skin capillaries to drugs and other stimuli. Am J Physiol 1022;61:528-47.

76. Martin GM, Roth GM et al. Cutaneous temperature of the extremities of normal subjects and patients with rheumatoid arthritis. Arch Phys Med Rehabil 1946;27:665.

77. Cuthbertson DP. Effect of massage on metabolism: a survey. Glasgow Med J 1933;2:200-13.

78. Schneider EC, Havens LC. Changes in the contents of haemoglobin and red corpuscles in the blood of men at high altitudes. Am J Physiol 1915;36:360.

79. Homewood AE. Neurodynamics of the vertebral subluxation. St. Petersburg, FL: Valkyrie Press; 1977.

80. Korr IM, editor. The neurobiologic mechanisms in manipulative therapy. New York: Plenum; 1978.

81. Sato A. The somatosympathetic reflexes: their physiologic and clinical significance. In: Goldstein M, editor. The research status of spinal manipulative therapy. DHEW Publication No. NIH 76-998. Washington, D.C.: U.S. Government Printing Office; 1975.

82. Leach RA. Somatoautonomic reflex hypothesis. In: The chiropractic theories. 2nd ed. Baltimore: Williams & Wilkins; 1986. p. 132-152.

83. Sato A. Spinal reflex physiology. In: Haldeman S, editor. Principles and practice of chiropractic. 2nd ed. East Norwalk, CT: Appleton and Lange; 1992.

84. Liebenson C. Active muscular relaxation techniques, Part 1. Basic principles and methods. J Manipulative Physiol Ther 1989;12:446-54.

85. Bogduk N, Twomey LT. Clinical anatomy of the lumbar spine. 2nd ed. Melbourne: Churchill Livingstone; 1991. p. 152.

86. Beal MC. Viscerosomatic reflexes: a review. J Am Osteopath Assoc 1985;85(12):53-68.

87. Van Buskirk RL. Nociceptive reflexes and the somatic dysfunction: a model. J Am Osteopath Assoc 1990; 90:792-809.

88. Sato A. The reflex effects of spinal somatic nerve stimulation on visceral function. Proceedings of the scientific symposium of the World Chiropractic Congress. Toronto; May 4-5, 1991.

89. Sato Y, Schaible HG, Schmidt RF. Reactions of cardiac postganglionic sympathetic neurons to movements of normal and inflamed knee joints. J Auton Nerv Syst 1985;12:1-13.

90. Korr IM. Osteopathic research: The needed paradigm shift. J Am Osteopath Assoc 1991;91:156-71.

91. Grainger HG. The somatic component in visceral disease. In: Academy of Applied Osteopathy 1958 Yearbook. Newark, OH: American Academy of Osteopathy; 1958.

92. Larson NJ. Summary of site and occurrence of paraspinal soft tissue changes of patients in the intensive care unit. J Am Osteopath Assoc 1976;75:840-2.

93. Kelso AF. A double blind clinical study of osteopathic findings in hospital patients. J Am Osteopath Assoc 1971;70:570-92.

94. Beal MC. Palpatory findings for somatic dysfunction in patients with cardiovascular disease. J Am Osteopath Assoc 1983;82:822-31.

95. Beal MC, Dvorak J. Palpatory examination of the spine: a comparison of the results of two methods and their relationship to visceral disease. Manual Med 1984;1:25-32.

96. Hofkosh JM. Classical massage. In: Basmajian JV, editor. Manipulation, traction, and massage. 3rd ed. Baltimore: Williams & Wilkins; 1985. p. 263.

97. Beard G, Wood EC. Massage: principles and techniques. Philadelphia: WB Saunders; 1964.

98. Nimmo RL. The receptor and tonus control method defined [self-published]. Receptor (undated);1:1-4.

99. Schneider MJ, Cohen JH. Nimmo receptor tonus technique: a chiropractic approach to trigger point therapy, In: Sweere JJ, editor. Chiropractic family practice. Gaithersburg, MD: Aspen Publishers; 1992. p. 1-18.

100. Cohen JH, Schneider MJ. Receptor-tonus technique: an overview. Chiro Tech 1990;2:13-6.

101. Travell JG, Simmons DG. Myofascial pain and dysfunction: the trigger point manual. Baltimore: Williams & Wilkins; 1983.

102. Ebner M. Connective tissue massage. Physiotherapy 1978;64(7):208-10.

103. Chaitow L. Soft-tissue manipulation. Rochester, VT: Healing Arts Press; 1988. p. 9.

104. Bennett TJ. Dynamics of correction of abnormal function. Sierra Madres, CA: RJ Martin; 1977.

105. Nelson WA. Diabetes mellitus: two case reports. Chiro Tech 1989;1:37-40.

106. Basmajian JV, Nyberg R, editors. Rational manual therapies. Baltimore: Williams & Wilkins; 1993. p. 21-47.

107. Logan HB. Textbook of Logan basic methods. St. Louis: Logan Basic College of Chiropractic; 1950.

108. Lawson DA. Logan basic technique: short and long lever, mechanical assisted. In: Proceedings of the 6th Annual CORE. Monterey, CA; 1991. p. 336-9.

109. Janse JJ. Principles and practice of chiropractic. Lombard, IL: National College of Chiropractic; 1947.
110. DeJarnene MB. Sacro-occipital technique. Nebraska City, NE: Major Bertrand DeJarnene; 1984.
111. Upledger JE, Vredevoogd JD. Craniosacral therapy. Chicago: Eastland Press; 1983.
112. Cottam C. Cranial and facial adjusting. Los Angeles: Self published; 1987.
113. Wakim KG. Physiologic effects of massage. In: Basmajian JV, editor. Manipulation, traction and massage. 3rd ed. Baltimore: Williams & Wilkins; 1985. p. 256.
114. Zucker A. Chapman's reflexes: medicine or metaphysics? J Am Osteopath Assoc 1993;93:346-52.

8

The Nonmanipulable Subluxation

Cynthia K. Peterson and
Meridel I. Gatterman

Key Words   Hypermobility, instability, nonmanipulable subluxation

After reading this chapter you should be able to answer the following questions:

Question 1   Is there a difference between hypermobility and instability?

Question 2   Are there any contraindications to manipulation noted on these radiographs?

Question 3   What procedural error did the practitioner make when taking this x-ray series?

The first problem confronting the clinician in the evaluation of a nonmanipulable subluxation is lack of consistency of terminology; the second problem is recognizing the associated clinical and radiologic signs. A nonmanipulable subluxation is a vertebral motion segment with radiologic or clinical features indicating that an adjustive force or osseous manipulation to this motion segment would be harmful or dangerous and is therefore contraindicated. Although it is well recognized that many pathologic processes affecting the skeletal system, such as malignant tumors and infections, are absolute contraindications to manipulation of the affected area, this chapter focuses on those conditions that may result in hypermobility, instability, or osseous fusion of the spinal motion segment. See Table 8-1 for criteria for defining nonmanipulable subluxations.

Table 8-1

Criteria for Defining Nonmanipulable Subluxations

Condition	Characteristics	Manipulation
Hypermobility	Excessive motion (reversible)	Nonrepetitive
Instability	Insufficient soft tissue (irreversible)	Contraindicated
Congenitally blocked segment	Motion absent (irreversible)	Contraindicated
Surgically fused segment	Motion absent (irreversible)	Contraindicated

Definitions of Instability and Hypermobility of the Cervical Spine

Clinical instability of the spine is defined as follows:

Loss of the ability of the spine under physiologic loads to maintain relationships between vertebrae in such a way that there is neither damage nor subsequent irritation to the spinal cord or nerve roots, and in addition, there is no development of incapacitating deformities or pain due to structural changes.[1]

The terms *instability* and *hypermobility* are often confused, both in practice and in the literature.[2-5] It is important to differentiate between these two conditions as they relate to the spine because the clinical significance and thus the therapeutic approaches to the these two entities are not the same. Segmental hypermobility has been defined as follows:

The mobility of a given motion unit (segment) which is excessive but not so extreme as to be life-threatening or require surgery.[5]

Several authors claim that hypermobility may be a precursor to the development of instability at a later date if not properly managed.[2,3,6] Some think that hypermobility is "...a distinct category along a continuum from normal joint motion to pathological movement."[5]

Chiropractic principles emphasize the importance of manipulating those motion segments that are fixed, or hypomobile, with the goal of restoring normal motion,[7,8] while avoiding motion segments that are already hypermobile, or unstable.[8,9] With this goal in mind, how are nonmanipulable subluxations recognized?

Excessive intersegmental motion to the degree that damage to the spinal cord or nerve roots becomes a potential hazard has several causes. These include acute trauma, repetitive microtraumas, congenital anomalies, degenerative and inflammatory arthropathies, surgical fusions and laminectomies, and compensatory phenomena caused by loss of motion in adjacent segments.[6,10-12]

Clinical Manifestations of Hypermobility and Instability in the Cervical Spine

Segmental hypermobility in children may simulate the symptoms of chronic rheumatic disease, making it difficult to properly diagnose.[5] Adult patients may complain of a variety of symptoms that seem to be slowly progressive, building over a period of years. The complaints include recurrent episodes of neck pain, which is often described as "dull" or "aching,"[5] with or without muscle spasm. The pain is either unilateral or bilateral and commonly located in the area of C5-C6. There may be associated crepitus in the neck at the end ranges of motion, and the patient often complains of "tight, tired, stressed" feelings throughout the neck. Headaches may be associated.[5] These clinical features are nonspecific and alone would not necessarily make the clinician think of excessive segmental motion. Some authors claim that cervical instability (they do not differentiate hypermobility from instability) is related to loss of the lordosis.[11] This finding alone, however, is insignificant because many factors may produce loss of cervical lordosis, including the fact that it can be normal and asymptomatic. Additional physical examination findings include hypertrophy of the anterior neck and anterior chest musculature with protraction of the scapula and elevation of the clavicles. Active and passive ranges of motion are usually limited. Segmental palpation may show hypermobility of the involved segments with restrictions above and below the affected levels.[5,11] Patients with segmental hypermobility are more likely to exhibit symptomatic degenerative joint disease (DJD) than those patients with DJD with no hypermobility.[5] Actual segmental instability may demonstrate similar clinical findings to hypermobility with the additional potential for neurologic signs and symptoms and progressive deterioration.[6,10]

Radiographic Evaluation of Hypermobility and Instability in the Cervical Spine

The definitive diagnosis of intersegmental hypermobility and instability has relied on the evaluation of kinematic radiographic studies of the cervical spine in the sagittal plane.[5,6,10,12-15] The chiropractic profession has used these radiographs for decades to assess global range of motion and intersegmental

range of motion and to attempt to objectify the effects of manipulation.[15,16] Neutral, flexion, and extension lateral radiographs are taken by various methods devised for assessing normal and abnormal motion.[6,7,12,14-17] These studies have traditionally been performed actively by the patient without reinforcement by the doctor. Dvorak et al.,[12] however, emphasize the value of obtaining functional radiographic studies of the cervical spine both with the patient actively moving the neck and passively, with the doctor forcing the patient's neck beyond the point where the patient actively ceases motion. They claim that many more hypermobile segments are discovered on the passive kinematic studies as compared with evaluating active flexion/extension radiographs only. Caution is advised when passively forcing the patient beyond the active range of motion since further damage may be caused to previously injured structures.

Spinal radiographs can be analyzed by hand, using templating procedures (see Chapter 6) or with the aid of computer digitizing. Digital video fluoroscopy is also used to assess the entire intersegmental motion.[13,14] (See Chapter 20.) The various assessment methods emphasize measuring translation in the sagittal plane, analyzing intervertebral angles, and calculating the axes of rotation.[6,17,18] There is consensus that the quantity of normal intersegmental motion varies considerably between the various motion segments of the cervical spine and that this intersegmental motion decreases with increasing age.[6,13,14,16] Some authors state that the "amount" of motion at an intervertebral segment is not as important as the "path" of the motion.[13]

Henderson and Dormon[6] developed a method of assessing intersegmental motion in the sagittal plane that can easily be applied to flexion and extension radiographs in clinical practice. Normal and abnormal intersegmental motion is defined in terms of a percentage of the sagittal body diameter (SBD). Absolute hypermobility is defined as intersegmental motion that falls between 61% and 72% of the sagittal body diameter, whereas instability is any motion exceeding 72% of the SBD. This is one of the only studies to attempt to objectively differentiate hypermobility from instability.

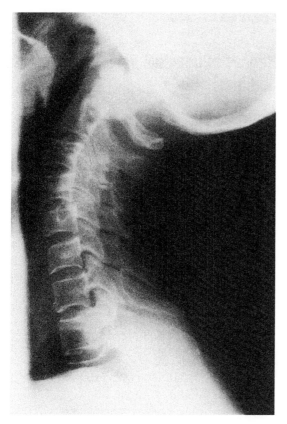

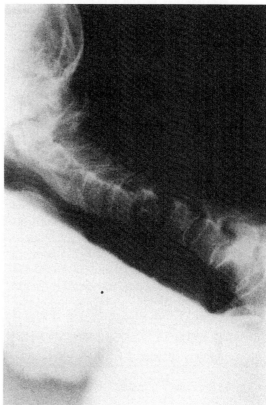

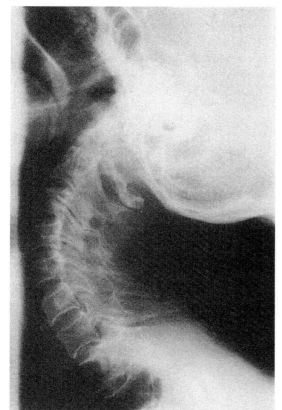

Figure 8-1 The slight anterolisthesis of C4 noted on the neutral radiograph demonstrates excessive translation in the sagittal plane during flexion and extension.

It is useful as a guide as long as the clinician keeps in mind that the range of normal segmental motion differs between and within subjects. Other studies have defined instability as a translation in the sagittal plane of one vertebra on another in excess of 3.5 mm during flexion to extension.[18] This is a useful and simple method for evaluation of excessive joint motion. Figure 8-1 demonstrates neutral, flexion, and extension lateral radiographs of a patient with an anterolisthesis of C3 (evident on neutral film) along with facet arthrosis between C2 and C3. Notice that the anterolisthesis increased during flexion and completely reduced during extension, giving an overall excursion of approximately 4 mm. This figure is consistent with a diagnosis of intersegmental instability, and this motion segment should not be manipulated.

Causes of Cervical Spine Hypermobility and Instability

Acute Trauma

Figure 8-2 represents the flexion and extension lateral radiographs of a teenage girl who fell onto her head while doing handstands at school. She complained of neck pain and stiffness immediately after the incident.

The flexion-extension radiographs of the young woman in Figure 8-2 demonstrate several of the classic signs of posttraumatic instability caused by ligamentous and discal injury at C4-5.

There is an acute kyphotic angulation between C4 and C5 with an anterolisthesis of C4, fanning of the spinous processes, gapping and overriding

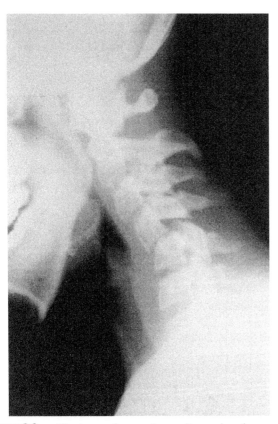
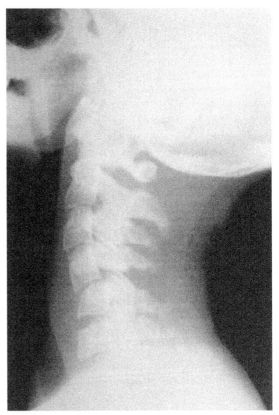

Figure 8-2   Flexion and extension radiographs of a teenage female who complained of neck pain and stiffness after falling onto her head during gymnastics class.

of the articular facets, and a loss of disc height at this level. The findings do not completely reduce on the extension film and would have been evident on a neutral lateral radiograph. The dangerous error made by the clinician responsible for this radiographic series was to have taken flexion-extension films in the first place because of the history of recent trauma.

In cases of acute cervical trauma, the neutral lateral radiograph must be taken first and scrutinized thoroughly for any signs of instability and ligamentous damage before subjecting the patient to motion studies.[10,12,19] If any signs of instability are noted, flexion-extension radiographs, as well as manipulation, are contraindicated. The patient should be placed carefully into a cervical collar and taken to the hospital. Halo bracing and surgical fusion are the appropriate treatments for acute traumatic instability. In addition to these signs, prevertebral swelling, displacement of the prevertebral fat stripe, and an increase in the ADI (atlantodental interval) may be noted in patients with acute posttraumatic instability.[19]

Latent or occult posttraumatic instability of the cervical spine is the physician's nightmare because the initial neutral lateral cervical radiograph may be seen as "normal." Reasons for this include technically inadequate radiographs; for example, the lower cervical spine may be obscured by the shoulders, muscle spasms may temporarily reduce a displaced vertebra, or hyperextension/hyperflexion dislocations may spontaneously reduce on recoil of the neck.[10,19] In such cases, careful analysis of the neutral lateral radiograph may show the warning signs of prevertebral soft tissue swelling and displacement of the prevertebral soft tissue stripe. An upright neutral lateral radiograph must be taken because subtle signs of posttraumatic instability may not be visible on supine cross-table lateral radiographs.[19]

This discussion focused on soft tissue injuries of the cervical spine associated with acute trauma. The myriad of fractures and fracture/dislocations of the cervical spine that also may be unstable are not covered, and the reader is referred to standard skeletal radiologic texts for this information. It must be noted that it is dangerous for chiropractors to manipulate new or recent fractures.

Anomalies

Look at the radiographs of the 60-year-old woman in Figure 8-3, A and B. This patient complained of neck pain and stiffness after an automobile accident.

Was her automobile accident responsible for the radiographic changes seen?

This type of question plagues clinicians daily and is one that usually has no definite answer. If you said that this patient has a dens fracture caused by her recent trauma, you are 100% wrong! There is definitely instability of C1 on C2 as noted by the marked translation in the sagittal plane during flexion and extension. Perhaps the accident caused her to rupture her transverse ligament? Wrong again. Posttraumatic rupture of the transverse ligament is very rare, and the patient is more likely to fracture the dens than to rupture this ligament.[19,20] The clue on the lateral views lies in the shape of the anterior tubercle of C1. Rather than the classic "D" shape with a straight posterior margin, this patient's anterior tubercle is rounded and hypertrophied. This important radiographic sign indicates an anomaly of the upper cervical complex.[20] You may have noticed that the dens was not visualized on the lateral view, and the open-mouth projection provides the evidence that the dens is absent (Figure 8-3, C). Other anomalies of the upper cervical spine that may result in instability include the os odontoideum and odontoid hypoplasia.[20] Flexion-extension views are indicated when anomalies are suggested to determine the presence or absence of instability. Translation in the sagittal plane of more than 3.5 mm[18] is considered instability, and these patients should be referred for surgical consultation.

Blocked Vertebrae

Figure 8-4 depicts the classic congenital blocked vertebra at C5-C6 with normal bone density, normal vertebral body height, wasp waist, and remnant disc. Congenital blocked vertebrae are common anomalies whose clinical significance

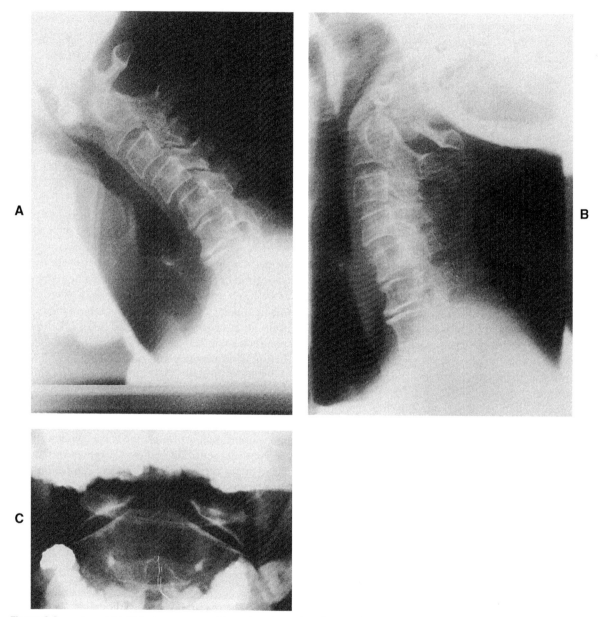

Figure 8-3   A and B, Elderly woman with neck pain and stiffness after a road traffic accident. In addition to the degenerative disc disease of the lower cervical spine, instability of C1 on C2 is present. The altered shape of the anterior tubercle of C1 is the clue to the cause. C, Agenesis of the dens is the cause of the instability of C1 on C2. This was not the result of the road traffic accident.

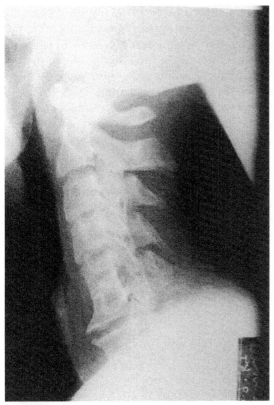

Figure 8-4   Classic congenital blocked vertebrae C5-6.

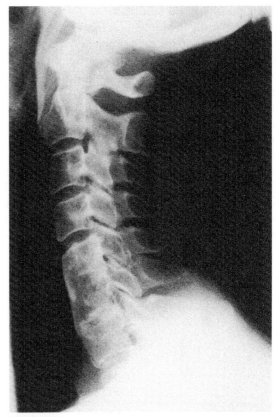

Figure 8-5   Surgically fused C5-7.

relates to the effect that this fusion has on adjacent mobile segments, and not to the fact that two segments are fused together.[6,20] Obviously, chiropractors do not attempt to manipulate blocked vertebra. What must be remembered, however, is that blocked vertebrae, whether they are congenital or surgical (Figure 8-5), can result in increased motion and potential instability at adjacent motion segments.[6,20] The patient in Figure 8-4 has large osteophytes at the adjacent anterior body margins between C6 and C7, indicating probable instability at some time. Whether this motion segment or the upper cervical motion segments are currently unstable cannot be determined on this neutral lateral film alone. Clinicians must be cognizant that the fused segments can cause adjacent hypermobilities or instabilities and must thoroughly evaluate these patients before manipulation.

Absence of the Transverse Ligament in Down Syndrome

Down syndrome, or mongolism, is a common congenital abnormality caused by trisomy of the twenty-first chromosome. The significance of this syndrome to chiropractors is that up to 20% of people with Down syndrome are born without a transverse ligament and are prone to instability of C1 on C2. Every patient with Down syndrome must be checked for this potentially life-threatening condition by taking a flexion lateral radiograph before manipulation of the upper cervical spine to evaluate the ADI.[20] A measurement of greater than 5 mm in the child or 3 mm in the adult is abnormal.[20,21]

Inflammatory Arthropathies

Now look at the flexion lateral film in Figure 8-6, B. The neutral lateral radiograph (Figure 8-6, A) demonstrates mild degenerative disc disease in the middle and lower cervical spine (C7 is not included on the film). The ADI is within normal limits. This is not the case, however, on the flexion lateral film of the same patient! The ADI now measures 6 mm, well above the maximum normal value of 3 mm. Note also the anterior displacement of the posterior spinal line, another indicator of C1-2 instability. Without the flexion lateral view, the clinician would not have realized that this patient, who has a history of rheumatoid arthritis (RA), has ruptured her transverse liga-ment and now has a potentially life-threatening instability. Obviously, manipulation is contraindi-cated in her upper cervical spine. Rheumatoid arthritis is notorious for affecting the upper cer-vical complex. As many as 40% of RA patients develop atlantoaxial subluxation in the course of the disease.[21] Other causes of instability with RA include erosion of the dens, posterior arch, and destruction of the alar ligaments.[21]

Although rheumatoid arthritis is the most common of the inflammatory arthropathies that cause rupture of the transverse ligament, it must be remembered that any of the inflammatory arthropathies, for example, ankylosing spondylitis, psoriatic arthritis, Reiter's syndrome, systemic

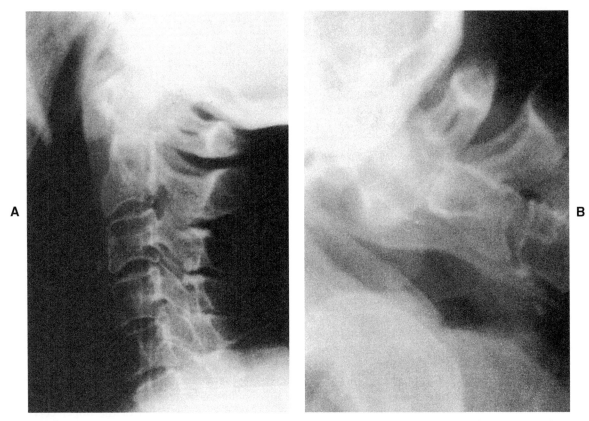

Figure 8-6   A, Neutral lateral radiograph of a middle-aged woman with a long history of rheumatoid arthritis. B, Spot flexion lateral upper cervical radiograph demonstrates an increased atlantodental interval consistent with rupture of the transverse ligament caused by rheumatoid arthritis.

lupus erythematosus, and juvenile rheumatoid arthritis, also can rupture this ligament and cause instability.[20,22]

Ankylosing spondylitis, as its name implies, can lead to osseous spinal fusion. Spinal manipulative therapy is not of benefit once these segments have become fused. However, as described under congenital and surgical blocked vertebrae, motion segments that are fused predispose nonfused segments to become hypermobile or unstable.[6,20]

Figure 8-7 depicts the lateral cervical radiograph of a man with longstanding ankylosing spondylitis with the typical appearance of the "bamboo spine." He suffered a minimal trauma recently and can suddenly move his neck better than he has been able to in years. He is thrilled and believes that the accident has helped his ankylosing spondylitis. Do you agree?

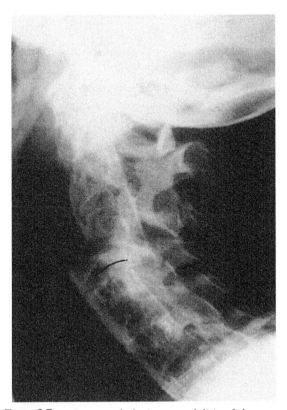

Figure 8-7   Severe ankylosing spondylitis of the cervical spine. The patient can suddenly move his neck, and he is thrilled!

Certainly not. This man has a "carrot stick fracture" at C3 with marked posterior displacement of the upper cervical spine. There is also marked prevertebral swelling noted. Amazingly, he suffered no neurologic deficits but is now at high risk for a spinal cord injury. He should be immediately transported by ambulance to the hospital with his neck carefully immobilized. Flexion-extension radiographs are obviously contraindicated, as is spinal manipulation.

Degenerative Arthritis

Degenerative joint disease (DJD) is the most common arthropathy seen by chiropractors and is certainly not in itself a contraindication to manipulation. In fact, many patients with this disorder benefit tremendously from spinal manipulation when it is applied judiciously. It is important, however, for the clinician treating the patient with DJD to recognize the association between degenerative changes in the spine and segmental hypermobilities or instabilities. Remember that hypermobility represents increased intersegmental motion, does not pose a threat to the nervous system, and is not considered a presurgical state. In contrast, instability, which is more severe, does threaten the neural elements and requires surgical intervention.

Just how is degenerative joint disease associated with segmental hypermobility and instability? There appear to be two main theories regarding this problem. The first suggests that hypermobility caused by repetitive microtraumas from occupational or sporting activities or a hereditary predisposition is the precursor to DJD.[3,5,6,10] The other purports that degenerative disc disease results in posterior capsular and ligamentous laxity, which then allows excessive intersegmental motion.[6,23] The importance to clinical practice, however, is to remember the association between these two entities rather than debating the actual causes after the fact.

Look at the radiographs of an elderly woman in Figure 8-8, A through C. The neutral lateral film shows an anterolisthesis of C4 on C5 of approximately 5 mm and a slight retrolisthesis of C3 on C4. Moderate to marked degenerative disc disease

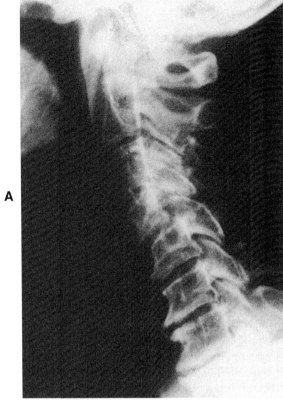

A

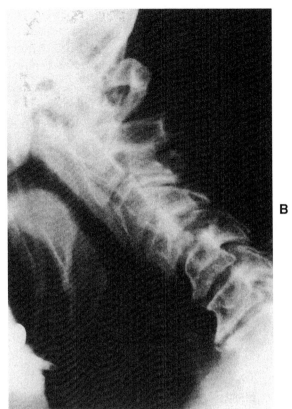

B

Figure 8-8   Degenerative hypermobility/
instability of the C3-5 motion segments.

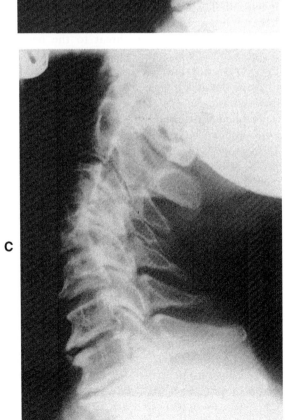

C

is present throughout the cervical spine. Flexion and extension radiographs were taken based on the findings noted on the neutral film. There is a slight increase in the forward translation of C4 during flexion and incomplete reduction in this subluxation during extension. The retrolisthesis of C3 is completely reduced during flexion and increases slightly during extension. Both of these motion segments demonstrate signs of intersegmental hypermobility on these kinematic studies.

A chiropractic technique that emphasizes the use of spinal manipulation to restore proper vertebral alignment without considering aberrant motion can prove detrimental to patients such as the woman in Figure 8-8.[5,7,10] A practitioner who adheres to the simplistic philosophy of replacing the "bone out of place" would adjust the spine, attempting to correct the anterolisthesis of C4 and retrolisthesis of C5 and, in effect, would be manipulating areas of hypermobility. Not only does this fail to correct the patient's problem, it may delay healing and create instability in already hypermobile articulations.[7,10]

Pain or tenderness alone is also not a sufficient criterion to justify a manipulative thrust into a motion segment. Hypermobile articulations are often painful,[5,7] with the symptoms frequently temporarily relieved by manipulation.[7] This relief is thought to be attributable to the reduction in local muscle spasm. Motion palpation of the involved segments is also often unrewarding, with difficulty arising in differentiating a "normal" motion segment from one that is hypermobile.[3,7]

Flexion-extension lateral radiographs are also the method employed to diagnose hypermobility associated with DJD. Should every patient with DJD of the cervical spine receive kinematic radiographic studies? Although there may be no clues on the neutral radiographs to differentiate patients with hypermobility,[5] the presence of an intersegmental anterolisthesis or a retrolisthesis, especially if associated with mild degenerative changes at the involved level or significant degenerative changes at the adjacent spinal levels, indicates inclusion of flexion-extension studies before manipulation.[3] Hypermobile or unstable motion segments related to degenerative joint disease frequently stabilize themselves through the formation of osteophytes,[5,23] but this process can take years. Severely degenerated motion segments that demonstrate hypomobility on kinematic radiographs may result in hypermobility in adjacent motion segments.

Chiropractic Management of Hypermobile and Unstable Cervical Segments

The treatment of the patient with hypermobile cervical motion segments is complex.[5] Chiropractors use many therapeutic approaches in addition to various manual procedures when treating their patients. As stated previously, manipulative thrusts into unstable articulations are contraindicated. However, it is possible that hypermobility and hypomobility or fixation may coexist in the same motion segment. Remember that an intervertebral motion segment is a three-joint complex consisting of the intervertebral disc and the two facet articulations; a fixation in one facet articulation might result in a compensatory hypermobility of the contralateral articular facet.[7] In such cases, adjusting the restricted side while leaving the hypermobile side alone would be logical as well as adjusting adjacent restricted motion segments. Additionally, hypermobility in one plane, for instance the sagittal plane, might be accompanied by restricted motion, such as lateroflexion or rotation,[3] in another plane; careful analysis and application of specific manipulative procedures are required. Various physical therapies can be employed, including electrical modalities. Specific exercise programs to stretch tight muscles and strengthen weak muscles should be incorporated. Trigger point therapy is also often beneficial.[7] Management of patients with unstable cervical motion segments requires conservative care and nonthrust procedures because of the danger of neurologic complications. Referral for neurologic and surgical consultation is recommended when the holding elements of the segment are damaged to the point of instability because of the threat of neurologic damage.

Hypermobility and Instability in the Lumbar Spine

The terms *hypermobility* and *instability* are used inconsistently and interchangeably when referring to the lumbar spine.[2,24,25] Several authors define lumbar segmental instability simply as an increase in segmental motion,[2,25] without differentiating between hypermobility and instability. Grieve[26] is clear in his definition of the two entities by stating that "hypermobility" represents "a little too much motion" and need not be painful, clinically significant, or unstable. On the other hand, "instability" occurs in a degenerating lumbar motion segment that is functionally incompetent because of insufficient soft tissue control. Paris[27] tends to agree with Grieve's differentiation of the two conditions, adding that "instability exists only when during the performance of an active motion, there is a sudden aberrant motion, such as a visible slip, catch, or shaking of the section."[27] In all of the definitions submitted for "instability" specifically relating to the lumbar spine, none includes the likelihood of resultant neurologic deficits as was so clearly the case for the cervical spine. This is most likely because acute posttraumatic instability caused by rupture of the ligaments of the lumbar spine, although occurring especially in the thoracolumbar junction, is not nearly as common as in the cervical spine.[19,28] Most unstable acute traumatic injuries to the lumbar spine also show evidence of fracture.[19] The terms *hypermobility* and *instability* should not be used interchangeably when referring to spinal mechanical lesions. Instability should be reserved for motion segments that produce neurologic effects, incapacitating deformities, or pain caused by structural defects.

Radiographic Evaluation

Static plain film radiographs cannot reliably detect lumbar intersegmental instability or hypermobility. The presence of an anterolisthesis, laterolisthesis, or retrolisthesis alone, although suggesting that hypermobility was most likely present at one time, does not indicate that the motion segment is currently unstable.[4,26] Degenerative and potentially unstable retrolistheses are more common at L5;

the most common level for anterolistheses[28] with similar characteristics is at L4 (Figure 8-9). The presence of the small traction spur is thought to be associated with instability, whereas the larger osteophyte indicates that the segment has stabilized itself.[24,26] This finding actually may be significant because the traction spur is one of the few radiographic findings to have a positive correlation with low back symptoms,[29] just as segmental instability is known to be symptomatic.[2,3,25,26,27]

As in the cervical spine, dynamic (kinematic) radiographic studies are the methods used to diagnose hypermobility and instability in the lumbar spine. The earliest procedure used flexion and

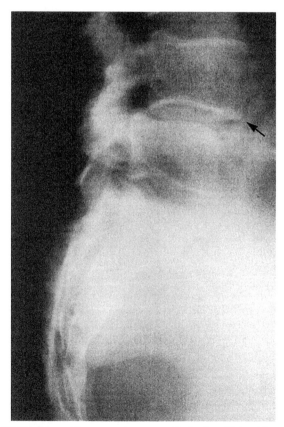

Figure 8-9   Degenerative anterolisthesis of L4 with decreased intervertebral disc space and sclerosis of the L4-5 facet articulations. It is not possible on this static neutral radiograph to determine the stability of this motion segment.

extension lateral lumbar views taken after the patients actively positioned themselves at the extreme of these ranges of motion.* This method is still widely used and, although incomplete in the assessment of intersegmental motion, gives valuable information as to intersegmental instability, along with being relatively easy to perform and interpret in the clinical setting.[2,26,30,34] Most proponents of flexion-extension radiographs have the patient perform the maneuvers actively in the standing position.[2,3,33,34] Hanley et al.[30] and Dupuis et al.,[25] however, recommend that flexion-extension views be performed with the patient recumbent in the lateral decubitus position. They state that recumbency increases the global range of motion by decreasing the effects of low back pain on the total excursion. Sitting flexion-extension radiographs also have been used, adding the effects of gravity while providing pelvic stabilization.[32] Dvorak et al.[31] are strong proponents of "passive" rather than "active" standing flexion-extension radiographs of the lumbar spine. They claim that the passive examination shows more intersegmental hypermobilities and instabilities than the active procedure because the patient with back pain will "not bend as far as the spine will permit." It is well recognized that the presence of low back pain influences the reliability of the findings obtained with flexion-extension radiography.[25,30,31,33]

Ora Friberg[4] in 1986 pioneered a new approach to diagnosing lumbar intersegmental instability. His study found that traction-compression lateral lumbar radiographs were superior to flexion-extension lateral radiographs for the diagnosis of instability in patients with anterolisthesis or retrolisthesis diagnosed on the neutral lateral films (Figure 8-10). Furthermore, he found that the severity of low back pain had no correlation with the severity of the listhesis noted on the neutral films but correlated significantly to the quantity of translatory movement found with traction-compression. This has been further substantiated by Sandoz.[3] Friberg's radiographic method appears to have two specific advantages over

flexion-extension radiographs, specifically that patients with back pain tolerate the procedure better with less motion artifact, and that reproducibility and comparability of traction-compression radiography in regard to patient positioning and measurement collection seems to be significantly better.[4]

Flexion-extension and traction-compression kinematic studies remain the primary methods used to diagnose intersegmental instabilities because of their accessibility and ease of interpretation. Several studies have stated that a translation of greater than 3 to 4 mm in the sagittal plane from full flexion to full extension is indicative of intersegmental instability.[24,26,28] When using these figures, however, one must remember that they are only a "rule of thumb" and that there remains a wide range of "normal" intersegmental motion within and between subjects.[25,30,32]

Digital videofluoroscopy (DVF) is much better than plain film for the detection of segmental instability.[24,35] DVF not only detects intersegmental translation and angular measurement, but it is also used to calculate the instantaneous centers of rotation (ICRs) for each motion segment. Although the radiation dose is considerably less than for plain film radiology of the lumbar spine, the expense of the procedure makes it impractical for routine use by the clinician in daily practice.

Lateral bending lumbar radiographs have been used in the past to detect aberrant and excessive intersegmental motion.[36-38] This radiographic procedure has fallen out of favor recently because of poor interrater reliability in interpretation of the intersegmental motion, in addition to the fact that "abnormal" motion patterns were shown to have no correlation with low back pain.[36,37]

Causes of Lumbar Spine Hypermobility and Instability

As previously mentioned, acute severe trauma is a fairly rare but possible cause of instability in a lumbar motion segment. Other causes include repetitive microtraumas, either work related or sports related, hereditary predisposition to hypermobility, spondylolytic spondylolisthesis, hormonal

---

*References 2-4, 8, 24, 26, 28, 30-34.

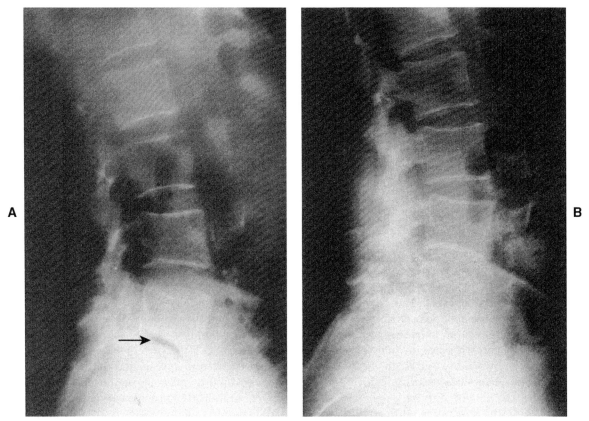

Figure 8-10   Traction (A) and compression (B) lateral lumbar radiographs. Note the vacuum phenomenon visible on the traction radiograph only. The sagittal plane translation of L5 measured approximately 3 mm from traction to compression.

influences (estrogen), adjacent hypomobilities or blocked vertebrae, spinal fusions, and wide laminectomies. However, the most common cause of lumbar spinal instability is undoubtedly degeneration of the intervertebral joints.[2,4,8,25-28]

Degenerative Disc Disease

Kirkaldy-Willis and Cassidy[2,8] identified three phases of the degenerative process affecting lumbar motion segments. The first phase is characterized by segmental dysfunction and decompensation presenting as a posterior joint syndrome or diminished functional capability of the back musculature. They claim that although there may be early pathologic changes in the intervertebral disc and facet joints in this first phase, these

changes are not readily apparent on radiographs. It is not until the second stage, referred to as the unstable phase of the degenerative process, that these radiographic changes become evident. They further state that the patient's symptoms are directly related to this abnormal increased intersegmental movement. Kinematic radiographic studies at this stage often show the increased intersegmental mobility,[2,28] suggesting that forceful manipulative procedures are contraindicated.[8] Sandoz[3] describes an additional phase characterized by episodic fixations of spinal motion segments. He notes that the unstable phase and the episodic joint-locking phase often coexist with much overlap. After the unstable phase, the spine stabilizes itself through the formation of osteophytes and pericapsular and intradiscal fibrosis (stage 3). This process may take many years with the end result being a fixed deformity and complete loss of intersegmental motion.[2,28] The clinical significance of this third phase of degeneration is that it alters the spinal canal dimensions because of the osteophytic formation resulting in potential lateral recess entrapment or spinal stenosis.[2,28]

Look at Figure 8-11 and evaluate the radiographic findings in the lumbar spine of this elderly man with longstanding low back pain. There is significant degenerative disc disease and facet arthrosis of the lower lumbar spine. Disc space narrowing is noted between L2 and L4 with anterolistheses at these levels. Additional findings include loss of lumbar lordosis, flexion between

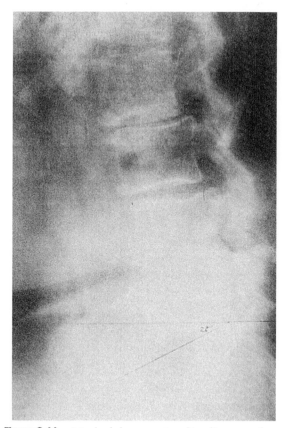

Figure 8-11 Marked degenerative disc disease and facet arthrosis of the lower lumbar spine resulting in anterolistheses of L2 and L3. Arteriosclerosis of the abdominal aorta and common iliac arteries is present.

L3 and L4, and calcification in the abdominal aorta and common iliac arteries.

Which if any of these findings are responsible for his low back pain? Although it may be hard to accept, the fact remains that there is little correlation between low back pain and the severity of degenerative arthritis seen radiographically.[29,39] The unstable phase of the degenerative process as just noted is usually symptomatic[2,25] but is associated with minimal radiographic findings of DJD. Therefore none of the findings found in the elderly gentleman's radiographs shown in Figure 8-11 may account for his symptoms.

The third phase of degeneration—that of "fixed deformity"—may be occurring in this patient, as evidenced by the significant anterior and posterior osteophytosis. Potential sequelae of this phase may be spinal stenosis of his lower lumbar spine and secondary hypermobilities or instabilities of the upper lumbar segments.[3,28] Clinical correlation is obviously indicated to detect lateral recess entrapment, central stenosis, or findings associated with hypermobility of L2 or L3. Based on the clinical findings in combination with the radiographic findings, flexion-extension or traction-compression radiographs may be indicated. However, these additional radiographs should only be taken with sufficient clinical justification and not as a routine procedure. If the patient does demonstrate evidence of nerve root entrapment or central stenosis, computed tomography (CT) or magnetic resonance imaging (MRI) images would be indicated.

Spondylolytic Spondylolisthesis
Defects in the pars interarticularis (spondylolysis) are present in approximately 5% to 7% of the population and involve the L5 vertebra in approximately 90% of cases.[20] The cause of these defects is now recognized to be stress fractures related to the upright posture. Much has been claimed about the clinical significance of spondylolysis and the often-resulting spondylolisthesis, with chiropractic and medical doctors offering inappropriate treatment and restricting the activities of these patients unnecessarily.[20] Pars interarticularis stress fractures usually occur in childhood and are an incidental

discovery on radiographs taken years later for other reasons.[4,20] Slippage usually occurs during the first 18 months to 2 years after the fracture and is therefore usually not unstable when discovered and, most likely, not the cause of the patient's low back pain.[26]

Friberg found that the severity of slippage of the vertebral body noted on neutral lateral lumbar radiographs had absolutely no correlation to low back pain.[4] Rather, back pain was significantly associated with the amount of translation in the sagittal plane found during traction-compression radiographs. Does this mean that every patient with radiographic evidence of spondylolysis should have flexion-extension or traction-compression radiographs done? Absolutely not! Most cases of spondylolytic spondylolisthesis are stable and of minimal clinical significance. If the patient does

not respond to conservative treatment and the clinician believes that instability may be present, traction-compression or flexion-extension radiographs are indicated. Excessive translation or angular motion in the sagittal plane is evidence of instability.

Figure 8-12 shows flexion and extension lateral lumbar radiographs of a patient with pars defects noted at L2. This is a rather unusual level for spondylolysis and correlated to the patient's area of complaint. The motion studies demonstrate translation of approximately 3 mm from full flexion to full extension and markedly increased intersegmental tilt (angular rotation) as compared with the adjacent levels. In this patient, forceful manipulative procedures to this motion segment would be contraindicated, and the clinician could claim that the spondylolytic spondylolisthesis was

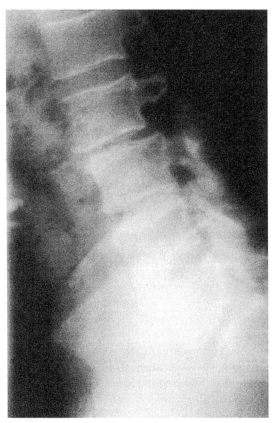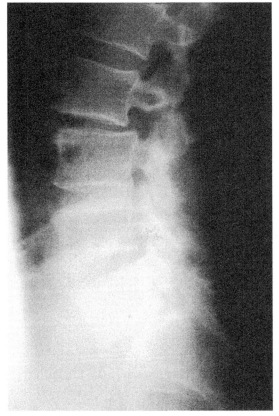

Figure 8-12   Spondylolysis with spondylolisthesis of L2, showing evidence of instability on flexion-extension radiographs.

most likely the cause of the back pain. Contrast this with the patient in Figure 8-13, who has pars defects at the common level of L5 but without any evidence of anterolisthesis. Flexion-extension radiographs were taken, and no evidence of instability is noted. These pars defects in this adult patient are therefore most likely not the cause of the low back pain and no contraindications to adjusting are noted on these radiographs.

Postsurgical Instability

The most common cause of postsurgical instability is the excessive removal of the supporting structures during decompression surgeries for nerve root entrapments.[28] The surgical removal of 30% to 50% of the articular facets may lead to instability. Plain film findings often show an anterolisthesis at the affected level that was not evident on the preoperative radiographs.[28] Even less radical spinal operations may lead to instability. Frymoyer and Selby[28] state that "20% of women who have undergone lumbar disc excision without removal of facet joints demonstrate signs of instability, usually at L4-5."

Look at the radiographs (Figure 8-14) of the middle-aged woman who presented with a long history of low back pain to a chiropractor. The most obvious finding is the absence of the spinous processes and laminae from L1 through L4 with no evidence of fusion. Additionally, note the moderate loss of disc height between L3 and L4 with anterolisthesis and left lateral listhesis at this level. The levoscoliosis also has its apex at the L3-4 level. All of these findings strongly suggest instability,

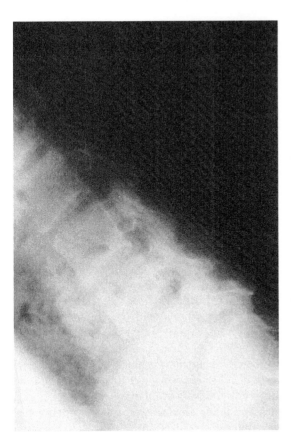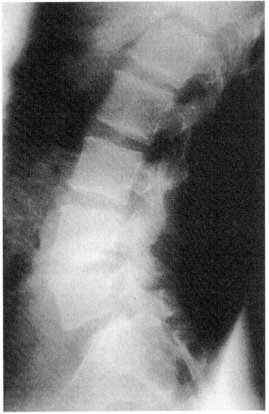

Figure 8-13 Flexion and extension lateral lumbar radiographs in a patient with spondylolysis of L5 but no evidence of instability.

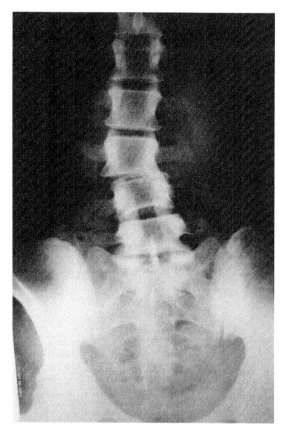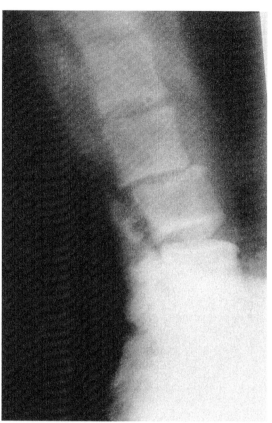

Figure 8-14   Laminectomy of L1 through L4 with no evidence of fusion. Loss of disc height is noted, along with both a laterolisthesis and retrolisthesis of L3. The levoscoliosis has its apex at the L3 level. Also noted is the diffuse bone sclerosis consistent with the patient's known osteopetrosis.

particularly at L3-4. You should have also noticed the diffuse marked increase in bone density. If you missed this significant finding, look at the "normal" L5 vertebra, which still possesses its posterior arch. This patient has osteopetrosis. Without this history, however, osteoblastic metastasis would be the first consideration. Osteopetrosis results in brittle bones that fracture easily, a factor very significant to the treating chiropractor. This case is a nice demonstration of the principle "The patient has the right to more than one condition."

Blocked Vertebrae

Surgically fused segments and congenitally blocked vertebrae may result in hypermobility or instability at the unfused motion segments above or below the block.[6,20] It has long been recognized that surgical fusion of one lumbar motion segment often causes eventual disc lesions at the adjacent superior motion segment caused by the excessive motion at that level induced by the surgical fusion. Not all surgical fusions, however, are successful at immobilizing the intended segments. Therefore assumptions cannot substitute for a careful clinical and radiologic examination of the area. Similarly, congenitally blocked vertebrae (Figure 8-15) lead to early degenerative disc disease at the adjacent levels, with these unfused motion segments passing through the unstable phase before osteophytic stabilization.[2,3,8] Just as in the cervical spine, there is no point in attempting to manipulate fused motion segments.

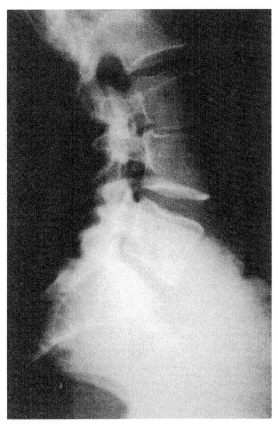

Figure 8-15 Classic congenital blocked vertebra L3-4.

Clinical Manifestations of Hypermobility and Instability in the Lumbar Spine

The clinical descriptions of patients presenting with hypermobility and instability are blurred and confusing because of the inconsistency in the use of the terminology. Those who do differentiate between these two conditions state that hypermobility is not necessarily symptomatic. It may be insignificant or reversible and, although it may lead to instability, this is not necessarily the case.[11,27]

In the early stages of the unstable phase, symptoms are often minor with the patient complaining of chronic, nagging, episodic low back pain.[2,25] This pain is often aggravated during specific movements such as extension or twisting—any movement that places strain on previously stretched ligaments.[25,28,40] However, movements in general may bring some temporary relief, and

these patients may have difficulty sitting still.[27,41] As the condition progresses, the interval between aggravating spinal movements and back pain becomes shorter and shorter to the point where any activity requiring axial pressure on the spine becomes symptomatic.[27,40] Several authors describe patient complaints of a "catching" sensation during specific spinal movements.[11,26,27] According to Dupuis et al.,[25] this is not a reliable or consistent finding.

Grieve[26] lists several clinical criteria that if present suggest lumbar instability. These include the following:

1. A history of much conservative treatment for low back pain and early morning stiffness
2. The presence of bilateral loin creases on observation from behind in nonobese or elderly patients
3. In earlier stages, surprisingly free, full, and painless movement, including straight leg raising (However, lumbar spine appears to "hinge" at one segment on extension.)
4. In some patients, a steadily increasing lumbosacral ache when extremes of spinal movement are sustained for 15 to 20 seconds
5. In later stages, cautious active movements, which often look rather precarious
6. A momentary catch or twinge distorting one or more lumbar movements—usually flexion, but sometimes others
7. A tendency to grasp the thighs for support when returning from flexion, with lordosis often maintained during flexion
8. Undue tenderness localized to one segment
9. A slight but unmistakable "boggy" feel on testing accessory movement with provocation of the lumbosacral ache or pain
10. Excessive movement on passive physiologic movement testing by comparison with adjacent segments

It is difficult for palpation alone to detect hypermobility.[3] A "boggy" end feel and overlying soft tissue edema are indicative of instability.[26,40] Palpation also may detect excessive segmental anteroposterior mobility by applying a posterior to anterior force to extend the patient's lumbar spine with the dorsum of the hand.[8] Uncoordinated muscle contractions or spasms during active forward flexion or localized deviations of motion may signify instability.[27]

Lumbar segmental hypermobility is too often overlooked, with incorrect interpretation of the clinical features leading to inappropriate therapeutic maneuvers. If the condition is not suggested, the confirming radiographic studies will not be done and the patient may receive a series of manipulative thrusts to the region. Although inappropriate, surprisingly, these adjustments may actually provide some temporary relief for the first few treatments,[26,41] after which they do not help and can actually worsen the condition.

Chiropractic Management of Lumbar Intersegmental Hypermobility/Instability

Conservative treatment begins by manipulating the adjacent fixed or hypomobile segments while avoiding hypermobile and unstable ones.[8] Sandoz[3] notes that dynamic instability is usually in the sagittal plane with concomitant fixation in lateroflexion and rotation. He emphasizes that the planes and directions of abnormal motion should always be mentioned. This should affect the types of manipulative procedures chosen. Muehlemann[41] emphasizes the importance of using "locking mechanisms" for adjacent hypermobile areas when adjusting fixations. He goes on to state that

> movement should be induced from the part of the spine that is not affected by hypermobilities, i.e., if a hypomobile L4-5 adjacent to a hypermobile L5-S1 is to be moved, movement should be induced from the superior part of the spine.

Furthermore, long-lever manipulative procedures should be avoided.[41]

Grieve[26] recommends "mobilization" of hypermobile (not unstable) segments within the normal range of accessory movement. He claims that this relieves the pain associated with the hypermobility and that in some cases no more need be done than to teach stabilization exercises. Stretching of the tight large muscles groups (iliopsoas, quadriceps, hamstrings, piriformis, quadratus lumborum) along

with trigger-point therapy in the smaller intersegmental muscles is helpful.[40]

Both Muehlemann[41] and Grieve[11,26] are strong proponents of progressive stabilization techniques, which require much dedication from both the patient and the physician. These stabilization techniques begin with short-lever isometric contractions, moving to continuously longer levers while avoiding trunk movements. These are started after 4 to 6 weeks of treatment of adjacent hypomobile segments. After 8 to 12 weeks of therapy, Muehlemann recommends guided and optimally measurable resistance exercises.[41] Posture should be improved by attempting to correct the tendency to hyperlordosis and by reducing obesity.[26,27] Activities that produce both compression and shear should be avoided. These include shoveling; lifting; playing handball, squash, racquetball, or tennis; cycling; and gardening.[27] Walking and swimming the backstroke or crawl are encouraged to increase overall fitness.[40]

It may be of comfort to both the patient and the doctor to remember that time alone will reduce hypermobility.[26,27] However, this may take years. Lumbosacral supports may be prescribed, but only if the doctor has a treatment plan intended to eliminate this support.[26]

Frymoyer and Selby[28] claim that although most standard conservative treatment programs are effective, there are some patients who have persistent symptoms. If the symptoms are exacerbated in extension and relieved by flexion, the patient may be helped by facet injection. If spinal fusion is contemplated, the specific area of segmental instability must be identified based on knowledge of coupled motion patterns and the surgical procedure must be tailored to it. By doing this, one may reduce the unacceptably high failure rate in the surgical management of degenerative spinal instability.[28]

Grieve summarizes the indications for surgical referral in those cases of lumbar segmental instability that fail to respond to appropriate conservative therapy.[26] These include the following:

1. The severity of symptoms
2. Lack of response to simple measures

3. The passage of time
4. Significant restriction of the patient's activities
5. Confidence as to the true origin of the pain

Lumbar segmental hypermobility is common and is often a transient stage affecting the lumbar spine; it frequently occurs as part of the degenerative process. Awareness of the frequency of this condition and the associated clinical features increases the diagnostic accuracy and the appropriateness of therapeutic choices for these patients.

Hypermobility and Instability of the Thoracic spine

Hypermobility and instability of the thoracic spine is less common than in the cervical and lumbar regions because of the stabilizing effect of the rib cage. Vertebral and costal joint dysfunction are often characterized by pain during respiration.[40] Diagnosis is more dependent on palpatory skills than through radiographic stress studies. Manual palpation of posterior to anterior (P-A) glide can test for excessive shear and instability, but has not been studied extensively.[42] With instability, there is a characteristic boggy sensation that indicates compromise of the segmental holding elements. As with other areas of the spine, areas of excessive motion in the thoracic region should be avoided when applying a manipulative thrust. Joint hypermobility in the thoracic region is difficult to stabilize due to respiratory excursion. Hypermobile subluxations of the costotransverse joints are not uncommon and occur secondarily to rotational trauma or a direct blow to the chest. The sympathetic chain may be affected by a change in the position of the head of the rib[43] or the sympathetic trunks may be compromised when spurring occurs on the anterolateral aspect of the vertebral bodies.[44] (See Chapter 14.)

Conclusion

The nonmanipulable subluxation is one in which manipulation is contraindicated because of excessive movement in the motion segment or the presence of fused or blocked segments make a forceful thrust useless. Stabilization of reversible hypermobility is desirable and manipulation is applied only occasionally to avoid aggravating the spinal segment. Instability that is not reversible may require surgery if severe and, in any case, contraindicates forceful manipulation. Segments above and below fused or blocked segments should be thoroughly evaluated for hypermobility that is often compensatory to a lack of segmental movement.

References

1. White AA, Panjabi MM. Clinical biomechanics of the spine. Philadelphia: JB Lippincott; 1978. p. 192.
2. Kirkaldy-Willis WH, Cassidy JD. Toward a more precise diagnosis of low back pain. In: Spine update 1984. San Francisco: Radiology Research and Education Foundation; 1983. p. 5-16.
3. Sandoz R. The natural history of a spinal degenerative lesion. Ann Swiss Chiro Assoc 1989;9:149-92.
4. Friberg O. Lumbar instability: a dynamic approach by traction-compression radiography. Spine 1987;12:119-29.
5. McGregor M, Mior SA. Anatomical and functional perspectives of the cervical spine. Part II. The "hypermobile" cervical spine. J Can Chiro Assoc 1989;33:177-83.
6. Henderson DJ, Dormon TM. Functional roentgenometric evaluation of the cervical spine in the sagittal plane. J Manipulative Physiol Ther 1985;8:219-27.
7. Gatterman MI. Indications for spinal manipulation in the treatment of back pain. ACA J Chiro 1982;16:51-66.
8. Cassidy JD, Potter GE. Motion examination of the lumbar spine. J Manipulative Physiol Ther 1979;2:151-8.
9. Lewit K. Manipulation: reflex therapy and/or restitution of impaired locomotor function. Manual Medicine 1986;2:99-100.
10. McGregor M, Mior S. Anatomical and functional perspectives of the cervical spine. Part III. The "unstable" cervical spine. J Can Chiro Assoc 1990;34:145-52.
11. Hertling D, Kessler RM. Management of common musculoskeletal disorders: physical therapy principles and methods. 2nd ed. Philadelphia: JB Lippincott; 1990. p. 522-3, 556-9.
12. Dvorak J, Froehlich D, Penning L, Baumgartner H, Panjabi MM. Functional radiographic diagnosis of the cervical spine: flexion/extension. Spine 1988;13:748-55.
13. Dvorak J, Panjabi MM, Grob D, Novotny JE, Antinnes JA. Clinical validation of functional flexion/extension radiographs of the cervical spine. Spine 1993;18:120-7.
14. Lind B, Sihlbom H, Nordwall A, Malchau H. Normal range of motion of the cervical spine. Arch Phys Med Rehabil 1989;70:692-5.
15. Hviid H. Functional radiography of the cervical spine. Ann Swiss Chiro Assoc 1965;3:37-65.

16. McGregor M, Mior S. Anatomical and functional perspectives of the cervical spine. Part I. The "normal" cervical spine. J Can Chiro Assoc 1989;33:123-9.

17. Amebo B, Worth D, Bogduk N. Instantaneous axis of rotation of the typical cervical motion segments. II. Optimization of technical errors. Clin Biomech 1991;6:38-46.

18. White AA, Johnson RM, Panjabi MM, Southwick WO. Biomechanical analysis of clinical stability in the cervical spine. Clin Orthop 1975;109:85-96.

19. Gehweiler JA, Osborne RL, Becker RF. The radiology of vertebral trauma. Philadelphia: WB Saunders; 1980. p. 99-100, 215-7, 229, 236, 267, 273.

20. Yochum TR, Rowe LJ. Essentials of skeletal radiology. Vols. 1 and 2. Baltimore: Williams & Wilkins; 1987. p. 100, 103-5, 176, 244-5, 269, 431, 434.

21. Reich C, Dvorak J. The functional evaluation of craniocervical ligaments in sidebending using x-rays. Manual Medicine 1986;2:108-13.

22. Chapman S, Nakielny R. Aids to radiological differential diagnosis. London: Bailliere Tindall; 1984. p. 53.

23. Resnick D, Niwayama G. Diagnosis of bone and joint disorders. Vol. 2. Philadelphia: WB Saunders; 1981. p. 1370-82.

24. Mick T, Phillips RB, Breen A. Spinal imaging and spinal biomechanics. In: Haldeman S, editor. Principles and practice of chiropractic. 2nd ed. East Norwalk, CT: Appleton and Lange; 1992. p. 402-12.

25. Dupuis PR, Yong-Hing K, Cassidy JD, Kirkaldy-Willis WH. Radiological diagnosis of degenerative lumbar spinal instability. Spine 1985;10:262-76.

26. Grieve GP. Lumbar instability. Physiotherapy 1982;68:2-9.

27. Paris SV. Physical signs of instability. Spine 1985;10:277-9.

28. Frymoyer JW, Selby DK. Segmental instability: rationale for treatment. Spine 1985;10:280-6.

29. Frymoyer JW, Newberg A, Pope MH, Wilder DG, Clements J, MacPherson B. Spine radiographs in patients with low back pain. J Bone Joint Surg 1984;66A:1048-55.

30. Hanley EN, Matteri RE, Frymoyer JW. Accurate roentgenographic determination of lumbar flexion-extension. Clin Orthop 1976;115:145-8.

31. Dvorak J, Panjabi MM, Chang DG, Theiler R, Gross D. Functional radiographic diagnosis of the lumbar spine: flexion-extension and lateral bending. Spine 1991;16:562-71.

32. Hayes MA, Howard TC, Gruel CR, Kopta JA. Roentgenographic evaluation of lumbar spine flexion-extension in asymptomatic individuals. Spine 1989;14:327-31.

33. Pearcy M, Portek I, Shapherd J. The effect of low back pain on lumbar spinal movements measured by three-dimensional x-ray analysis. Spine 1985;10:150-3.

34. Sandoz R. Technique and interpretation of functional radiography of the lumbar spine. Ann Swiss Chiro Assoc 1965;3:66-110.

35. Shalen PR. Radiological techniques for diagnosis of lumbar disc degeneration. Spine: State of the Art Reviews 1989;3(1):27-48.

36. Haas M, Nyiendo J, Peterson C, Thiel H, Sellers T, Dal Mas E et al. Lumbar motion trends and correlation with low back pain. Part I. A roentgenological evaluation of coupled lumbar motion in lateral bending. J Manipulative Physiol Ther 1992;15:145-58.

37. Haas M, Nyiendo J, Peterson C, Thiel H, Sellers T, Cassidy D et al. Interrater reliability of roentgenological evaluation of the lumbar spine in lateral bending. J Manipulative Physiol Ther 1990;13:179-89.

38. Weitz EM. The lateral bending sign. Spine 1981;6:388-97.

39. Magora A, Schwartz A. Relation between the low back pain syndrome and x-ray findings. I. Degenerative osteoarthritis. Scand J Rehabil Med 1976;8:115-25.

40. Panzer DM, Gatterman MI. Disorders of the lumbar spine. In: Gatterman MI. Chiropractic management of spine related disorders. Baltimore: Williams & Wilkins; 2003. p. 191-3.

41. Muehlemann D, Zahnd F. Die lumbale segmentale hypermobilitaet. Manuelle Medizin 1993;31:47-54.

42. Pope M, Frymoyer JW, Krag MH. Diagnosing instability. Clin Orthop 1992;269:60.

43. Giles LGF, Singer KP. Clinical anatomy and management of thoracic pain. Oxford: Butterworth-Heinemann; 2000. p. 280.

44. Gatterman MI, Panzer DM. Disorders of the thoracic spine. In: Gatterman MI. Chiropractic management of spine related disorders. Baltimore: Williams & Wilkins; 2003. p. 208.

Part TWO

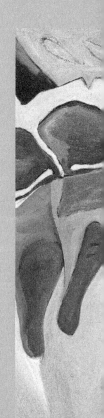

The Subluxation Complex

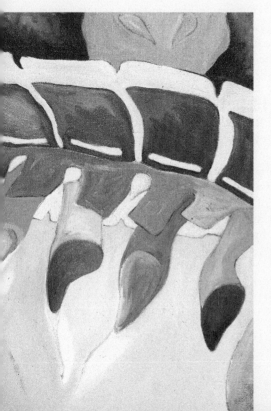

T he subluxation complex is a theoretical model of motion segment dysfunction (subluxation) that incorporates the complex interactions of pathologic changes in nerve, muscle, ligamentous, vascular, and connective tissues. First described by Faye as a paradigm shift from the static misalignment or "bone out of place" concept of subluxation, the vertebral subluxation complex has served as a more dynamic and inclusive teaching and research model for the chiropractic profession. According to Kuhn, a paradigm prepares students for membership in the scientific community with which they will later practice. By joining a group who learned the bases of their field from the same model, subsequent practice provides a basis for agreement over fundamentals. An accepted paradigm must seem better than alternatives but does not necessarily explain all the facts with which it can be confronted. It suggests which experiments are worth performing and selects phenomena in more detail for more rigorous study. Supporting Palmer's concept that the neurologic component of the subluxation is the cornerstone of chiropractic theory, the subluxation complex provides a structure to better understand the foundation principles of chiropractic theory and provides a paradigm for chiropractic education and research.

Chapter 9 "The Vertebral Subluxation Complex" presents an overview of the subluxation complex paradigm, outlining the areas affected by the articular subluxation. The interaction of the pathologic changes of the nerve, muscle, ligamentous, vascular, and connective tissue components is discussed. Taking the subluxation concept beyond that of a biomechanical lesion, this chapter explores the functional manifestations associated with the articular lesion.

Chapter 10 "Theoretic Models of Subluxation" discusses the proposed causative agents put forth to explain the misalignment, aberrant movement, and dysfunction characteristic of the subluxation. Articular adhesions, ligamentous shortening, meniscoid entrapment and extrapment, muscle spasm, and mechanical locking have all been implicated as causative agents of the subluxation. The rationale and supporting evidence for these suggested causes are presented.

Chapter 11 "Kinesiology: An Essential Approach toward Understanding the Chiropractic Subluxation" emphasizes the aberrant movement component of the subluxation. Considered the primary element in the hierarchy of the subluxation complex, the kinesiopathology that both causes and results from altered movement in the spinal motion segment is examined. Both normal and abnormal movement are considered, and the role the muscle spindle plays in each is presented.

Chapter 12 "Buckling: A Biomedical Model of Subluxation" presents original research that goes beyond the traditional theories of chiropractic. The biomechanics of spinal motion segment buckling are presented with supporting evidence for this model.

Chapter 13 "Three Neurophysiologic Theories on the Chiropractic Subluxation" reviews three theories that explain the proposed effects of the subluxation on the nervous system. Used to visualize the abstract principles involved, models of intervertebral encroachment, altered somatic afferent input, and dentate ligament and cord distortion are discussed. These theories present the neurologic foundations of chiropractic theory in light of current supporting evidence.

Chapter 14 "Vertebral Subluxation and the Anatomic Relationships of the Autonomic Nervous System" emphasizes the important association of the autonomic nervous system with the effects of the subluxation complex. The potential for widespread changes in the parasympathetic and sympathetic nervous systems caused by vertebral subluxation is a controversial topic fundamental to the foundations of chiropractic principles. The anatomic relationships relative to this debate are documented, with the physiologic implications for somatic dysfunction outlined.

Chapter 15 The neuroimmunologic implications of spinal manipulation are presented in "Review of the Systemic Effects of Spinal Manipulation." Observed changes in the immune system after manipulation support the theory that improved neurologic function has beneficial effects on overall health. The possible role of manipulation in modulating neuroimmunologic function is discussed.

Chapter 16 "Spinal Cord Mechanisms of Referred Pain and Related Neuroplasticity" explores the scientific evidence that convergent input onto spinal neurons produces widespread neurologic activity. Studies evaluating the nociceptive "traffic flow" involved in spinal pain are discussed. Theories of somatosensory input with neuronal responses to mechanical and sympathetic stimuli produced by manipulation are proposed.

9

The Vertebral Subluxation Complex

David R. Seaman and

L. John Faye

Key Words   Subluxation complex, kinesiopathology, histopathology, pro-inflammatory biochemical changes

After reading this chapter you should be able to answer the following questions:

Question 1   How are homeostatic neural mechanisms altered by the subluxation complex?

Question 2   What methods do chiropractors use to assess the subluxation complex?

Question 3   How do chiropractors reduce the effects of subluxation complex?

Many chiropractors maintain clinical practices for 40 or 50 years, and they do so because of the profound effects they have witnessed after patients receive a chiropractic adjustment. Patients return again and again because they feel the chiropractor offers something special, something different from the classic medical encounter. In this regard, we believe that there are vitalistic, psychospiritual aspects of patient care that occur during the hands-on chiropractic encounter. While science cannot describe this immaterial aspect of chiropractic care, much data now exist regarding spinal dysfunction that can help to describe the positive physiological outcomes related to pain relief, reduction of visceral symptoms, and feelings of wellness.[1,2] Readers should be aware that such research does not validate the existence of subluxation or that subluxations are corrected by the adjustment. We can only say with certainty that the chiropractic clinical encounter offers positive outcomes, which is the likely reason why chiropractic has lived on despite attempts to sanction and eliminate the profession.

This chapter represents an attempt to describe the subluxation complex in a pathological and pathophysiological context and begins with the history and development of the subluxation complex as a theory. Key terminology and conceptual issues are also examined, such as why the subluxation complex is a pathological process, one that is not synonymous with pain. This leads to a discussion about how the subluxation complex is likely to be a condition that affects a significant percentage of our populace. The remainder of the chapter focuses on the relationship between the subluxation complex and the nervous system. For example, contemporary research suggests that the subluxation complex stimulates the nociceptive afferent system, which can lead to a variety of symptomatic presentations. Additionally, research suggests that the subluxation complex alters neural homeostatic mechanisms such that the nervous system actually malfunctions in a manner that perpetuates the subluxation complex. Finally, various treatment options are briefly discussed; their application is based on the pathophysiologic changes that are known to occur in the spine.

This chapter is written on a level that will challenge students and clinicians to apply basic science knowledge so that they can expand their clinical understanding of the subluxation complex. On a practical level, this can translate into improved patient care and an enhanced ability to communicate with other health care professionals and legislative bodies.

Subluxation Complex History and Development

When Faye first proposed the subluxation complex in 1967, much of the chiropractic world still viewed subluxation as a misaligned vertebra; that is, a vertebra that had moved out of alignment with respect to supraadjacent and infraadjacent segments. Subluxation was considered an entity that existed somewhere between normal function and disease, a concept that was and still is difficult for those outside the chiropractic profession to understand.

To describe the nature of the effect of subluxation on human beings, the chiropractic profession put forth the term "dis-ease," which connotes a lack of "ease," wellness, or normal function within the body. The theory goes on to suggest that if this state of "dis-ease" induced by spinal subluxation is allowed to persist, then the body's natural adaptive, recuperative, or homeostatic powers (referred to in chiropractic terminology as innate intelligence) will be compromised and disease will develop within some organ system of the body.

Subluxations were thought to block the flow of innate intelligence at the intervertebral foramen of the subluxated vertebra, which would be most compromising for the organs and tissues related to that spinal level. Another belief was that subluxations at the atlas would be most devastating to an individual because the flow of innate intelligence would be blocked at the atlas, thereby depriving the entire body of the organizational energy needed to function normally and rendering it susceptible to diseases.

It was believed that, due to birth trauma and normal childhood injuries, most people had atlas subluxations. Clearly, this theory places spinal subluxation as the cause of most diseases. To date, this theory has yet to be supported by objective evidence and essentially creates an incongruent educational scenario for chiropractic students. The result is that they learn about chiropractic technique and theory in one classroom and then learn about basic sciences in another classroom without any perceivable connection between the two. In essence, chiropractic students would begin college and enter two different educational tracks, the subluxation and adjusting track that trains one to be a chiropractor who adjusts the spine, and the separate and distinct basic science track that allows one to pass boards and obtain a chiropractic license.

This educational disconnect was obvious to Faye while he was teaching at Anglo-European College during the 1960s. He also realized that chiropractors were essentially left with no conceptual model of subluxation to utilize in clinical practice, save for the bone-out-of-place theory. After much thought and study, in 1967 Faye presented his students with the term *subluxation complex* and the associated heuristic model that was eventually popularized in the late 1970s and early 1980s in the United States by the Motion Palpation Institute (Figure 9-1).

Faye's original intent was to create a heuristic model of subluxation, that is, a speculative formulation to serve as a guide for the investigation of the subluxation. The original subluxation complex was to serve three main purposes: (1) that chiropractors would be able to relate subluxation to the world in kinesiologic, physiologic, and pathophysiologic terms that are already accepted, (2) that chiropractic would have a dynamic and scientific model of subluxation that could be appropriately researched, and (3) that chiropractors could properly function as holistic, vitalistic doctors with a strong scientific foundation. To date, none of these original intents have been widely understood or practically realized. In fact, the original dynamic subluxation complex has been converted by some into a static so-called component model[3-5] that has been utilized for describing a condition that can only be affected by an adjustment.

Readers should be aware that Figure 9-1 was utilized throughout the 1970s and 1980s prior to publication in Schafer and Faye's 1989 text.[6] Notice the components of the chiropractic therapeutic approach for subluxation reduction include the following:
1. Adjustive procedures
2. Reflex techniques
3. Exercise
4. Diet, supplementation
5. Postural advice
6. Modalities
7. Socio-occupational advice
8. Other (open-ended to include for new techniques in patient care that fall within the scope of chiropractic care)

This armamentarium of treatments was recommended because the adjustment cannot magically resolve all the components of the subluxation complex, such as inflammation, the stress reaction, or atrophic muscles. In fact, it is entirely possible that the profound analgesic effect of the adjustment can mask the presence of underlying pathologies.[7] This is certainly inconsistent with the goals of a holistic, vitalistic doctor of the type that Faye envisioned chiropractors to be. Seaman[8] considered this problem and also thought the terms *subluxation* and *subluxation complex* might be too strongly associated in the minds of chiropractors with an "adjustment only" treatment approach. He proposed the term *joint complex dysfunction* and also listed causes and treatments that turned out to be consistent with Faye's original model. Thereafter, Seaman emphasized getting at the biochemical causes,[9,10] while others, including DeFranca,[11] Liebenson,[12] Murphy,[13] Stude,[14] and Troyanovich,[15] focused on addressing the deconditioned myopathological spine with exercise. Each of the authors subsequent to Faye also understood that the subluxation complex, or spinal dysfunction, could not be effectively addressed with the adjustment alone.

As outlined in Figure 9-1, the adjustment is thought to affect the movement component directly and may have an indirect effect on the other components. Thorough resolution of the subluxation complex depends on maintaining

THE SUBLUXATION COMPLEX

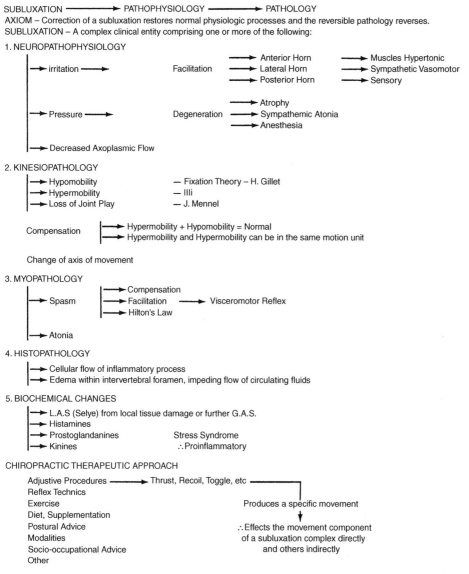

SUBLUXATION ————————► PATHOPHYSIOLOGY ————————► PATHOLOGY

AXIOM – Correction of a subluxation restores normal physiologic processes and the reversible pathology reverses.

SUBLUXATION – A complex clinical entity comprising one or more of the following:

1. NEUROPATHOPHYSIOLOGY

────► irritation ───────►   Facilitation ────► Anterior Horn   ────► Muscles Hypertonic
                                              ────► Lateral Horn   ────► Sympathetic Vasomotor
                                              ────► Posterior Horn   ────► Sensory

────► Pressure ───────►   Degeneration ────► Atrophy
                                              ────► Sympathemic Atonia
                                              ────► Anesthesia

────► Decreased Axoplasmic Flow

2. KINESIOPATHOLOGY

────► Hypomobility   — Fixation Theory – H. Gillet
────► Hypermobility   — IIIi
────► Loss of Joint Play   — J. Mennel

Compensation   ────► Hypermobility + Hypomobility = Normal
                ────► Hypermobility and Hypermobility can be in the same motion unit

Change of axis of movement

3. MYOPATHOLOGY

────► Spasm   ────► Compensation
                ────► Facilitation ────► Visceromotor Reflex
                ────► Hilton's Law

────► Atonia

4. HISTOPATHOLOGY

────► Cellular flow of inflammatory process
────► Edema within intervertebral foramen, impeding flow of circulating fluids

5. BIOCHEMICAL CHANGES

────► L.A.S (Selye) from local tissue damage or further G.A.S.
────► Histamines
────► Prostoglandanines   Stress Syndrome
────► Kinines   ∴ Proinflammatory

CHIROPRACTIC THERAPEUTIC APPROACH

Adjustive Procedures ————————► Thrust, Recoil, Toggle, etc
Reflex Technics
Exercise   Produces a specific movement
Diet, Supplementation
Postural Advice   ∴ Effects the movement component
Modalities   of a subluxation complex directly
Socio-occupational Advice   and others indirectly
Other

RATIONALE FOR THE ADJUSTMENT

(A) Find the hypomobility; (B) use adjustive procedure to mobilize the fixation; (C) recheck to confirm that movement has improved. Therapeutic approach is then applied to other components of the subluxation complex and their causes; therefore, a holistic, multicausal interdisciplinary approach for each patient's health problems. The progosis depends on the reversibility of the pathology, the restoration of normal function, and the ability to keep the joints free of subluxation-fixations and other causes of malfunction.

PREVENTION – Regular motion palpation examinations to discover early aberrant motion, especially fixations to prevent the subluxation complex from developing.

Figure 9-1   The original subluxation complex theory.

joint motion with adjustment and other passive forms of therapy, such as myofascial care and various electrical modalities, and on removing the other causes of disease, such as poor nutrition, sedentary lifestyle, smoking, and other unhealthy factors. Without utilizing this holistic, vitalistic approach, the chiropractor functions exactly like the medical doctors we criticize for not getting at the cause of the patient's problem. These may be hard words to swallow for some, but the assessment is nonetheless accurate.

Consider a patient who develops the subluxation complex and back pain (a symptom of some of the subluxation syndromes) due to bad posture, a lack of exercise, and a proinflammatory diet. Medical doctors will medicate or perform surgery on dysfunctional joints, while chiropractors adjust them. If neither addresses the causes, then there is no philosophical difference between medical and chiropractic doctors, just different methods of treating a disease. We use the term *disease* because certain components of the subluxation complex (histopathology and biochemical changes) are found in all diseases.[16,17]

How should we view the subluxation complex? First, it should be considered a concept or conceptual model, not as a definitive entity that exists only if all components are present. Second, the subluxation complex should be viewed as a pathology, which by definition is represented by cell and/or tissue changes or adaptations that are no longer considered normal in the context of biomechanics, biochemistry, physiology, or anatomy.[17] Like other diseases, the subluxation complex has no definitive or measurable beginning point, and we cannot arbitrarily state that we have cleared our patients of this condition with an adjustment or a combination of treatments mentioned in Figure 9-1. Third, the subluxation complex should be viewed as a generator of symptoms, such as pain and visceral or autonomic symptoms.[2] The subluxation complex is also likely to act as a stressor that participates in driving Selye's general adaptation syndrome.[2,18] Fourth, the subluxation complex should be viewed as a local condition that is a reflection and/or a component of systemic

body dysfunction or deconditioning, i.e., ill health. The term *deconditioning syndrome* describes patients with (1) the degeneration and atrophy that occurs in hypomobile and hypermobile spinal tissues, referred to in this chapter as the subluxation complex, (2) a reduction in cardiovascular fitness, (3) pain, and (4) subclinical chronic inflammation that drives both the subluxation complex and other chronic diseases.[8,10,19] It should be clear that the deconditioning syndrome is not a synonym for the subluxation complex; rather, the subluxation complex is a component of the deconditioning syndrome.

With these four perspectives of the subluxation complex in mind, the chiropractor has to make a choice. We can manipulate joints to theoretically "put bones back in place" or to "treat" mechanical low back pain, which can result in positive clinical outcomes. Or we can strive to be holistic, vitalistic doctors who offer multiple therapeutic approaches to improve both spinal and systemic function and bring the body closer to a state of optimal physical, mental, and social well-being, i.e., health. Figure 9-2 illustrates the deconditioning process and related treatments.

The remainder of this chapter will focus on the nature of the subluxation complex, the local spinal problem. However, we should not forget the bigger picture. Although the subluxation complex can generate various symptoms, we must remember that the subluxation complex is a component of the systemic deconditioning syndrome.

Subluxation Complex: A Term of Convention

Faye proposed the term *subluxation complex* because the classic chiropractic subluxation that conceptually eludes other practitioners and is only amenable to chiropractic care has not been demonstrated to exist. The question of whether bones do move out of place by themselves, occlude the intervertebral foramen, press on spinal nerves, and interfere with the transmission of mental impulses has not been resolved by the

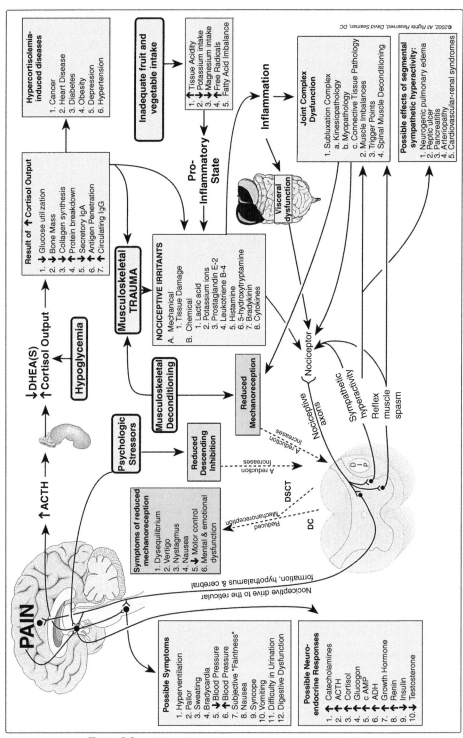

Figure 9-2   The subluxation complex causes and effects.

publication of any credible evidence that lends support to this theory, nor is there proof that this type of lesion can be corrected with an adjustment. We are *not saying definitively* that this historical variety of subluxation does not exist; only that convincing evidence does not support its existence or postadjustment correction. Further, our view is consistent with that of Langworthy, Smith, and Paxon, who published a text in 1906 entitled *Modernized Chiropractic,* wherein they proposed that chiropractic adjustments address motion restriction, not bones out of place.[20]

To date, a significant body of literature has demonstrated that injury and sedentary lifestyles will produce changes in spinal mobility,[21-24] alterations in neurological activity,[2,8,25-27] spinal muscle atrophy,[28-30] histopathological changes,[21,22,24] and proinflammatory biochemical changes,[8,10,17] i.e., the subluxation complex. Clearly, the articular subluxation (see Part One) and the subluxation complex are different concepts about spinal dysfunction. The only similarity is the word *subluxation;* the modifying word *complex* changes the character of the lesion as outlined in Figure 9-1.

Faye would have preferred to drop the word *subluxation.* He knew, however, that simply trying to change the subluxation paradigm from a static and mechanistic model to a dynamic and vitalistic one would be difficult enough, much less simultaneously suggesting that we no longer utilize the word subluxation at all. The term *subluxation complex* was selected as a matter of convention that included a dynamic model dating back to 1906. Faye's hope was that the chiropractic profession would move smoothly toward a dynamic model consistent with physiological and pathophysiological evidence of the day. Regrettably, this has not happened to an adequate degree, exemplified by the fact that different chiropractors, different chiropractic colleges, and different chiropractic associations define subluxation in very dissimilar fashions. (See Chapter 1.) Some still advocate the notion that subluxation is solely a bony misalignment that can be corrected by replacing the malpositioned vertebra while others embrace the "subluxation complex" but do not comprehend that it is a heuristic model.

The Subluxation Complex Is Not Synonymous with Back Pain

We have chosen to emphasize that the subluxation complex is not synonymous with back pain because this seems to be a misunderstood topic. Ultimately, debates about whether the subluxation complex is associated with pain and debates about the existence of the subluxation complex illustrate that our profession has not adequately applied the principles of pathology and neuroscience to the spine.

Pain is a symptom that is considered a component of subluxation syndromes, but it need not be present for the subluxation complex to exist. Similarly, heart disease, cancer, diabetes, Alzheimer's disease, cirrhosis, osteoporosis, and all other chronic diseases are known to exist long before symptoms appear. Why should this be any different for the subluxation complex? Research has clearly demonstrated that pathologic changes of the spinal column, which we call the subluxation complex, may exist without symptoms. Consider that significant disc herniations can be present in individuals without back pain[31] and that atrophic changes and fatty infiltration of spinal muscles exist in 45% of asymptomatic individuals.[29]

Strained and biomechanically stressed tissues will release chemical mediators of inflammation that constitute the biochemical changes of the subluxation complex. It is known that the cells of injured discs and joint tissue release chemical mediators, such as proinflammatory eicosanoids (prostaglandin-E2, leukotriene-B4, thromboxane-A2) and proinflammatory cytokines, such as interleukin-1 and tumor necrosis factor.[32,33] These biochemical changes that we associate with the subluxation complex can stimulate spinal nociceptors and generate the back pain we commonly encounter.[2,9,10] Initially, such biochemical changes can occur without obvious signs of degeneration, inflammation, and nociception and without the generation of symptoms—the way that every chronic disease begins.[17]

In summary, it is clearly inappropriate to equate the subluxation complex with low back pain; rather, the subluxation complex should be viewed as a promoter of low back dysfunction and as component of the deconditioning syndrome. Moreover, it is important to understand that treatment of the subluxation complex and the deconditioning syndrome does not end merely because back pain resolves.

Who Suffers with the Subluxation Complex?

Due to the various definitions and notions that chiropractors harbor regarding "subluxation," the answer to the question posed in this heading will result in a wide variety of responses. To adequately consider the existence of the subluxation complex, we must examine what is known about the pathological and pathophysiological changes that occur in the spine.

It is important to recall that the subluxation complex was originally defined as a spinal condition characterized by neuropathophysiology, kinesiopathology, myopathology, histopathology, and biochemical abnormalities, pathological changes that occur in most diseases/dysfunctional tissues.[17] We must further remember that the subluxation complex is merely the word chiropractors use to describe pathological changes that occur in the spine and extremities; it is not an entity that is peculiar to the chiropractic profession.

If we were to say that loss of function or motion, altered visual appearance, focal tenderness, warmth, instability, and neurovascular dysfunction are all clues that reveal the subluxation complex, most chiropractors would agree. However, such examination findings were listed in an article about sports injuries of the elbow that stated these findings "are all clues to elbow injury."[34] If a chiropractor trained in extremities were to encounter these findings, he or she might reasonably refer to the condition as a subluxation complex of the elbow.

Waddell[23] explains that the key concept for osteopathy, chiropractic, manual medicine, and physical therapy is painful musculoskeletal dysfunction. This painful dysfunction arises in response to abnormal forces imposed on or generated within the musculoskeletal system that relate to abnormal posture or abnormal joint movement. He advances the term *musculoskeletal dysfunction,* which includes several components, such as abnormalities of posture, abnormal joint movement (hypermobility and hypomobility), muscle dysfunction, connective tissue dysfunction, muscle imbalances, and neurophysiologic changes that include abnormal sensory input and abnormal neurophysiologic processing.[23] Clearly, Waddell's description of musculoskeletal dysfunction is nearly identical to our subluxation complex. Additionally, Kirkaldy-Willis[24] provides a similar description of pathological changes that occur in the spines of patients with back pain. The work of Waddell and Kirkaldy-Willis gives the distinct impression that anyone with back pain must suffer from pathological changes in the spine that chiropractors call the subluxation complex. In other words, the subluxation complex is a collection of pathologies and pain is a potential symptom.

Concerning the terminology used to describe the subluxation complex, readers should be aware that pain is an outcome of neuropathophysiology as are visceral symptoms.[1,2] Consider that under normal circumstances, nociceptors are not activated. They have very high thresholds for activation, requiring a noxious, injurious stimulus. Accordingly, pain is due to tissue injury or abnormalities that initiate the firing of the normally quiescent nociceptive system. This equates with the terms *neuropathophysiology* or *nervous system irritation* when put in the context of historical subluxation complex terminology. *Nerve interference* is an inappropriate term when we are dealing with an increased level of nervous system activity in the presence of pain. Palmer wrote that the "transmission of physiological impulses, which by augmentation or diminution, become pathological."[35]

Just how common is back pain, a neuropathophysiologic manifestation of the subluxation complex? In a study commissioned by the Merck Corporation, we are told that 9 out of 10 Americans suffer with some sort of pain.[36] Low back pain remains the leading cause of lost work days and the sixth most costly medical condition with a recurrence rate of 70% to 90%,[37] which suggests that the subluxation complex is a quite a common condition.

How common is the myopathology component of the subluxation complex? Lumbar paraspinal muscles in 74 so-called healthy volunteers ranging in age from 19 to 74 years were examined with MRI. Subjects in all age groups demonstrated paraspinal muscle degeneration, the degree of which increased with age. Muscle degeneration was characterized by diminished muscle size and infiltration of fat. Muscle degeneration is stated to be as common as disc degeneration in the lumbar area.[28] In a follow-up study, the authors evaluated the trunk muscles in chronic low back pain patients and in matched control subjects; all participants ranged in age from 30 to 47 years. A total of 45% of so-called healthy controls were deemed to have paraspinal muscle degeneration. The percentage rises for those in the moderate and severe pain groups and actually reaches 100% in the severe pain group.[29]

Evidence indicates that all first-time low back pain sufferers will experience multifidus inhibition and atrophy that does not resolve spontaneously after resolution of the pain.[30] Such myopathology is thought to be a reason why low back pain recurrence is so common. Exercise training to promote co-contraction of the multifidus and transverse abdominis resulted in significantly less recurrence of low back pain in the exercise group compared to controls. One year after treatment, there was a 30% recurrence of low back pain in the exercise group and an 84% recurrence in control group. Two to three years after treatment, there was a 35% recurrence in the exercise group and a 75% recurrence for controls.[38]

As stated above, paraspinal muscle degeneration in the lumbar spine is as common as lumbar disc degeneration. When computed tomography was utilized to study 52 "normal" subjects, it was determined that herniated discs were present in 20% of those under the age of 40 and in 27% of subjects over 40. In another study, 67 "normal" subjects were evaluated with MRI. Herniated discs were found in 20% of those younger than 60 years of age and in 36% in those older than 60 years. Degenerated discs were present in 46% of those younger than 60 years of age and in 93% in those older than 60 years.[31]

We should mention that we do not consider these degenerative changes in the disc to be normal merely because the patients were symptom free; rather, they represent spinal pathology, i.e., the subluxation complex, which had yet to manifest symptomatically in this cohort. Such pathological changes in the disc represent degeneration of part of the three-joint complex of the spine (two zygapophyseal joints and the intervertebral disc). This condition can lead to progressive deterioration of the spine, raising the likelihood that pain will manifest at some point in the future.[24] We offer this view of disc disease for the purpose of comparing it with other degenerative diseases, such as atherosclerosis and cancer. Such diseases do not manifest symptoms for most of their course of development until the end, when it is usually too late. No one would suggest that asymptomatic cancer or atherosclerosis are not real conditions or problems that should be addressed; we believe the same holds true for the subluxation complex.

The term *histopathology* refers to microscopic tissue changes that occur when spinal muscles, joints, and discs undergo degeneration; it is known that all tissue degeneration is associated with histopathological changes[17] and the reduced mobility promotes histopathological changes.[21,22] Recent animal research by Cramer et al.[39] has demonstrated that zygapophyseal joints undergo degenerative histopathological changes within four weeks of spinal immobilization. Osteophytes developed in the articular processes and degenerative changes occurred on the articular surfaces. (See Chapter 4.) We cannot clinically visualize histopathology in the spinal joint complex; however, it is important to realize that it is present in degenerated tissues and is intimately associated with biochemical abnormalities.

Herniated discs and arthritic joints are characterized by biochemical abnormalities because they produce a variety of inflammatory/nociceptive mediators including proinflammatory cytokines such as tumor necrosis factor (TNF) and interleukin-1, -6, and -8 (IL-1, IL-6, IL-8), prostaglandin E2 (PGE2), leukotriene B4 (LTB4), thromboxane A2 (TXA2), nitric oxide, histamine, and bradykinin. These mediators are produced by infiltrating macrophages and also by resident cells of the injured tissues including histiocytes, fibroblasts, myofibroblasts, endothelial cells, and chondrocytes.[32,33]

One outcome of inflammatory mediator release is nociception and pain. In this sense, inflammation drives the experience of pain. Because inflammation and nociception are so common in the joint complex, the use of antiinflammatory medications is significant. In the United States, more than 30 billion nonprescription NSAIDs and more than 70 million prescription NSAIDs are sold each year.[40] During a 12-month period, the prescription volume for the COX2-inhibitors, Celebrex and Vioxx, exceeded 100 million.[41]

As described above, all of the various aspects of the subluxation complex are commonly found in the population from which our patients are derived. For this reason, it is rational to state that the subluxation complex as defined in this chapter is a common condition. We know that most people have back pain (neuropathophysiology)[36,37,40,41]; most people have spinal muscle degeneration (myopathology)[19,28-30,38]; most people have spinal disc/connective tissue degeneration (histopathology)[21,22,31,39]; and most people have problems with inflammation (biochemical abnormalities).[32,33,40,41] Finally, movement restrictions (kinesiopathology) are a natural outcome of such degenerative changes in the joint complex, and it is agreed that reduced spinal joint motion is a common clinical finding.[21-24] Additionally, spinal histopathology, myopathology, and biochemical changes are regularly discussed in refereed journals including *Spine, The Spine Journal, European Spine Journal,* and *Journal of Spinal Disorders.* Also routinely discussed are related alterations in spinal mobility (kinesiopathology) and neurological changes (neuropathophysiology), such as increased nociception, that typically lead to the experience of pain.

In summary, it is important to appreciate that, each and every day, patients with the subluxation complex literally "walk" into the offices of chiropractors, medical doctors, and physical therapists. The only difference is the name we give to the pathological changes that occur in spinal tissues. Chiropractors most commonly use the terms *joint dysfunction* or *subluxation complex.*

Bone-out-of-Place Subluxation versus Mechanical Low Back Pain

With the information in the previous section in mind, it is important to comment on the bone-out-of-place idea of subluxation and mechanical low back pain. Each concept fails to take into consideration that altered biochemistry plays a role in the related concepts of spinal dysfunction and further leads one to believe that the effective care involves either replacing a displaced bone or fixing some type of mechanical dysfunction and nothing more.

Although our bodies are the vehicles that convey us through life, we cannot equate them with other machines such as bicycles and cars that can have purely mechanical problems. Human beings cannot suffer from a mechanical problem. We suffer with biomechanical problems. Unfortunately, those who view spinal problems as a bone out of place or as mechanical low back pain fail to consider the nature of the prefix *bio-* in the word *biomechanical.* The prefix demands that we consider "mechanical" dysfunction in the context of the biological sciences, such as physiology and biochemistry. In short, spinal dysfunction cannot occur in a "mechanical" vacuum. Reducing spinal dysfunction to a bone out of place or a mechanical dysfunction is absolutely inconsistent with how biological tissues express pathophysiological changes, which will be outlined in detail in the following section.

The reductionist approach to back pain has recently been modified, and we are now told that back pain has mechanical, chemical, and psychological causes,[42] echoing the words of D.D. Palmer some 100 years ago when he wrote that disease is cause by trauma, toxins, and autosuggestion.[35]

The Subluxation Complex as a Pathological Process

On a practical level "pathology deals with the study of deviations from normal structure, physiology, biochemistry, and cellular and molecular biology."[16] The subluxation complex generally refers to pathological changes that occur in the spine,[4-6] and its clinical character depends on the combination of injured tissues and the extent of injury.

As stated earlier, Palmer[35] explained that trauma, toxins, and autosuggestion are the determining causes of disease. We are exposed to such injurious stimuli over a lifespan and, sooner or later, the outcome is pathology; when this occurs in the spine and extremities, we refer to it as the subluxation complex. Back pain researchers agree and indicate that the risk of developing low back pain is greater when there is a lack of fitness or the person is in poor health (a predisposition to trauma), when there are psychosocial issues (autosuggestion), and if one is a smoker (i.e., toxins),[43] which dispels the foolish idea that back pain is solely mechanical.

D.D. Palmer's view of disease is also consistent with the writings of modern pathology. Pathology is known to be caused by diverse agents, including oxygen deprivation, physical agents, chemical agents and drugs, infectious agents, immunologic reactions, genetic derangements, and nutritional imbalance.[17] These injurious agents are known to express injury potential in the same fashion. No matter if the cause of the initial injury was physical, hypoxic, or infectious, five stereotypical biochemical themes will mediate the expression of cell injury and cell death, including (1) defects in cell membrane permeability, (2) free radicals, (3) ATP depletion, (4) intracellular calcium and loss of calcium homeostasis, and (5) irreversible mitochondrial damage.[17] These biochemical themes apply to all pathologies, suggesting that we must consider them in the context of the subluxation complex.

When applied to musculoskeletal tissues, the pathomechanics we encounter are initially expressed via *biochemical themes,* which are often difficult to conceptualize for both chiropractic and medical doctors. General biochemistry and the biochemistry of pathology are commonly taught early in our educations and with far too few clinical correlations. Accordingly, we typically deliver our treatment approaches without due consideration of the biochemical changes that occur in injured tissues. Complicating this problem further is the lack of in-depth nutrition training in both chiropractic and medical education, for it is with nutrition that the biochemical changes are best addressed. The information presented in this section will alert us to deficiencies in the concepts of subluxation solely as a bone out of place or as mechanical low back pain, considering the fact that we cannot artificially separate biochemistry from biomechanics.

Biochemical Injury Theme 1: Defects in the Cell Membrane

Each cell type found in the spine contains an external limiting membrane called the plasma membrane, or cell membrane, a dynamic structure consisting of various lipids, proteins, and carbohydrates. It is intimately connected with the extracellular compartment by numerous membrane receptors that signal the intracellular compartment. The lipid component of the cell membrane is extremely important for membrane fluidity and in the context of creating inflammatory potential. Phospholipids and cholesterol are the lipid substances that make up the cell membrane and generally are present in a 1 to 1 ratio.[44]

Phospholipids are built on a glycerol backbone, a three-carbon molecule to which a phosphatide component, a saturated fatty acid, and a polyunsaturated fatty acid are attached. Two sheets of phospholipids make a cell membrane, referred to as a lipid bilayer membrane. The hydrophilic phosphatide components face the fluid-rich extracellular and intracellular spaces, while the hydrophobic fatty acids face each other in the center of the lipid bilayer.

The phosphatide portion and saturated fatty acid are assembled within the body. The polyunsaturated fatty acid is obtained from our diets and is referred to as an essential fatty acid, either an omega-6 (n6) or omega-3 (n3) fatty acid. Omega-6 and omega-3 fatty acids are found in both vegetable and animal foods, and a 1:1 dietary ratio is thought to be ideal for promoting appropriate inflammatory and healing responses.[45] Ratios greater than 3:1 are thought to promote excessive inflammatory responses.

Linoleic acid is the n6 fatty acid that our bodies convert into the proinflammatory arachidonic acid, which is then inserted into the phospholipid. Arachidonic acid is the precursor to proinflammatory eicosanoids (prostaglandin E2, leukotriene B4, and thromboxane A2), which are part of the large family of chemical mediators of inflammation that constitute the biochemical changes associated with the subluxation complex (mentioned earlier in this chapter).

Linoleic acid is found in all grains and grain products, such as cereal, pasta, and bread; the average n6:n3 ratio is 20:1 for these foods.[46] Seeds contain almost exclusively n6 fatty acids, as do their oils including corn, sunflower, and safflower oils. This creates a ratio that exceeds 100:1. Peanuts, a legume and not a nut, have ratios that also exceed 100:1.[47] Processed foods that have n6 oils added to them have very high ratios, such as potato chips that boast 60:1.[46] Meat and eggs from grain-fed animals have ratios well above 3:1.[48,49]

Linolenic acid is the n3 fatty acid that we convert into eicosapentaenoic acid (EPA), which is then inserted into the cell membrane phospholipid. EPA is the precursor to antiinflammatory eicosanoids (prostaglandin E3, leukotriene B5, and thromboxane A3). In foods such as fruits and vegetables, the n6:n3 ratio is quite favorable, ranging from about 3:1 to 1:3.[46] Fish, grass-fed beef, and wild game range from about 3:1 to 1:7.[46,48,49]

With a 1:1 dietary ratio of linoleic (n6) to linolenic acid (n3), we would get a similar ratio of arachidonic acid to eicosapentaenoic acid, allowing for an appropriate inflammatory response. However, the dietary ratio of n6 to n3 fatty acids has been maintained at about 20:1 or greater for the past half-century or longer,[45] resulting in an excessive and persistent inflammatory response and an increased incidence of inflammatory diseases such as cancer, heart disease, Alzheimer's disease, and arthritis.[10,45]

In the context of cells and tissues directly related to the subluxation complex, research has shown that normal cartilage has low levels of proinflammatory n6 fatty acids. As we age, concentrations steadily increase—a trend that is especially pronounced in osteoarthritic cartilage. Lipid accumulation in chondrocytes generally precedes local tissue degeneration in several models of degenerative arthritis. Histological severity of osteoarthritis has been related to accumulation of arachidonic acid,[50] an n6 acid and a precursor of the previously mentioned proinflammatory eicosanoids.

Biochemical Injury Theme 2: Free Radicals

Contained within the cell membrane is the cytoplasm of the cell, composed of cellular fluids and various organelles, such as lysosomes and mitochondria. Moving closer to the nucleus we encounter the Golgi apparatus and endoplasmic reticulum, an extension of the nuclear envelope that houses the nucleus. While this in no way is a review of histology, we can safely say that these are some major structures common to all cells, and it is these structures that are at risk for injury.

Pathology texts tell us that cell membranes, enzymes, circulating lipids, and DNA are at risk of injury from free radicals.[17] In particular, consider that free radicals can damage cell membranes, resulting in the release of arachidonic acid and its subsequent conversion to proinflammatory eicosanoids. Thus there is interplay between biochemical injury themes 1 and 2.

Free radicals are generated by many normal body reactions. The free radicals that are most compromising to us are the ones produced by our own bodies. Consider that immune cells fend off invaders by releasing free radicals that can also damage cell membranes. Internal biological processes, including ATP synthesis, liver detoxification processes, prostaglandin synthesis, phagocytosis, xanthine oxidase, and the normal degradation of catecholamines,[51] also generate free radicals. Even at rest we produce free radicals; production increases during exercise.[52]

Although free radicals are produced by our bodies, we need outside support if we are to mount an effective defense against them. Only through the liberal consumption of fruits and vegetables are we able to provide our bodies with the antioxidant nutrients needed to fight free radical activity. The consumption of olive oil and red wine also provides powerful antioxidants.[53] Additionally, recent research has demonstrated that restricting caloric intake is an effective way to reduce the body's generation of free radicals.[54,55]

It is thought that free radical attack may be one of the final common denominators of cell injury. Such attacks may be responsible for the progression of all diseases,[56] including conditions that are considered to be components of or related to the subluxation complex, such as disc herniation. Lipofuscin, known as the aging pigment, is produced by the oxidation of lipids or lipoprotein. At the time of disc surgery, lipofuscin has been found in regions associated with strong histologic degeneration, including the nucleus pulposus and the inner and middle layers of the anulus fibrosis. Lipofuscin was found in the discs of individuals older than 20 years of age.[57]

Free radicals are also involved in articular cartilage degeneration and arthritis, with chondrocytes playing a significant role. Although we typically view them as producers of cartilage, we saw earlier that their cell membranes concentrate arachidonic acid and become proinflammatory.[50] These small cells are also able to generate abnormal production of a hydrogen peroxide free radical that can damage joint cartilage proteoglycans, hyaluronic acid, and collagen.[50,58] Chondrocytes from osteoarthritic cartilage also release proinflammatory inducible nitric oxide, which acts as a potent free radical.[59] It is also known that a chondrocyte-derived lipid peroxidation product called malondialdehyde (MDA) mediates oxidation of cartilage collagens. White cells such as macrophages are a likely source of the free radicals that induce the production of MDA via oxidization of the fatty acids within the phospholipids of chondrocyte cell membranes.[60]

Free radical mechanisms are thought to play a role in the pathogenesis of most diseases. As described previously, evidence suggests that free radical mechanisms are involved in cartilage and disc degeneration and therefore should be viewed as promoters of the subluxation complex.

Biochemical Injury Themes 3 to 5: Related to ATP Synthesis

The final three themes that mediate the expression of cell injury include ATP depletion, intracellular calcium and loss of calcium homeostasis, and irreversible mitochondrial damage. They are described collectively because they are interrelated. For example, mitochondrial damage will deplete ATP, which can disrupt calcium homeostasis. Calcium ions are highly concentrated in the extracellular compartment. Without adequate mitochondrial function and ATP synthesis, excess calcium may enter the cell and cause cell injury and death.[17] The seriousness of this relationship should not be taken lightly because most diseases are likely to be driven at least in part by this process, including the normal aging process.[17,61-64]

A histological view of any cell quickly reveals the presence of numerous mitochondria, the organelles responsible for ATP synthesis. ATP is required for countless body reactions, as most chiropractors have learned in biochemistry classes. Germane to chiropractic practice is the fact that ATP is required for contraction and relaxation of sarcomeres, functional units of a muscle fiber.

The cellular synthesis of ATP utilizes three biochemical pathways. Glycolysis occurs in the cytoplasm; the Krebs cycle and electron transport occur in the mitochondria. Tissues highly dependent on oxygen and ATP, such as the cardiac muscle, skeletal and smooth muscle, the central and peripheral nervous system, the kidney, and pancreatic beta cells are especially susceptible to defective mitochondrial function. There is evidence that mitochondrial dysfunction and reduced ATP synthesis play an important role in atherosclerosis, Alzheimer's disease, Parkinson's disease, diabetes, and aging.[62]

The interrelationship among the biochemical themes of injury continues here because it is known that free radicals damage mitochondria. During a lifetime, mitochondrial DNA (mtDNA) undergoes a variety of mutations. The bioenergetic decline associated with mitochondrial mutations, often coupled with nuclear DNA damage, are thought to contribute to the reduced function of cells and organs, especially in postmitotic tissues.[63] On a histological level, postmitotic tissues such as skeletal muscle develop what has been referred to as a "damage mosaic."[63] Skeletal muscle atrophy and muscle fiber type changes occur.[63] Between the ages of 20 to 80, there is about a 40% decrease in skeletal muscle mass.[64] Such changes clearly have an impact in the manner in which we view the subluxation complex as our patients age.

Summary of Biochemical Injury Themes

We need to appreciate that various biochemical injury themes are responsible for driving the sub-clinical pathological changes that result in clinical biomechanical expressions of altered function equated with the subluxation complex. While our primary subluxation complex intervention is biomechanical, i.e., the chiropractic adjustment, we must remember that altered biomechanics is ultimately a macroscopic expression of altered biochemistry at the microscopic cellular and tissue level.

Upon reaching a certain threshold, altered bio-chemistry in spinal tissues will alert the nervous system, usually in the form of pain or an altered sensation. This is the case with most diseases. Accordingly, understanding nervous system function in the context of the biochemical injury themes and the subluxation complex is very important.

The Relationship between the Subluxation Complex and the Nervous System

Neuroanatomy tends to be a confusing subject for specialists in fields other than neurology, as well as for doctors trained as generalists, including internists, general medical practitioners, and chiropractors. However, we chiropractors have "staked a claim" in the study of the nervous system, contending that the subluxation complex and the adjustment can dramatically influence the function of peripheral and central nervous systems, as well as the autonomic nervous system. Such a claim demands that we understand the nervous system better than other practitioners. This chapter does not permit adequate space for an in-depth review of the nervous system; however, pertinent details will be highlighted.

Generally lost in conversations about the sub-luxation complex is the manner in which spinal tissues are innervated. How are joints, muscles, ligaments, and discs innervated? How does this pattern of innervation relate to spinal function and the subluxation complex? How does the sub-luxation complex generate symptoms? How does the adjustment influence the subluxation complex and the nervous system? These are four very important questions to answer and key areas for future research.

Innervation of Joints, Muscles, Ligaments, and Discs

Outside the intervertebral foramen, the spinal nerve divides into ventral and dorsal rami. Nearly every posterior spinal structure is innervated by the dorsal ramus. All palpable spinal muscles, the posterior spinal ligaments, and the zygapophyseal joint capsule are innervated by the dorsal ramus. The dura of the spinal cord, posterior longitudinal ligament, and the posterior and posterolateral portions of the intervertebral disc are innervated by the recurrent meningeal or sinuvertebral nerve. (See Chapter 3.)

We should recollect that nerves themselves do not innervate spinal, cranial, or appendicular structures. Nerves are merely the connective tissue "tubes" that contain the nerve fibers that inner-vate all of our body's structures, a very important distinction. While we have hundreds of different names for the different tubes, such as ulnar nerve, axillary nerve, and femoral nerve, there are only four types of motor nerve fibers and four types of sensory nerve fibers that innervate muscu-loskeletal tissues. Even though there are a small number of nerve fiber types, nerve fiber nomencla-ture can be confusing because both letters and

BOX 9-1 ■ Nerve Fibers Innervating Spinal Structures

Motor

- Aα-motoneurons to extrafusal muscle fibers
- Aβ-motoneurons to intrafusal muscle fibers
- Aγ-motoneurons to intrafusal muscle fibers
- Postganglionic (sympathetic) C-fibers
- Preganglionic (sympathetic) B-fibers*

Sensory

- Group I (Ia and Ib) afferents (Aα size)
- Group II afferents (Aβ size)
- Group III afferents (Aδ size)
- Group IV afferents (C-fiber size)

*B-fibers represent the fifth type of motor fiber, but they do not innervate musculoskeletal tissues.

Roman numerals are used to classify nerve fibers. Box 9-1 lists the main nerve fibers that innervate spinal tissues.

Understanding nerve fiber types is often confusing because afferent and efferent fibers are of similar size. If we were to examine a cross section of a nerve at mid-length, it would be impossible to tell if a given fiber is afferent or efferent unless we know the origin or termination of the fiber. All fibers are one of the following sizes: Aα, Aβ, Aγ, Aδ, B, or C. Postganglionic B-fibers travel from the intermediolateral column of the T1-L2 spinal cord levels and synapse in either the paravertebral ganglia or prevertebral ganglia, making no direct connection with musculoskeletal tissues. Only Aγ- and B-fibers are exclusively motor, and Aδ-fibers are exclusively sensory. All other fiber sizes may be motor or sensory. To differentiate among afferent and efferent fibers, a Roman numeral classification was devised. When we read about group I, II, III, and IV fibers, we are reading about afferent fibers only.

To understand the neurology of the subluxation complex, we need to have a thorough understanding of the afferent fibers that innervate the structures of the joint complex. From a clinical perspective, we can easily argue that the sensory system should be our focus because patients go to a doctor's office almost exclusively when they feel that something is wrong. Abnormal feelings or symptoms can only occur if our afferent system alerts us to a problem, pain being the most obvious example. Consider further that it is mostly the afferent/sensory system we challenge during the physical exam. Most orthopedic tests are considered positive when pain is elicited. Pain and tenderness upon spinal palpation alerts us to areas of dysfunction. It is important to realize that pain could not occur in these instances unless there is increased activity of group III and IV afferents, which constitute our nociceptive fibers.

As indicated in Box 9-1, there are only four different types of afferent fibers that innervate structures in the human body, including the spinal column, and these are group I, II, III, IV afferents. In any given peripheral nerve, such as the dorsal ramus that innervates our posterior spinal structures, we only have group I through IV afferents, no more and no less. Keeping this information in mind is important as a neuroscience foundation.

The division of afferent fibers into groups is determined by the size of the nerve fiber. Group I fibers have the largest diameter (12 to 20 μm) and are heavily myelinated, which provides them with the ability to conduct action potentials faster than all other afferent fibers (70 to 120 m/sec). Group II afferents are also myelinated; their diameter ranges from 6 to 12 μm, and conduction velocities range from 30 to 70 m/sec. Group III fibers are thinly myelinated with diameters ranging from 1 to 6 μm and conduction velocities that range from 5 to 30 m/sec. Group IV fibers are the smallest and are unmyelinated. Their diameter ranges from 0.1 to less than 2 μm, and they have the slowest conduction velocities of all afferents (0.5 to 2 m/sec).

Group I and II Afferents

Group I afferents have two subcategories, group Ia afferents from muscle spindles, the so-called annulospiral endings, and group Ib afferents from Golgi tendon organs. Group II afferents also come from muscle spindles and are typically referred to as secondary or flower spray endings. Group II afferents also provide innervation to the CNS from all corpuscular mechanoreceptors, such as Ruffini endings, Pacinian corpuscles, and Meissner's corpuscles, which are found in skin, joints, and muscles.

Groups I and II afferents are referred to as mechanoreceptive afferents because they arise from mechanoreceptors (muscle spindles, Golgi tendon organs, and corpuscular mechanoreceptors). A mechanoreceptor is defined as a receptor that responds to normal movements or physical stimuli, such as touch, vibration, joint position, and joint motion. Under normal circumstances, mechanoreceptors are not activated by noxious stimuli and so do not induce the experience of pain. While there is some evidence that mechanoreceptive input can play a role in pain generation, it remains unclear how this occurs in the clinical setting.[2,65]

There are many central nervous responses or outcomes associated with mechanoreceptor activation, such as the inhibition of nociception that can reduce the experience of pain. Mechanoreceptors also reduce segmental sympathetic outflow that is induced by nociceptive input. Suprasegmental responses from mechanoreception include proprioception and motor control.[66] In the clinical setting, many chiropractors activate mechanoreceptors via the adjustment and soft tissue manipulation, as well as by using a mechanically induced motion apparatus to cause repeated passive joint motion.

Group III and IV Afferents

In contrast with group I and II afferents, group III and IV afferents are typically characterized as nociceptors; however, there are group III and IV fibers that respond to innocuous input. The number of these nonnociceptive group III and IV fibers and their functional significance are not well characterized. Accordingly, for the purpose of this chapter, we will view group III and IV afferents as nociceptors unless otherwise stated. Nociceptors are best described as injury or tissue damage receptors; they are not pain receptors. Pain is the limbic or emotional response to tissue damage and nociception. There are also well known auto-

nomic and endocrine responses to nociception, such as cardiovascular, respiratory, and gastrointestinal symptoms.[1,2]

We should be alerted to the inappropriate term *pain generator* that is often used interchangeably with nociceptor and sometimes as a stand-alone term; *nociceptor* is the appropriate and accurate word. This distinction should not be taken lightly; Bonica, the founder of the International Association for the Study of Pain, made it clear that nociceptors are not to be referred to as pain receptors.[67] No receptor in the human body encodes *pain*, defined as *a nociceptive-induced sensory and emotional experience that occurs in the limbic sectors of the cerebral cortex*.[65,67] Consider that the transmission of noxious/injurious stimuli must pass through a first-order sensory neuron (group III and IV afferents), a second-order projection neuron (spinothalamic fiber), and a third-order thalamocortical projection neuron prior to reaching the limbic cortex where pain is experienced. In short, pain should be viewed as one potential outcome of nociceptive activity.

Standard physiology or neurology texts do not apprise us of the distribution of receptors and afferent fibers within musculoskeletal tissues, presenting a problem to practitioners whose lives are devoted to caring for the musculoskeletal system. Many chiropractic and medical clinicians are surprised to discover that nociceptive afferents significantly outnumber mechanoreceptive afferents. In a recent review of the literature, Leach and Pickar indicate that up to 95% of joint afferents can be group III and group IV,[68] which, as stated earlier, are generally viewed as nociceptors.

Schmidt et al.[69] list the fiber distribution in both the medial articular nerve (MAN) and posterior articular nerve (PAN) of the cat knee joint. A total of 630 afferent fibers were found in the MAN; no group I afferents (0%), 59 group II afferents (9%), 131 group III afferents (21%), and 440 group IV afferents (70%). Of the 630 afferents in the MAN, 91% belong to the nociceptive category. A total of 680 afferents was found in the PAN; 27 group I afferents that were thought to be stray muscle spindle afferents from the popliteus muscle (4%), 149 group II afferents (22%), 94 group III afferents

(14%), and 410 group IV afferents (60%). Of the 680 afferents in the PAN, at least 74% belong to the nociceptive category. There were also 500 sympathetic efferent fibers in the MAN and 515 in the PAN.[69] The predominance of nociceptive and sympathetic innervation of joints has the potential to augment healing or inflammation, which will be discussed later in this chapter.

Few studies have examined human spinal joint innervation; however, those that have reflect the outcome of animal studies. In human cervical spine joint capsules, mechanoreceptors were found in only 17 of 21 joint capsules, while nociceptors were plentiful.[70] A similar pattern of innervation exists in the thoracolumbar spine. Only 5 mechanoreceptors were found in 10 thoracic joint capsules, and 12 mechanoreceptors in 13 lumbar joint capsules, while nociceptors were abundant in all specimens.[71]

At present we do not have details about the innervation patterns of small intrinsic spinal muscles, such as the intertransversarii, interspinalis, rotatores, multifidus, and the suboccipital muscles; however, it is likely that they may have a balance of afferents that favors mechanoreceptors. The spinal intrinsic muscles possess a heavy concentration of muscle spindles, compared to muscles elsewhere in the body.[2] Unlike spinal muscles, patterns of innervation have been characterized in appendicular muscles, and it turns out that patterns of muscle innervation are not dissimilar from joints, save for significantly more group I afferents that are associated with muscle spindles and Golgi tendon organs, which are not found in joints. The nerve to the lateral gastrocnemius muscle was examined and found to contain 1480 afferents. About 25% of afferents are group I and II, while the remaining 75% are group III and IV afferents that are typically associated with nociceptive afferents[72]; however, the breakdown of fiber types is more discrete. Mense studied cat muscle and tendons and determined that of group III afferents, 33% were nociceptive, 23% were thermosensitive, and 44% were low-threshold mechanosensitive. Within the family of group IV afferents, the following distribution was observed: 43% nociceptive, 19% thermosensitive, 19% con-

traction sensitive, and 19% low-threshold mechanosensitive.[72]

The group III and IV afferents innervate tendons, fascia, the area between muscle fibers, and blood vessels.[73] The number of postganglionic sympathetic efferents approximately equaled that of the nociceptive afferents,[72] once again reflecting the predominance of nociceptive and sympathetic innervation in peripheral musculoskeletal tissues. In spinal tissues, it is thought that nociceptors are located in skin, subcutaneous and adipose tissue, fibrous capsules of apophyseal and sacroiliac joints, spinal ligaments, periosteum covering vertebral bodies and arches (and attached fascia, tendons and aponeurosis), dura mater and epidural fibroadipose tissue, walls of blood vessels supplying the spinal joints, sacroiliac joints, and the vertebral cancellous bone, walls of epidural and paravertebral veins, walls of intramuscular arteries, and at least the outer third of the annulus fibrosis.[74-83]

Wyke[81] provided a vivid anatomical description of the nociceptive receptor system, contrasting interstitial and perivascular nociceptors. He described interstitial nociceptors as "a continuous tridemensional plexus of unmyelinated nerve fibers that weaves (like chicken-wire) in all directions throughout the tissue." A similar plexus of unmyelinated nerve fibers is embedded in the adventitial sheath that encircles each blood vessel.[81] Charman[77] states that the "network of each C-fibre innervates a three-dimensional receptive field of between 6 and 15 mm in diameter and of variable depth with extensive field overlapping between adjacent C-fibres." Thus we can envision the presence of an almost unending meshwork of nociceptors within the various tissues.

All nociceptors are typically described as unmyelinated "free nerve endings," a misnomer because they represent the beginning of the nerve fiber in peripheral tissues, such as the disc or facet joint, so they are really unmyelinated "free nerve beginnings." Once the unmyelinated beginnings of Aδ-fibers (group III afferents) enter the perineurial sheath of the respective peripheral nerve, they become lightly myelinated and are recognized as Aδ-fibers. However, once the unmyelinated beginnings of C-fibers enter the perineurial sheath, they remain unmyelinated and are recognized as C-fibers. Recall that the peripheral nerves that provide nociceptive innervation to spinal structures are the dorsal ramus (joints, muscles, and ligaments), sinuvertebral nerve, a.k.a., the recurrent meningeal nerve (dura, posterolateral disc, and posterior longitudinal ligament), and branches of the so-called sympathetic nerves (lateral and anterior disc, and anterior longitudinal ligament).

The details of nociceptor anatomy and physiology are quite complex and not fully understood even by the experts, requiring that our descriptions herein will need to be modified when more details are discovered. For our purposes, we will describe what appear to be the main three categories of nociceptors, which include specific nociceptors, silent nociceptors, and polymodal nociceptors, all of which are group III afferents (Aδ-fibers) and/or the more common group IV afferents (C-fibers). In some cases the larger group II afferents (Aβ-fibers) are associated with nociceptors, but this is not that common.[73]

Functional Nociceptor Classification

Examples of specific nociceptors include mechanical nociceptors, mechanothermal nociceptors, and thermal nociceptors, corresponding to noxious mechanical stimulation, noxious mechanical and/or thermal stimulation, or noxious thermal stimulation, respectively. Specific nociceptors are mostly represented as group III afferents (Aδ-fibers) that quickly alert us about noxious stimuli that impact the surfaces of our bodies.[73,84] Silent or sleeping nociceptors are found in all tissues. They remain inactive in healthy tissues, are not activated by noxious mechanical stimuli, and begin firing when tissues become increasingly inflamed. Silent nociceptors might best be classified as inflammation detectors because inflammatory chemicals activate them. Silent nociceptors are typically C-fibers and referred to as group IV afferents.[73]

Polymodal nociceptors are the third category of nociceptor to be discussed herein. They are an extremely interesting cell type that can be Aδ-fibers (group III afferents) but are mostly C-fibers (group IV afferents). Not surprisingly, they are found in somatic and visceral tissues, and their properties and proportion match the defense and homeostatic needs of the anatomical structure or region. Polymodal nociceptors have been well studied in joints.[73] Recently researchers have begun to refer to polymodal nociceptors as polymodal *receptors* or *neuroeffectors* because they have diverse functions beyond nociception. Consider for example, that "polymodals" are activated by chemical, thermal, and mechanical stimuli that may be nonnoxious or noxious, which allows them to regulate inflammation, wound healing, and tissue homeostasis.[73] Because polymodals are activated by a wide range of stimuli, we must maintain a flexible view of group IV afferents; some act as mechanoreceptors, others as thermoreceptors, some as tissue homeostats, and others as nociceptors. It is likely that polymodals alter their phenotypes depending on the nature of the local tissue milieu. The fact that living cells such as nociceptors display such dynamic adaptive properties should be a concept that is easily comprehended by chiropractors.

As described earlier, there is almost an equal balance of group IV afferents and sympathetic innervation of our spinal structures. The purpose of this balance is to orchestrate local tissue homeostasis in conjunction with the suprasegmental autonomic and neuroendocrine systems.[73] As bodily homeostasis has been a historically important subject for chiropractors, it is intriguing to note that the so-called pain literature is a source of information about the homeostatic nature of the nervous system, the last place that most chiropractors would look for information to support a vitalistic chiropractic view of body function. Most practitioners of medicine and chiropractic are unaware of the homeostatic functions of group IV afferents because only specialty texts devoted to pain and nociception discuss this topic.[73] In standard physiology and neuroscience texts, only the group IV-nociceptor-pain relationship is described, which leads practitioners to develop an inaccurate perception of group IV afferents and nociceptor function, unless specialty texts are considered.

It is important to understand that the innate programming goal of the polymodal receptor is to monitor and facilitate local physiology and to shift neural behavior in ways that promote health, prevent or reduce injury, and enhance healing.[73] However, something goes wrong; rather than effective healing and symptom reduction, chronic pain and inflammation commonly develop and plague millions of people.

As stated earlier, polymodal receptors are highly adaptable cells that have a wide phenotypic range; that is, polymodal receptors adapt their functional activity to match the tissue environment. It seems that when a proinflammatory environment is encountered, polymodal receptors and silent nociceptors team up to drive chronic nociceptive and neuropathic pain.[73] This unique function of polymodal receptors occurs because individual polymodal receptors express a variety of chemoreceptors on their axolemmae, i.e., cell membranes, which allows them to respond differently to various antiinflammatory and proinflammatory chemical mediators; the concentration of which can vary within the same tissue and among various tissues. Consider that polymodals have receptors for bradykinin, hydrogen ions, prostaglandin E2, leukotriene B4, serotonin, histamine, interleukin-1, interleukin-6, and tumor necrosis factor, all mediators typically associated with inflammation and pain. Polymodals also have receptors for ligands including glutamate, GABA, acetylcholine, norepinephrine, adenosine, ATP, estrogen, glucocorticoids, corticotrophin releasing factor, substance P, neurokinin A, cholecystokinin, somatostatin, bombesin, angiotensin II, neuropeptide Y, endorphins, enkephalin, dynorphin, nerve growth factor, brain-derived neurotrophic factor, glial-derived neurotrophic factor, and fibroblast growth factor.[73]

In general, noxious mediators, such as prostaglandin E2 and bradykinin, promote polymodal and silent nociceptor firing, while other agents, such as opioids and interleukin-10 produced by local white blood cells reduce their activation and augment tissue healing.[73,85] In this context, it is important to understand that polymodals and silent nociceptors in the spinal joint complex can only respond to the chemical nature of the tissue milieu; it seems that our modern proinflammatory lifestyles result in the production of inflammatory mediators that tell polymodals and silent nociceptors to maintain their noxious, painful, and inflammatory activity. The manner in which inappropriate dietary habits and sedentary living promote inflammation and chronic inflammatory disease is reviewed elsewhere.[9,10,86] Amidst the business of living our proinflammatory lives, at some point most of us will get injured to a degree that is significant enough to activate our nociceptive systems, leading to a cascade of events that can cause pain and inflammation, which in part characterizes the subluxation complex.

In summary, peripheral sensory neuroanatomy of the musculoskeletal systems begins with two types of somatosensory receptors, mechanoreceptors and nociceptors, and four groups of sensory neurons. In total, the neuromusculoskeletal system has only four motor neurons and four sensory neurons. (See Box 9-1.) When considering musculoskeletal tissues such as the spine, our focus should be drawn to the neurons that predominate, which includes group IV afferents and postganglionic sympathetic efferents. How does this pattern of innervation relate to the subluxation complex? This is an important question to answer from both a clinical and research perspective.

Group IV Afferents and Postganglionic Sympathetic Fibers in Relation to the Subluxation Complex

In standard physiology and neuroanatomy books, we are presented with a basic description of group III and IV afferents, most commonly called pain fibers. We also get basic descriptions of the spinothalamic or anterolateral system, the so-called pain pathway, and the sympathetic nervous system is only described as the motor system to our viscera. These descriptions do not allow us to perceive that the nervous system may reduce or augment clinical syndromes, such as arthritis, allergic rhinitis, atopic dermatitis, psoriasis, inflammatory bowel disease, or asthma,[87-89] or the chiropractic subluxation complex.[2,8] In this section, the putative relationship between the nervous system and the subluxation complex will be described.

There are three likely mechanisms by which nociceptive processes drive the subluxation complex. The first and most obvious mechanism involves pain. If it hurts to move, we consciously immobilize the painful joint complex, which can lead to pathological changes we associate with the subluxation complex.[8] The second mechanism involves segmental spinal cord reflexes induced by nociceptive input. Nociceptive input is able to stimulate both segmental somatomotor and sympathetic neurons that can alter muscle activity and contribute to joint hypomobility and the subluxation complex.[8] The third mechanism is related to chronic inflammation that is perpetuated by nociceptors and sympathetic terminals, a process referred to as neurogenic inflammation. In the remainder of this section, each of these processes will be discussed in detail.

Pain and Segmental Reflexes as Promoters of the Subluxation Complex

As described earlier, the subluxation complex is likely to begin as subtle proinflammatory changes related to cell membrane–derived eicosanoids, free radicals, and altered ATP synthesis, which can eventually promote altered biomechanics. Such proinflammatory and biomechanical changes, in conjunction with microtraumatic or macrotraumatic injury, will eventually lead to the stimulation of local joint complex nociceptors and polymodal receptors. It is not possible to define the exact timing or sequence of this process; it develops microscopically and asymptomatically, which is consistent with other diseases. Patients and clinicians eventually meet when this pathophysiological process becomes symptomatic, pain and discomfort being the most common example. Such symptoms develop due to nociceptor stimulation.

Normally, polymodal receptors and silent nociceptors are not actively driving nociceptive processes. They only begin transmitting noxious information when tissues are injured and inflammation begins. In other words, our nociceptive receptors have a high-threshold for activation; they are not normally activated by innocuous stimuli such as light touch or normal movements. After injury and with persistent inflammation, nociceptors undergo a sensitizing process. The constant stimulation by inflammatory chemicals brings nociceptors and polymodals closer to threshold, so that light touch and normal movements are now able to stimulate nociceptors. This change in polymodal and silent nociceptor sensitivity is called "sensitization."[73,90] Sensitized nociceptors often fire spontaneously and develop what is referred to as background discharge. It is likely that chiropractors encounter a sensitized nociceptive system when patients experience pain upon palpation and passive movement that are normally part of the physical exam and chiropractic treatment procedures. The term *allodynia* is used to describe pain caused by innocuous input such as normal palpation,[90] which is a common finding in clinical practice and should lead chiropractors to think about nutrition and exercise to help reduce inflammation.

The sensitization process has been studied in cat knee joints by comparing the firing pattern of afferents during normal and inflamed conditions. The resting discharge of the normal medial articular nerve of the cat knee joint was 1800 impulses per 30-second interval. The rate increased to 11,000 impulses during inflammation of the joint, a 6.2-fold increase in action potentials. During normal movements, there were 4400 impulses in 30 seconds; however, with inflammation this rose to 30,900 impulses, a 7-fold increase in action potentials during joint inflammation.[69] This increase in discharge from inflamed joints is predominantly due to the activation and sensitization of polymodals and silent nociceptors resulting in excessive nociceptive bombardment into the spinal cord,[69,73] which then drives central nociceptive sensitization.

The central terminals of nociceptive afferents release substance P and excitatory amino acids, i.e., glutamate and aspartate, which then stimulate second-order neurons and glial cells related to the synapse between nociceptive afferents and their second-order neurons. The constant bombardment of second-order neurons by sensitized nociceptive afferents induces neuroplastic changes in second-order neurons, bringing them closer to threshold and making them more readily activated.[2,65,90]

Glial cells, which are found throughout the gray matter of the cord, are also stimulated by nociceptive afferents. Nociceptive input causes glial cells to release interleukin-1, interleukin-6, tumor necrosis factor, free radicals, nitric oxide, prostaglandins, excitatory amino acids, and ATP. All of these can enhance the excitability of second-order neurons and stimulate an exaggerated release of substance P, glutamate, and aspartate from group IV afferents, further exciting second-order neurons, promoting central sensitization.[91]

These central sensitizing mechanisms are also thought to apply to the activation of α-motoneurons and γ-motoneurons located within the ventral horn, which leads to a segmental increase in somatomotor outflow that can manifest as increased muscle tension, a common finding during spinal palpation. Segmental sympathetic preganglionic outflow may also become sensitized. Preganglionic sympathetic neurons are located in the intermediolateral cell column and they are also activated by peripheral nociceptive bombardment. Increased sympathetic outflow is also a likely promoter of the subluxation complex because postganglionic sympathetic fibers release mediators that perpetuate inflammation and nociception,[8] which will be discussed later in the chapter.

Inflammation and nociception have an additional important effect on spinal cord function, about which chiropractors need to be aware. Normally, group II afferents (Aβ-fibers) from mechanoreceptors enter the dorsal horn at lamina III and IV. In contrast, group III (Aδ-fibers) and IV (C-fibers) nociceptive afferents mainly terminate in lamina I, the outer half of lamina II (referred to as lamina II-external [IIe]), and lamina V, from which second-order nociceptive tracts emanate such as the spinothalamic tracts). Clearly, there are distinctly different termination points for mechanoreceptive and nociceptive afferents, extremely important in the context of pain generation.

If mechanoreceptive afferents were to terminate in laminae I, IIe, and V, then light touch and normal movements would activate spinothalamic pathways and promote pain with the outcome being constant and unending pain. Fortunately, we are not normally wired in this fashion; however, researchers have demonstrated that inflammation can cause group II afferent terminals in the dorsal to sprout collateral branches that migrate superficially into lamina IIe and make synaptic contacts with spinothalamic neurons.[73,92] This process is referred to as dorsal horn reorganization and allows normally innocuous stimuli to be painful. Presumably, this reorganization is restored to normal after inflammation resolves and healing takes place. More research is needed in this area to determine what role this reorganization process may play in chronic pain syndromes. Perhaps the spinal cords of certain chronic pain patients are genetically disposed to undergo this reorganization process, which does not resolve after the initial injury. To date, we do not know why certain patients develop chronic pain after normal injuries, while others do not.

In summary, it is likely that nociceptive input will increase somatomotor activity, which will promote muscle tension (myopathology) and reduce joint mobility (kinesiopathological component of the subluxation complex). Pain is also an outcome of nociception and can also promote kinesiopathology, so that patients with pain are likely to be psychologically motivated to reduce joint motion in an effort to avoid pain. It is easy to see why it is likely that nociception functions as a driver of the subluxation complex.

Neurogenic Inflammation as a Promoter of the Subluxation Complex

While inflammation can lead to tissue healing, chronic inflammation can promote diseases such as cancer, heart disease, Alzheimer's disease, and most other chronic degenerative diseases.[10,17,45] Chronic inflammation also drives musculoskeletal degeneration and chronic pain, which suggests the term *mechanical* low back pain is inaccurate and inappropriate.[10] Indeed, it is known that chronic inflammation can lead to scarring/fibrosis, intraarticular and extraarticular adhesions, continued pain, loss of function, loss of range of motion, loss of power due to atrophy, and a tendency for reinjury,[93] factors we associate with the subluxation complex. Of interest to chiropractors is the fact that nociceptors and sympathetic terminals are responsible for driving the local inflammatory process, referred to as neurogenic inflammation.

Polymodal receptors perpetuate the inflammatory process by releasing numerous mediators that can modulate the local tissue environment, including substance P, calcitonin gene-related peptide (CGRP), glutamate, glycine, GABA, acetylcholine, serotonin, bombesin, neuropeptide Y, and neurotrophins.[73] The most studied mediators are substance P and CGRP, which are released by polymodals in response to tissue injury and inflammation. Substance P and CGRP function to influence local cells, such as fibroblasts and mast cells, as well as the various cells that migrate into the area of injury, such as platelets and macrophages. Substance P stimulates all of these cells to further release inflammatory mediators, which serve to (1) perpetuate the inflammatory process and (2) continue to activate the nociceptor, which in turn, releases more substance P.[94,95] In summary, we can see how this neuroeffector activity of local nociceptors will serve to increase their own stimulation.

Nociceptors are also stimulated by local sympathetic activity. As mentioned in a previous section, nociceptive afferents enter the cord and simulate segmental autonomic outflow. This leads to sympathetic discharge back into the area of the activated nociceptor, such that the terminals of postganglionic sympathetic fibers have a direct interaction with nociceptive afferents. Sympathetic terminals release numerous mediators that interact with local cells and nociceptors including norepinephrine, neuropeptide Y, ATP, adenosine, prostaglandin E2, prostacyclin, 5-HETE, 12-HETE, and endothelium-derived relaxing factor.[96] The release of these mediators can further excite inflammatory and nociceptive processes, which is thought to contribute to the development, severity, and possibly the prolongation of tissue injury.[96] As an example, sympathetic postganglionic fiber activity is necessary for bradykinin and other inflammatory mediators to fully express their inflammatory and nociceptor-sensitizing properties.[97]

Pain, an outcome of nociceptive input, can also influence the sympathetic nervous system and perpetuate local neurogenic inflammation. This is because both the experience of pain and nociceptive input autonomic centers in the hypothalamus and brainstem are capable of inducing epinephrine release from the adrenal medulla. Circulating epinephrine can stimulate sympathetic terminals in the area of injury or dysfunction and perpetuate inflammation.[96,98,99]

In summary, we suggest that the subluxation complex may develop insidiously due to the development of a low-grade, chronic proinflammatory state that leads to tissue degeneration and inflammation. Such a condition can be magnified by microtraumatic or macrotraumatic injuries that occur throughout the normal course of living. The inflammatory process is likely to be actively maintained by the nociceptive and sympathetic systems (neurogenic inflammation); we should view these components of our nervous systems as promoters and perpetuators of the subluxation complex. Neurogenic inflammation is the likely mechanism that causes tissues to remain tender and dysfunctional and may be the reason why pain persists in many of the patients we see.

The Subluxation Complex and Symptom Generation

Dysafferentation

It is important to remember that we typically "feel" symptoms. Abnormal feelings that are generated by dysfunctional spinal tissues can only become feelings if musculoskeletal receptors are abnormally activated. While we may experience a variety of symptoms due to spinal dysfunction, such as local pain, referred pain, and visceral symptoms, we can help to make diagnostic sense of such symptoms if we remember that there are only two categories of receptors found in skeletal tissues that are capable of generating feelings or symptoms that we can perceive; those include nociceptors and mechanoreceptors.

Recall 75% to 95% of joint afferents are related to nociceptors and polymodal receptors, but 5% to 25% of afferents are related to mechanoreceptors. In muscles, up to 75% of afferents are nociceptors and polymodal receptors, and 25% are related to mechanoreceptors. When one considers the abundance of nociceptive and polymodal innervation, it should not be at all surprising that pain is an almost universal complaint. Accordingly, back pain and headaches are the most common symptoms encountered by chiropractors.

Consider that, in part, local inflammation and hypomobile joints characterize the subluxation complex. This relates directly to what we encounter during an examination: areas of pain and tenderness, and reduced mobility. Pain and tenderness are due to increased nociceptive activity. In contrast, reduced mobility would result in reduced mechanoreceptor activity, and this is because the adequate stimulus for a mechanoreceptor in the joint complex is movement.[2,8]

In the past, researchers have performed studies that provide us with insight into the potential symptoms that can be generated by such dysafferentation, i.e., increased nociception and reduced mechanoreception.[2] Researchers preferentially activate nociceptors by injecting hypertonic saline into spinal joints and muscles. In contrast, injecting substances such as lidocaine can reduce nociception and mechanoreception. Feinstein et al.[100] injected hypertonic saline into dorsal ramus–innervated tissues, including interspinous tissues and paraspinal muscles of normal volunteers, for the purpose of characterizing local and referred pain patterns that might develop. Pain was typically elicited at the sites of injection and stereotypical patterns of referred pain also developed, the extent and intensity of which corresponded to the amount of saline injected. The pain referral patterns were very similar to those of patients who enter chiropractic offices; that is, diffuse achy pain that is not dermatomal in nature and not associated with abnormalities in the standard sensory and motor exams.

The type of pain caused by hypertonic saline injections, whether the pain is local or referred, is known as nociceptive pain, the appropriate descriptor for any pain that is induced by injury to musculoskeletal tissues. Neuropathic pain is the appropriate term to describe any pain that is generated by injury to the peripheral or central nervous system. In short, we suffer from nociceptive, neuropathic, and/or psychogenic pain syndromes.[65]

Hypertonic saline injections into spinal tissues also proved to cause a variety of visceral manifestations. Pallor, sweating, bradycardia, fall in blood pressure, subjective "faintness," nausea, and syncope were observed. Feinstein et al.[100] referred to these symptoms as "autonomic concomitants." They explained that these visceral manifestations "were not proportional to the severity of or to the extent of radiation; to the contrary, they seemed to dominate the experience of subjects who complained of little pain, but who were overwhelmed by this distressing complex of symptoms." It was also reported that "this is an example of the ability of deep noxious stimulation to activate generalized autonomic responses independently of the relay of pain to conscious levels,"[100] which should alert us to the possibility that the subluxation complex may cause local pain, referred autonomic symptoms, or no symptoms at all. Autonomic concomitants are most likely caused by nociceptive stimulation of autonomic centers in the brainstem, particularly the medulla and hypothalamus.[2,101] While segmental sympathetic mechanisms are possible, it seems that suprasegmental mechanisms are more likely to be involved. Detailed reviews of these mechanisms are described elsewhere.[1,2]

Of note is that malaise and flu-like and cold-like symptoms, which represent the acute phase response, may be driven by nociceptive stimulation of the medulla and hypothalamus. Most practicing chiropractors have witnessed acute-phase symptoms improve after chiropractic adjustments. A natural interpretation would be that the adjustment somehow increased the activity of a depressed immune system. In fact, research suggests the opposite. Injection of inflammatory cytokines into experimental animals produces an acute phase response; that is, inducing the inflammatory process results in flu-like symptoms.[102] It is believed that such noxious peripheral stimulation leads to excitation of the nucleus tractus solitarius and hypothalamus and promotes CNS cytokine release that drives the flu-like response.[102] It is possible that, by inhibiting nociception, the adjustment may reduce cold and flu symptoms if such symptoms are induced by nociception in the treated musculoskeletal tissues.

Instead of using hypertonic saline and inflammatory agents, de Jong et al.[103] utilized lidocaine and injected human subjects in the area halfway between the mastoid process and carotid tubercle at the level of the second and third cervical vertebrae. Injections were made unilaterally. Immediately after injection symptoms of dysequilibrium began to appear, which included ataxia, hypotonia of the ipsilateral arm and leg, and a strong sensation of ipsilateral falling or tilting. Symptoms were more pronounced on the side of injection and lasted for about an hour. The authors suggested that the injection of local anesthetics "interrupted the flow of afferent information from neck and muscle receptors," which can affect vestibular nuclei function and promote a variety of vestibular and cerebellar symptoms.[103]

While patients with dramatic cerebellovestibular symptoms do regularly present in chiropractic offices, it is not uncommon for chiropractors to treat patients with dizziness and vertigo. For example, cervicogenic vertigo is not uncommon, and chiropractic adjustments have demonstrated to provide positive outcomes.[104] (See Chapter 18.) The subluxation complex appears to be related to altered spinal receptor function and dysafferentation, which may promote a variety of pain, autonomic, and sensorimotor symptoms. More research is needed in this area, and we suggest replicating the work of Feinstein et al.[100] and de Jong et al.[103]

Segmental Sympathetic Dysfunction

The Meric System of adjusting was developed by B.J. Palmer and James Wishart (circa 1910) and was the first attempt to relate vertebral segments with specific organs. It was based on the classic anatomical connections between spinal nerves and specific viscera.[105] Accordingly, if a patient presented with stomach complaints, the chiropractor would focus on the mid dorsal vertebrae in an effort to remove the subluxation responsible for causing the stomach ailment. The concept was that subluxations would impinge on spinal nerves and reduce the mental impulse force or nerve energy that is delivered to the organ, with disease of that organ being the final outcome. This simplistic theory fails to include any physiological rationale. Indeed, Masarsky's text that reviews somatovisceral manifestations provides no evidence to support such simplistic segmental relationships between the subluxation complex and visceral disease.[106]

Osteopathic researcher Irvin Korr was the first to provide a reasonable theory for how pathologic changes in the spinal column, called the osteopathic lesion by osteopaths and subluxation by chiropractors, may influence visceral disease.[107,108] He posited that aberrant afferent input, i.e., dysafferentation, from spinal dysfunction would promote segmental sympathetic hyperactivity, which he referred to as sympatheticotonia. In particular, Korr advanced the notion that the vasomotor changes, particularly vasoconstriction, induced by heightened sympathetic activity would help promote visceral disease. He provided an impressive review of the literature of this subject in 1978 and illustrated that increasing segmental sympathetic tone could advance visceral disease, which could be reversed by sympatheticotonia.[108] The disease processes reviewed by Korr included neurogenic pulmonary edema, peptic ulcer, pancreatitis, arteriosclerosis, and hypertension. Korr theorized that over time, sustained segmental sympatheticotonia, which is induced by a facilitated spinal cord segment, may promote these and other conditions.[108] The facilitated segment is currently known as central nociceptive sensitization. Korr was led to advance the concept of the facilitated segment based on the earlier work of Denslow and colleagues in the late 1930s and early 1940s.[109,110] For more details about their work, see the collected papers of Korr[111] and Denslow.[112]

Korr retired from active research in the 1970s, and since that time few efforts have been made to further examine his original work relating spinal lesions to segmental sympatheticotonia. In 1995, Nansel and Szlazak suggested that the regulation of segmental sympathetic functions is tightly controlled and that sustained segmental sympatheticotonia does not seem to be a likely promoter of visceral disease. Instead, they suggested that the subluxation complex is likely to create visceral symptoms that mimic true visceral disease via mechanisms similar to those described earlier in the dysafferentation section of this chapter.[1]

The current knowledge about the regulation of autonomic function is far from complete, and in the context of the subluxation complex, our knowledge of autonomic regulation remains in its infancy. However, the balance of evidence suggests that a combination of segmental and suprasegmental mechanisms are likely to be involved.[113,114] It is time we begin investigating these potential mechanisms at our chiropractic college research centers.

The General Adaptation Syndrome

The general adaptation syndrome (GAS) was included as a component of the original subluxation complex model. (See Figure 9-1.) It was Faye's perception that many of the systemic manifestations of the local subluxation complex are likely to be driven by the GAS. In other words, Faye proposed that the subluxation complex would act as a stressor that would induce the GAS. This concept was lost in a number of subsequent reviews regarding subluxation theory.[3-5,106,115]

For details regarding the GAS see reviews by Selye and others.[18,116-127] In part, the GAS, or the stress response, is characterized as an increased release of the stress hormones cortisol and catecholamines that occurs in response to numerous and varying stressors. This is referred to as the alarm reaction. As we adapt to a stressor, we enter the resistance stage, during which cortisol and catecholamine secretion lessens but maintains a higher than normal level. Finally, we enter the stage of exhaustion, in which we are unable to effectively produce stress hormones. Selye made it clear that the GAS is "stress" and that numerous stressors are capable of promoting stress.

Pain, nociception, fear, apprehension, anxiety, prolonged and strenuous exercise, and hypoglycemia are all stressors and known to increase cortisol release.[116-118] Pain and nociception are components of the subluxation complex, and it is possible that the subluxation complex can play a role in promoting the GAS. (See Figure 9-2.) Indeed, pain is one of the stressors used in the research setting to study stress.[123]

In short, all psychological, physical, and biochemical stressors drive the GAS. Whereas cortisol release in normal amounts is physiologically beneficial, a continuous exposure to excess cortisol can produce a continuous drain on body protein stores, especially in muscle, bone, connective tissue, and skin.[116] Excess endogenous cortisol can also reduce REM sleep, reduce cell-mediated immunity by inhibiting the production of interleukin-1, interleukin-2 and gamma interferon, decrease the proliferation of osteoblasts, decrease calcium absorption, reduce collagen synthesis, and reduce glucose utilization.[116]

While we would be typically led to believe that increased cortisol output would suppress inflammation, it is known that glucocorticoid release can also lead to an increased production of inflammatory cells and proinflammatory cytokine release.[124] Additionally, as cortisol release is blunted due to chronic stress, the body begins to lose its endogenous ability to reduce inflammation. This leads to an increase in proinflammatory cytokine release,[122] which can augment the proinflammatory state that is created by a proinflammatory diet[10] and a lack of exercise.[86]

Over the span of a lifetime, the pathophysiologic outcomes of stress, which disrupt tissue homeostasis, are thought to drive numerous diseases including hypertension, depression, atherosclerosis, ischemic heart disease, obesity, syndrome X, cancer, osteoporosis, aging and most other diseases, including the subluxation complex.[18,116-127] This information should lead us to understand why the treatment of chronic disease has failed; there is no one cause of disease. Stress is driven by physical, biochemical, and psychological stressors, which means that the prevention and treatment of chronic disease requires a holistic approach.

Patients must take charge with appropriate lifestyle modifications.

The holistic approach to care illustrated in Figures 9-1 and 9-2 is likely to positively impact upon the general adaptation syndrome, so that chiropractors could play a very positive role in reducing the development of stress-driven diseases. With the advent of salivary adrenal hormone testing in the last decade, it is now possible to measure a component of the stress response in a noninvasive fashion. We can also measure blood levels of acute phase mediators associated with subclinical chronic inflammation, such as interleukin-6 and high sensitivity C-reactive protein. By applying chiropractic care and various lifestyle modifications, we can measure the degree to which we may have an impact on the general adaptation syndrome and the proinflammatory state. Through such measures we can determine how we may impact upon the progression of chronic disease; however, the same measures can be used as markers of wellness.

Chiropractic Care for the Subluxation Complex

Historically, many chiropractors have maintained that adjustments correct subluxations (a bone out of place), and since 1967, some claim the adjustment corrects the subluxation complex, which refers to various pathologic changes in the spine.

The subluxation complex as presented in this text is defined as follows:

A theoretical model of motion segment dysfunction (subluxation) that incorporates the complex interaction of pathologic changes in nerve, muscle, ligamentous, vascular, and connective tissues.

The subluxation complex is a useful model for teaching concepts central to chiropractic theory. To date, extrapolation of related data supports these concepts but should not be construed as "proving" that adjustment actually corrects the subluxation complex.

With this view of the subluxation complex in mind, we know that spinal mobility improves after an adjustment,[128,129] which Faye mentioned in Figure 9-1. We know that neurological changes occur after an adjustment, and that pain diminishes,[128-130] vertebrogenic visceral symptoms may abate,[1,2] and proprioception and motor control may improve.[2,104] We do not know if, and to what extent, myopathology, histopathology, and biochemical changes may improve after an adjustment. We simply do not have the data to make conclusive statements. In theory, myopathology and histopathology would improve as a consequence of the increased movement within the motion segment, assuming the joint remains mobile, which is likely to depend directly on exercise[12,13,131] and indirectly on antiinflammatory nutrition.[10,50]

It is also possible that the analgesic and symptom-reducing effects of the adjustment may not make any corrections and actually mask ongoing pathologies. The first documented case was published in 1981, involving the masking of appendicitis,[132] but little has been written since that time.[7]

Coming to grips with these important issues will be of great benefit to our profession. We need to face where we are with subluxation complex research and accept potential adverse effects of the adjustment, while simultaneously embracing the many potential benefits through appropriate documentation. In this regard, case histories are an excellent way to demonstrate the utility of the chiropractic encounter and an easy way for the private practitioner to publish.

Conceptual Issues to Guide Treatment Approach: The Bigger Picture

The subluxation complex is neither a bone out of place nor a solely mechanical disorder that causes mechanical low back pain. Accordingly, appropriate care of the subluxation complex involves more than a mechanical thrust into the spine, as described previously, and as illustrated in Figures 9-1 and 9-2. The subluxation complex can be viewed as a component of two systemic conditions that are not mutually exclusive. The first is the deconditioning syndrome, which reflects general physical and cardiovascular deconditioning, and the second is the general adaptation syndrome that serves to act as a driver of most chronic degenerative visceral diseases.

After ruling out red flag conditions that require immediate medical referral,[23,133,134] we suggest that chiropractors provide a consultation, provide an examination, and conduct special tests when necessary for the purpose of arriving at a double diagnosis. A biomechanical assessment of the subluxation complex in spinal and extremity joint function would require manipulative, myofascial, and rehabilitative procedures.[6,12-15] This assessment should also include a careful examination of the spine for allodynia, i.e., pain produced by normal palpation, which develops as a consequence of inflammation and nociceptor sensitization that speaks to the need of utilizing an antiinflammatory nutritional approach.[8-10]

Care should be taken to palpate spinous processes, interspinous tissues, and paraspinal muscles. It is not uncommon to find numerous sensitive areas in the spine that are distant from the area of pain complaint. This is particularly true of patients who complain only of low back or sacroiliac pain, yet have allodynia in cervical and upper thoracic tissues. We believe this to be a reflection of chronic subclinical systemic inflammation and not just a local spinal phenomenon. This should lead the chiropractor to be judicious and thoughtful in consideration of the second component of the double diagnosis, which involves a classic yet functional diagnosis that ascertains the general health status of the patient.

Despite the existence of spinal allodynia and chronic inflammation, it is often common for patients to present with no classic diagnostic entities. This is why we elected to use the phrase "classic yet functional diagnosis." The deconditioning syndrome and the GAS should be viewed as "gray areas" in classic diagnosis; we know something is wrong, we just do not know what it is yet in the context of ICD-9 codes. Regarding deconditioning issues, numerous functional assessment procedures that are not part of the classic diagnostic paradigm are available to determine spinal, appendicular, and cardiovascular deconditioning.[12-14,131] Outcome assessment tools are also useful in this regard.[135]

Assessing the GAS is more complicated; however, we can screen for cortisol levels and various inflammatory markers, such as hsCRP and interleukin-6. Carbohydrate or glucose tolerance tests can be used to assess prediabetic states that are known to be proinflammatory. Even if one chooses not to perform biochemical assessments that are not part of the classic diagnostic paradigm, it is possible to therapeutically impact upon the GAS. This is because we can assume that most suffer with the GAS to varying degrees,[18,116-127] which is likely why Selye titled his text, *The Stress of Life*.[18] The following are examples of things we can promote to reduce the GAS: becoming pain free, eating to prevent hypoglycemia, not overeating, eating only antiinflammatory foods, regularly performing moderate to moderately intense exercise, severing unhealthy relationships, reading inspiring or spiritual works, and listening to inspiring music and motivational tapes. In other words, we should urge our patients to pursue health and wellness and we should act as examples.

While practitioners can elect to offer only mechanical care to the spine via the adjustment, we need to appreciate that this approach cannot create a state of optimal physical, mental, and social well-being, i.e., health. A state of health is ultimately an ideal that must be continuously pursued from several angles, and we believe that spinal adjusting is one. There are numerous lifestyle factors related to combating the deconditioning syndrome and the GAS about which patients require guidance from a competent practitioner—hopefully a chiropractor.

Conclusion

Despite the efforts of Langworthy and others who promoted a dynamic model of subluxation some 100 years ago, the segmental bone-out-of-place model of subluxation is still embraced by many current-day chiropractors. Hart presents a case in which a patient was followed and adjusted for four years.[136] Pretreatment and posttreatment cervical x-rays (AP open mouth and neutral lateral cervical) were identical; that is, no changes occurred in the segmental misalignments despite four years of care. Intriguingly, positive changes were noted in motion palpation, leg length, and paraspinal thermographic coupling, suggesting that spinal tissue function improves while static misalignments remain the same. Hart indicates that his findings are consistent with work published by B.J. Palmer in 1938.[136]

Moving away from a static model of subluxation represents a paradigm shift for our profession, even for those who do not perceive subluxation to be a segmental bone out of place. Faye initiated an organized paradigm shift in 1967 when he developed the dynamic, physiological model of the subluxation complex. Since that time, several attempts have been made to advance the concept,[3-5,137,138] each of which essentially views the subluxation complex as a local lesion that requires an adjustment as the only approach to correction. In essence, this misinterpretation of the subluxation complex represents a more contemporary and sophisticated bone-out-of-place model; it is not consistent with physiological mechanisms, pathophysiological mechanisms, and their related treatments, and it represents a continuation of the static chiropractic paradigm.

Clearly, we as a profession are still shifting from a static paradigm to one that is dynamic and integrated in terms of physiology, and pathophysiology and communication among professionals.[139] We hope this chapter helps to further intraprofessional and interprofessional communication.

References

1. Nansel D, Szlazak M. Somatic dysfunction and the phenomenon of visceral disease simulation: a probable explanation for the apparent effectiveness of somatic therapy in patients presumed to be suffering from true visceral disease. J Manipulative Physiol Ther 1995;18:379-97.
2. Seaman DR, Winterstein JF. Dysafferentation, a novel term to describe the neuropathophysiological effects of joint complex dysfunction: a look at likely mechanisms of symptom generation. J Manipulative Physiol Ther 1998;21:267-80.
3. Kent C. Models of vertebral subluxation: a review. J Vert Subluxation Res 1996;1:1-7.
4. Lantz C The vertebral subluxation complex. ICA Review 1989;(Sep/Oct):37-61.
5. Lantz C. The vertebral subluxation complex. In: Gatterman M, editor. Foundations of chiropractic: subluxation. St. Louis: Mosby; 1995. p. 149-74.
6. Schafer R, Faye L. Motion palpation and chiropractic technique. 2nd ed. Huntington Beach, CA: Motion Palpation Institute; 1990.
7. Seaman DR. Do spinal adjustments/manipulation mask ongoing pathologic conditions? J Manipulative Physiol Ther 1999;22:171-9.
8. Seaman DR. Joint complex dysfunction, a novel term to replace subluxation/subluxation complex: etiological and treatment considerations. J Manipulative Physiol Ther 1997;20:634-44.
9. Seaman DR. Clinical nutrition for pain, inflammation, and tissue healing. Hendersonville, NC: NutrAnalysis, Inc; 1998.
10. Seaman DR. The diet-induced pro-inflammatory state: a cause of chronic pain and other degenerative diseases. J Manipulative Physiol Ther 2002;5:168-79.
11. DeFranca GG. Pelvic locomotor dysfunction: a clinical approach. Gaithersburg, MD: Aspen; 1996.
12. Liebenson C, editor. Rehabilitation of the spine: a practitioner's manual. Baltimore: Williams & Wilkins; 1996.
13. Murphy DR, editor. Conservative management of cervical spine syndromes. New York: McGraw-Hill; 2000.
14. Stude DE. Spinal rehabilitation. Stamford, CT: Appleton & Lange; 1999.
15. Troyanovich SJ. Structural rehabilitation of the spine and posture: a practical approach. Huntington Beach, CA: MPAmedia; 2001.
16. Robbins S. Pathologic basis of disease. Philadelphia: WB Saunders; 1974. p. 21-2.
17. Cotran RS, Kumar V, Collins T. Robbins' pathologic basis of disease. 6th ed. Philadelphia: WB Saunders; 1999. p. 1-112.
18. Selye H. The stress of life. New York: McGraw-Hill; 1978.
19. Mayer T, Gatchel R. Functional restoration for spinal disorders: the sports medicine approach. Philadelphia: Lea & Febiger; 1988.
20. Leach RA. History of chiropractic theories. In: Leach RA, editor. The chiropractic theories: a textbook of scientific research. 4th ed. Philadelphia: Lippincott Williams & Wilkins; 2004. p. 13-27.
21. Liebenson C. Pathogenesis of chronic back pain. J Manipulative Physiol Ther 1992;15(5):299-308.
22. Norkin CC, Levangie PK. Joint structure and function: a comprehensive analysis. Philadelphia: FA Davis; 1992. p. 87-8, 120.
23. Waddell G. The back pain revolution. New York: Churchill Livingstone; 1998. p. 9-25, 135-54.
24. Kirkaldy-Willis WH. Pathology and pathogenesis of low back pain. In: Kirkaldy-Willis WH, Burton CV, editors. Managing low back pain. 3rd ed. New York: Churchill Livingstone, 1992; p. 49-79.

25. Slosberg M. Effects of altered afferent input on sensation, proprioception, muscle tone, and sympathetic reflex response. J Manipulative Physiol Ther 1988;11:400-8.

26. Peterson D. Principles of adjustive technique. In: Bergmann T, Peterson D, Lawrence D. Chiropractic technique. New York: Churchill Livingstone; 1993. p. 123-95.

27. Janse J. The integrative purpose and function of the nervous system: a review of classical literature. J Manipulative Physiol Ther 1978;1:182-91.

28. Parkkola R, Kormano M. Lumbar disc and muscle degeneration on MRI: correlation to age and body mass. J Spinal Disord 1992;5:86-92.

29. Parkkola R, Rytokoski U, Kormano M. Magnetic resonance imaging of the discs and trunk muscles in patients with chronic low back pain and healthy control subjects. Spine 1993;18:830-6.

30. Hides JA, Richardson CA, Jull GA. Multifidus muscle recovery is not automatic after resolution of acute, first-episode low back pain. Spine 1996;21:2763-9.

31. Deyo RA. Understanding the accuracy of diagnostic tests. In: Weinstein JN, Rydevik BL, Sonntag VK, editors. Essentials of the spine. New York: Raven Press; 1995. p. 55-69.

32. Schmidt RF. The articular polymodal nociceptor in health and disease. Prog Brain Res 1996;113:53-81.

33. Watkins LR, Maier SF. Beyond neurons: evidence that immune and glial cells contribute to pathological pain states. Physiol Rev 2002;82:981-1011.

34. Nirschl RP, Kraushaar B, Ashman ES. Common sports-related injuries of the elbow. J Musculoskeletal Med 2003;20:324-34.

35. Palmer DD. The chiropractor's adjustor: the science, art, and philosophy of chiropractic. Portland, OR: Portland Printing House Company; 1910. p. 359.

36. Pain in America. A Research Report Prepared for Merck. Ogilvy Public Relations Worldwide; 2000.

37. Patel RK, Everett CR. Low back pain: 20 clinical pearls. J Musculoskeletal Med 2003;20:324-34.

38. Hides JA, Jull GA, Richardson CA. Long-term effects of specific stabilizing exercises for first-episode low back pain. Spine 2001;26:E243-8.

39. Cramer G, Fournier J, Henderson C. Degenerative changes of the articular processes following spinal fixation. J Chiropractic Education 2002:16(1):7.

40. Rich M, Scheiman JM. Nonsteroidal anti-inflammatory drug gastropathy at the new millennium: mechanisms and prevention. Sem Arth Rheum 2000;30:167-79.

41. Mukherjee D, Nissen SE, Topol EJ. Risk of cardiovascular events associated with selective COX-2 inhibitors. J Am Med Assoc 2001;286:954-9.

42. Kirkaldy-Willis WH, Bernard TN. A new look at an old problem. In: Kirkaldy-Willis WH, Bernard TN, editors. Managing low back pain. 4th ed. New York: Churchill Livingstone; 1999. p. 3-9.

43. Burton CV, Cassidy JD. Economics, epidemiology, and risk factors. In: Kirkaldy-Willis WH, Burton CV, editors. Managing low back pain. 3rd ed. New York: Churchill Livingstone; 1992. p. 1-6.

44. Young B, Heath JW. Wheater's functional histology: a color atlas. New York: Churchill Livingstone; 2000.

45. Simopoulos AP. Essential fatty acids in health and chronic disease. Am J Clin Nutr 1999;70(3 Suppl):560S-9S.

46. Hand ES. Nutrients in food. Philadelphia: Lippincott Williams & Wilkins; 2000.

47. Enig MG. Know your fats. Silver Spring, MD: Bethesda Press; 2000.

48. Rule DC, Broughton KS, Shellito SM, Maiorano G. Comparison of muscle fatty acid profiles and cholesterol concentrations of bison, beef cattle, elk, and chicken. J Animal Sci 2002;80:1202-11.

49. Cordain L, Watkins BA, Florant GL, Kelher M, Rogers L, Li Y. Fatty acid analysis of wild ruminant tissues: evolutionary implications for reducing diet-related chronic diseases. Eur J Clin Nutr 2002;56:181-91.

50. Tiku ML, Shah R, Allison GT. Evidence linking chondrocyte lipid peroxidation to cartilage matrix protein degradation: possible role in cartilage aging and the pathogenesis of osteoarthritis. J Biol Chem 2000; 275:20069-76.

51. Demopouolos HB, Pietronigro DD, Seligman ML. The development of secondary pathology with free radical reactions as a threshold mechanism. J Am Coll Toxicol 1983;2:173-84.

52. Sen CK, Packer L. Thiol homeostasis and supplements in physical exercise. Am J Clin Nutr 2000;72(Suppl): 653S-69S.

53. Visioli F, Galli C. The role of antioxidants in the Mediterranean diet. Lipids 2001;36:S49-S52.

54. Chung HY, Kim HJ, Kim JW, Yu BP. The inflammation hypothesis of aging molecular modulation by calorie restriction. Ann NY Acad Sci 2001;928:327-35.

55. Olgun A, Akman S, Serdar MA, Kutluay T. Oxidative phosphorylation enzyme complexes in caloric restriction. Exp Gerontol 2002;37:639-45.

56. Halliwell B, Evans P, Kaur H, Aruoma O. Free radicals, tissue injury, and human disease: a potential of therapeutic use of antioxidants? In: Kinney J, Tucker H, editors. Organ metabolism and nutrition: ideas for future critical care. New York: Raven Press; 1994. p. 425-45.

57. Yasuma T, Arai K, Suzuki F. Age-related phenomena in the lumbar intervertebral discs: lipofuscin and amyloid deposition. Spine 1992;17:1194-8.

58. Tiku ML, Liesch JB, Robertson FM. Production of hydrogen peroxide by rabbit articular chondrocytes: enhancement by cytokines. J Immunol 1990;145:690-6.

59. Grigolo B, Roseti L, Fiorini M, Facchini A. Enhanced lipid peroxidation in synoviocytes from patients with osteoarthritis. J Rheumatol 2003;30:345-7.

60. Tiku ML, Allison GT, Naik K, Karry SK. Malondialdehyde oxidation of cartilage collagen by chondrocytes. Osteoarthritis Cartilage 2003;11:159-66.

61. Brown GC, Nicholls DG, Cooper CE, editors. Mitochondria and cell death. Princeton, NJ: Princeton University Press; 1999.

62. Fosslien E. Mitochondrial medicine—molecular pathology of defective oxidative phosphorylation. Ann Clin Lab Sci 2001;31:25-67.

63. Linnane AW, Zhang C, Yarovaya N, Kopsidas G, Kovalenko S, Papakostopoulos P et al. Human aging and global function of coenzyme Q10. Ann NY Acad Sci 2002;959:396-411.

64. McKenzie D, Bua E, McKiernan S, Cao Z, Wanagat J, Aiken JM. Mitochondrial DNA deletion mutations: a causal role in sarcopenia. Eur J Biochem 2002;269: 2010-15.

65. Seaman DR, Cleveland C. Spinal pain syndromes: nociceptive, neuropathic, and psychologic mechanisms. J Manipulative Physiol Ther 1999;22:458-72.

66. Seaman DR. Proprioceptor: an obsolete, inaccurate word. J Manipulative Physiol Ther 1997;20(4): 279-84.

67. Bonica JJ. Definitions and taxonomy of pain. In: Bonica JJ, editor. The management of pain. 2nd ed. Philadelphia: Lea & Febiger; 1990. p. 18-27.

68. Leach RA, Pickar JG. Segmental dysfunction hypothesis: joint and muscle pathology and facilitation. In: Leach RA, editor. The chiropractic theories: a textbook of scientific research. Baltimore: Lippincott Williams & Wilkins; 2004. p. 137-205.

69. Schmidt R, Schaible H, Messlinger K, Heppelmann B, Hanesch U, Pawlak M. Silent and active nociceptors: structure, functions, and clinical implications. In: Gebhart GF, Hammond DL, Jensen TS, editors. Proc 7th World Congress Pain, 1993, Paris, France. Seattle; 1994. p. 213-250.

70. McLain RF. Mechanoreceptor endings in human cervical facet joints. Spine 1994;19:495-501.

71. McLain RF, Pickar JG. Mechanoreceptor endings in human thoracic and lumbar facet joints. Spine 1998; 23:168-73.

72. Mense S, Simmons DG. Muscle pain: understanding its nature, diagnosis and treatment. Philadelphia: Lippincott, Williams & Wilkins; 2001. p. 26-30.

73. Byers MR, Bonica JJ. Peripheral pain mechanisms and nociceptor plasticity. In: Loeser JD, editor. Bonica's management of pain. 3rd ed. Philadelphia: Lippincott, Williams & Wilkins; 2001. p. 26-72.

74. Bogduk N. Innervation patterns of the cervical spine. In: Grant R, editor. Physical therapy of the cervical and thoracic spine. 2nd ed. New York: Churchill Livingstone; 1994. p. 65-76.

75. Bogduk N, Valencia F. Innervation patterns of the thoracic spine. In: Grant R, editor. Physical therapy of the cervical and thoracic spine. 2nd ed. New York: Churchill Livingstone; 1994. p. 77-87.

76. Bogduk N. Innervation, pain patterns, and mechanisms of pain production. In: Twomey L, Taylor J, editors. Physical therapy of the low back. 2nd ed. New York: Churchill Livingstone; 1994. p. 93-109.

77. Charman R. Pain and nociception: mechanisms and modulation in sensory context. In: Boyling J, Palastanga N, editors. Grieve's modern manual therapy: the vertebral column. 2nd ed. New York: Churchill Livingstone; 1994. p. 253-70.

78. Grieve G. Common vertebral joint problems. 2nd ed. New York: Churchill Livingstone; 1988. p. 51-2.

79. Haldeman S. The neurophysiology of pain. In: Haldeman S, editor. Principles and practice of chiropractic. 2nd ed. Norwalk, CT: Appleton-Century-Crofts; 1992. p. 165-84.

80. Wyke B. The neurological basis of thoracic pain. Rheum Phys Med 1970;10(7):356-67.

81. Wyke BD. Neurological aspects of pain therapy. In: Swerdlow M, editor. The therapy of pain. Philadelphia: Lippincott; 1980. p. 1-30.

82. Bove GM, Light AR. Unmyelinated nociceptors of rat paraspinal tissues. J Neurophysiol 1995;73:1752-62.

83. Bove GM. Nociceptors, pain, and chiropractic. In: Redwood D, editor. Contemporary chiropatic. New York: Churchill Livingstone; 1997. p. 205-17.

84. Price DD. Psychological and neural mechanisms of pain. New York: Raven Press; 1988.

85. Brack A, Rittner HL, Machelska H, Shaqura M, Mousa SA, Labuz D et al. Endogenous peripheral antinociception in early inflammation is not limited by the number of opioid-containing leukocytes but by opioid receptor expression. Pain 2004;108:67-75.

86. Booth FW, Chakravarthy MV, Spangenburg EE. Exercise and gene expression: physiological regulation of the human genome through physical activity. J Physiol 2002;543:399-411.

87. Granstein RD. Neuropeptides in inflammation and immunity. In: Gallin JI, Snyderman R, editors. Inflammation: basic principles and clinical correlates. 3rd ed. Philadelphia: Lippincott, Williams & Wilkins; 1999. p. 397-404.

88. Barnes PJ. Neurogenic inflammation and asthma. J Asthma 1992;29:165-80.

89. Joos GF, Germonpre PR, Pauwels RA. Role of tachykinins in asthma. Allergy 2000;55:321-37.

90. Willis WD. Hyperalgesia and allodynia. New York: Raven Press; 1992.

91. Watkins LR, Milligan ED, Maier SF. Glial activation: a driving force for pathological pain. Trends Neurosci 2001;24:450-5.

92. Baba H, Doubell TP, Woolf CJ. Peripheral inflammation facilitates A fiber-mediated synaptic input to the substantia gelatinosa of the adult rat spinal cord. J Neurosci 1999;19:859-67.

93. Reid DC. Sports injury assessment and rehabilitation. New York: Churchill Livingstone; 1992. p. 13-29.

94. Rang HP, Bevan S, Dray A. Chemical activation of nociceptive peripheral neurones. Brit Med Bull 1991;47(3): 534-48.

95. Rang HP, Bevan S, Dray A. Nociceptive peripheral neurons: cellular properties. In: Wall PD, Melzack R, editors. Textbook of pain. 3rd ed. New York: Churchill Livingstone; 1994. p. 57-78.

96. Basbaum AI, Levine JD. The contribution of the nervous system to inflammation and inflammatory disease. Can J Physiol Pharmacol 1991;69:647-51.

97. Levine J, Taiwo Y, Heller P. Hyperalgesic pain: inflammatory and neuropathic. In: Willis W, editor. Hyperalgesia and allodynia. New York: Raven Press; 1992. p. 117-23.

98. Heller PH, Green PG, Tanner KD, Miao FJP, Levine JD. Peripheral neural contributions to inflammation. In: Fields HL, Liebeskind JC, editors. Pharmacological approaches to the treatment of chronic pain: new concepts and critical issues: progress in pain research and management; Seattle: IASP Press; 1994. p. 31-42.

99. Coderre TJ, Basbaum AI, Dallman MF, Helms C, Levine JD. Epinephrine exacerbates arthritis by an action at presynaptic β2-adrenoceptors. Neuroscience 1990;34:521-3.

100. Feinstein B, Langton J, Jameson R, Schiller F. Experiments on pain referred from deep somatic tissues. J Bone Joint Surg 1954; 36A(5):981-97.

101. Bonica J. Clinical importance of hyperalgesia. In: Willis W, editor. Hyperalgesia and allodynia. New York: Raven Press; 1992. p. 17-43.

102. Watkins LR, Maier SF. The pain of being sick: implications of immune-to-brain communication for understanding pain. Annu Rev Psychol 2000;51:29-57.

103. de Jong P, de Jong J, Cohen B, Jongkees L. Ataxia and nystagmus induced by injection of local anesthetics in the neck. Ann Neurol 1977;1:240-6.

104. Fitz-Ritson D. Cervicogenic vertigo. J Manipulative Physiol Ther 1991;14(3):193-8.

105. Peterson D, Wiese G. Chiropractic: an illustrated history. St. Louis: Mosby; 1995. p. 247.

106. Masarsky CS, Todres-Masarsky M. Somatovisceral aspects of chiropractic: an evidence-based approach. New York: Churchill Livingstone; 2001.

107. Korr IM. Clinical significance of the facilitated state. J Am Osteo Assoc 1955;54:277-82.

108. Korr IM. Sustained sympathicotonia as a factor in disease. In: Korr IM, editor. The neurobiologic mechanisms of manipulative therapy. New York: Plenum Press; 1978. p. 229-68.

109. Denslow J, Hassett C. The central excitatory state associated with postural abnormalities. J Neurophysiol 1942;5:393-402.

110. Denslow J, Korr I, Krems A. Quantitative studies of chronic facilitation in human motoneurons. Am J Physiol 1947;150(2):229-38.

111. The collected papers of Irvin M. Korr. American Acad Osteopathy; 1978.

112. Selected papers of John Stedman Denslow. 1993 Yearbook. Indianapolis: American Acad Osteopathy; 1993.

113. Sato A. Reflex modulation of visceral functions by somatic afferent activity. In: Patterson MM, Howell JN, editors. The central connection: somatovisceral/viscerosomatic interaction. Athens, OH: American Academy of Osteopathy; 1992. p. 53-72.

114. Blessing WW. The lower brainstem and bodily homeostasis. New York: Oxford University Press; 1997.

115. Leach RA, editor. The chiropractic theories: a textbook of scientific research. 4th ed. Philadelphia: Lippincott Williams & Wilkins; 2004.

116. Berne R, Matthew L. Physiology. 3rd ed. St. Louis: Mosby; 1993. p. 949-79.

117. Dilman V, Dean W. The neuroendocrine theory of aging and degenerative disease. Pensacola, FL: Center for Bio-Gerontology; 1992. p. 26-7.

118. Asterita M. The physiology of stress. New York: Human Sciences Press; 1985. p. 176.

119. Sapolsky R. Why zebras don't get ulcers. New York: WH Freeman and Company; 1994.

120. Sapolsky R. Stress, the aging brain, and the mechanisms of neuron death. Cambridge, MA: MIT Press; 1992. p. 6, 265, 267.

121. Csermely P, editor. Stress of life: from molecules to man. Ann NY Acad Sci 1998;851:1-547.

122. McEwen BS. Protective and damaging effects of stress mediators. New J Med 1998;338:171-9.

123. Pacak K, Palkovits M. Stressor specificity of central neuroendocrine responses: implications for stress-related disorders. Endocr Rev 2001;22:502-48.

124. Sapolsky RM, Romero LM, Munck AU. How do glucocorticoids influence stress responses? Integrating permissive, suppressive, stimulatory, and preparative actions. Endocr Rev 2000;21(1):55-89.

125. Sapolsky RM. Glucocorticoids, stress, and their adverse neurological effects: relevance to aging. Exp Gerontol 1999;34(6):721-32.

126. Szabo S. Hans Selye and the development of the stress concept. Special reference to gastroduodenal ulcerogenesis. Ann N Y Acad Sci 1998;851:19-27.

127. Chrousos GP. Stressors, stress, and neuroendocrine integration of the adaptive response: the 1997 Hans Selye Memorial lecture. Ann NY Acad Sci 1998;851:311-35.

128. Cassidy JD. Kirkaldy-Willis WH, Thiel HW. Manipulation. In: Kirkaldy-Willis WH, Burton CV, editors. Managing low back pain. 3rd ed. New York: Churchill Livingstone; 1992. p. 283-96.

129. Carrick FR. Cervical radiculopathy: the diagnosis and treatment of pathomechanics in the cervical spine. J Manipulative Physiol Ther 1983;6:129-37.

130. Kirkaldy-Willis WH, Cassidy JD. Spinal manipulation in the treatment of low back pain. Can Fam Phys 1985;31:535-40.

131. McGill SM. Low back disorders: evidence-based prevention and rehabilitation. Champaign, IL: Human Kinetics; 2002.

132. Dyck VG, Embree BE. The enigma of referred abdominal pain in chiropractic practice: a literature review and case report. J Manipulative Physiol Ther 1981;4:11-4.

133. Souza TA. Differential diagnosis and management for the chiropractor: protocols and algorithms. Gaithersburg, MD: Aspen Publishers; 2001.

134. Nelson C, Murphy DR, Fowler J, Wilterdink J, Tabamo R. Headache. In: Murphy DR, editor. Conservative management of cervical spine syndromes. New York: McGraw-Hill; 2000.

135. Yeomans SG. The clinical applications of outcomes assessment. Stamford, CT: Appleton & Lange; 2000.

136. Hart JF. Persistence of vertebral misalignments detected on radiographs of cervical spine during chiropractic care: a case study. J Vertebral Sublux Res 1997;1:1-5.

137. Dishman RW. Static and dynamic components of the chiropractic subluxation complex: a literature review. J Manipulative Physiol Ther 1988;11:98-107.

138. Dishman RW. Review of the literature supporting a scientific basis for the chiropractic subluxation complex. J Manipulative Physiol Ther 1985;8:163-74.

139. Gatterman MI. Principles of chiropractic. In: Gatterman MI. Chiropractic management of spine related disorders. 2nd ed. Baltimore: Lippincott, Williams and Wilkins; 2003. p. 49-68.

10

Theoretic Models of Subluxation

Robert D. Mootz

Key Words   Vertebral malposition, joint fixation, meniscoid entrapment, somatic dysfunctional adhesion, nuclear fragmentation, facet tropism, motion segment buckling, somatic reflexes

After reading this chapter you should be able to answer the following questions:

Question 1   How does the early model of chiropractic subluxation differ from the model of osteopathic lesion?

Question 2   How can one tell if a chiropractic theory is of high quality?

Question 3   What are the strengths and weaknesses of using subluxation models as a scientific theory, a professional identity, a clinical finding, and a diagnosis?

Question 4   What is *motion segment buckling* and how might it be best classified (e.g., as a biomechanical, neurologic, or trophic model)?

Question 5   How might chiropractors use the placebo effect to benefit their patients?

This discussion offers an overview of models of chiropractic subluxation along with an approach for classification (Box 10-1). The "chiropractic vertebral subluxation" remains a controversial concept. Its nature remains elusive, and its diagnostic and political values have been vigorously debated.[1-3] Numerous reviews, discussions, definitions, and justifications abound,[4-7] but the ability to discuss, support, critically evaluate, and differentiate between what is known, what is only supported, and what is purely conjecture regarding the subluxation remains an emotional issue within the profession. A lack of agreement on standardization in definitions and classifications has permeated discussions on adjusting and subluxation.[8,9] This lack of agreement has stimulated a study for the development of chiropractic nomenclature through consensus. In addition to chiropractors, other health care providers manipulate the spine, including some osteopaths, physical therapists, and physical medicine practitioners. Each professional group has developed and perpetuated a philosophically trademarked "brand name" for the spinal lesion it manipulates. Historically, each has offered its own explanations of the lesion and any physiologic implications. These are summarized in Box 10-2.

BOX 10-1 ■ Criteria for Plausible and Acceptable Theory

- Systematic set of interrelated concepts, definitions, and propositions that formulates explanation of relationships
- Components are orderly and based on data
- Derived from empirical observations and facts (as opposed to speculations)
- Contributes to classification of concepts and constructs
- Empirical generalizations may inform conceptual frameworks
- Informs research hypotheses about predicted relationships that are scientifically testable
- Evolves and is refined based on new knowledge

BOX 10-2 ■ Historical Development of Manipulable Spinal Lesion Concepts

Chiropractic vertebral subluxation

- Early conception (1910): Structural disrelationship of spinal joints causing nerve impingement at the intervertebral foramen.
- Modern conception (1979): Abnormal physical relationship between adjacent articular structures eliciting neurologic responses.

Osteopathic concepts

- Early conception of osteopathic lesion (1899): Altered relationship of zygapophyseal joints affecting flow of vital body fluids (blood, lymph, nerve).
- Modern conception of somatic dysfunction (1973): Impaired or altered function of related somatic components (musculoskeletal, arthrodial, and myofascial) and related vascular, lymphatic, and neural elements.

Medical manipulable spinal lesion concepts

- Early conceptions (1930s): Facet fixation due to mechanical derangement of the posterior joints may cause pain; intervertebral disc dysfunction may cause pain and/or radiculopathy.
- Modern conception (1978): Joint dysfunction contributes to complex neurologic reflexes that affect the neuromusculoskeletal system.

From Mootz RD. Chiropractic models: current understanding of vertebral subluxation and manipulable spinal lesions. In: Sweere J, editor. Chiropractic family practice. Gaithersburg, MD: Aspen Publishers; 1992.

The Palmers originally described and defined the chiropractic subluxation by a number of clinically observable characteristics.[10,11] They proposed that subluxation was a structural disrelation that resulted in altered or impeded neurologic function.[12,13] The American Chiropractic Association has established that a subluxation represents an abnormal physical relationship between adjacent anatomic structures whose contiguous tissues elicit neurologic responses.[7] Although the sophistication of hypothetical mechanisms has increased,[5,14,15] chiropractors have continually emphasized the proposed neurologic component of the subluxation. This emphasis on the neurologic components of the subluxation has led to development[16] and refinement of the vertebral subluxation complex.[17] (See Chapter 9.)

Osteopathy describes a different lesion altogether. A.T. Still[18] coined the term *osteopathic lesion* to describe an altered relationship of the zygapophyseal joints affecting the flow of "vital body fluids," especially blood and lymph. In recent years the osteopathic profession has agreed on a name change to *somatic dysfunction*. This has been defined as "impaired or altered function of related components of the somatic system: musculoskeletal, arthrodial and myofascial structures, and related vascular, lymphatic, and neural elements."[19,20] Throughout its history, the osteopathic world has speculated on the ischemic and trophic qualities of spinal disrelation as well as neurologic aberration.

Manual medicine also has recognized manipulable spinal lesions. However, medicine's terminology has been based on strict anatomic diagnoses. Mennell[21] was convinced that a mechanical posterior joint derangement was responsible for loss of joint play. Cyriax[22] emphasized the contribution of "intervertebral disc dysfunction." Other manual medicine practitioners and physical therapists have theorized an important role for loss of soft tissue elasticity.[23] Although medical manipulators' opinions differ as to what the manipulable lesion is, they have tended to be skeptical of any significant neurologic component other than pain being associated with it. With recent English-language works of East European neurologists such as Lewit[24] and Janda,[25,26] medical thought is beginning to appreciate more complex neurologic ramifications of spinal joint dysfunction. Organized medicine as a whole has only recently begun to acknowledge benefits from spinal manipulation.

Conceptual Models and Controversy

Although the medical and osteopathic professions have a small number of proponents for manipula-

---

BOX 10-3 ■ Conceptual Uses of Subluxation Models

- As chiropractic theory—explanatory of physical effects of adjustment
- As professional identity—basis for practice and defining profession
- As a clinical finding—target for localizing adjustive interventions
- As a clinical diagnosis—a distinct clinical condition or syndrome

---

tion and models of spinal lesion, in the chiropractic profession attention to subluxation is found in virtually every dimension of its existence, be it clinical, political, philosophical, or scientific. Although few chiropractors dispute that manipulative and adjustive interventions in the spine are targeted at some kind of physical dysfunction, chiropractors have varied substantially in the rationale, importance, and use of the syntax surrounding that dysfunction. Subluxation has been used at least four distinct ways by chiropractors (Box 10-3). All four uses of subluxation have merits and liabilities within different contexts.

- Subluxation as Chiropractic Theory: Subluxation is used as an explanatory mechanism for physical effects of chiropractic intervention.[5]
- Subluxation as Professional Identity: Subluxation forms the entire basis of and for chiropractic practice.[27]
- Subluxation as a Clinical Finding: Subluxation serves as target for localizing manipulative and adjustive intervention.[28]
- Subluxation as a Clinical Diagnosis: Subluxation represents a distinct clinical condition or syndrome.[10]

Use as Theory

As a theory, subluxation has merit in that the kinds of models and contentions proposed for subluxation are consistent with how models are developed within the greater scientific and health communities. Using subluxation in this way is understandable by nonchiropractors and experimental verification and refinement are enhanced as more information is learned. Subluxation theory remains poorly developed, however. Most models are primarily conceptual and explanatory. Although basic science research, particularly in biomechanics, has grown dramatically in recent years, experimental evolution of models remains in its infancy. Underdeveloped theory also has potential for "mis-use" or "misguided" use when promulgated as a justification to avoid accountability to conventional medical or health care constraints (e.g., appropriateness of care determinations, duration, and frequency of care issues). Chiropractic theory represents the primary context in which subluxation is used in this chapter.

Use as Professional Identity

Subluxation as a concept has been used in attempts to distinguish chiropractic practice from what other health providers do. The merit of this approach is that "self-identity" is enhanced, permitting a concise way to differentiate roles and services provided by doctors of chiropractic. Using "subluxation" as a basis for practice can also focus care strategies. Consistent with a specialist model typical of other health professions is identification of the chiropractic profession with something like "spinal health." It is a general concept with a positive image that centers on something of concern and interest to patients. Dentists, for example, tend to identify their place in health care with "oral health" more so than a particular theoretical model or syntax related to dental caries. In addition to inconsistency with social norms, identifying with a theoretical pathophysiological condition is very doctor-centric and may convey perceptions of lack of interest in patients, i.e., if the chiropractic profession fits patients to its needs rather than the other way around. [Editor's note: A broader and more patient-centered professional identity is that of chiropractors as wellness doctors who do not subtract the patient from the subluxation or from the spine.]

When an identity becomes codified in laws and policies, updating them is difficult once conventions or knowledge changes. The x-ray requirement to document subluxation radiographically for Medicare coverage in the United States is a classic example. After studies reported problems with demonstrating subluxation on x-ray, new and better dynamic models of subluxation were developed, and alternative clinical methods for detection became standard. Chiropractors and their representatives spent countless dollars and hours trying to change laws and had to practice for decades under outdated conventions that they themselves had championed at one point. It is not surprising that all other health professions aim to "legislate as broadly as possible" and "practice as narrowly" as they choose. When this is superimposed on a lack of professional consensus about subluxation as well, it contributes to substantial confusion in the minds of policy makers and the public.[29]

Use as a Clinical Finding

As a clinical tool for helping a doctor of chiropractic localize and target his or her intervention, subluxation has many strengths. Having profession-unique syntax and models that might not be readily conceptualized by others is not a problem when used as a clinical tool. All professions have their corollaries. Because standard clinical evaluation methods allow manifestations of subluxation to be operationalized by indirect means (e.g., localized tenderness, muscle spasm, asymmetrical or limited gait or motion, neurological radiation patterns), the lesion per se need only be conceptualized, not specifically demonstrated.

Use as a Clinical Diagnosis

Subluxation is also used as a clinical diagnosis. Frequently modified to be a complex or syndrome, the idea here is to actually label a patient's condition with this. Some feel a unique diagnostic term confers legitimacy to practice models, and just focusing on a single diagnostic term simplifies initial insurance reporting. However, diagnostic conditions that lack accepted case definitions (e.g., presentation, progression) are sources of controversy in policymaking, and coverage decisions can become problematic. For example, if a condition is to be covered by many payers, the health consequences need to be well established. A "diagnosis" of subluxation further lacks specificity to drive intervention or even a systematic approach to options for intervention. The single diagnosis of subluxation really implies that any chiropractic technique is appropriate for any subluxation. Techniques must be modified to the area of complaint and the uniqueness of the individual. In addition, clustering around a single diagnostic entity for actuarial purposes can be a problem. Diagnostic categorization of all chiropractic patients who have subluxation reveals dramatic practice variation and serves as policy justification for arbitrary cost containment policies. If subluxation can be fixed in three visits with some patients, why can it not be fixed that quickly in all patients? Consideration of the aggregate of signs and symptoms that commonly occur with subluxation of different regions of the spine along with concomitant pathology is necessary to describe and document the true status of the patient's condition. (See Chapters 17 to 27.)

Overall, as a theory, model, or clinical finding, subluxation offers significant utility and does so in a fashion that is not out of step with the greater health care community. Implementing subluxation as a professional identity per se or as a simple clinical diagnosis without concomitant findings, however, can be fraught with unintended social reactions that can engender more arbitrary treatment and lead to greater scrutiny and administrative burden.

Clinical Rationale Provides Logical Method for Model Classification

Development of clinical theories and models are typically the result of attempts to rationally explain empirically observable clinical phenomena. Such is the case with manipulable subluxations. The historical models discussed earlier represent isolated attempts to do so. Research in this arena originally occurred primarily within the osteopathic profession.[30,31] In recent years, advances in understanding of spinal cord neural behavior, pain generation, reflex effects, and biomechanics have generated a substantial amount of scientific litera-

ture that is shedding light on how chiropractors approach subluxation models.[32-34] It is worthwhile to characterize some clinical issues in attempting to classify subluxation models. All practitioners tend to follow similar clinical processes in attempting to identify the site of a manipulable subluxation. Box 10-4 lists some common clinical characteristics looked for by manipulators. This approach provides the basis for organizing the various models of subluxation presented here.

After a thorough history and physical examination, practitioners perform a mechanical evaluation. The manipulator may look for contributing mechanical causes (nature of injury, repetitive postural activities), static asymmetries (e.g., high shoulder, altered curves, externally rotated hip or foot), dynamic asymmetries (gait, other movements), as well as passive and active individual joint ranges of motion (static and motion palpation). Some practitioners try to image these altered mechanics radiographically.[35]

Most practitioners also look for changes in neurologic activity, often identified by patient symptomatology. Pain distribution patterns provide historic cues. Palpating for tenderness and muscle spasm or altered tone also may suggest neurologic

---

BOX 10-4 ■ Evaluation for Manipulable Subluxations

General health assessment

- History
- Physical examination
- Special studies (radiographic imaging, clinical laboratory tests, etc.)

Mechanical assessment

- History of mechanical etiologies
- Static structural asymmetries
- Dynamic structural/mechanical asymmetries
- Static palpation
- Motion palpation
- Imaging of structural alterations (radiographic, functional capacity testing, motion analysis, etc.)

activity. Some look for indirect indications of neurologic involvement by assessing vasoconstriction or dilation (thermography), and sudomotor activity (galvanic skin response). Standard neurologic indicators including hyperreflexia or hyporeflexia, sensory changes, and motor changes also may suggest spinal dysfunctions. Some consider altered tissue texture and edema as indications of aberrant local tissue metabolism or vascularization (e.g., rubor, tumor, dolor, calor).

All healers recognize the role the patient's psyche and lifestyle play in the function of the body's somatic structures. Mental attitude, social interactions, lifestyle habits, and stress may induce muscular tightness that leads to more anxiety and contributes to abnormal muscle tension. Attempting to break the cycle with a spinal adjustment has been a clinical option taken by many manipulators.

When assessing the purposes of manipulation, it is clear that aberrant mechanics, neurologic activity, trophic function, or psychosocial problems are addressed. The argument then is made that a classification system for models of subluxation as a manipulable spinal lesion should be based on commonalities of generic clinical practice rather than "brand-name" theories. Specific explanations of the vertebral subluxation within each of these four general categories of biomechanical, neurologic, trophic, and psychosocial models are presented and summarized in Box 10-5. Rationale, explanations, and brief reviews of relevant literature of these clinically derived models are presented in the following discussion.

BOX 10-5 ■ Models of Chiropractic Subluxation

Biomechanical models

- Vertebral malposition
- Fixation caused by adhesion
- Fixation caused by nuclear fragmentation
- Disc deformation caused by tissue creep
- Hypermobility and ligamentous laxity
- Mechanical joint locking
- Motion segment buckling

Neurologic models

- Nerve, root, DRG compression or traction
- Spinal cord compression and traction
- Somatosomatic reflexes
- Autonomic reflexes
- Motor system degeneration
- Psychoneuroimmunology

Trophic models

- Aberrant axoplasmic transport
- Intraneural microcirculation ischemia
- Macrocirculation ischemia
- Altered cerebrospinal fluid flow

Psychosocial models

- Placebo effects
- Stress reduction
- Lifestyle modification

Models of Chiropractic Subluxation

Biomechanical Models

Vertebral Malposition

One of the oldest concepts of subluxation considers trauma to be a major cause of altered joint position. Palmer[12] and Still[36] both discussed this model, and Leach's chapter[5] on intervertebral subluxation reviews medical literature regarding radiographically demonstrable articular disrelationships. Trauma, disc degeneration, erosive arthritides, and congenital factors all have been shown to cause such radiographic changes. However, reduction of such mechanical alterations has not been demonstrated with manipulation. More subtle mechanical alterations are probably what chiropractors adjust; these are difficult to demonstrate radiographically.[35] The clinical value of radiography for such assessments has been questioned.[37,38] (See Chapters 6 and 8.)

The concept of a static misalignment, although promising initially, seems difficult to support. Chiropractic studies have thus far shown interobserver and intraobserver agreement of many technique-based x-ray markings to be relatively poor.[38] Some radiographic mensuration methods indicating disc wedging and overall articular contours can be evaluated consistently and are sometimes used as indications for mechanical therapies. However, good quantitative outcome studies clearly identifying usefulness remain to be done. Although this mechanical approach may potentially indicate aberrant segmental position, it also may be representative of activity of surrounding musculature. Discussion of the latter lies within the domain of neurologic models, specifically somatosomatic reflexes. Mechanically, the "out-of-place bone" is not likely to be the sole explanation for chiropractic subluxation.

Fixation Caused by Adhesion

Adhesion in and around synovial joints may arise in two ways. It may result from trauma that results in extracellular accumulation of inflammatory exudate and blood.[39] Platelets then release thrombin-converting fibrinogen into fibrin, which organizes into collagenous scar tissue, resulting in a variety of soft tissue and articular adhesions. A second type of adhesion results from the dehydration associated with immobilization. Extensibility of connective tissue is caused by infusion of water between layers of proteoglycan molecules. This provides lubrication, allowing for a more parallel configuration and greater stretch under longitudinal tension.[40] Immobilization leads to dehydration with resultant approximation of the proteoglycans, which tend to stick together, creating movement restrictions.[41,42] Another by-product of prolonged immobilization can be intraarticular fatty adhesion within synovial joints.[43] The relevance to spinal lesion models is that both trauma and immobilization are frequently implicated causes in patients with subluxation. Manipulation increases movement in dehydrated tissues, promoting the imbibition of fluid, or the actual mechanical shearing or breakdown of newly deposited adhesions. This model explains many clinical phenomena and is supportable based on the literature.[44]

Fixation Caused by Meniscoid Entrapment

Bogduk and Engel[45] and Giles and Taylor[46,47] have reported on the presence of intraarticular synovial tabs, or meniscoids. These tabs may cause fixation when the fibrocartilaginous edge of a tab gets caught between the articular surfaces.[48] The resultant deformation and restriction, especially at end range, is also thought to stress the joint capsule from which the meniscoid originates. This may result in irritation of the capsular nerve endings and may contribute to pain and spasm. Meniscoids appear to be present throughout the spinal facet joints.[48,49] However, problems with this model have been identified:[42] Meniscoids may not be present in fixed joints, and most meniscoids may actually be softer than the joint cartilage and therefore may be more likely to be deformed or cleaved by the joint.[44] Disorders such as rheumatoid arthritis appear to have associated proliferation of synovial tabs,[48] yet there does not seem to be any reporting of increased likelihood of fixation in these individuals. Although the potential is promising for some kind of role of synovial tabs, particularly as instigators of muscle spasm,[45] or perhaps through extrampment where the meniscoid becomes trapped beyond the articular facets, they do not seem likely to be the primary cause of subluxation.

Fixation Caused by Nuclear Fragments

This model suggests that, through movement, a portion of the disc's nucleus pulposus pushes through weakened sections of the anulus fibrosis. The concept of disc fragmentation is fairly well established, and its role in creating stresses in the nucleus that lead to fissures appears plausible.[50] The phenomenon that such fragments may impede normal movement between the end plates and that spinal manipulation may obviate resultant dysfunction is the model considered here. Dysfunction or restriction in normal movement (as well as resultant muscle spasm) may result in fixation.[51] Disc derangements have been implicated in manipulable spinal lesions for some time.[52-54] Sandoz[55] suggests that long axis manipulation coupled with rotation could suction the fragment centrally. It has been suggested by Farfan et al.[56] that the layers of the anulus migrate, permitting the disc to withstand large amounts of compression before a second rupture. However, manipulators report fixation in joints without discs (for example, the atlanto-occipital junction, or the sacroiliac joints).[24,57] Fixations seem to occur in younger individuals for whom disc degeneration is not a likely contributing factor. Further contradicting this model are arguments pointing out that the earliest degenerative anular changes begin at the periphery and work centrally.[58] Additionally, there seems to be little evidence of nuclear fragmentation on autopsy.[58]

Disc Deformity as a Manipulable Lesion

Radiographically observable changes in intervertebral disc alignment have been used as an indicator of subluxation.[59,60] Prolonged compressive loading of a disc has been shown to lead to tissue creep[61] that results in degenerative changes in anular composition. Manipulation of such discs has not been shown to alter either configuration or composition of structures having undergone such tissue creep, However, it is reasonable to suggest that mechanical stresses (manipulation, stretch, exercise) directed in an opposing manner may help slow progressive degenerative changes. In light of Weisel's report[62] of a significant incidence of disc herniation in asymptomatic patients, the clinical role such trophic and biomechanical changes play remains speculative.

Hypermobility and Laxity as Manipulable Lesions

It is obvious that a lax joint is not likely to be mechanically benefited by manipulation. It can be argued, however, that hypermobility and the resultant irritation may lead to muscle spasm and symptomatology that could respond to mechanical stimuli. Manipulation of an unstable segment seems unlikely to promote greater instability, provided such manipulation is properly applied within the joint's physiologic range. However, this approach would probably be temporary and palliative. Some have suggested that hypermobile segments result from fixed or fused segments at an adjacent level.[58] Instability then may be an indicator for assessment of surrounding areas. (See Chapter 8.)

Mechanical Joint Locking

From a purely mechanical point of view, Steindler[63] noted that tropism in the lumbar spine,

in which one facet has a more coronal orientation while the other is oriented more sagittally, can lead to the sagittal facets mutually locking on each other. Farfan and Sullivan[64] describe this locking as the "cam" effect of the facets when one facet is rotated against its "fellow." They contend that the more coronal-facing facet fails to resist sheer force created by torsion. High magnitude strain falls directly on the disc corresponding to the level of disc pathology and the side of disc herniation.

Coplens[65] suggests that tropism or asymmetry of the apophyseal joint causes diminished mechanical efficiency, leading to limitation of motion that may be readily relieved by manipulation. A change in the axis of rotation allowed by the slight translation in the spinal motion segment can screw down the inferior facets, twisting them like an eccentric cam and jamming them against the cup-like superior facets.[66] Gravity and muscle spasm then continue to hold the facets in a locked position. Mechanical locking from a slight shift in the rotational axis of the sacroiliac joints has also been described by Turek.[67] (See Chapter 26.) The immediate relief often experienced after manipulation makes this theory appealing.

Motion Segment Buckling

Triano[33,34] has proposed that a mechanical phenomenon associated with a local, uncontrolled mechanical response to spinal loading results in a confluence of tissue reactions that can become symptomatic. The concept of motion segment buckling is that empirically, the "lesions" practitioners manipulate are often structurally undefined. They might be best characterized as "functional spinal lesions" that alter the expected behavior of functional spinal units (similar to motion segments) or larger function spinal regions. As a joint or system of joints is confronted with unacceptable deformation, a local uncontrolled mechanical response occurs that may irritate surrounding tissues and lead to motion changes, altered tone, pain and paresthesia, swelling, tissue degenerative changes (consistent with stress or immobilization reactions), radicular or scleratogenous referral, and/or spasm. Forces from manipulation can then alter the dynamics of the buckled region. (See Chapter 13.)

Neurologic Models

Nerve, Nerve Root, and Dorsal Root Ganglion Compression or Traction

Nerve compression is of historical note as Palmer's "foot on the hose" theory.[12] He suggested that nerve energy could be reduced or increased from pressure applied by the vertebra. Leach[5] summarizes the debate on this model in his chapter on nerve compression. Early work by Hadley[68,69] suggested that nerve root compression could result from radiographically demonstrated intervertebral subluxation. However, Crelin[70] tried to refute this. He attempted to close an electric circuit between wires placed along the nerve and inside of the intervertebral foramen in cadavers. Manual forces applied along all ranges of motion were unable to close the circuit. Both his methodology and conclusions could hardly be considered unbiased and do not account for structural variants such as transforaminal ligaments or functional alterations such as edema.[71]

Given that there are other structures within the foramen (e.g., blood and lymphatic vessels, fat, connective tissue), the possibility exists that other kinds of mechanical stresses may affect the nervous system. Luttges et al.,[72,73] Triano and Luttges,[74] and MacGregor et al.[75] have demonstrated that mechanical pressures and tensions may create a myriad of subclinical neurophysiologic alterations. These range from changes in intraneural protein composition to altered nerve conduction characteristics. The dorsal root seems to be more sensitive to small amounts of pressure and tension than the efferent anterior root or the nerve itself.[76] The magnitude of tension on the posterior root required to effect a change may be within the scope of mechanical distortion possible from traction or edema around the foramen or capsule, but this has not been experimentally verified.

The dorsal root ganglion (DRG) is a distinct structure also in the vicinity of the intervertebral foramen. Lantz[77] points out the exquisite sensitivity of the DRG to mechanical stresses. DRG compression has been implicated as a cause of pain in stenosis, disc bulge, fibrosis, and other conditions. The distinction between nerve root and DRG is primarily anatomic, but Lantz notes that a significant aspect of DRG physiology is that the cell bodies of the DRG undergo trophic changes when the nerve is injured peripherally.[78] Concerns regarding the kinds of mechanical forces needed to affect the DRG are the same as those outlined previously for nerve root compression and traction.

Spinal Cord Compression or Traction

B.J. Palmer was perhaps the first proponent of this model of subluxation.[79] It has served as a basis for upper cervical chiropractic techniques[80] and has been implicated in post-birth trauma leading to sudden infant death.[81] Additionally, cord and thecal sac compression are well recognized as complications of spinal canal pathology.[82] Cord and neural element distortion caused by traction also provide a rationale for craniosacral techniques.[83] Breig et al.[84,85] have investigated the mechanical relationship of the meninges with the spinal cord and the osseous vertebral column. Distortion of the cervical spinal cord caused by stabilizing attachments of the dentate ligaments has been observed with normal cervical flexion.[83,86] The rationale for this hypothesis appears to be sound, but no evidence exists to show that mechanical vertebral or cranial restriction is capable of placing the kinds of force on cord structures that create altered neurophysiology.

Somatosomatic Reflexes

Sometimes referred to as the proprioceptive insult hypothesis,[14,87] the somatosomatic reflex model suggests that the highly innervated soft tissues around joints may become irritated, which may lead to reflex modifications in postural tone and neural integration of postural activities. Wyke[88,89] has suggested that spinal manipulation stretches mechanoreceptors in the joint capsule. This stimulus has an inhibitory effect (mediated through cord interneurons) on nociceptive activity. This mechanism has been called the pain gate.[90] Gillette[91] has expanded on this model by providing a detailed accounting of the various somatic mechanoreceptor populations in the lumbar fascia. Although Wyke[88] has documented that joint capsule stretch can inhibit pain, Gillette[91] speculates that this phenomenon has the potential to be initiated by other nerve ending populations as well.

Another example of a somatosomatic reflex involves reflex muscle spasm.[92,93] This is a positive-feedback cycle mediated by the gamma motor loop in which a spasmed muscle may result from and contribute to proprioceptive irritation. This has been referred to as the "facilitated segment." It appears that spinal cord segments in the vicinity of a spinal fixation have a lower threshold for firing.[27,28,92] There is some evidence for the reduction of muscle spasm as measured by electromyography after spinal adjusting.[94,95] Perhaps one of the most promising models of the manipulable subluxation, somatosomatic reflex pathways seem to explain many of the clinical observations seen with spinal adjusting. In and of itself, this model does not represent any kind of pathologic lesion; rather it suggests a mechanism by which spinal adjusting and manipulation has an effect on reduction of pain and spasm in the absence of any specific spinal lesion.

A confluence of many mechanical and neurological events into hyperfacilitated segments, reflex muscle spasm, aberrant movement, and the like has been described as vertebral subluxation complex.[96,97] The idea that altered sensory and proprioceptive inputs lead to aberrant segmental motion or vice versa has been central to experimental modeling and efforts to assess how altered sensory input affect the vertebral column.[32] (See Chapter 9.)

Autonomic Reflexes

This model is frequently cited to explain apparent effects manipulation might have with organic disorders.[98] Early osteopathic research in this area concluded that vertebral lesions in animals may affect vascular supply to various glands and viscera.[5] Sato and Swenson[99] demonstrated sympathetic discharge in rats by placing mechanical stresses into the spinal joints. Somatic stimulation by

manipulation has been shown to affect gastric function[100] and angina pain.[101] Early work by Speransky[102] suggested that somatic blockade injections at segmental spinal levels have a beneficial effect on the progression of lobar pneumonia.

Spinal lesions have been clinically associated with deep visceral pain.[103] In addition, physiologic effects of somatic stimulation by mechanical means have some early experimental support.[104,105] It is reasonable to consider that certain organic disorders may contribute to development of segmental somatic muscle tone changes. Some early osteopathic animal research provides evidence that somatic interventions (e.g. adjustment, injection) may influence the progression of a small number of organic conditions. Mechanical movement of the thoracic and lumbar segments has been shown to produce short-lived differential reflex responses in renal and adrenal sympathetic nerves in rats.[106]

What is clearly speculative at this point is the role that spinal lesions have in the development of these organic disorders. Clear manipulative treatment protocols and quantitative outcome studies for different kinds of conditions are also lacking. Although both chiropractic and osteopathic practitioners report anecdotal successes with various organic disorders, most patients who present to chiropractors self-select for neuromusculoskeletal conditions.[107,108] The outcome literature for somatic interventions on organic problems is limited, dated, or anecdotal.

Motor System Degeneration

The Eastern European manual medicine movement has theorized a model of peripheral and somatic "blockages" and their role in affecting integrated function of the motor system from cortex to periphery.[24,26,109] This model offers a considerably different role for spinal or extremity dysfunction than other neurologic models. Two kinds of nervous system integration can be described. The first is termed *vertical integration,* which refers to the relationship between four vertical components: the central nervous system (CNS) structures, the spinal cord, peripheral nerves, and musculoskeletal structures. The second term, *horizontal integration,* refers to the relationship between anatomically adjacent or related structures within any of the four vertical components (e.g., motor cortex and cerebellum from the CNS structures, knee and hip from the musculoskeletal structures).

It is well known that in upper motor neuron lesions degeneration of function follows in both horizontal and vertical directions and that loss of function becomes more permanent over time. For example, after a cerebrovascular accident, neurologic firing patterns change in the vicinity of the lesion, leading to reorganization and changes in related CNS structures (horizontal degeneration). In addition, there is a gradual cumulative functional vertical change in the cord and peripheral nerves, which eventually leads to muscular atrophy in the affected peripheral structures. The motor system degeneration model argues that a lesion in any of the four vertical levels (including a peripheral joint lesion) leads to subtle and gradual functional alterations vertically and horizontally throughout the motor system. Treatment and rehabilitation programs by modern manual medicine and physical therapy practitioners have centered on distinctions between active (patient-performed) care and passive (doctor-performed) care.[110] It is thought that treatment of peripheral joint lesions (including spinal dysfunction) needs to be more than passive mechanical work (e.g., spinal adjustment). Because of the holistic nature of the entire motor system, care must include exercise and retraining along lines similar to those involved in rehabilitation of other motor system pathologic conditions (such as upper motor neuron lesions). The longer the condition is left to progress, the greater the likelihood that recruitment (vertical and horizontal) of other areas of the motor system will occur, leading to recurrence of the peripheral lesion.[22]

Psychoneuroimmunology

Just as somatosomatic reflexes may be considered a component part of the motor system degeneration model, somatoautonomic and viscerosomatic reflexes may be considered a component part of psychoneuroimmunology. Attempts to quantify the relationship of psychological considerations with immune system function mediated through the endocrine and nervous systems are being made. Because of the intimate relationship between the nervous and endocrine systems, the specialty of behavioral medicine has taken a particular interest in psychoneuroimmunology.[111] Ader's text[112] on the subject reviews literature and concepts that support the role that various psychologic and behavioral factors play in physiologic function.

The field, although controversial,[113] has a rational basis and a large literature base that seems to correlate behavioral syndromes and interventions with clinical phenomena and outcomes.[114] In the previous discussion of the motor system it was suggested that somatic injury can provide sensory input to the nervous system, leading to horizontal and vertical integration with resultant long-term patterning. It is reasonable to speculate that a chiropractic adjustment, which might influence somatoautonomic activity, could also contribute input to higher CNS centers that may be important in psychoneuroimmunology relationships. With increasing interest in neuroimmunology research, this model is likely to develop greatly. Exact neural pathways and neurophysiologic responses are neither well identified nor understood, and chiropractic applications of this model remain speculative. (See Chapter 15.)

Trophic Models

Aberrant Axoplasmic Transport

It is known that axonal transport can be affected chemically,[115,116] and mechanical stresses have been shown to alter intracellular protein metabolism.[76] This model suggests that mechanical or chemical stresses (from metabolism of traumatized tissue) may alter nervous system physiology. Singer[117] describes how nerves provide trophic sustenance for muscle growth and maintenance. He further states that axoplasmic flow can be affected without damage to nerve conduction. The suggested role of manipulation would be to free up mechanical pressure, perhaps in the soft tissues, which may impede axonal transport. However, no studies exist that demonstrate changes in axoplasmic flow with spinal or soft tissue manipulation. Also unclarified are the details regarding the extent and kinds of mechanical pressure possible with spinal or soft tissue lesions.

Intraneural Microcirculation Ischemia

Because the blood vessels supplying nerve tissue are softer and more susceptible to compression than are the nerves, a likely candidate for a spinal lesion is localized neuroischemia. The symptoms of neurapraxia are understood clinically[118] and often manifest as paresthesias. This model is closely related to the axoplasmic transport model in that one of the major consequences of neural ischemia is altered intracellular metabolism of the nerve and resultant aberrant axoplasmic flow. A detailed review of the experimental literature in this area has been provided by Sjostrand et al.[119] This model has been a favorite of the osteopathic profession but suffers the same limitations as the previous model—absence of documentation regarding the kinds of pathoanatomic lesions that could lead to ischemia.

Macrocirculation Ischemia (Aberrant Vascular and Lymphatic Supply)

This model serves as an extension of microcirculation ischemia as it applies to larger blood vessels and lymphatics. Many clinical syndromes involving tissue contracture or space-occupying lesions can impede larger vessels. To what extent spinal dysfunction can influence larger vessel flow is debatable. Although mechanical stresses can impact cerebral blood flow, many documented cases of mechanical impingement are secondary to excessive trauma and may not be manipulable.

Vertebrobasilar arterial insufficiency after cervical manipulation has been implicated as a cause of stroke.[120] Therefore predisposition to vascular insufficiency is a possible contraindication to certain kinds of cervical adjusting.[121] Because functional mechanical stresses associated with spinal manipulation may significantly affect cephalic circulation, it is reasoned that manipulation may have beneficial effects as well as negative ones. The significance of this model is that chiropractic adjusting has been implicated in the resolution of a wide variety of cephalic symptomatology.[122,123] Although neurologic explanations may account

for some of these effects, possible vascular consequences have not been adequately considered. Although most of the literature regarding this mechanism centers on cervical vasculature, this model might be extrapolated to other anatomic regions where mechanical intrusions on vascular elements may occur.

Altered Cerebrospinal Fluid Flow

Improper circulation of the cerebrospinal fluid (CSF) has been suggested as a mechanism in spinal dysfunction that is amenable to manipulation.[85,124] Movement of the cranial bones secondary to pressure changes within the cranium may be responsible for a pumping action that circulates CSF.[85,125] Craniopelvic manipulation is thought by some to normalize aberrations of this movement. It is unclear what the exact clinical consequences of impaired CSF flow would be, but speculation based on clinical experience has suggested the value of this approach for a wide variety of head symptoms and postural disorders. Much of the literature surrounding the biomechanical model of cord compression and traction is applicable here. This speculative rationale suggests that a condition of CSF stasis or aberrant flow leads to decreased nutritional supply to those CNS components bathed by the fluid. Surgical case studies can be found showing that a complete obliteration of the subarachnoid space can lead to obstructed CSF flow and resultant atrophy of neural elements.[126] However, this is far removed from minute, manipulable mechanical stresses allegedly causing subtle alterations in the nutritive capacity of CSF. The exact mechanisms of this model are perhaps best discarded in favor of direct subtle mechanical effects of meningeal traction on CNS components.

Psychosocial Models

Placebo Effect

The placebo effect has often been cited as a source of the effectiveness of spinal manipulation by its detractors.[127] Yet the therapeutic value of the placebo effect should not be overlooked.[128] It is important for providers to recognize the mind-body relationship and the role that the patient-doctor relationship has in healing. Placebo has too often been used to explain away the unknown while confounding psychological responses with sources of experimental design variability, such as measurement error, sampling error, and so forth.[129] Cherkin and MacCornack[130] have compared patient satisfaction with family practitioners and chiropractors in back pain patients and noted higher degrees of confidence and satisfaction with chiropractors. This was attributed to the chiropractors' ability to communicate clearly and believably with their patients. Although Cherkin and MacCornack did not attribute any portion of patient satisfaction to adjustive care, the point is demonstrated that the patient's belief in both the practitioner and the treatment plays an important role in the healing process. Interestingly, another report noted that almost half of the family practitioners stated that they use the placebo effect therapeutically with their back pain patients.[131] Fewer than 5% of the chiropractors stated that they did so. Part of a placebo's effectiveness may come from the practitioner's lack of awareness of, or unwillingness to acknowledge, placebo effects.

Placebo certainly constitutes a portion of the therapeutic effect of any health care approach.[132] The extent to which it has an effect in chiropractic practice is not clearly quantified, but it does serve as one of the possible models or explanations of the effectiveness of spinal manipulation. Practitioners need not be fearful or belittled by elucidation of its extent in chiropractic. Placebo is perhaps the most noninvasive of approaches, and its role should be maximized because it truly uses the patient's own recuperative ability. The only caveat is that this should not serve as a justification to avoid seeking understanding of other possible physical mechanisms.

Stress Reduction
Selye[133] articulated the role that emotional stress plays with the endocrine system and muscle tension. High anxiety and stress levels have been implicated in a number of muscle tension and other clinical syndromes.[134] Spinal adjusting may help relax tense muscles as outlined in the somatosomatic reflex model, yet many chiropractors go

further with relaxation exercise, biofeedback, lifestyle counseling, nutritional guidance, and related procedures. For the sake of completeness, stress needs to be considered as a possible mechanism in the mediation of spinal dysfunction, especially for cases in which muscle tension and joint fixation fail to resolve with a reasonable amount of care.

Lifestyle Modification
In addition to stress, many of the activities of daily living are likely contributors to spinal and joint dysfunction. Repetitive and prolonged postural activity, either static or dynamic, nutritional neglect, inadequate or improper exercise, and toxic exposure are examples of numerous areas that manipulative practitioners might address clinically by education on environmental and lifestyle modification. Although many of these problems may not always be considered as the primary instigators of joint dysfunction, chiropractors have recognized the importance of trauma, toxicity, and autosuggestion in health and disease since the time of D.D. Palmer.[12] Often the doctor's recommendations for changes in lifestyle can be the active ingredient in a therapeutic response. The chiropractor who casually suggests a change in posture or activity at the work station may very well give full therapeutic credit to the passive component (spinal adjustment) while neglecting to consider the role played by the lifestyle modification.

Conclusions
Whether it is called chiropractic subluxation, manipulable subluxation, manipulable lesion, somatic dysfunction, fixation, or "bump in the back," this clinical phenomenon brings millions of patients to doctors. Perhaps communication and collaboration among various interested parties will advance our understanding in this area. D.D. Palmer[135] first noted the problem of multifactorial terminology when he wrote the following:

> Too many manufacture their own definition of terms....What would be the result if each banker and broker should invent and persist in using his own devised addition and multiplication table. Herein

arises the discordant, inharmonious jangling among chiropractors regarding what constitutes the principles of science.

As chiropractors continue to integrate into the health care mainstream, chiropractic theory must become mainstream as well. Opinionated historically and politically motivated definitions of subluxation (or other terms) are no longer adequate to explain the myriad effects that spinal adjusting is thought to have.[27,29] Meeker[136] has challenged us to embrace evidence-based approaches standard in science for developing, describing, and refining the theoretical basis of chiropractic. He proposes that one can determine the quality of a theory by a number of characteristics that can be assessed by asking questions about a theory's ability to explain relationships, be tested, and be refined (Box 10-6).

As this review and the text in which it appears attest, great strides are being made in moving beyond the speculative into the descriptive. The purpose of theory is to both explain the observable and set the stage for scientific inquiry. Theory is not static; rather, it is ever evolving. Our concepts, procedures, and professional identity need to be clarified not only so others may understand what we offer, but so we can refine our clinical science and practices to better serve our patients.

BOX 10-6 ■ Questions for Assessing Quality of Scientific Theory

- Is the theory consistent with and does it provide a thorough and rational explanation of observed facts?
- Does the theory help to classify relevant variables and predict the effect of relationships?
- Does the theory permit deductions that form testable hypotheses?
- Can the theory incorporate new knowledge into its conceptual framework?
- Will the theory withstand revision without collapse?
- Is the theory important and does it reflect a profession's values and identity?

References

1. Brantingham JW. A survey of the literature regarding the behavior, pathology, etiology, and nomenclature of the chiropractic lesion. ACAJ Chiropractic 1985;19(8):65-70.
2. Brantingham JW. A critical look at the subluxation hypothesis. In: Hodgson M et al., editors. Current topics in chiropractic: reviews of the literature. Sunnyvale, CA: Palmer College of Chiropractic-West; 1987. D1:1-6.
3. Keating JC. Science and politics and the subluxation. Am J Chiropractic Med 1988;1(3):107-10.
4. Dishman RW. Review of the literature supporting a scientific basis for the chiropractic subluxation complex. J Manipulative Physiol Ther 1985;8:163-74.
5. Leach RA. The chiropractic theories: a textbook of scientific research. 4th ed. Baltimore: Lippincott, Williams & Wilkins; 2003.
6. Mootz RD, CiRullo BL, Haney PL. The existence of the manipulable spinal lesion. In: Coyle BA, editor. Current topics in chiropractic: reviews of the literature. Sunnyvale, CA: Palmer College of Chiropractic-West; 1984. B4:1-16.
7. Schafer RC, editor. The ACA basic procedural manual. 4th ed. Arlington, VA: American Chiropractic Association; 1984.
8. Mootz RD. Chiropractic models: current understanding of vertebral subluxation and manipulable spinal lesions. In: Sweere J, editor. Chiropractic family practice. Gaithersburg, MD: Aspen; 1992. 2-2:1-12.
9. Leach RA. Chiropractic theories: an introduction. In: Sweere J, editor. Chiropractic family practice. Gaithersburg, MD: Aspen; 1992. 2-1:1-4.
10. Gatterman MI, Hansen DT. The development of chiropractic nomenclature through consensus. J Manipulative Physiol Ther 1994;17:302-9.
11. Lomax EL. Manipulative therapy: an historical perspective from ancient times. In: Goldstein M, editor. The research status of spinal manipulative therapy. NINCDS Monograph No. 15. Washington, D.C.: U.S. Government Printing Office; 1975. p. 11-15.
12. Palmer DD. The science, art, and philosophy of chiropractic. Portland, OR: Portland Printing House; 1910.
13. Palmer BJ. Fight to climb. Davenport, IA: Palmer School of Chiropractic; 1950.
14. Homewood AE. The neurodynamics of the vertebral subluxation. 3rd ed. St. Petersberg, FL: Valkyrie; 1979.
15. Janse J. Principles and practice of chiropractic. Lombard, IL: National College of Chiropractic; 1976.
16. Faye LJ. Motion palpation of the spine. Huntington Beach, CA: Motion Palpation Institute; 1983.
17. Lantz CA. The vertebral subluxation complex. ICA Review 1989;(Sept/Oct):37-61.
18. Still AT. Philosophy of osteopathy. Kirksville, MO: Author; 1899.
19. HICDA. Hospital adaptation of ICDA. 2nd ed. Ann Arbor, MI: Commission on Professional and Hospital Activities; 1973.

20. Greenman PE. Principles of manual medicine. Baltimore: Williams & Wilkins; 1989.
21. Mennell JM. History of the development of medical manipulation concepts: medical terminology. In: Goldstein M, editor. The research status of spinal manipulative therapy. NINCDS Monograph No. 15. Washington, D.C.: U.S. Government Printing Office; 1975. p. 19.
22. Cyriax J. Treatment of pain by manipulation. In: Goldstein M, editor. The research status of spinal manipulative therapy. NINCDS Monograph No. 15. Washington, D.C.: U.S. Government Printing Office; 1975. p. 19.
23. Paris SV. Spinal manipulative therapy. Clin Orthop 1983;179:55.
24. Lewit K. Manipulative therapy in the rehabilitation of the motor system. 2nd ed. London: Butterworths; 1991.
25. Janda V. Muscles, central nervous regulation and back problems. In: Korr IM, editor. Neurobiologic mechanisms in manipulative therapy. New York: Plenum Press; 1978. p. 27-42.
26. Janda V. On the concept of postural muscles and posture. Aust J Physiother 1983;29:83.
27. Mootz RD. Professional identity: the role of chiropractic theory. Top Clin Chiropr 2001;8(1):1-8.
28. Lantz CA. A review of the evolution of chiropractic concepts of subluxation. Top Clin Chiropr 1995;2(2):1-10.
29. Terwilleger KJ. The view from the outside. Top Clin Chiropr 2000;7(1):80-3.
30. Korr IM, editor. The neurobiologic mechanisms in manipulative therapy. New York: Plenum Press; 1978.
31. Korr IM. The collected papers of Irvin M. Korr. Colorado Springs, CO: American Academy of Osteopathy; 1979.
32. Pickar JG. Neurophysiological effects of spinal manipulation. Spine J 2002;2:357-71.
33. Triano JJ The functional spinal lesion: An evidence-based model of subluxation. Top Clin Chiropr 2001;8(1): 16-28.
34. Triano JJ. Biomechanics of spinal manipulative therapy. Spine J 2001;1:121-30.
35. Meeker WC, Mootz RD. Evaluating the validity, reliability, and clinical role of spinal radiography. In: Coyle et al., editors. Current topics in chiropractic: reviews of the literature. Sunnyvale, CA: Palmer College of Chiropractic-West; 1985. E5:1-20.
36. Still AT. Osteopathic research and practice. Kirksville, MO: Author; 1910.
37. Wyatt LH, Schultz GD. The diagnostic efficacy of lumbar spine radiography: a review of the literature. In: Hodgson et al., editors. Current topics in chiropractic: reviews of the literature. Sunnyvale, CA: Palmer College of Chiropractic-West; 1987. A2:1-14.
38. Mootz RD, Meeker WC. Minimizing radiation exposure to patients in chiropractic practice. J Chiropractic 1989;26(4):65-70.
39. Robbins SL, Cotran RS, Kumar V. Inflammation and repair. In: Pathologic basis of disease. Philadelphia: WB Saunders; 1984. p. 55-106.
40. La Vigne A, Watkins R. Preliminary results on immobilization induced stiffness on monkey knee joints and posterior capsule: perspectives in biomedical engineering. In: Proceedings of the Symposium of Biomedical Engineering Society, U Strathclyde, Glasgow. Baltimore: Baltimore University; 1973.
41. Akeson WH, Amiel D, Mechanic GL, Woo SL, Harwood FL, Hamer ML. Collagen crosslinking alterations in joint contractures: changes in reducible crosslinks in periarticular connective tissue after nine weeks of immobilization. Connect Tissue Res 1977;5:15-9.
42. Akeson WH, Amiel D, Woo S. Immobility effects of synovial joints: the pathomechanics of joint contracture. Biorheology 1980;17:95.
43. Emmeking W, Horowitz M. The intra-articular effects of immobilization on the human knee. J Bone Joint Surg 1972;54A:973.
44. Rahlmann JF. Intervertebral joint fixation. J Manipulative Physiol Ther 1987;10(4):177-87.
45. Bogduk N, Engle R. The menisci of the lumbar zygapophyseal joints: a review of their anatomy and their clinical significance. Spine 1984;9:454-60.
46. Giles LGF, Taylor JR. Histological preparation of large vertebral specimens. Stain Technol 1983;58:45-9.
47. Giles LGF. Lumbar apophyseal joint arthrography. J Manipulative Physiol Ther 1984;7:21-4.
48. Wolf J. The reversible deformation of joint cartilage surface and its possible role in joint blockage. In: Lewit K et al., eds. Proceedings of the 4th Congress International Federation of Manual Medicine. Bratislava, Slovakia: Orbis; 1975. p. 30-4.
49. Rauschning W. Detailed sectional anatomy of the spine. In: Rothman S, et al. Multiplanar CT of the spine. Baltimore: University Park Press; 1985.
50. Aspden RM, Porter RW. Localized stresses in the intervertebral disc resulting from a loose fragment. A theory for fissure and fragment. Spine 1999;24:2214-8.
51. Sandoz R. Newer trends in the pathogenesis of spinal disorders. Ann Swiss Chiropractic Assoc 1971; 5:93-180.
52. Maigne R. Orthopaedic medicine: a new approach to vertebral manipulations. Springfield, IL: Charles C Thomas; 1972.
53. Cyriax J. Textbook of orthopaedic medicine. 9th ed., Vol. 2. London: Balliere Tindall; 1974.
54. Cox JM. Low back pain: mechanism, diagnosis, and treatment. 6th ed. Baltimore: Williams & Wilkins; 1999.
55. Sandoz R. Some physical mechanisms and effects of spinal adjustments. Ann Swiss Chiropractic Assoc 1976;6:91-141.
56. Farfan HF, Cosserte JW, Robertson GH, Wells RV. The effects of torsion on the lumbar intervertebral joints: the role of torsion in the production of disc degeneration. J Bone Joint Surg 1970;52A:468.
57. Good AB. Spinal joint blocking. J Manipulative Physiol Ther 1985;8:1-8.

58. Kirkaldy-Willis WH, Bernard TM, editors. Managing low back pain. 4th ed. New York: Churchill Livingstone; 1999.

59. Sweere J. Predisposing factors to lower spinal instability: an illustrated guide. Bloomington, MN: Northwestern College of Chiropractic; 1987.

60. Goldstein M. The research status of spinal manipulative therapy. NINCDS Monograph No. 15. Washington, D.C.: U.S. Government Printing Office; 1975.

61. White AA, Panjabi MM. Clinical biomechanics of the spine. 2nd ed. Philadelphia: JB Lippincott; 1990. p. 3-10.

62. Weisel SW, Tsourmas N, Feffer HL, Citrin CM, Patronas N. A study of computer-assisted tomography. I. The incidence of positive CT scans in an asymptomatic group of patients. Spine 1984;9:549-51.

63. Steindler A. Kinesiology of the human body under normal and pathological conditions. Springfield, IL: Charles C Thomas; 1973.

64. Farfan NHF, Sullivan JB. The relation of facet orientation to intervertebral disc failure. Can J Surg 1967; 10:179-85.

65. Coplens CW. The conservative treatment of low back pain. In: Helfet AJ, Grubel Lee DM, editors. Disorders of the lumbar spine. Philadelphia: JB Lippincott; 1978. p. 161.

66. Gatterman MI. Chiropractic management of spine related disorders. Baltimore: Lippincott, Williams & Wilkins; 2003. p. 173-4.

67. Turek SL. Orthopaedics principles and their application. 3rd ed. Philadelphia: JB Lippincott; 1977. p. 1469.

68. Hadley LA. Intervertebral joint subluxation, bony impingement, and foramen encroachment with nerve root changes. Am J Roentgenol Radiat Ther 1951; 65:377-402.

69. Hadley LA. Anatomico-roentgenographic studies of the spine. Springfield, IL: Charles C Thomas; 1964.

70. Crelin ES. A scientific test of the chiropractic theory. Am Sci 1973;61:574-80.

71. Golub BS, Silverman B. Transforaminal ligaments of the lumbar spine. J Bone Joint Surg 1969;51A:947-56.

72. Luttges MW, Kelly PT, Gerren RA. Degenerative changes in mouse sciatic nerves: electrophoretic and electrophysiologic characterizations. Exp Neurol 1976;50:706-33.

73. Luttges MW, Stodiek LS, Beel JA. Post injury changes in the biomechanics of nerves and roots in mice. J Manipulative Physiol Ther 1986;9(2):89-98.

74. Triano II, Luttges MW. Nerve irritation: a possible model of sciatic neuritis. Spine 1982;7:129-36.

75. MacGregor RI, Sharpless SK, Lunges MW. A pressure vessel model for nerve compression. J Neurol Sci 1975;24:299-304.

76. Sharpless SK. Susceptibility of spinal roots to compression block. In: Goldstein M, editor. The research status of spinal manipulative therapy. NINCDS Monograph No. 15. Washington, D.C.: U.S. Government Printing Office; 1975. p. 155.

77. Lantz CA. The role of dorsal root ganglia in the development of chiropractic subluxations. In: Keene KI, et al., editors. Current topics in chiropractic: reviews of the literature. Sunnyvale, CA: Palmer College of Chiropractic-West; 1986. C2:1-12.

78. Carmel PW, Stein BM. Cell changes in sensory ganglia following proximal and distal nerve section in the monkey. J Comp Neurol 1969;135:145-66.

79. Palmer BI. The subluxation specific: the adjustment specific. Davenport, IA: Palmer School of Chiropractic; 1934. p. 205.

80. Grostic ID. Dentate ligament: cord distortion hypothesis. Chiro Res 1988;1(1):47-55.

81. Banks BD, Beck RW, Columbus M, Gold PM, Kinsinger FS, Lalonde MA. Sudden infant death syndrome: a literature review with chiropractic implications. J Manipulative Physiol Ther 1987;10(5):246-52.

82. Dyck P, Homer CP, Doyle IB, Rieder II. Intermittent cauda equina compression syndrome. Spine 1977;2(1): 75-80.

83. Upledger IE, Vredevoogd ID. Cranio-sacral therapy. Chicago: Eastland Press; 1983.

84. Brieg A, Turnbull I, Hassler D. Effects of mechanical stress on the spinal cord in cervical spondylosis. J Neurosurg 1960;25:45-56.

85. Brieg A. Adverse mechanical tension in the central nervous system. New York: John Wiley and Sons; 1978.

86. Tunturi AR. Elasticity of the spinal cord, pia, and dentate ligament in the dog. J Neurosurg 1978;48: 975-9.

87. Spencer I. The neurophysiological relationships between asymmetrical spinal proprioception and postural muscle asynergism. In: Proceedings of the 13th Biomechanics Conference on the Spine. Sunnyvale, CA: Palmer College Chiropractic-West; 1982. p. 227-38.

88. Wyke BD. Articular neurology: a review. Physiotherapy 1972;58:94-9.

89. Wyke BD. Articular neurology and manipulative therapy. In: Glasgow EF, Twomey LT, Scull ER, Kleynhans AM, editors. Aspects of manipulative therapy. 2nd ed. Melbourne: Churchill Livingstone: 1985.

90. Wall PD. The gate control theory of pain mechanism: a reexamination and restatement. Brain 1978;101:1-18.

91. Gillette RG. A speculative argument for the coactivation of diverse somatic receptor populations by a chiropractic adjustment: review of the evidence from human and animal research. In: Keene et al. Current topics in chiropractic: review of the literature. Sunnyvale, CA: Palmer College of Chiropractic-West; 1986. El:1-28.

92. Korr IM. Proprioceptors and the behavior of lesioned segments. In: Stark EH, editor. Osteopathic medicine. Acton, MA: Publication Sciences Group; 1975.

93. Coote JH. Somatic sources of afferent input as factors in aberrant in autonomic, sensory, and motor function. In: Korr IM, editor. The neurobiologic mechanisms in manipulative therapy. New York: Plenum Press; 1978.

94. Grice A. Muscle tone changes following manipulation. J Can Chiro Assoc 1975;18(4):29.

95. England R, Deibert P. Electromyographic studies. Part 1. Consideration in the evaluation of osteopathic therapy. J Am Osteopath Assoc 1972;72:162-9.

96. Faye LJ. Motion palpation of the spine. Huntington Beach, CA: Motion Palpation Institute; 1983.

97. Lantz CA. Immobilization degeneration and the fixation hypothesis of chiropractic subluxation. Chiro Res J 1988;1:21-46.

98. Nansel D, Szlazak M. Somatic dysfunction and the phenomenon of visceral disease stimulation: a probable explanation for the apparent effectiveness of somatic therapy in patients presumed to be suffering from visceral disease. J Manipulative Physiol Ther 1995; 18(6):379-97.

99. Sato A, Swenson R. Sympathetic nervous system response to mechanical stress of spinal columns in rats. J Manipulative Physiol Ther 1984;7:141-8.

100. Sato A, Schmidt RF. Somato-sympathetic reflexes: afferent fibers, central pathways, discharge characteristics. Physiol Rev 1973;53:916-47.

101. Rogers JT, Rogers JC. The role of osteopathic manipulative therapy in the treatment of coronary heart disease. J Am Osteopath Assoc 1976;76:71-81.

102. Speransky AD. Experimental and clinical lobar pneumonia. Dolevni Pneumoni 1942;3:17.

103. Rinzler SH, Travell J. Therapy directed at the somatic component of cardiac pain. Am Heart J 1948;35:248.

104. Pengra CA, Alexander GA. Effects of spondylotherapic and osteopathic stimulation on the secretion of urine. Still Res Inst Bull 1916;2:128-32.

105. Deason J, Doron CL. Some immediate effects of bony lesions on vascular reflexes. Still Res Inst Bull 1916; 2:99-101.

106. Budgell B, Hotta H, Sato A. Spinovisceral reflexes evoked by noxious and innocuous stimulation of the lumbar spine. J Neuromusculoskel Sys 1995;3(3): 122-30.

107. Burns L. Immediate effects of certain manipulations upon the secretion of hydrochloric acid. Still Res Inst Bull 1931;7:70-3.

108. Briggs L, Boone WR. Effects of a chiropractic adjustment on changes in pupillary diameter: a model for evaluating somatovisceral response. J Manipulative Physiol Ther 1988;11(3):181-9.

109. Dvorak J. Neurologic and biomechanical aspects of back pain. In: Beurger AA, Greenman PE, editors. Empirical approaches to the validation of spinal manipulative therapy. Springfield, IL: Charles C Thomas; 1985.

110. Saal JA. General principles and guidelines for rehabilitation of the injured athlete. Phys Med Rehabil: state of art reviews. Philadelphia: Hanley & Belfus; 1987.

111. Soloman GF. The emerging field of psychoneuroimmunology with a special note on AIDS. Advances 1985; 2(1):6-19.

112. Ader R, editor. Psychoneuroimmunology. New York: Academic Press; 1981.

113. Melnechuk T. Why has psychoneuroimmunology been so controversial? Proponents and skeptics at a scientific conference. Advances 1985;2(4):22-38.

114. Locke SE, Hornig-Rohan M. Mind and immunity: an annotated bibliography. New York: Institute for the Advancement of Health; 1983.

115. Sampson F. Axonal transport: the mechanisms and their susceptibility to derangement; anterograde transport. In: Korr IM, editor. The neurobiologic mechanisms in manipulative therapy. New York: Plenum Press; 1978.

116. Thoenen H, Schwab M, Barde Y. Transfer of information to innervating neurons by retrograde axonal transport of macromolecules. In: Korr IM, editor. The neurobiologic mechanisms in manipulative therapy. New York: Plenum Press; 1978.

117. Singer M. Discussion of the trophic functions of nerves and their mechanisms in relation to manipulative therapy. In: Korr IM, editor. The neurobiologic mechanisms in manipulative therapy. New York: Plenum Press; 1978.

118. Lundborg G. Ischemic nerve injury: experimental studies on intraneural microvascular pathophysiology and nerve function in a limb subjected to temporary circulatory arrest. Scand J Plast Reconstr Surg Suppl 1970;6:3-113.

119. Sjostrand J, Rydevik B, Lundborg G, McLean W. Impairment of intraneural microcirculation, blood nerve barrier, and axonal transport in experimental ischemia and compression. In: Korr IM, editor. The neurobiologic mechanisms in manipulative therapy. New York: Plenum Press; 1978.

120. Mueller S, Sahs A. Brain stem dysfunction related to cervical manipulation. Neurology 1976;26:547-50.

121. Kleynhans AM. Complications and contraindications to spinal manipulative therapy. In: Haldeman S, editor. Modern developments in the principles and practice of chiropractic. New York: Appleton-Century-Crofts; 1980.

122. Haldeman S. The influence of the autonomic nervous system on cerebral blood flow. J Can Chiro Assoc 1974;19:6-14.

123. Jackson R. The cervical syndrome. Springfield, IL: Charles C Thomas; 1978.

124. DeJarnette M. Sacro-occipital technique. Nebraska City, NE: Author; 1984.

125. Bering EA. Choroid plexus and arterial pulsations of cerebrospinal fluid: demonstration of choroid plexus as a cerebrospinal fluid pump. Arch Neur Psychiatry 1955;73:165.

126. Heilbrun MP, Davis DO. Spastic paraplegia secondary to cord constriction by the dura. J Neurosurg 1973;39: 645-7.

127. Haldeman S. Basic principle in establishing a chiropractic clinical trial. J Am Chiro Assoc 1978;12(Suppl):33-7.

128. Bennett P. Placebo and the art of medicine. Placebo 1988;1:1-21.

129. Keating JC. The placebo issue and clinical research. J Manipulative Physiol Ther 1897;10(6):329-32.
130. Cherkin DC, MacCornack FA. Patient evaluations of low back pain care from family physicians and chiropractors. Western J Med 1989;150(3):351-5.
131. Cherkin DC, MacCornack FA, Berg AO. Managing low back pain: a comparison of the beliefs and behaviors of family physicians and chiropractors. Western J Med 1988;149(4):475-80.
132. Evans FJ. Expectations and the placebo response. Advances 1984;1(3):11-20.
133. Selye H. Stress in health and disease. London: Butterworth; 1975.
134. Monjan AA. Stress and immunologic competence: studies in animals. In: Ader R, editor. Psychoneuroimmunology. New York: Academic Press; 1981.
135. Palmer DD. The chiropractor. Los Angeles: Press of Beacon Light; 1914.
136. Meeker WC. Concepts germane to an evidence-based application of chiropractic theory. Top Clin Chiropr 2000;7(1):67-73.

Kinesiology: An Essential Approach toward Understanding the Chiropractic Subluxation

Brian A. Enebo and Meridel I. Gatterman

Key Words   Kinesiology, spinal motion segment, three-joint complex, six degrees of freedom, coupled motion, hypomobility, hypermobility, aberrant motion, instability, instantaneous axis of rotation

After reading this chapter you should be able to answer the following questions:

Question 1   What contributes to the coupled motion of spinal motion segments?

Question 2   What is the function of muscle spindles?

Question 3   What are the stages of spinal joint degeneration and how do they affect segmental spinal motion?

Kinesiology is the study of movement (*kinesis*—to move; *ology*—to study). Under this broad definition, kinesiology includes the specialized areas of biomechanics, motor control, and exercise physiology. Although each of these areas has relevance to the student and doctor, a detailed discussion of each area is beyond the scope of this chapter. Instead we will focus our discussion of kinesiology on the study of human movement with particular interest in the anatomic and clinical biomechanical interactions of the musculoskeletal system. The purpose of limiting our definition is so that we may better understand articular motion (i.e., kinematics) and the forces acting at the motion segment (i.e., kinetics). *Kinematics* describes the position and motion of the body (i.e., limb, trunk, joint, spinal motion segment) without consideration of the forces acting on the body. Kinematics is quantified using measurements for displacement (e.g., range of motion), velocity, and acceleration. *Kinetics* is the description of forces that maintain equilibrium in the body or that produce, stop, or modify body motion. In application, these principles of motion and force are used therapeutically through the chiropractic adjustment to normalize, restore, and enhance function in the patient's interest (Table 11-1).

Chiropractic students and the profession[1] often use the term *kinesiology* in reference to Applied Kinesiology Technique (AK). The academic discipline of kinesiology, however, is not synonymous with the chiropractic technique system of AK. George Goodheart originated this technique system in 1964, associating muscle function with the diagnosis of various conditions. He noted a close association between specific muscle weaknesses and related organ or gland dysfunction.[2] Neither the technique system nor the "diagnostic" procedures it employs should be considered the academic discipline of kinesiology. The ensuing confusion is unfortunate and subsequently the term *biomechanics* has been emphasized when the more encompassing term is *kinesiology.*

This chapter focuses primarily on the kinesiopathology of the subluxation complex by applying fundamental principles that govern human motion to the spinal motion segment. In this chapter, *kinesiopathology* refers to spinal motion segment dysfunction presenting as hypomobility, hypermobility, or aberrant motion. In this context the subluxation complex is described according to principles of motion or kinesiology. In doing so, a continuum of abnormal motion from hypomobility to hypermobility and instability is discussed. In addition, aberrant motion and compensatory hypermobility are presented. We begin by first describing features of normal regional and intersegmental spinal motion. Through this exploration, we provide the basis for understanding how deviation from normal motion can be used to characterize a subluxation complex.

We conclude with an outline of a mechanistic model of subluxation, linking mechanical effects with the neurophysiologic. We review studies that address manipulable subluxation response to the chiropractic adjustment. Finally, pathologic changes that occur with degeneration of the three-joint complex are discussed relative to the effects on segmental spinal movement.

Characteristics of Normal Motion

The anatomic position, with the erect body facing forward, the elbows and fingers extended at the sides of the body, with the palms and the feet facing forward, is the standard position of reference to describe any human motion (Figure 11-1). It should be apparent that not all motion or activities that we perform on a daily basis begin or end in this reference position. Additionally, we know that it is possible to perform motions in combination; for example, flexion and rotation occur together when bending forward to touch your right hand to your left foot. An accurate description of the characteristics of normal motion includes discussion on a central coordinate system and planar motion (Figure 11-2).

The fundamental unit of spinal movement referred to as the motion segment[3] is a three-joint complex.[4] This unit consists of an intervertebral disc surrounded by two adjacent vertebrae, the two posterior joints, and the surrounding contiguous

Table 11-1

Criteria for the Kinesiologic Evaluation of the Subluxation

Kinesiologic descriptors of normal joint function	Kinesiopathology: criteria for subluxation*	Symptoms related to the subluxation
Kinetic		
• Equilibrium of forces at a joint	• Disruption of joint force equilibrium	Local and/or regional:
	• A change in the way forces move across a motion segment during functional activities	• Joint pain and tenderness
	• Altered joint function above and/or below the level of subluxation to compensate for altered transmission of forces	• Periarticular muscle spasm and/or redness
		• Articular swelling
Kinematic		
• Regional spinal range of motion	• Decreased regional range of motion	• Asymmetrical movement occurring regionally to compensate for altered segmental movement
• Segmental range of motion	• Altered segmental range of motion at the spinal motion segment (i.e., hypomobility, hypermobility, or aberrant motion)	• Asymmetrical and/or aberrant range of motion at the level of subluxation
• Motor control or movement accuracy	• Decreased movement accuracy	• Altered spatial and/or temporal accuracy during active movements in response to a change in mechanoreceptor feedback
	• Altered feedback from mechanoreceptors	

*The term *subluxation* is characterized and defined according to principles of kinesiology. In this model, contact between joint surfaces is assumed to remain partially intact and changes in joint function are mechanically related to a change in function of articular and periarticular soft tissue structures.

ligaments including capsules (Figure 11-3). The three-joint complex is the functional unit of spinal motion. Additionally, given the unique anatomy of the spinal motion segment, it is important to discuss coupled motion and an instantaneous axis of rotation (Figure 11-4) with respect to the potential for six degrees of freedom at this three-joint complex.

Central Coordinate System

The central coordinate system describes three-dimensional motion in the human body. In this system, motion and forces are defined as acting along any combination of three axes, X, Y, and Z. The X, Y, and Z axes are orientated at right angles to one another (see Figures 11-1 and 11-2) and define or locate the extent of two general types of

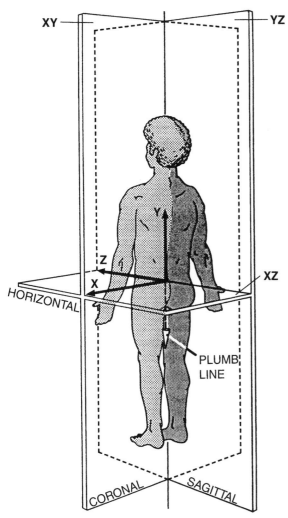

Figure 11-1 Central coordinate system with its origin between the cornua of the sacrum. The human body is shown in anatomic position. The planes are as shown: The sagittal plane is the YZ plane; the frontal plane is the YX plane; the horizontal plane is the XZ plane. The −Y axis is described by the plumb line dropped from the origin, and the +X axis points to the left at 90 degrees to the Y axis. The +Z axis points forward at a 90-degree angle to both the Y axis and the X axis. Movements are described in relation to the origin of the coordinate system. *(From White AA, Panjabi MM. Clinical biomechanics of the spine. 2nd ed. Philadelphia: JB Lippincott; 1990. p. 87.)*

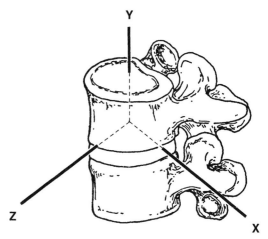

Figure 11-2 The spatial orientation of the superior vertebra relative to the inferior vertebra can be plotted using the central coordinate system with the origin placed at the center of the superior vertebra. Motion then can be described in relation to translation along or rotation around any of the three axes. These six components of vertebral motion give six degrees of freedom to the vertebral motion segment. *(From Gatterman MI. Chiropractic management of spine related disorders. Baltimore: Williams & Wilkins; 1990. p. 25.)*

movement—linear motion and angular or rotational motion.[5,6] All movements that occur about an axis are considered rotational, whereas translational movements along an axis and through a plane are linear movements.[5] Note then, that linear motion can occur along a straight or curved line (curvilinear). Curvilinear motion occurs when a rotational movement is accompanied by a translational movement.[5]

With three axes orientated 90 degrees to one another, any point in space can be exactly defined. Two of these axes may already look familiar. You may recall from geometry that the X and Y axes provide a two-dimensional description of a plane (or piece of graph paper) that has been divided into four quadrants. The center of these quadrants is located at the junction of the perpendicular lines and labeled the origin. The line running horizontally through the origin is the X axis (i.e., abscissa) and the line running vertically through the origin

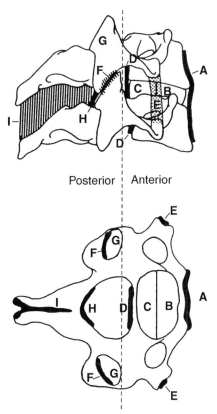

Posterior | Anterior

Figure 11-3 Three-joint complex of the lower cervical spine. Anterior elements: **A,** anterior longitudinal ligament; **B,** anterior anulus fibrosus; **C,** posterior anulus fibrosus; **D,** posterior longitudinal ligament. Posterior elements: **E,** costotransverse ligament; **F,** capsular ligament; **G,** articular facet; **H,** ligamentum flavin; **I,** interspinous and supraspinous ligaments. *(From White AA, Johnson RM, Panjabi MM, Southwick WO. Clin Orthop 1975;109:87.)*

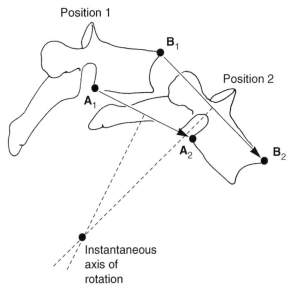

Figure 11-4 Instantaneous axis of rotation. Graphical technique for determining the instantaneous axis of rotation when a body moves from position 1 to position 2. The axis is located at the intersection of the two perpendicular bisectors of translation vectors A_1-A_2 and B_1-B_2 of any two points A and B on the body. *(From White AA, Panjabi MM. Clinical biomechanics of the spine. 2nd ed. Philadelphia: JB Lippincott; 1990. p. 659-60.)*

is the Y axis (i.e., ordinate). To describe motion in three dimensions, a third axis must be introduced. This is the Z axis, and it is perpendicular to both the X and Y axes. By convention, the origin of the three-dimensional coordinate system is placed at the body's center of mass (approximately 2 cm anterior to the second sacral vertebra for the standing human). However, for many body motions, it is not always convenient to reference the center of mass. It is acceptable to reference any

point from which movement can be defined. For example, when describing movement at a spinal motion segment, the origin of the three-axis coordinate system is placed at the center of the superior vertebral body with the lower vertebra regarded as fixed. (See Figure 11-2.) Motion at the three-joint complex is then described by translation along or rotation around any of the three axes.

Some chiropractic authors suggest using the central coordinate system as a spinal listing method to describe fixation or subluxation of the spinal motion segment. For researchers, the coordinate system is useful for plotting vertebral displacement during a manipulative thrust; however, it can be confusing when used clinically to determine the direction for application of thrust in comparison to the common kinesiology terms of flexion, extension, lateral flexion, and rotation.[7-10]

Planar Motion

Planar motion is another way to characterize motions we are already familiar with, namely, flexion, extension, abduction, adduction, lateral flexion, and rotation (medial/lateral and right/left). Specifically, planar motion describes structural position and direction of functional movement. To move in a specific plane is to move a body segment parallel to that plane. (See Figure 11-1.) For example, flexion and extension occur in the sagittal plane; abduction, adduction, and lateral flexion occur in the coronal or frontal plane; and rotation occurs in the transverse or horizontal plane. What are these three planes of movement, and how do they relate to the central coordinate system? The three planes of human motion, horizontal or transverse, coronal or frontal, and sagittal, are illustrated in Figure 11-1. Each of these planes is defined according to the central coordinate system. Additionally, the body planes are derived from dimensions in space and are arranged perpendicular to one another. (See Figure 11-1.) The midsagittal and sagittal plane divides the body into right and left halves and is made up of the Y and Z axes, thereby forming the YZ plane. The coronal plane, also called the frontal plane, is at right angles to the sagittal plane and divides the body into anterior and posterior portions. It is defined by the X and Y axes, forming the XY plane. The transverse plane is a horizontal plane, dividing the body into upper and lower components and is defined by the X and Z axes forming the XZ plane.

The central coordinate system and planar motion are not mutually exclusive when it comes to the description of motion. In fact, specific motions are defined by the axis around which movement takes place (i.e., central coordinate system) and the plane through which movement occurs (i.e., planar motion). The motions of flexion and extension occur around the X axis and parallel to the sagittal plane. Lateral flexion, abduction, and adduction occur around the Z axis, parallel to the coronal plane. Axial rotation (medial/lateral and right/left) occurs around the vertically orientated Y axis and parallel to the transverse plane. For the spinal motion segment,

the origin of motion is the intersection of the three planes and is conventionally placed in the center of the superior vertebral body. Therefore motion at the three-joint complex is described in terms relative to the superior vertebrae.

Six Degrees of Freedom

Six degrees of freedom or directions of motion are available at the three-joint complex. These motions are described in relation to the central coordinate system. (See Figure 11-2.) The potential exists for a spinal joint to exhibit translational and rotational movements along and around each of the X, Y, and Z axes. Thus we characterize a motion segment as a viscoelastic, energy-absorbing entity possessing six degrees of motion.[11-14] As we will see, rotation around these three axes is restricted by the plane that articular facet lies in and occurs in different amounts according to the region of the spine.[15]

The potential for six degrees of freedom originates from the unique arrangement of the three-joint complex. The separation of the vertebral bodies by the intervertebral disc allows for translation in all directions. Although the amount of motion permitted in each segment is slight and restricted by the plane of the joint surface and anatomy of the posterior facet joint, this multi-linked mechanical system of motion segments allows for a wide range of overall spinal motion.

Coupled Motion

Coupled motion is defined as vertebral movement around one axis (e.g., X axis), being consistently and automatically associated with movement around a second but different axis (e.g., Y axis).[16] A sound understanding of coupled motion is important for understanding potential mechanisms of injury and in the appropriate application of rehabilitation methods. The concept of coupled motion is especially relevant during the chiropractic adjustment because vertebral motion can occur parallel to a plane of motion that is different from the plane in which force was applied. For example, during a rotational mobilization, Lee[17] noted vertebral movement in all three anatomic planes. Additionally, coupled motion helps the chiropractic student better understand the rationale behind different preadjustment patient positioning techniques. Positioning the patient appropriately assists the doctor in isolating the spinal motion segment to be adjusted and improves the chance for success while minimizing patient discomfort and the possibility of injury.[18]

Coupled motion can also be thought of in terms of the six degrees of freedom available to the spinal motion segment. Coupling of more than one degree of freedom occurs when rotation or translation of the vertebra about one axis is consistently associated with rotation or translation of that same vertebra about another axis.[15] Jofe et al.[19] stated that coupling is primarily caused by the geometry of the regional facet articulations with the connecting ligaments and curvature of the spine having a secondary role. Coupled motions in the spine include flexion with axial rotation, lateral flexion with contralateral rotation and lateral flexion with ipsilateral rotation.[16,20] It is important to note that when we discuss coupled motions, we are referencing the spinal motion segment such that gross movements occur independently of coupled motion.[21] Imagine then, coupling occurring at the level of a single spinal motion segment. As we will see, spinal curvature and specific regional anatomical properties[21-23] contribute to coupled motions such that coupling patterns will vary by spinal region. Altered and asymmetrical coupling of motions have been noted in persons with low back pain.[21] Despite our attention to the concept of coupled motion, keep in mind that motion coupling differs across individuals and the clinical importance of normal and abnormal motion is still being debated.[16,21] Instead, think of coupled motion as a guideline for patient positioning and force application rather than absolute truth for clinical application. As such, coupled motion will vary by spinal region, adding to the confusion and controversy regarding actual motion couplings.

Instantaneous Axis of Rotation

Recall the description of motion as occurring around a particular axis. For example, the axis of rotation for flexion and extension is the X axis.

This definition would hold in the human body if all of our joints were designed like the wheel of a bicycle. For the wheel, the axis of rotation is at the center (i.e., axle). A wheel is perfectly round (or at least very close to round); joints of the human body, however, are not symmetrically round. Because of this, small changes in the axis of rotation occur. The changing axis of rotation is referred to as the instantaneous axis of rotation (IAR). Interestingly, a vertebral body's IAR may shift as different forces are applied.[15]

A rigid body's motion can be described with reference to the IAR or helical axis of motion. At every instant of planar motion, there is a line through the body (or hypothetical extension of it) that does not move. This line is perpendicular to the motion plane and is defined as the IAR.[15] (See Figure 11-4.) A helical axis of motion is defined as the unique axis in space that completely defines the three-dimensional motion of a rigid body from position 1 to position 2.[24] It is analogous to the instantaneous axis of rotation for plane motion. According to the laws of mechanics, a rigid body may always be moved from position 1 to position 2 by a rotation about a certain axis and a translation along the same axis.[24] This constitutes helical motion. The motion of a screw is an example of helical motion. A given instantaneous axis of rotation depends on the structure as well as the type of loading. The calculation for a particular vertebra differs as a result of various combinations of force and movement.[15]

Due to the incongruence between the curved surfaces of a joint, motion at the three-joint complex can occur through several axes at once. This concept is relevant to chiropractors with respect to defining a subluxation as having some component of aberrant motion. Changes to the IAR resulting in decreased aberrant motion have been reported following manipulation of the lumbar spine.[7]

Analysis of Motion

Before the advent of x-rays, range of motion was studied in cadavers.[11,12,25,26] This posed difficulties because of postmortem changes that occur with cadaveric specimens and thus did not accurately reflect spinal mobility. Today, in vitro studies continue and attempt to simulate motion without consideration for the influence of muscle force (i.e., kinematics). Although in vivo procedures have been developed, they are too complex to perform clinically in a practical manner.

The analysis of normal and abnormal motion requires a system of measurement that can produce a reliable description of motion in a simple, accurate, and repeatable manner. Radiographic studies are often the initial imaging modality of choice. However, standard radiographic series provide static information only, capturing the structural status of the spine in one plane. "Functional" radiographs depict the instantaneous positions of a vertebra at the extremes of global range of motion. This imaging procedure is not truly "functional" and although individual segmental movement cannot be assessed, aberrant motion may be identified as restricted or increased, or as abnormal vertebral alignment at the end of a given range of motion. (See Chapter 6.) Various authors have used template analysis[27] and "motor diagrams" from these radiographs to quantify motion (Figure 11-5).[28-31] Dimnet et al.[32,33]

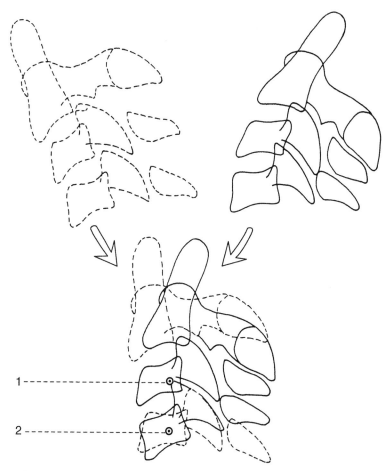

Figure 11-5   Movement diagram or template analysis. The solid lines represent extension of C2-C4, and the interrupted lines depict flexion of C2-C4. These can be superimposed onto an image of C2-C4 in neutral (not shown). Analysis of intersegmental translation and rotation can then be performed. *(From Penning L. Am J Roentgenol 1978;130:317-26.)*

studied lateral cervical radiographs in full flexion, full extension, and three intermediate motions to detect angles and centers of movement for each vertebra.[32] This same procedure was used earlier in the lumbar spine to observe lumbar sagittal plane motion.[33] Coupled motions outside of the sagittal plane, however, have not be observed.

The dynamic evaluation of spinal motion has been advocated by many authors[34] using stress radiographs. Stress radiographs consist of frontal radiographic views of the spine while the patient is placed in maximum right and left lateral bending, and lateral views of the spine while the patient is positioned in maximum lumbar flexion and extension.[34] Stress radiographs, like functional radiographs, are not truly dynamic. Both still capture a single static moment in time. While the findings from these studies can be extrapolated to truly dynamic situations, their predictive validity should be used cautiously.

More sophisticated and costly imaging techniques are now available, such as biplanar orthogonal radiography. Radiographs are taken simultaneously through two x-ray tubes arranged at right angles to one another (Figure 11-6). Movement in all three planes can be detected and quantified.[35-40]

A year after Roentgen's discovery of the x-ray in 1895, fluoroscopic screens were introduced, allowing for x-ray observation of dynamic events.[41] In 1921, investigators began using cineradiography. This process documents fluoroscopic examinations by photographing a fluoroscopic screen with 16-mm or 35-mm motion picture film.[41] The film can later be viewed at real-time, slow motion, or freeze-frame speeds. By the late 1950s, several researchers began to apply cineradiography to the skeletal system to evaluate joint motion.[42-44] This technique allows for the study of dynamic motion with the contribution of the joints, disc, ligaments, and muscles. Cineradiography requires increased radiation dosages and poses difficulty to the investigator in quantifying the enormous amount of data.

The widespread availability of video recording systems in the 1970s and 1980s led to the inevitable replacement of cineradiography by videofluoroscopy. Serial x-ray images were digitized from an image intensifier and directly interfaced to a

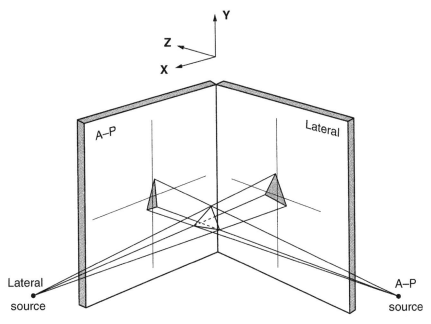

Figure 11-6 Biplanar radiographic technique. Geometric construction showing the projection of points on a body onto two orthogonal planes. *(From Pearcy M, Burrough S. J Bone Joint Surg 1982;64B:228-32.)*

computerized image processor. This digitized and displayed selected fluoroscopic images on a computer monitor. This spinal imaging modality is subject to observer variation in measuring angles and operator inconsistency.[45] It has potential in evaluating asymmetrical or paradoxical motion and intersegmental motion with lower radiation exposures. Newer techniques such as dynamic computed tomography (CT) and magnetic resonance imaging (MRI) are being used to visualize three-dimensional moving images.[41] In conclusion, the cost, dose, and yield must be evaluated before choosing a method of imaging to assess spinal kinematics.

Normal Intersegmental Motion by Spinal Region

The physiologic range of translation and rotation of a vertebra for each of the six degrees of freedom are explored in the cervical, thoracic, and lumbar spine. The reader should be aware that the literature spans a wide range of techniques used to evaluate and describe ranges of motion. This will inherently cause conflicting data when quantifying and qualifying motion. In addition to this factor, biologic variation is always at play. Regardless of the spinal location, the quantity and quality of motion are determined by normal variation in sagittal curvature and segmental orientation,[46,47] muscular control,[48,49] facet orientation,[50] and degenerative changes of the motion segments.[51,52] For example, in the cervical spine, facets are orientated primarily in the coronal plane and provide resistance to translatory movements.[53] Facets in the thoracic spine tend to be orientated between the coronal and sagittal planes while the lumbar facets are orientated more in the sagittal plane and provide greater resistance to rotation.[53] The facets between L5 and the sacrum are an exception, being orientated mostly in the coronal plane.[53]

Cervical Spine

The functional role of the cervical spine is both complex and intricate owing to seemingly contradictory roles for function. The cervical spine allows for the entrance, exit and protection of neu-

rovascular structures. The cervical spine provides strong support to the skull yet remains flexible to provide shock absorption to help protect the brain. Similarly, the vertebrae of the cervical spine provide rigid attachment points for muscle and yet still must maintain flexibility for movement.

Atlantooccipital Joints

The atlantooccipital joint (i.e., C0 and C1) is formed by the articulation of the convex occipital condyle with the concave facet of the atlas. This is a symmetrical and mechanically linked joint.[54] Movement at the atlantooccipital joint occurs predominately in the sagittal plane, producing flexion and extension as the condyles slide in the corresponding lateral masses of the atlas (Figure 11-7). Significant controversy exists as to the amount of flexion and extension available at this joint. Findings from radiographic studies have suggested as little as 13 degrees[14,55] while cineradiographic studies have found sagittal plane motion of 35 degrees.[43] Penning[56] performed overlay studies on 20 healthy adults and found an average of 30 degrees sagittal motion, with a range of 25 to 45 degrees. In later studies, Panjabi et al.[57] observed an average range of 24.5 degrees, approximately 21 degrees of extension and 3.5 degrees flexion. Differences in reported segmental motion may be related to head position. For example, Jones[58] suggested two different patterns of total cervical flexion exist and differentially affect motion at the atlantooccipital joints. Cervical flexion initiated with the chin retracted produces greater motion at the C0-C1 segment compared to flexion starting with the head erect.

Most authors agree that pure rotation does not occur at the atlantooccipital joints.[15,19,55,58] However, Kapandji[54] believes that rotation between C0 and C1 (3 degrees) occurs secondary to rotation of the atlas about the odontoid and is accompanied by secondary minimal linear displacement to the same side of rotation and lateral flexion on the opposite side (Figure 11-8). Dvorak et al.,[59] using computed tomography (CT), found the maximal rotational excursion of this joint to be 10.25 degrees while Penning and Wilmink[60] reported a mean value of 1 degree rotation at this level using

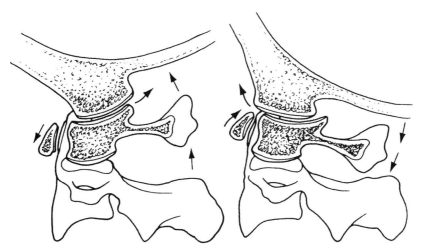

Figure 11-7   Flexion and extension of the occiput on the atlas. During flexion (left diagram) the occipital condyles glide posteriorly and superiorly on the lateral masses of the atlas, as the occipital bone separates from the posterior arch. During extension (right diagram) the condyles slide anteriorly on the lateral masses of atlas, while the occipital bone approximates the posterior arch of atlas. *(From Bergmann TF, Peterson DH, Lawrence DJ. Chiropractic technique. New York: Churchill Livingstone; 1993. p. 219.)*

CT scans. Using stereophotogrammetry (measurements derived from three-dimensional photographs), Panjabi et al.[57] reported as much as 7.2 degrees of ipsilateral axial rotation. (See Figure 11-8.)

Lateral flexion of the atlantooccipital articulation is limited not only by the osseous geometry but by the alar ligament attachment (Figure 11-9).[24] Werne[55] in his early studies on cadavers contended 11.9 degrees lateral bending with slightly less (7.8 degrees) on radiographs. Based on a review of the literature and their own analysis, White and Panjabi[15] reported approximately 8 degrees of lateral flexion. Later, Panjabi et al.[57] found lateral bending of 5.5 degrees using stereophotogrammetry.

Due to the convex shape of the occipital condyles and concave shape of the atlas's articular surfaces, movement in the coronal plane is coupled with opposite movement in the transverse plane. Thus lateral flexion is coupled with rotation of the head to the opposite side.[24,43,61] Additionally, with lateral flexion to the left, C1 translates to the left to adjust the position of the left lateral mass of C1, which otherwise would prevent lateral flexion to the left side (Figure 11-10). During left lateral flexion, the right alar ligament is pulled tight by this movement, pulling on the dens and rotating

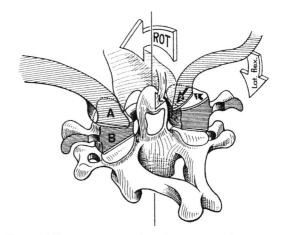

Figure 11-8   Rotation at the atlantooccipital joint. Rotation of the occiput to the left is associated with anterior displacement of the right occipital condyle on the right lateral mass of the atlas *(arrow 1)*. At the same time, tension develops in the atlantooccipital ligament, pulling the right occipital condyle to the left *(arrow 2)*. Rotation of the occiput to the left is associated with a linear displacement of 2 to 3 mm to the left and lateral flexion to the right. *(From Kapandji IA. The physiology of the joints. Vol. 3. The trunk and the vertebral column. Edinburgh: Churchill Livingstone; 1982. p. 182-3.)*

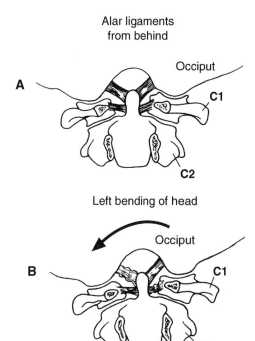

Alar ligaments
from behind

Figure 11-9   The role of the alar ligaments with the atlantooccipital articulation in lateral flexion: **A**, posterior view in the neutral position; **B**, left lateral flexion. Motion is limited by the right upper portion and the left lower portion of the alar ligaments. *(From Bergmann TF, Peterson DH, Lawrence DJ. Chiropractic technique. New York: Churchill Livingstone; 1993. p. 220.)*

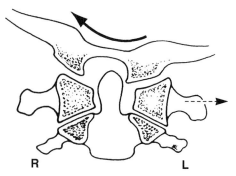

Figure 11-10   Left lateral flexion of the upper cervical spine *(solid arrow)* with translation of the atlas *(broken arrow)* toward the left. *(From Bergmann TF, Peterson DH, Lawrence DJ. Chiropractic technique. New York: Churchill Livingstone; 1993. p. 223.)*

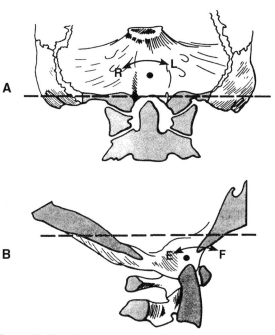

Figure 11-11   The approximate location of the instantaneous axis of rotation (IAR) *(dot)* for the atlantooccipital joint in the frontal plane during right and left lateral flexion (**A**). The location of the IAR in the sagittal plane during flexion and extension (**B**). *(From White AA, Panjabi MM. Clinical biomechanics of the spine. 2nd ed. Philadelphia: JB Lippincott; 1990. p. 96.)*

the C2 spinous process to the right. Penning[56] contends that lateral bending of the atlantooccipital segment is always combined with lateral bending and slight rotation of the C1-C2 joint. Jirout,[61] however, suggests that rotation of the atlas from the side of inclination cannot be looked on as normal and constant because it does not occur.

The instantaneous axis of rotation for flexion/extension is located in a sagittal axis 2 to 3 cm above the apex of the dens.[24] For lateral bending, the axis appears to be located in the midline, slightly more distant from the tip of the dens.[62] Because there is very little or no axial rotation at the occipitoatlantal articulation, the instantaneous axis of rotation for this plane is not considered (Figure 11-11).

Atlantoaxial Joints

The mechanically linked four-joint complex between C1 and C2 lacks the disc of the typical vertebral motion segment.[63] Thus the pattern of motion is primarily controlled by the geometry of the osseous and ligamentous articulations. There are two paired atlantoaxial joints, one central atlantoodontoid joint, and one joint between the transverse ligament and the posterior aspect of the odontoid process.

The predominate motion at the atlantoaxial joints is rotation of the atlas around the Y axis of the odontoid process. Werne[55] reported rotational movement of 47 degrees, accounting for 40% to 50% of the total axial rotation available in the cervical spine and making the atlantoaxial joints the most mobile segment of the cervical spine. Similar values for rotation have been reported by Panjabi and White.[15] Compared to the atlantooccipital joints, there is less discrepancy in the degree of rotation occurring at the atlantoaxial joints. Penning and Wilmink[60] report 40.5 degrees of rotational motion to either side, with a range of 29 to 46 degrees. Work by Dvorak et al.[59] as well as Panjabi et al.[57] support findings that a range of

rotational motion likely exists at the atlantoaxial joints; the researchers found an average of 32.2 degrees and 38.9 degrees, respectively.

The coupled motion during rotation is a "screwlike" mechanism, allowing the atlas to drop 2 to 3 mm because of the biconvexity of the joint surfaces (Figure 11-12). With rotation, there is also an associated coupling of ipsilateral lateral bending to a small degree.[56] This vertical approximation was confirmed by Hohl[64] using cineradiographs. Werne[55] concluded that vertical displacement or amount that the atlas drops depends on the extent to which the longitudinal axis of the dens correlates with the imaginary longitudinal axis of the body. The more parallel the two are, the more distinctive the vertical displacement.[55] Jirout[65] used x-ray analysis to formulate conclusions regarding rotation and linear displacement. In his model, rotation had two phases. The initial phase involved a symmetrical rotation of C2 around the longitudinal axis of the cervical spine (attributable to the facet joints), followed by an asymmetrical phase of further rotation (influenced by the addition of muscle traction) with pronounced lateral translation of the axis against the atlas.

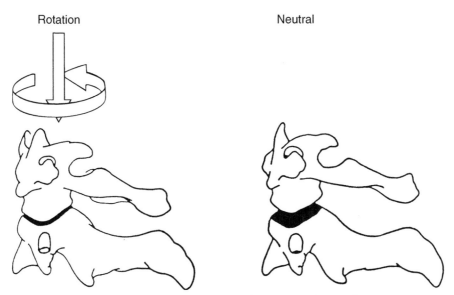

Figure 11-12   Coupled motion: vertical translation of C1 with axial translation of C1 on C2. *(From Bergmann TF, Peterson DH, Lawrence DJ. Chiropractic technique. New York: Churchill Livingstone; 1993. p. 222.)*

During flexion and extension, the anterior arch of C1 slides superiorly and inferiorly on the odontoid process as the inferior facets of C1 roll and slide on the superior facets of C2. In flexion, the posterior joint capsule and posterior arches separate and the articular surface of the atlas glides forward. In extension, the posterior joint capsule and posterior arches approximate and the articular surface of the atlas glides posteriorly.[66] Panjabi et al.[57] report 11.5 degrees flexion and 10.9 degrees extension at the atlantoaxial joint. Similar measurements have been reported by Werne[55] and Hohl,[64] who demonstrated 10 degrees of flexion and extension. Penning[56] used movement diagrams from functional radiographs during flexion and extension and found an average 30 degrees of motion

with a range of 25 to 45 degrees. Although it is generally accepted that there is little measurable lateral flexion at the atlantoaxial joint,[19] Penning[56] reports a mean value of 10 degrees to each side while Panjabi et al.[57] report 6.7 degrees of lateral flexion to one side at the atlantoaxial segment.

Flexion and extension movements of the atlantoaxial joint are coupled with small translational movements from 2 to 3 mm in the adult and up to 4.5 mm in the child.[24] The atlantodental interspace also diminishes during flexion, creating a V-shaped appearance.[43] Although there is still controversy as to whether lateral (X axis) translation of the atlantoaxial joint occurs, most of the literature suggests that a displacement of 0 to 4 mm is normal.[19]

The instantaneous axis of rotation for the atlantoaxial joint has been located through cineradiographic studies to the middle third of the dens during flexion and extension (Figure 11-13).[55] For axial rotation, the axis may be assumed to lie in the center portion of the axis (Figure 11-14).[19] Because lateral flexion at this joint is small or nonexistent, the location of an axis for this motion may be deemed irrelevant.[62]

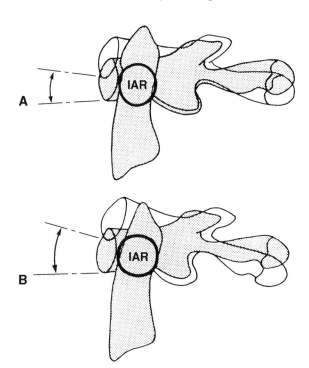

Figure 11-13   **A,** Representation of sagittal plane motion of C1 on C2, with approximate instantaneous axis of rotation also indicated. **B,** The anterior curvature of the dens may permit some degree of additional sagittal plane motion in both rotation and translation. *(From White AA, Panjabi MM. Clinical biomechanics of the spine. 2nd ed. Philadelphia: JB Lippincott; 1990. p. 93.)*

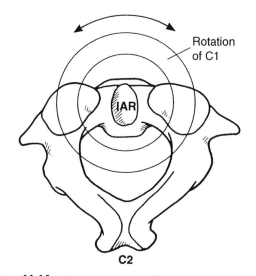

Figure 11-14   Representation of the approximate location of the instantaneous axis of rotation for axial rotation of C1 on C2. *(From White AA, Panjabi MM. Clinical biomechanics of the spine. 2nd ed. Philadelphia: JB Lippincott; 1990. p. 96.)*

Lower Cervical Spine

The lower cervical spine from the second to the seventh vertebra possesses six degrees of motion: flexion, extension, rotation (right and left), and lateral flexion (right and left). Range of motion for the typical vertebrae of the cervical spine is determined by osseous geometry and the stiffness of the disc.[14] Additional variations in motion can occur due to age because younger individuals may possess general ligamentous laxity, demonstrating disproportionately greater motion at C2-C3 compared to adults who tend to show the greatest amount of flexion at C4-C5 or C5-C6.[67]

Cervical spine flexion and extension predominately occur in the lower cervical spine and are coupled with translation and rotation (Table 11-2). Figure 11-15 depicts movement of the spinal motion segment with the superior vertebrae tilting and gliding on the articular surfaces of the lower facet joints, producing the total motion required by the head and neck. The coupled translation that occurs with flexion and extension has been measured at approximately 2 mm per segment.[19,68] In the sagittal plane, translation along the Z axis occurs in decreasing magnitude approaching the C7 vertebra,[15] producing a "stair-step" effect. In addition, for every degree of sagittal plane rotation, more translation occurs in the upper cervical

segments than in the lower cervical segments.[66] This translation has been attributed to the inclination of the facet joints.[43] Conversely, the caudal segments tend to have a larger amount of tilt.[28]

Lateral flexion averages approximately 10 degrees (segmentally) to each side in the mid cervical segments, with decreasing flexibility in the caudal segments.[66] (See Table 11-2.) Lateral flexion in the lower cervical spine is coupled with rotation such that ipsilateral lateral bending is coupled with rotation of the spinous process to the contralateral side (or convexity of the curve) (Figure 11-16). The degree of coupled motion decreases in a caudal direction.[66] For example, at the second cervical vertebra, there are 2 degrees of coupled axial rotation for every 3 degrees of lateral bending, a ratio of 2:3.[19] At the seventh vertebra, there is 1 degree of coupled axial rotation for every 7.5 degrees of lateral bending, a ratio of 1:7.5. Jofe[19] theorizes that the gradual change in coupling ratio may be related to the change in inclination of the facet joints. The greatest obliquity of the facet joints is at C2-C3 (40 to 45 degrees), progressively decreasing to 10 degrees at C7-T1.[54] Kapandji[54] also believes that during lateral flexion some degree of extension occurs as a result of anatomic structure.

Using CT, Penning and Wilmink[60] found during lateral flexion that the superior vertebra translated

Table 11-2

Limits and Representative Values of Rotation of the Cervical Spine

Interspace	Combined flexion/extension (±x-axis rotation)		One side lateral bending (z-axis rotation)		One side axial rotation (y-axis rotation)	
	Limits of ranges (degrees)	Representative angle (degrees)	Limits of ranges (degrees)	Representative angle (degrees)	Limits of ranges (degrees)	Representative angle (degrees)
Middle						
C2-3	5-16	10	11-20	10	0-10	3
C3-4	7-26	15	9-15	11	3-10	7
C4-5	13-29	20	0-16	11	1-12	7
Lower						
C5-6	13-29	20	0-16	8	2-12	7
C6-7	6-26	17	0-17	7	2-10	6
C7-T1	4-7	9	0-17	4	0-7	2

Modified from White AA III, Panjabi MM, editors. Clinical biomechanics of the spine. 2nd ed. Philadelphia: JB Lippincott; 1990.

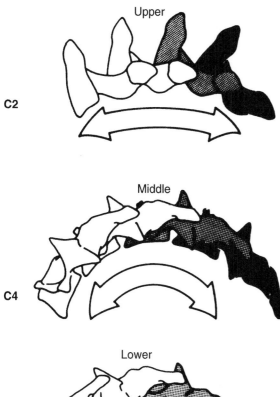

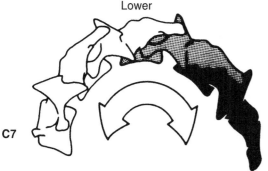

Figure 11-15 A diagrammatic approximation of the relative regional cephalocaudal variations in radii of curvature of the arches, defined by the cervical vertebrae as they rotate and translate in the sagittal plane. *(From White AA, Panjabi MM. Clinical biomechanics of the spine. 2nd ed. Philadelphia: JB Lippincott; 1990. p. 99.)*

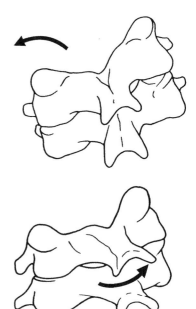

Figure 11-16 Movement of the facet surfaces in the lower cervical spine causes coupled rotation with lateral flexion. *(From Bergmann TF, Peterson DH, Lawrence DJ. Chiropractic technique. New York: Churchill Livingstone; 1993. p. 233.)*

in a contralateral direction to avoid imbrication with the uncinate process. Because the uncinate process is located posteriorly on the edges of the vertebral bodies, this mechanism takes place only posteriorly.[63] With posterior translation of the upper vertebra with respect to the lower vertebra in the opposite direction during lateral flexion, simultaneous rotation must occur.[63] Fielding[43] adds that because of the inclination of the intervertebral joints, during lateral flexion, the inferior articular processes on the concave side glide downward and backward, whereas those on the convex side glide upward and forward, thus producing the motion of rotation.

Rotation in the lower cervical spine is coupled by some degree of lateral flexion.[54] (See Table 11-2.) Ranges of motion for segmental axial rotation on average are slightly less than those for lateral flexion, with a similar tendency for decreased movement in the lower cervical segments.[66]

Few studies give indication of the location of instantaneous axes of rotation in the cervical region. Lysell[68] postulates these locations based on judgment from observations of patterns of motion rather than on quantitative assessment. The

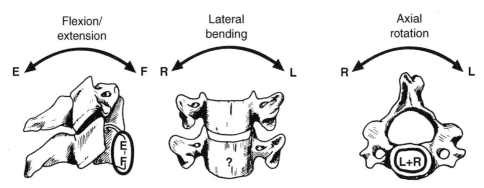

Figure 11-17   The approximate locations of the instantaneous axes of rotation (IAR) in the lower cervical spine. *F* is the location in going from a neutral to a flexed position. *E* is the location of the IAR in going from a neutral to extended position. *L* shows the approximate location of the axis in left axial rotation and *R* shows the axis in right axial rotation. The question mark indicates that there are no convincing estimates of the IAR for lateral bending in the cervical spine. *(From White AA, Panjabi MM. Clinical biomechanics of the spine. 2nd ed. Philadelphia: JB Lippincott; 1990. p. 102.)*

IAR for sagittal and horizontal plane motion is located in the anterior portions of the subadjacent vertebrae.[68] The instantaneous axis of rotation for lateral flexion has not been determined (Figure 11-17).[68]

Thoracic Spine

The thoracic spine is an area of transition from the coronally situated facets of the cervical spine to the sagitally orientated facets of the lumbar spine. Although the thoracic spine is capable of performing flexion, extension, rotation and lateral flexion, motion is limited in all planes because of the ribs, narrowed discs, and elongated spinous processes. Additional anatomical constraints to motion include thickening of the anterior longitudinal ligament and the ligamentum flavum as well as tighter facet capsules.

Globally, less flexion and extension occurs in the upper thoracic spine (T1-T6) compared to the lower half of the thoracic spine (T9-T12). The average combined flexion and extension in the thoracic spine is approximately 6 degrees per motion segment and increases in a cephalocaudad direction.[66] Movement averages 4 degrees in the upper thoracic spine, 6 degrees in the midsegments, and 12 degrees in the lower two motion segments (Table 11-3).[24] Axial rotation of the thoracic spine is encouraged in the

upper segments because of the more transverse orientation of the facet joints. Segmental axial rotation averages 8 to 9 degrees in the upper thoracic spine.[24] Rotational movement decreases in the cephalocaudad direction, approximating 2 degrees in the lower two or three thoracic segments.[24] (See Table 11-3.) Rotation is also limited by the anterior attachment of the ribs to the sternum. Lateral flexion averages approximately 6 degrees to each side, with the lower two segments averaging 7 to 9 degrees.[66] (See Table 11-3.)

As in the lower cervical spine, flexion and extension of the thoracic spine (i.e., sagittal plane motion) is accompanied by axial rotation (transverse plane) and small amounts of translation (sagittal plane). Translation is uniform but markedly less than that of the cervical spine.[24] Data on the coupled motion of rotation and lateral flexion in the thoracic spine is less convincing because the results have been somewhat varied depending on the segments studied.[14] In general, coupled motion in the upper thoracic region mimics that seen in the lower cervical spine. For example, lateral flexion is coupled with ipsilateral rotation (i.e., the vertebral body rotates into the concavity and the spinous process deviates to the convexity). The degree of lateral bending produces somewhat less axial rotation than it did in the

Table 11-3

Limits and Representative Values of Rotation of the Thoracic Spine

Interspace	Combined flexion/extension (±x-axis rotation)		One side lateral bending (z-axis rotation)		One side axial rotation (y-axis rotation)	
	Limits of ranges (degrees)	Representative angle (degrees)	Limits of ranges (degrees)	Representative angle (degrees)	Limits of ranges (degrees)	Representative angle (degrees)
T1-T2	3-5	4	5	5	14	9
T2-T3	3-5	4	5-7	6	4-12	8
T3-T4	2-5	4	3-7	5	5-11	8
T4-T5	2-5	4	5-6	6	5-11	8
T5-T6	3-5	4	5-6	6	5-11	8
T6-T7	2-7	5	6	6	4-11	7
T7-T8	3-8	6	3-8	6	4-11	7
T8-T9	3-8	6	4-7	6	6-7	6
T9-T10	3-8	6	4-7	6	3-5	4
T10-T11	4-14	9	3-10	7	2-3	2
T11-T12	6-20	12	4-13	9	2-3	2
T12-L1	6-20	12	5-10	8	2-3	2

From White AA III, Panjabi MM, editors. Clinical biomechanics of the spine. 2nd ed. Philadelphia: JB Lippincott; 1990. p. 103.

cervical spine.[15] In the middle and lower thoracic spine, the coupling is less distinct and may occur in any direction, but it is generally assumed that the lower thoracic segments have a tendency to follow the coupling pattern of the lumbar spine.[66] Average IARs for the thoracic spine are presented in Figure 11-18.

Lumbar Spine

In addition to discussing the principal movements of lumbar spine flexion, extension, axial rotation, and lateral flexion, axial compression and axial distraction will be discussed because of their clinical relevance. Flexion and extension occur about the X axis with small amounts of translation. The facet joints guide rotation and resist translation allowing for 8 to 13 degrees of rotation about the X axis[69] and 1 to 3 mm of translation.[39,69,70] Segmentally, flexion and extension are the predominant motions of the lumbar spine. With motion increasing from the thoracolumbar junction to the lumbosacral junction (Table 11-4), the combined sagittal plane motion averages from 14 to 15 degrees per segment.[24,38]

Compared to flexion and extension, axial rotation in the lumbar spine is extremely limited and further hindered by the intervertebral joints (Figure 11-19). Segmental rotation is relatively uniform throughout the lumbar spine and averages between 2 and 3 degrees.[24,38,69] (See Table 11-4.) Segmental lateral flexion averages approximately 6 degrees to each side uniformly throughout the lumbar spine, with the exception of the L5-S1 motion segment. (See Table 11-4.) The lumbosacral junction demonstrates half of this motion.[24] Pearcy and Tibrewal[46] found the same pattern of lateral flexion, with approximately 10 degrees occurring in the upper three levels but there was significantly less movement at L4-L5 (6 degrees) and L5-S1 (3 degrees).

Axial rotation is variably coupled with flexion and extension with either flexion or extension occurring during left or right rotation, but neither occurs consistently.[69] Lateral flexion may be accompanied by either flexion or extension of the same joint, but extension occurs more frequently and to a greater degree.[69] Lumbar lateral flexion involves a complex coupled movement of lateral tilting and rotatory motion that is open for much

Table 11-4

Limits and Representative Values of Ranges of Motion of the Lumbar Spine

Interspace	Combined flexion/extension (±x-axis rotation)		One side lateral bending (z-axis rotation)		One side axial rotation (y-axis rotation)	
	Limits of ranges (degrees)	Representative angle (degrees)	Limits of ranges (degrees)	Representative angle (degrees)	Limits of ranges (degrees)	Representative angle (degrees)
L1-L2	5-16	12	3-8	6	1-3	2
L2-L3	8-18	14	3-10	6	1-3	2
L3-L4	6-17	15	4-12	8	1-3	2
L4-L5	9-21	16	3-9	6	1-3	2
L5-S1	10-24	17	2-6	3	0-2	1

Modified from White AA III, Panjabi MM, editors. Clinical biomechanics of the spine. 2nd ed. Philadelphia: JB Lippincott; 1990. p. 107.

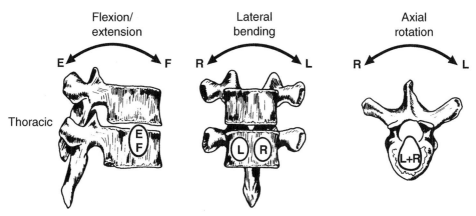

Figure 11-18   The approximate locations of the instantaneous axes of rotation in the thoracic spine. *(From White AA, Panjabi MM. Clinical biomechanics of the spine. 2nd ed. Philadelphia: JB Lippincott; 1990. p. 105.)*

debate regarding the precise biomechanical motion. During lateral bending, some authors describe the "normal" lumbar vertebral bodies as rotating toward the concavity, with the spinous processes rotating toward the convexity.[71-73] Unfortunately, this may not always be the case. Cassidy[48] and Grice[74] were the first to classify three patterns of coupled motion with lateral flexion in the lumbar spine. These patterns included type I, lateral flexion associated with contralateral vertebral body rotation (spinous processes rotate toward the side of lateral flexion); type II, ipsilateral vertebral body tipping with ipsilateral body rotation (spinous process toward

the convexity); and type III, reversal or lack of vertebral body tipping with contralateral body rotation.[48] Grice later expanded on these classifications by adding a type IV, reversal of lack of segmental tilt and rotation of the vertebral body toward the side of trunk bending (Figure 11-20).[49] These patterns are primarily determined by evaluation of lateral bending functional x-ray studies. Type I has been suggested to be the normal coupled movement of the lumbar spine with types II, III, and IV indicating aberrant motion patterns.[48,49] Other authors took this a step further by stating that coupled motion mechanics at various regions of the lumbar spine are different. That is, L1, L2,

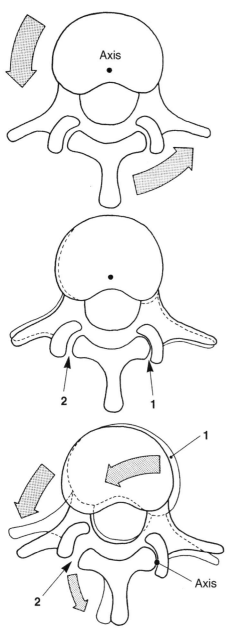

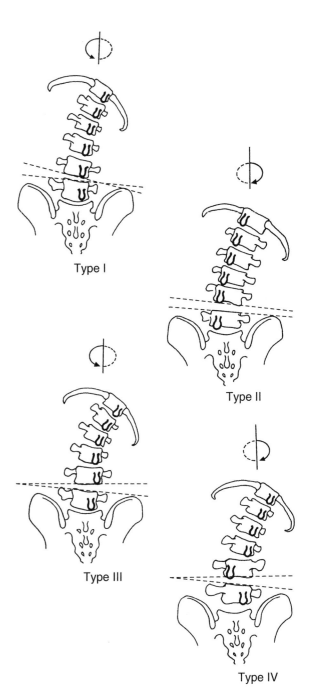

Figure 11-19 The mechanism of left axial rotation for a lumbar intervertebral joint. Two consecutive vertebrae superimposed on one another are viewed from above. The lower vertebra is depicted by a dotted line. *1,* Initially, rotation occurs about an axis in the vertebral body. *2,* As the posterior elements swing around, the right inferior articular process of the upper vertebra impacts the superior articular process of the lower vertebra. *(From Bodguk N, Twomey LT. Clinical anatomy of the lumbar spine. Edinburgh: Churchill Livingstone; 1987. p. 66.)*

Figure 11-20 The classifications of motion patterns during lumbar lateral flexion. *(From Grice AS. J Manipulative Physiol Ther 1979;2(1):26-34.)*

and L3 demonstrate axial rotation accompanied by lateral flexion to the contralateral side.[46,47,69] In contrast, the L5-S1 joint demonstrates axial rotation accompanied by lateral flexion to the same side and L4-L5 shows no particular preference; both coupling patterns can exist.[46,47,69] Haas et al.[75] have shown that 40% to 60% of asymptomatic and symptomatic subjects demonstrate type II motion at various levels of the lumbar spine (L1-L4). It is possible that much of the type II motion is a consequence of normal asymmetries in facet anatomy, soft tissue orientation and normal variation in cooperative muscle activity.[76] More research is necessary to verify "normal" and "normal variant" coupling mechanics in the lumbar spine.

The IAR for axial rotation and lateral flexion is placed within the posterior nucleus and anulus of the subadjacent disc space.[24] The IAR for flexion and extension is most commonly placed within the intervertebral disc of the subadjacent vertebra, with flexion located toward the anterior portion and extension toward the posterior portion (Figure 11-21).[24]

The human spine is exposed frequently to compressive forces. The sagittal alignment of spinal curves aids in resisting compressive forces we experience during physical activity and activities of daily living. The lordosis of the lumbar spine and anterior ligaments participate in the axial load-bearing mechanism with risk of injury increasing as the lumbar lordosis flattens.[77] Compared to the cervical spine, the lumbar spine has a greater ability to resist compressive forces because of the increasing size of vertebral bodies. Normally, the nuclear portion of the intervertebral disc will bear more compressive force compared to the outer annular fibers. However, degenerative spinal changes cause a shift in the normal load bearing characteristics of the spine with the anulus fibrosus and the zygapophyseal joints being subjected to greater strain.[78] Facet joint strain also increases as the orientation of their surfaces shifts out of the coronal plane. These joints also share a greater portion of compressive loads by the impaction of the inferior articular process with the superior articular facet of the vertebra below during extension,[69] accounting for increased pain

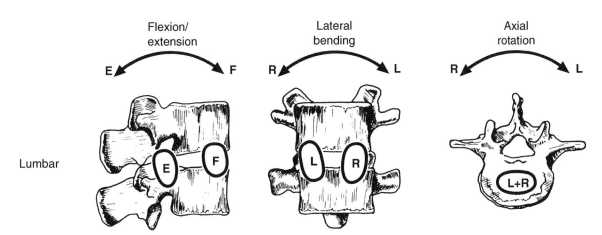

Figure 11-21 The approximate locations of the instantaneous axes of rotation in the lumbar spine. *(From White AA, Panjabi MM. Clinical biomechanics of the spine. 2nd ed. Philadelphia: JB Lippincott; 1990. p. 112.)*

associated with a lumbar facet syndrome during hyperextension.

In axial distraction, tensile or distractive forces usually occur in combination with other primary motions. For example, complex loads that combine flexion, extension, and rotation as well as axial distraction are often responsible for spinal injuries.[79] The capsules of the zygapophyseal joints are a significant element resisting this motion. For example, during forward flexion, the posterior elements of the spine are subjected to stress from distraction. Recognizing what anatomical structures are sensitive to tensile forces is important for understanding mechanisms of injury and for the safe and effective application of traction therapies (e.g., flexion-distraction therapy). For example, patient positioning is an important element of axial distraction. Specifically, axial distraction of the lumbar spine can be coupled with other motions depending on patient positioning.[80] Additionally, the distractive force needed to stretch posterior elements decreases depending on patient position (e.g., supine with knees and hips flexed).[80]

Abnormal Joint Motion

Abnormal joint motion can be characterized into three categories: hypomobility, or restriction of normal motion; hypermobility, or motion in excess of normal; and aberrant mobility, or motion in which there is a change in the axis or rotation, including paradoxical or reversed motion.

Hypomobility

Hypomobility ranges from a slight restriction of joint motion to a total absence of motion or joint locking. Based on the idea that the intervertebral joint was capable of a certain field of motion and a certain axis of motion, the term hypomobility was introduced into the chiropractic literature in 1906.[81] Since that time, a plethora of other terms have been proposed to describe hypomobility including malalignment.

Early chiropractic paradigms viewed the subluxation complex as a malalignment wherein normal motion was not possible because the vertebrae had been restrained in an abnormal position. This model suggested that a vertebra was pulled out of its ideal neutral position by alterations in articular and periarticular soft tissues. Additionally, a malaligned vertebra was restricted in movements away from the direction of the malposition.[82] Note, however, that the concept of a malaligned vertebra is not contained in the definition of hypomobility or restricted motion as applied in current theory and research. In a study by Howe,[44] estimates of intervertebral malposition from plain film radiographs did not correlate with motion studies that might indicate dysfunction in the form of hypomobility, hypermobility, erratic movement, or even reversal of normal motion. Conversely, apparently well-aligned vertebrae may exhibit abnormal motion. Additionally, the premise that the direction of malposition can predict the direction of movement restrictions has been refuted by Haas and Peterson.[82] In this same study, segmental malalignment was universal in the population studied.[82] Schram and Hosek[83] could not demonstrate the effects (change in position) of chiropractic manipulation using prestatic and poststatic radiographic technology.

In the more recent literature, synonyms for hypomobility have included interarticular dyskinesia,[84] spinal articular dysfunction,[85] manipulable lesion,[85] and joint fixation.[86] These later terms help to define hypomobility with respect to the chiropractic subluxation and the subluxation complex. However, the restriction or hypomobility of joint movement, which is thought to be a principal component of the manipulable subluxation, should be reversible for manipulation to be of benefit. This last point raises another interesting question—should the presence of hypomobility by itself represent an indication for chiropractic adjusting? For example, in a study of the sacroiliac joints, asymmetry of motion between the right and left sacroiliac joints occurred in the absence of symptoms.[87] Although there is no direct answer, the question itself suggests current limitations in what we know about the subluxation and subluxation complex and highlights the importance of clinical judgment and experience when applying the skilled art of chiropractic.

Hypermobility

Clinically, hypermobility ranges from a slight but reversible increase in joint motion to instability, where the stabilizing elements of the spinal motion segment are no longer intact. In the latter instance, usually a traumatic or congenital anomaly has altered the integrity or properties of the restraining tissue, permitting excessive joint movement. Conversely, segmental hypermobility has been defined by McGregor and Mior[88] in the cervical spine as "the mobility of a given motion segment which is excessive and is accompanied by local and/or peripheral symptoms, but not so extreme as to be life-threatening or require surgery." Three main factors determine segmental hypermobility: congruency of the joint surfaces in close-packed position; structural integrity of the collagen that contributes to joint capsule, tendons and overlying tissues; and neuromuscular tone that stabilizes the spine under physiologic conditions. Differences exist then between hypermobility that is a contraindication to manipulation and segmental hypermobility. For example, motion that slightly exceeds normal range of motion, if reversible, may not be an absolute contraindication to manipulation. Additionally, excess joint motion may shift the joint axis of rotation, resulting in an abnormal pattern of movement. In this example, a manipulable subluxation may occur for a motion segment in which the passive stabilizing elements have been moderately stretched. However, clinical judgment is warranted as repeated thrusting into such a joint may not produce optimal results and could prolong the healing time of the stretched elements.

In contrast to segmental hypermobility, instability represents extreme hypermobility whereby the holding elements of the three-joint complex have been damaged in such a way that the pattern of abnormal motion is not reversible through manipulation. In such cases, the subluxation of the joint is considered nonmanipulable and may require surgical repair especially if neurologic deficits are apparent. Sandoz[89] refers to this as a surgical subluxation as opposed to a reversible fixation characterized by a vertebral body, a zygapophyseal joint, or both that have moved into a position that they can never occupy during normal spinal movement. (See Chapter 8.) Additionally, clinical instability in the cervical spine has been defined as "the pathological state of motion at an intervertebral level...that results in clinically intolerable symptoms, as in cord or root damage, requiring prolonged bracing or surgery."[90] By tracking the instantaneous axes of rotation through the entire range of motion for the hypermobile segment, relative amounts of segmental translation and rotation can be evaluated.[91] Mechanical irregularity or instability at a joint may be indicated by inconsistencies in the distribution of translation and rotation.[91] Clinically, a loss of normal end play resistance ("empty end feel") is a potential manifestation of joint hypermobility or instability.[66]

Interestingly, hypermobility need not have a negative connotation. For example, in a study of joint hypermobility in musicians, hypermobility had clear advantages and disadvantages. Specifically, hypermobility of those joints used repetitively when playing a musical instrument may be of benefit while hypermobility of joints not moved repetitively (e.g., knee or spine) may be of detriment.[92] Similar benefits of spinal hypermobility have been reported for ballet dancers.[93]

Aberrant Motion

Aberrant motion has been described as both motion in which a change in the axis of rotation has occurred or a paradoxical reversal of normal motion. Paradoxical motion has been observed at the atlantooccipital joint, for example, with the occiput moving into extension on the atlas during cervical flexion.[58] Lane considered this motion to be a normal variant.[94]

Smith et al.[81] described aberrant motion as a change in the field of vertebral motion; a subluxation is like a "wheel whose hub was off center" (eccentric in contrast to concentric). A normal change in the instantaneous axis of rotation has also been described by White and Panjabi[24] when referring to changes that occur with coupled motion. For example, with flexion of a vertebra, translation along the Z axis coupled with rotation around the X axis produces an instantaneous change in the axis of rotation as flexion proceeds. Conceptually, a restriction at one joint in the three-joint complex may produce a change in the axis of rotation resulting in an abnormal pattern of motion. Physiologic consequences of aberrant segmental mechanics can lead to unnatural load distributions. It is postulated that manipulation can effectively change the instantaneous axis of rotation in a motion segment where movement has been demonstrated to be pathologic in reference to the normal coupling mechanism.[95] Thus the quality of motion, not the quantity, has changed.

Compensatory Hypermobility

Global motion of the spine is dependent on the combined movement of 24 spinal motion segments. It has been proposed that restriction of movement at one level will be compensated for by hypermobility in other areas.[27,96] Compensatory hypermobility often occurs adjacent to a restricted segment or surgically fused segment.[97-101] Using biplanar radiography, Stokes et al.[102] studied the behavior of spinal segments adjacent to surgical fusions and found segments in the lower lumbar spine to be hypermobile during flexion and lateral bending. In addition, these primary motions were accompanied by an increase in coupled motion that resulted in increased shear on the disc and posterior facet joints.[102] In dogs, immobilization of multiple spinal segments influenced the remaining mobile segments by increasing the load and motion, not only at the immediately adjacent segment, but also at the distal segments.[103] Increased motion can occur above a fused segment as well as above an unstable segment.[90] Goel et al.[104] observed an increase in the relative motion of segments above an induced instability. These compensatory mechanical effects have also been observed across spinal regions. For example, sagittal lumbar movement was found to be significantly reduced with increasing sacroiliac restriction.[105] This relation, however, reversed at a certain level of sacroiliac restriction. At this point, lumbar mobility increased with increasing sacroiliac restriction but never to "normal" sagittal lumbar mobility.

Mechanistic Model of Intervertebral Joint Restriction

Restricted segmental movement, a component of the chiropractic subluxation complex, has been discussed in Chapter 10. However, determining the mechanism by which manipulation could positively affect characteristics of movement via feedback from the motion segment remains a challenge. Clouding this issue is that the relative contribution of muscle spindles, Golgi tendon organs (GTO), mechanoreceptors, and skin receptors to movement remains unknown.[106] Further, while both muscle spindles and mechanoreceptors contribute proprioceptive information during active movement, the contribution of these joint afferents is also mediated by deformation of the joint capsule from muscular contraction.[107] Heikkila and Wenngren[108] suggested that injury to cervical zygapophyseal joints was responsible for altered proprioceptive feedback. While mechanoreceptors of the zygapophyseal joints could certainly be injured during trauma to the cervical spine, the literature suggests that these mechanoreceptors are most active nearer the end range of joint movement.[109-111] Similarly, while joint manipulation may affect mechanoreceptors, the importance of this effect on movement accuracy during normal ranges of motion remains uncertain.

It remains possible that there are indirect effects of mechanoreceptors on movement. Specifically, they may reflexively alter GTO firing[107] and may reflexively stimulate nearby muscles.[107,110,112] Conversely, mechanoreceptors can be stimulated by activation of articular nerves,[110] pressure applied to the joint capsule,[107,112] and contraction of muscles crossing the joint.[110] As such, the firing pattern of joint receptors is dependent on more than one variable, requires additional study for clarification, and is probably not the primary afferent means of monitoring joint movement and position.[107,110,111]

This section presents one theory of motion restriction first described by Korr.[113] Korr's theory for the kinesiopathologic aspect of the "osteopathic lesion" or "somatic dysfunction" is based on the premise that muscle spindles can participate in the development of muscular resistance. From a mechanical viewpoint, the osteopathic lesion is synonymous with the chiropractic subluxation. Palpation of decreased mobility and increased resistance in one or more planes of motion is used to identify and evaluate the subluxation. Korr[113] perceived this resisted motion to be caused by one or more hypertonic muscles that traverse a vertebra. A discussion of muscle spindles follows to help in understanding Korr's theory.

The Muscle Spindle

The muscle spindle is a proprioceptor found throughout skeletal muscle that generates length and velocity information. The muscle spindle lies parallel with skeletal muscle fibers (extrafusal fibers) and contains specialized fibers called intrafusal fibers. These intrafusal fibers are encapsulated by connective tissue that joins either with the fascia of the skeletal muscle fibers or at the musculotendon junction.

There are two types of afferent fibers responsible for sensory output. Type Ia afferent endings (primary endings) innervate all of the intrafusal fibers, whereas type II afferent endings (secondary endings) innervate mostly the nuclear chain fibers. The primary and secondary afferent endings of each spindle provide monosynaptic feedback to the dorsal root and ultimately synapse on the alpha-motor neurons that supply the muscle containing the spindle. These spindles may also provide feedback to alpha-motor neurons that supply muscles in the vicinity of the activated spindle. Group Ia afferent fibers are velocity- and length-sensitive nerves. That is, they signal the rate at which muscle length is changing (velocity) and also signal absolute changes in muscle length. Group II primarily signals length sensitivity. In reference to Korr's theory, only the primary type Ia afferent nerve endings are considered.

The muscle spindle is controlled efferently by the central nervous system through the gamma

neuron system. These gamma fibers originate alongside of the alpha-motor neurons in the anterior horn of the spinal gray matter. They descend directly to innervate the polar (contractile) regions of the intrafusal fibers so that with gamma activation, a contraction of both polar regions of each intrafusal fiber occurs. This in turn generates elongation of the central region of the intrafusal fibers. As the central region of the spindle becomes stretched, so do the membranes encasing the Ia afferent nerve endings. This leads to an actual opening of the pores of these membranes, creating ionic exchanges and leading to an action potential that travels along the Ia afferent fibers.

There are two ways to stretch the spindle's central region to increase its discharge: stretching the overall muscle and contracting the polar regions of the spindle through the gamma system. Both methods increase the firing of the Ia afferent output. This introduces one final point regarding spindle structure—gamma dynamic and gamma static efferent nerve endings. The gamma fibers have acquired their names from their functions. If you activate the gamma dynamic efferents, this affects the sense of velocity or rate of muscle shortening. If the gamma static efferents are activated in isolation, then only the sense of absolute muscle length is affected. The reasons for this observation are discussed in the next section.

Muscle Spindle Function

Muscle spindles are the only receptors known to be activated with respect to limb position and velocity.[114] Additionally, muscle spindles have been shown to exhibit altered perceptions of muscle length and force following eccentric loading injury.[115] Also of interest to human movement, especially with respect to accuracy of movement and force production, is the sensitivity of muscle spindles to stretch and contraction.[116] Electrical discharge of the muscle spindle can continue following the termination of active contraction or stretch.[116-120] These same studies, involving the extremities, suggest that the muscle spindle discharge rate can extend over a long period of time and should theoretically have a negative effect on spatial accuracy and muscle force production during movement via altered afference to the central nervous system. The short-term excitability of muscle spindles, resulting in an increased firing discharge during subsequent muscle contraction has been attributed to the activation of gamma neurons of the Ia afferents.[120]

Understanding the function of the muscle spindle requires a better understanding of the gamma system. In isolation, the purpose of the gamma system is to regulate the length or stiffness of the polar regions of specific types of intrafusal fibers. This in turn modifies the length or stretch characteristics of the central region where the sensory Ia afferent nerve endings are located. Furthermore, because the muscle spindles lie parallel with the extrafusal fibers, the spindles and thus the central region change in length as the whole muscle changes in length. Thus the output of the spindle is dependent on the length of the muscle only when there is no gamma involvement. In vivo, however, this is not the case. Both the gamma system and overall muscle length work in concert to generate accurate proprioceptive sensations regarding the rate of change in muscle length and absolute length.

The gamma dynamic system is especially important in the maintenance of posture. Any time a limb is moved rapidly out of the intended posture, the muscle spindle will produce a very high discharge with a subsequent large downward creep of Ia afferent output. From higher centers, this large downward creep will activate appropriate alpha-motor neuron pools to restore adequate limb posture. If a situation arose in which one required a greater perception of muscle length change to perform a given task, the CNS would turn up the gamma dynamic efferents. With this in mind, the gamma dynamic efferents are somewhat like an amplifier, amplifying our perception of rate of stretch and respective reflexive responses.

If, however, you stimulate the gamma static efferents alone, you would see a significant increase in the steady-state output of the Ia afferent nerve endings. This is attributable to the shortening of the polar regions of the nuclear chain fibers where there are well-developed myofibrils allowing no downward creep. The importance of the static system is to maintain the Ia afferent output (sensitivity) of the spindle during the course of muscle shortening. For example, flexing the elbow shortens the biceps and therefore shortens the muscle spindles. This potentially unloads the sensory region of the involved spindles if it were not for the gamma static efferents. Therefore if you apply a resistance to the biceps in a shortened position, you are likely to see less Ia output of the spindle, indicating that the spindles are not operating optimally throughout the full range of muscle shortening or lengthening.

During the initiation of limb movement, output from higher centers simultaneously activates the gamma-motor and alpha-motor neurons, eliciting both intrafusal and extrafusal fiber contraction. This alpha gamma coactivation is referred to as servo-assistance control.[121] As the muscle shortens, the overall length of the spindle shortens but the length of the equatorial region is maintained because of the contraction of the polar regions from the gamma activation. Therefore the gamma static system maintains a constant amount of stretch on the equatorial (sensory) region of the spindle as the muscle undergoes length change.

Korr's Theory of Joint Fixation

As previously discussed, the gamma static efferents in conjunction with the alpha neuron system can modulate Ia afferent output. During muscle shortening, there is a "canceling effect" between the extrafusal fiber shortening and the intrafusal fiber polar region shortening, creating a constant spindle equatorial length and thus a steady-state spindle Ia output throughout all ranges of muscle length. Korr termed this *gamma gain*. The greater the gain, the greater the steady state spindle output at all muscle lengths. Now, let us apply this to the chiropractic subluxation.

Korr hypothesized that segmental muscles of the spine may have acquired an increased gamma gain. During this high gamma activity, the spindles may be encouraging their homonymous muscle, already in a shortened state, to contract, creating restriction of the involved motion segment. The spindle reports the extrafusal fiber length relative to the polar region length of the intrafusal fibers, not absolute extrafusal fiber length. This means that increased gamma gain is really an increased steady state in spindle discharge through all ranges in muscle length. The greater this gamma gain, with its increased spindle afferent output and corresponding facilitated alpha motor neurons, the greater the extrafusal contraction in an attempt to shorten the extrafusal fibers and silence the spindle output.

Korr mentions two causes for this increased setting in gamma gain: (1) an unanticipated "giving way" of a load during an isometric contraction, or (2) the abrupt approximation of two muscular attachments as with two vertebrae. Both of these situations yield a sudden slackening of the equatorial region of the spindle, creating spindle silencing. In response, the CNS would demand feedback from the spindle by increasing the gamma discharge to the intrafusal fibers and subsequently restore the spindle afferent output discharge. After recovery from these external forces, the two muscular attachments would then be in opposition to regain their normal anatomic relationship because of the continued gamma discharge exiting the alpha-motor neurons of the resisting muscle(s). The more stretch applied to the muscle, the greater the resistance to stretch caused by the increased spindle afferent output.

Korr theorized that when an external force (e.g., the palpating hand of a chiropractor) is applied to a spinous process stretching the hypertonic musculature, muscle spindles of the involved muscles increase their already heightened output, promoting more contraction and further resistance to stretch, creating a "blocked" end feel. If such an event were to happen, how would the chiropractic adjustment help?

The high velocity, low amplitude thrust, when applied to restore normal physiologic motion of a specific vertebra, would be stretching the hypertonic muscles responsible for this restricted movement. Korr explained that rapid stretch of these extrafusal fibers generates a rapid stretch of the intrafusal fiber's equatorial region, which is already under significant tension as previously set by the gamma efferents. The subsequent spindle stretch would potentially generate such an immense barrage of afferent impulses that the CNS would appropriately respond by "turning down" the gamma efferents. Normal gamma gain would therefore be reestablished with concomitant return of normal muscle tonus.

Edin and Vallbo[117] have demonstrated that after rapid muscle stretching, elevated Ia firing decreases. They and others have suggested that stable attachments of actin-myosin crossbridges in intrafusal muscle fibers (after fusimotor stimulation) are formed, generating an elevated level of Ia afferent output.[117,122-124] A rapid stretch to the involved muscles could potentially break the "stuck" bonds of the actin-myosin filaments in the intrafusal fibers and consequently decrease the once elevated Ia afferent discharge. Decreases in muscle activity following manipulation have been demonstrated.[125,126] Whether this is a result of muscle spindle pathways remains controversial.

Assessment of Abnormal Motion

As chiropractors we rely on numerous measures to diagnose spinal dysfunction, beginning with regional and intersegmental joint range of motion. Unfortunately, there is currently no singular gold standard for detecting the manipulable subluxation.

Although interobserver and intraobserver reliability studies have somewhat supported the use of passive and active gross or regional motion procedures,[127-130] testing of intersegmental motion has resulted in contradictory findings.[131,132] Intersegmental motion assessed using motion palpation is defined as the palpatory diagnosis of the quality and quantity of passive and active intersegmental joint ranges of motion. Keating completed a literature review of the interexaminer reliability of motion of the lumbar spine and concluded weak evidence of reliability.[133] Nansel et al.[134] found poor interexaminer reliability detecting cervical spine asymmetries in asymptomatic subjects. On a more positive note, researchers have found good sensitivity and specificity in the manual detection of cervical joint dysfunction[135] (see Chapter 17) and lumbar joint dysfunction[136] and good intraexaminer and interexaminer agreement using motion palpation of the sacroiliac joint.[137] Using anesthetic blocks to the facet joints as the gold standard, Jull and coworkers[135,138-140] have demonstrated both validity and reliability of motion palpation procedures in the cervical spine. The possible reasons for discrepancies between the different studies are interpretation of the degree of fixation by the examiner, improper standardization of methodology, increase in spinal mobility after the first examination, improper statistical analysis and discrepancy in the definition of fixation, and the use of asymptomatic subjects.

In addition to assessing active motion in the three planes of physiologic movement (i.e., flexion-extension, lateral flexion, and rotation) and passive segmental motion of the joint (i.e., using motion palpation), there is also end play and joint play. End play is assessed by applying additional overpressure to the specified joint at the end range of passive movement.[66] Each spinal region has characteristic end play qualities that are determined by the local bony and soft tissue anatomy.[66] Evaluation of end feel encompasses detection of the point at which resistance is encountered, with assessment for the quality of resistance as well as associated tenderness. Loss of anticipated end play elasticity is thought to be indicative of disorders within the joint, its capsule, or periarticular soft tissue.[66] The overall clinical utility of end play assessment remains under debate. Historically, end play resistance has been taught as a significant finding in the determination of joint dysfunction and adjustive vector orientation (along the planes of encountered resistance).[66] However, a recent study comparing the use of end play assessment prior to spinal manipulation in the cervical spine did not show a difference with respect to pain or stiffness outcomes compared to individuals where end play assessment was not used to target the manipulation.[141]

In the 1930s, John Mennell described another form of physiologic motion he called joint play, which cannot be produced by voluntary muscles.[142] It is a qualitative evaluation of the joint's resistance to movement when it is in a neutral or loose-packed position.[66] Joint play assessment is advantageous to differentiate articular-based pain and

dysfunction from nonarticular soft tissue disorders. As with end play, you check for the presence or absence of pain, the quality of movement, and the degree of encountered resistance.[66] Joint play procedures attempt to isolate a particular plane of increased or restricted glide. This procedure has been proposed as a method for determining the direction of appropriate adjustment.[66]

Triano[143] summarizes the outcome measures used to diagnose and treat the subluxation complex as (1) regional mobility, (2) pain reporting instruments, (3) self-care activities, and (4) limited performance measures. Additionally, objective measures of joint pain can be achieved using algometry. Algometry measures the patient's perceived pressure-pain threshold; when applied correctly, it has been shown to be reliable and valid with respect to quantifying joint pain.[144,145] Chiropractic researchers have used algometers to measure pressure-pain thresholds as a means of identifying segmental dysfunction associated with a manipulable spinal lesion[146] and to document improvement (outcome measure) after a chiropractic adjustment.[147,148]

Other methods for the assessment of abnormal motion include palpation for bony and soft tissue tenderness[149] and postural assessment[150] and have demonstrated satisfactory reliability. Chiropractors also palpate for tissue texture changes (weak interexaminer reliability) and muscle tonus (little significant agreement between examiners) to establish a clinical picture in the determination of segmental dysfunction.[149] Leg-length assessments for the detection of spinal motion segment mobility have demonstrated poor to satisfactory reliability.[151-153] Chiropractic functional leg-length tests, which should not be confused with radiographic procedures used to determine an anatomically short leg, are suspect in the area of validity and correlation with clinical findings.

More sophisticated measures of spinal segmental motion abnormalities include surface electromyography,[154,155] infrared and liquid crystal thermography, videofluoroscopy, motion radiography,[48,49] and physical performance evaluation (strength testing). Although these methods employ newer and often more expensive technology, their role in documenting the chiropractic subluxation remains under study. With the advent of digitized radiographs and computer-aided measurement analysis, improved documentation of aberrant motion at the three-joint complex may be possible.[156] However, improved technologies still need to be weighed against cost benefits, clinical utility, and risk to patient (e.g., radiation dose).

Effects of the Chiropractic Adjustment: The Kinesiology of the Manipulable Subluxation

It is the purpose of this section to review some of the research that has studied the behavior of the spinal motion segment, specifically its motion characteristics after the application of chiropractic manipulation.

Cervical Spine

Nansel et al.[157,158] investigated the effectiveness of cervical spine manipulation to correct end-range asymmetries of lateral flexion. The results of the first experiment demonstrated that a single lower cervical adjustment delivered to the most restricted side of end range did provide a short-term (30 minutes) decrease in the magnitude of cervical lateral flexion passive end-range asymmetries.[158] In a follow-up study, two groups with left versus right cervical lateral flexion passive end-range asymmetries (defined as 10 degrees or greater with a goniometer) were compared.[158] The groups consisted of individuals who had previously traumatized their necks and individuals with no history of neck trauma. Both groups demonstrated a significant reduction in lateral flexion asymmetry up to 4 hours. By 24 hours, 100% of the group members with no previous neck trauma maintained their lateral flexion symmetries, whereas only 56% of the previous trauma group members maintained their symmetries. By 48 hours, 75% of the previous neck trauma group members had regained their asymmetries to the point of no significant difference from their preadjustive values. However, 88% of the subjects with no history of neck trauma still continued to exhibit left

versus right lateral flexion symmetries of less than 10 degrees. It is important to note that both studies measured global, not segmental, range of motion.

In addition to improving spinal regional range of motion, manipulation may also improve the quality of motion. In a preliminary study, Enebo[159] compared the short-term benefits on the accuracy of cervical spine rotation in two groups of healthy individuals. Cervical spine joint manipulation increased overall movement accuracy and decreased overall movement variability but did not improve intraparticipant variability compared to a nonmanipulation control.

Thoracic Spine

Gal et al.[160] used unembalmed human cadavers to study the subsequent segmental translational and rotational movements that occurred between the vertebrae T10, T11, and T12 after a posterior to anterior adjustment to the right transverse process of T11. This direct approach on cadavers allowed for accurate measurements that are difficult to perform on living subjects.

During the adjustive thrust, posterior to anterior translation was only slightly greater for T11, the contact vertebra, compared with the adjacent vertebra. Rotational movements were also found, even though the line of drive was from posterior to anterior. All three vertebrae rotated in a right axial direction; however, the greatest significant rotation was measured at T12. Right translation was shown to be greatest at T11. The most striking data demonstrated sagittal rotation of T10 and T11 inferiorly, while T12 rotated in a superior direction.

Immediately following the adjustment, changes in the relative sagittal position of T11 and T12 remained, implying some permanent or semipermanent change in relative vertebral position with respect to its neighboring one. This experiment demonstrated the potential for small relative movements among vertebrae after adjustments, but it was not designed to make direct predictions about the mechanical responses of the vertebral column in live patients. However, the authors believe that similar trends in relative vertebral movements would be observed in live patients following the same adjustive procedure.

Lumbar Spine and Pelvis

Cramer et al.[161,162] used MRI to document mechanical changes at the zygapophyseal joints following chiropractic side-posture manipulation. The effects of side-posture manipulation, side-posture positioning only, and control group were compared for their ability to produce gapping at the zygapophyseal joints measured using MRI. Side-posture manipulation resulted in greater gapping of the zygapophyseal joints compared to either side-posture positioning or control. Also of interest, side-posture positioning alone resulted in gapping of the zygapophyseal joints compared to the control group.

The work by Gal et al.[163] on cadavers represented a unique method of evaluating vertebral movements during a manipulative thrust. Until recently, it has not been possible to use this methodology in live participants. In vivo measurements of lumbar vertebral movement during impulsive manipulation has demonstrated coupling of motion[163] and greater displacement compared to a sham treatment.[164]

Herzog et al.[165,166] demonstrated indirect effects of chiropractic manipulation on movement. The application of six manipulative therapy sessions (over 12 days) for a unilateral sacroiliac syndrome resulted in significant changes in ground reaction forces during walking.[166] The sacroiliac joint motion was tested using the Gillet motion palpation procedure and indicated improved mobility in all patients. This improvement remained without treatment for at least 14 to 17 days.

Spinal Pain

From a clinical standpoint, does improved mechanical function equate to pain reduction? There is little, if any, doubt that spinal manipulation has a significant effect on the reduction of mechanical low back pain.[167] Cassidy et al.[168,169] demonstrated a significant reduction in pain levels after a single cervical rotary adjustment directed to the same side of pain.

Conversely, spinal motion aberrations are not always directly related to presenting symptomatology.[82] Studies investigating the relation between pain and segmental spinal movement have not demonstrated any significant differences between symptomatic and nonsymptomatic groups.[75,76] In fact, there tends to be a low correlation between functional disability and self reported pain levels.[170] However, Vernon[171] used static and dynamic roentgenography to conclude that there is a higher prevalence of abnormal motion patterns and pathologic changes in symptomatic subjects. Conversely, Phillips et al.[34] failed to demonstrate a relation between abnormal clinical findings and abnormal spinal motion in patients suffering from low back pain. Haas and Nyiendo[76] stated that lumbar motion cannot be used with any accuracy to diagnose or prognosticate a patient's low back pain status or be used to characterize a patient's lumbar segmental motion in lateral bending. Therefore as clinicians, we must be cautious in deducing abnormal segmental motion as the sole cause for the presenting pain. Nansel et al.[159] demonstrated that asymmetry magnitudes in cervical passive end-range motion did not distinguish between subjects who had previous neck trauma and those who did not.

Kinesiopathology of Spinal Joint Degeneration

The relation between spinal motion and pathologic changes in the three-joint complex is of interest to chiropractors. Whether from the aging process, unhealthy lifestyle, or microtrauma and macrotrauma, degenerative changes produce changes in spinal movement patterns. Spinal degeneration with associated manipulable subluxations may produce both increased motion (hypermobility) and decreased motion (hypomobility). Both may occur simultaneously in the same individual and result from a pattern of degeneration.

In 1965, Hall[172] described a pattern of degeneration in the cervical spine. He noted that in the early stage of degeneration, cavities formed at the lateral margin of the anular fibers of the intervertebral disc that spread from one side to the other with accompanying loss of disc height. In the final stage, the intervertebral distance was greatly reduced and the bone structure became distorted by osteophyte formation. Kirkaldy-Willis[173] later outlined three stages of degenerative changes in the lumbar spine as a working model for the management of low back pain. Like the stages of cervical spine degeneration described by Hall, each phase of lumbar spine degeneration blended into the other. The earliest stage is characterized mainly by abnormal function with only slight anatomical and kinesiopathology changes. At the end of this phase, the changes in the three-joint complex may progress to the unstable phase or proceed directly to those changes described in the stabilization phase.

The unstable phase is characterized by increased abnormal motion, recognized radiographically as an increase in translation most commonly seen as retrolistheses. Spondylolisthesis and abnormal opening of the disc can be seen in flexion. Retrospondylolisthesis, narrowing of the intervertebral foramen and abnormal discal wedging, can be seen in extension. As the degree of degeneration increases, so does the degree of movement.

The third phase is one of restabilization occurring when motion in the apophyseal joints and disc become restricted from degeneration of cartilage, loss of disc substance, fibrosis, and the formation of osteophytes around the posterior joints and disc. This process leads to stabilization of the hypermobile motion segment that furthers the degenerative process and hypermobility in adjacent segments as the spine attempts to maintain an optimal global range of motion.

Building on the work of Kirkaldy-Willis, Sandoz[174] introduces a fourth phase of episodic fixations that correspond to manipulable subluxations. He describes these episodic fixations as acute, reversible, and usually occurring at the extremes of movement. In contrast, he notes that chronic fixations (nonmanipulable subluxations) encountered in the final stage of stabilization, as a rule, occur at or near the neutral position and are not reversible.

In light of the above work, Good and Mikkelsen[52] studied the correlation between discogenic spondylosis and sagittal plane motion of the intervertebral motion segments in the lower cervical spine. In global cervical flexion when little or no degenerative change was present, most cases of abnormal motion were hypermobile in character, not hypomobile. This contradicts the hypothesis in the Kirkaldy-Willis model, which suggests that in the face of this type of degenerative change, hypomobility is usually present. In a similar contradiction, when there were moderate degenerative changes, normal motion or hypomobility was often present, not hypermobility. Finally, hypermobility was as common as hypomobility when severe degenerative changes existed. In global cervical extension, the high incidence of hypomobility occurring with absent or mild discogenic spondylosis agrees with the Kirkaldy-Willis model. However, hypermobility was still somewhat common. Additionally, when discogenic spondylosis was classified in the moderate or severe stages, hypomobility was the rule and hypermobility was very uncommon.

These findings, however, do not describe the degenerative condition of the posterior column (facet joints) in conjunction with discogenic or anterior spondylosis, which would most likely influence the movements associated with flexion. McNab[175] suggested that in the first stage of cervical disc degeneration the involved segment became unstable and the movement of the related vertebra became excessive and irregular. This was another contradiction to the Kirkaldy-Willis model. More recently, decreased strength of the posterior lumbar spine ligaments was positively correlated with increasing age or with facet degeneration.[176] Additionally, Borenstein[177] suggested that osteoarthritis of the lumbar spine is a precipitating cause for low back pain.

Despite the controversy surrounding the description of degenerative changes, pathologic changes that upset the intrinsic equilibrium of the spinal motion segment are thought to contribute to the production of a manipulable subluxation. In this light, Triano[178] has suggested a list of comorbidities associated with the manipulable subluxation that include costovertebral joint disorders, degenerative disc disease, disc bulge/protrusion/herniation, facet syndrome, and sprain/strains. (See Chapter 12.)

Pathologic Effects of Joint Immobilization

Poor vascularity of both the intervertebral disc and the articular cartilage of the posterior zygapophyseal joints has deleterious consequences on the three-joint complex. Both structures are dependent on joint motion for exchange of nutrients and removal of waste products. Compressive loading and unloading of the intervertebral disc and articular cartilage of the posterior synovial joints is dependent on segmental spinal motion and is necessary for a healthy three-joint complex. Grieve[179] documented that without mobility, lack of nutrition leads to joint and tissue breakdown, producing inflammation and the earliest stages of degenerative joint disease.

Based on studies of rabbit knees immobilized for a 3-week period, Salter[180] demonstrated that irreparable lesions occur in the articular cartilage when normal movement is restricted. In addition to the restriction of synovial fluid flow, the mechanical stress led to damage and death of chondrocytes from continuous compression of the articular cartilage. The irreversibility of the degenerative changes observed led Salter to conclude that prolonged immobilization of joints prevents healing and increases disability. In addition to the deleterious effect on the joint, the adjacent bone and surrounding muscles also deteriorate.[181]

Spinal motion segment hypomobility resulting from spinal fusion or intervertebral degeneration affects adjacent motion segments and may accelerate the spinal degenerative process.[182,183] Woo et al.[184] found excessive tissue depositions on gross inspection of the synovial joints after immobilization. This excessive fatty fibrous connective tissue formed mature scar tissue and created intraarticular adhesions. Immobilization resulted in a loss of water and glycosaminoglycans along with collagen changes. Using a small animal model, collaborative work by researchers from two chiropractic colleges has documented degenerative changes at the zygapophyseal joints following spinal fixation.[185] (See Chapter 4.) This recent work is relevant to chiropractors and represents the first published documentation of changes to the articular surfaces of zygapophyseal joints due to hypomobility.

Conclusion

This chapter has focused on defining and analyzing expected motion in each region of the spine as a basis for understanding abnormal motion. We suggest that a change in normal joint function helps to characterize a kinesiopathologic component of the subluxation complex. Examining the kinesiopathologic component of the chiropractic subluxation in isolation, however, may be misleading because any movement modification may very well be the result of both biomechanical and neurogenic reflexes working in concert. Whether the restoration of normal movement to the three-joint complex and concomitant therapeutic effects transpire as a direct consequence of the forces exerted onto the joints themselves, through neuromuscular mechanisms, or through a combination of both is still under study.

In this chapter we have left some questions unanswered. This ambiguity may leave some readers questioning whether any certainty exists with regard to the mechanical properties of the manipulable subluxation or the mechanisms involved in the therapeutic effects of chiropractic manipulation. However, one who seeks understanding must never forget that as with all academic quests to gain knowledge and certainty, more questions will inevitably remain unanswered.

References

1. Scoop A. An experimental evaluation of kinesiology in allergy and deficiency disease diagnosis. Orthomolecular Psychiatry 1978;7(2):137-8.
2. Lee HK, Gatterman M. Chiropractic adjusting techniques. In: Peterson D, Weis G. Chiropractic: an illustrated history. St. Louis: Mosby; 1995. p. 251.
3. Farfan Hl. Biomechanics of the lumbar spine. In: Kirkaldy-Willis, editor. Managing low back pain. New York: Churchill Livingstone; 1988. p. 27-37.
4. Nachemson AF, Schultz AB, Berkson MH. Mechanical properties of human lumbar spine motion segments: influences of age, sex, disc level, and degeneration. Spine 1979;4(1):1-8.
5. Lawrence DJ, Bergmann TF. Joint anatomy and basic mechanics. In: Bergmann TF, Peterson DH, Lawrence DJ,

editors. Chiropractic technique. New York: Churchill Livingstone; 1993. p. 11-50.

6. Whiting WC, Zernicke RF. Biomechanics of musculoskeletal injury. Champaign, IL: Human Kinetics; 1998. p. 41-85.

7. Carrick FR. Treatment of pathomechanics of the lumbar spine by manipulation. J Manipulative Physiol Ther 1981;4:173-8.

8. Gilford SR, Dano CJ. Let's speak the same language. Dynamic Chiropractic. MPI: November 1985. p. 35-36.

9. Simmon J. A more precise listing system—the "international." J Am Chiropractic Assoc 1986;23:62.

10. Gal J, Herzog W, Kawchuk G, Conway PJ, Zhang YT. Movements of vertebrae during manipulative thrusts to unembalmed human cadavers. J Manipulative Physiol Ther 1997;20:30-40.

11. Farfan HF, Cossette JW, Robertson GH, Wells RV, Kraus H. The effects of torsion on the lumbar intervertebral joints: the role of torsion in the production of disc degeneration. J Bone Joint Surg 1970;52A:468-97.

12. Kazarian LE. Dynamic response characteristics of the human spine. Acta Orthop Scand Suppl 1972;146:1-86.

13. Laborde JM, Burstein AH, Song K, Brown RH, Bahniuk E. A method of analyzing the three-dimensional stiffness properties of the intact human lumbar spine. ASME J Biomech Eng 1981;103:299-300.

14. Panjabi MM, White AA III. Physical properties and functional biomechanics of the spine. In: White AA III, Panjabi MM, editors. Clinical biomechanics of the spine. Philadelphia: JB Lippincott; 1978. p. 1-83.

15. White AA III, Panjabi MM. The basic kinematics of the human spine: a review of past and current knowledge. Spine 1978;3(1):12-20.

16. Dreyer SJ, Dreyfuss PH. Low back pain and the zygapophysial (facet) joints. Arch Phys Med Rehabil 1996;77:290-300.

17. Lee RYW. Kinematics of rotational mobilization of the lumbar spine. Clin Biomech 2001;16:481-8.

18. Gibbons P, Tehan P. Patient positioning and spinal locking for lumbar spine rotation manipulation. Man Ther 2001;6(3):130-8.

19. Jofe MH, White AA, Panjabi MM. Physiology and biomechanics. In: The cervical spine. Philadelphia: JB Lippincott; 1983. p. 23-35.

20. Panjabi MM, Crisco JJ, Vasavada A, Oda T, Cholewicki J, Nibu K et al. Mechanical properties of the human cervical spine as shown by three-dimensional load-displacement curves. Spine 2001;26:2692-700.

21. Cholewicki J, Crisco JJ, Oxland TR, Yamamoto I, Panjabi MM. Effects of posture and structure on three-dimensional coupled rotations in the lumbar spine. Spine 1996;21:2421-8.

22. Clausen JD, Goel VK, Traynelis VC, Scifert J. Uncinate processes and Luschka joints influence the biomechanics of the cervical spine: quantification using a finite element model of the C5-C6 segment. J Orthop Res 1997;15:342-7.

23. Takeuchi T, Abumi K, Shono Y, Oda I, Kaneda K. Biomechanical role of the intervertebral disc and costovertebral joint in stability of the thoracic spine: a canine model study. Spine 1999;24:1414-20.

24. White AA III, Panjabi MM, editors. Clinical biomechanics of the spine. 2nd ed. Philadelphia: JB Lippincott; 1990.

25. Brown T, Hansen RJ, Yorra AJ. Some mechanical tests on the lumbosacral spine with particular reference to the intervertebral discs. J Bone Joint Surg 1957;39A:73-6.

26. King AE, Vulcan AP. Elastic deformation characteristics of the spine. J Biomech 1971;4:413-29.

27. Hviid H. Functional radiography of the cervical spine. Ann Swiss Chiro Assoc 1965;3:37-65.

28. Henderson DJ, Dorman TM. Functional roentgenometric evaluation of the cervical spine in the sagittal plane. J Manipulative Physiol Ther 1985;8:219-27.

29. Penning L. Nonpathologic and pathologic relationships between the lower cervical vertebrae. Am J Roentgenol 1964;91:1036-50.

30. Prancl K. X-ray examination and functional analysis of the cervical spine. Manual Med 1985;2(1):5-15.

31. Grice AS. Preliminary evaluation of 50 sagittal cervical motion radiographic examinations. J Can Chiro Assoc 1977;21:33-4.

32. Dimnet J, Pasquet A, Krag MH, Panjabi MM. Cervical spine motion in the sagittal plane: kinematic and geometric parameters. J Biomech 1982;15:959-69.

33. Dimnet J, Fischer LP, Gonon G, Carret JP. Radiographic studies of lateral flexion in the lumbar spine. J Biomech 1978;11:143-50.

34. Phillips RB, Howe JW, Bustin G, Mick TJ, Rosenfeld I, Mills T. Stress x-rays and the low back pain patient. J Manipulative Physiol Ther 1990;13:127-33.

35. Brown RH, Burnstein AH, Nash CL, Schock CC. Spinal analysis using three-dimensional radiographic technique. J Biomech 1976;9:355-65.

36. Frymoyer JW, Frymoyer WW, Wilder DG, Pope MH. The mechanical and kinematic analysis of the lumbar spine in normal living human subjects in vivo. J Biomech 1979;12:165-72.

37. Matteri RE, Pope MH, Frymoyer JW. A biplane radiographic method of determining vertebral rotation in post-mortem specimens. Chiropractic Orthop 1976;116:95-8.

38. Pearcy M, Portek I, Shepherd J. Three-dimensional x-ray analysis of normal movement in the lumbar spine. Spine 1984;9:294-7.

39. Pearcy MJ. Stereo radiography of normal lumbar spine motion. Acta Orthop Scand (Suppl) 1985;56:212.

40. Benson DR, Schultz AB, Dewald RL. Roentgenographic evaluation of vertebral rotation. J Bone Joint Surg Am 1976;58:1125-9.

41. Bell GD. Skeletal applications of videofluoroscopy. J Manipulative Physiol Ther 1990;13:396-405.

42. Buonocore E, Hartman JT, Nelson CL. Cineradiograms of the cervical spine in diagnosis of soft-tissue injuries. JAMA 1966;198:143-7.

43. Fielding JW. Cineradiography of the normal cervical spine. J Bone Joint Surg 1957;39A:1280-8.

44. Howe JW. Observations from cineroentgenological studies of the spinal column. J Am Chiropractic Assoc 1970;7:65-70.

45. Humphreys K, Breen A, Saxton D. Incremental lumbar spine motion in the coronal plane: an observer variation study using digital videofluoroscopy. Eur J Chiropractic 1990;38:56-62.

46. Pearcy MJ, Timbrewal SB. Axial rotation and lateral bending in the normal lumbar spine measured by three-dimensional radiography. Spine 1984;9:582-7.

47. Panjabi M, Yamamoto I, Oxland T, Crisco J. How does posture affect coupling in the lumbar spine? Spine 1989;14:1002-11.

48. Cassidy JD. Roentgenological examination of the functional mechanics of the lumbar spine in lateral flexion. JCCA 1976;(July):13-6.

49. Grice AS. Radiographic, biomechanical, and clinical factors in lumbar lateral flexion. Part 1. J Manipulative Physiol Ther 1979;2(1):26-34.

50. Scholten PJ, Veldhuizen AG. The influence of spine geometry on the coupling between lateral bending and axial rotation. Eng Med 1985;14:167-71.

51. Hohl M, Brummett SW. Cinefluorography in the diagnosis of the diseased or damaged cervical vertebral disc. J Bone Joint Surg 1968;50A:1060.

52. Good CJ, Mikkelsen GB. Intersegmental sagittal motion in the lower cervical spine and discogenic spondylosis: a preliminary study. J Manipulative Physiol Ther 1992; 15:556-64.

53. Resnick DK, Weller SJ, Benzel EC. Biomechanics of the thoracolumbar spine. Neurosurg Clin N Am 1997; 8:455-69.

54. Kapandji IA. The physiology of the joints. Vol. 3. The trunk and the vertebral column. London: Churchill Livingstone; 1982.

55. Werne S. Studies in spontaneous atlas dislocation. Acta Orthop Scand 1957;Suppl 23:1-150.

56. Penning L. Normal movements of the cervical spine. Am J Roentgenol 1978;130:317-26.

57. Panjabi M, Dvorak J, Duranceau J, Yamamoto I, Gerber M, Rauschning W et al. Three-dimensional movements of the upper cervical spine. Spine 1988;13:726-30.

58. Jones MD. Cineradiographic studies of the normal cervical spine. Calif Med 1960;63:293-6.

59. Dvorak J, Panjabi M, Gerber M, Wichmann W. CT-functional diagnostics of the rotatory instability of upper cervical spine. Part 1. An experimental study on cadavers. Spine 1987;12(3):197-205.

60. Penning L, Wilmink JT. Rotation of the cervical spine. Spine 1987;12:732-8.

61. Jirout J. Rotational synkinesis of occiput and atlas on lateral inclination. Neuroradiology 1981;21:1-4.

62. Soderberg GL. Kinesiology: application to pathological motion. Baltimore: Williams & Wilkins; 1986. p. 287.

63. Gatterman MI, Panzer DM. Disorders of the cervical spine. In: Gatterman MI, editor. Chiropractic management of spine related disorders. Baltimore: Williams & Wilkins; 1990. p. 205-55.

64. Hohl M, Baker HR. The atlanto-axial joints: roentgenographic and anatomical study of normal and abnormal motion. J Bone Joint Surg 1964;46A:1739-52.

65. Jirout J. Changes in the atlas-axis relations on lateral flexion of the head and neck. Neuroradiology 1973; 6:215-8.

66. Peterson DH, Bergmann TF. The spine: anatomy, biomechanics, assessment, and adjustive techniques. In: Bergmann TF, Peterson DH, Lawrence DJ. Chiropractic technique. New York: Churchill Livingstone; 1993. p. 197-521.

67. Lind B, Sihlbom H, Nordwall A, Malchau H. Normal range of motion of the cervical spine. Arch Phys Med Rehabil 1989;70:692-5.

68. Lysell E. Motion in the cervical spine. Acta Orthop Scand 1969;Suppl 123:1+.

69. Bogduk N, Twomey LT. Clinical anatomy of the lumbar spine. Edinburgh: Churchill Livingstone; 1987.

70. Posner I, White AA, Edwards WT, Hayes WC. A biomechanical analysis of the clinical stability of the lumbar and lumbosacral spine. Spine 1982;7:374-89.

71. Gatterman MI, Panzer D. Disorders of the lumbar spine. In: Gatterman MI, editor. Chiropractic management of spine related disorders. Baltimore: Williams & Wilkins; 1990. p. 129-75.

72. Frieberg O. Clinical symptoms and biomechanics of lumbar spine and hip joints in leg length inequality. Spine 1983;8:643-51.

73. Lovett RW. A contribution to the study of the mechanics of the spine. Am J Anat 1903;2:457-62.

74. Grice AS. Harmony of joint and muscle function in the prevention of lower back syndromes. JCCA 1976; (July):7-11.

75. Haas M, Nyiendo J, Peterson C, Thiel H, Sellers T, Dal Mas E et al. Lumbar motion trends and correlation with low back pain. Part 1. A roentgenological evaluation of coupled lumbar motion in lateral bending. J Manipulative Physiol Ther 1992;15:145-58.

76. Haas M, Nyiendo J. Lumbar motion trends and correlation with low back pain. Part II. A roentgenological evaluation of quantitative segmental motion in lateral bending. J Manipulative Physiol Ther 1992;15:224-34.

77. Shirazi-Adl A, Parnianpour M. Effect of changes in lordosis on mechanics of the lumbar spine-lumbar curvature in lifting. J Spinal Disord 1999;12(5):436-47.

78. Yang KH, King AI. Mechanism of facet load transmission as a hypothesis of low-back pain. Spine 1984; 9:557-65.

79. Yoganandan N, Pintar FA, Maiman DJ, Cusick JF, Sances Jr A, Walsh PR. Human head-neck biomechanics under axial tension. Med Eng Phys 1996;18:289-94.

80. Lee RYW, Evans JH. Loads in the lumbar spine during traction therapy. Aust J Physiother 2001;47:102-8.

81. Smith OG, Langeworthy SM, Paxson MC. Modernized chiropractic. Cedar Rapids, IA: Laurence Press; 1906.

82. Haas M, Peterson D. A roentgenological evaluation of the relationship between segmental motion and malalignment in lateral bending. J Manipulative Physiol Ther 1992;15:350-60.

83. Schram S, Hosek R. Error limitations in x-ray kinematics of the spine. J Manipulative Physiol Ther 1982;5:5-10.

84. Dishman RW. Review of the literature supporting a scientific basis for the chiropractic subluxation complex. J Manipulative Physiol Ther 1985;8:163-74.

85. Brantingham JW. A critical look at the subluxation hypothesis. J Manipulative Physiol Ther 1988;11(2): 130-2.

86. Rahlmann JF. Mechanisms of intervertebral joint fixation: a literature review. J Manipulative Physiol Ther 1987;10:177-87.

87. Dreyfuss P, Dryer S, Griffin J, Hoffman J, Walsh N. Positive sacroiliac screening tests in asymptomatic adults. Spine 1994;19:1138-43.

88. McGregor M, Mior SA. Anatomical and functional perspectives of the cervical spine. Part II. The "hypermobile" cervical spine. JCCA 1989;33(4):177-83.

89. Sandoz R. Some physical mechanisms and effects of spinal adjustments. Ann Swiss Assoc 1976;6:90-138.

90. McGregor M, Mior S. Anatomical and functional perspectives of the cervical spine. Part II. The "unstable" cervical spine. JCCA 1990;34(3):145-52.

91. Ogston NG, King GJ, Getzbein SD, Tile M, Kapasouri A, Rubenstein JD. Centrode patterns in the lumbar spine: baseline studies in normal subjects. Spine 1986; 11:591-5.

92. Larsson LG, Baum J, Mudholkar GS, Kollia GD. Benefits and disadvantages of joint hypermobility among musicians. N Engl J Med 1993;329:1079-82.

93. Nilsson C, Wykman A, Leanderson J. Spinal sagittal mobility and joint laxity in young ballet dancers. A comparative study between first-year students at the Swedish Ballet School and a control group. Knee Surg Sports Traumatol Arthrosc 1993;1(3-4):206-8.

94. Lane G. Cervical spine: its movement and symptomatology. J Clin Chiro Arch Ed 1971;1:128-45.

95. Carrick FR. Treatment of pathomechanics of the lumbar spine by manipulation. J Manipulative Physiol Ther 1981;4:173-8.

96. Jirout J. Studies in the dynamics of the spine. Acta Radiol 1965;46:55-60.

97. Luk KDK, Lee RBI, Leong JCY, Hsu LCS. The effect on the lumbosacral spine of the Ing spinal fusion for idiopathic scoliosis. Spine 1987;12:996-1000.

98. Frymoyer JW. Failed lumbar disc surgery requiring a second operation. Spine 1978;3:7-11.

99. Lee CK, Langrana NA. Lumbosacral spinal fusion: a biomechanical study. Spine 1984;9:574-81.

100. Pearcy M, Burrough S. Assessment of bony union after interbody fusion of the lumbar spine using biplanar radiographic technique. J Bone Joint Surg 1982; 64B:228-32.

101. Woesner ME, Mitts MG. The evaluation of cervical spine motion below C2: a comparison of cineroentgenographic and conventional roentgenographic methods. Am J Radiogr 1972;(May):148-52.

102. Stokes IAF, Wilder DG, Fymoyer JW, Pope MH. Assessment of patients with low-back pain by biplanar radiographic measurement of intervertebral motion. Spine 1981;6:233-40.

103. Nagata H, Schendel MJ, Transfeldt EE, Lewis JL. The effects of immobilization of long segments of the spine on adjacent and distal facet force and lumbosacral motion. Spine 1993;18:2471-9.

104. Goel VK, Clark CR, McGowan D, Goyal S. An in-vitro study of the kinematics of the normal, injured and stabilized cervical spine. J Biomech 1984;17:363-76.

105. Bishop RG, Byfield D, Bolton JE. A preliminary investigation into the relationship between lumbar sagittal mobility and pelvic mobility. Eur J Chiro 1991;39: 3-11.

106. Laszlo JI, Bairstow PJ. Kinaesthesis: its measurement, training, and relationship to motor control. Q J Exp Psychol 1983;35A:411-21.

107. Newton RA. Joint receptor contributions to reflexive and kinesthetic responses. Phys Ther 1982;62(1):22-9.

108. Heikkila HV, Wenngren B. Cervicocephalic kinesthetic sensibility, active range of cervical motion, and oculomotor function in patients with injury. Arch Phys Med Rehabil 1998;79:1089-94.

109. Brumagne S, Cordo P, Lysens R, Verschueren S, Swinnen S. The role of paraspinal muscle spindles in lumbosacral position sense in individuals with and without low back pain. Spine 2000;25:989-94.

110. McLain RF. Mechanoreceptor endings in human cervical facet joints. Spine 1994;19(5):495-501.

111. Schmidt RA, Lee TD. Motor control and learning: a behavioral emphasis. 3rd ed. Champaign, IL: Human Kinetics, 1999:110-4.

112. Slosberg M. Effects of altered afferent articular input on sensation, proprioception, muscle tone, and sympathetic reflex responses. J Manipulative Physiol Ther 1988; 11:400-8.

113. Korr IM. Proprioceptors and somatic dysfunction. J Am Osteopathic Assoc 1975;74:638-50.

114. Cordo P, Bevan L, Gurfinkel V, Carlton L, Carlton M, Kerr G. Proprioceptive coordination of discrete movement sequences: mechanism and generality. Can J Physiol Pharmacal 1995;73:305-15.

115. Brockett C, Warren N, Gregory JE, Morgan DL, Proske U. A comparison of the effects of concentric versus eccentric exercise on force and position sense at the human elbow joint. Brain Res 1997;771:251-8.

116. Wilson LR, Gandevia SC, Burke D. Increased resting discharge of human spindle afferents following voluntary contractions. J Physiol 1995;488:833-40.

117. Edin B, Vallbo A. Stretch sensitization of human muscle spindles. J Physiol 1988;400:101-11.

118. Edin B, Vallbo A. Dynamic response of human muscle spindle afferents to stretch. J Neurophysiol 1990;63:1297-1306.

119. Edin B, Vallbo A. Muscle afferent responses to isometric contraction and relaxations in humans. J Neurophysiol 1990;63:1307-13.

120. Hutton RS, Atwater SW. Acute and chronic adaptations of muscle proprioceptors in response to increased use. Sports Med 1992;14:406-21.

121. Ackermann U. Essentials of human physiology. St. Louis: Mosby; 1992. p. 190.

122. Brown MC, Goodwin GM, Matthew PBC. After-effects of fusimotor stimulation on the response of muscle spindle primary afferent endings. J Physiol 1969;205:677-94.

123. Poppele RE, Quick D. Stretch-induced contraction of intrafusal muscle in cat muscle spindles. J Neurosci 1981;1:1069-74.

124. Morgan DL, Prochazka A, Proske U. The after-effects of stretch and fusimotor stimulation on the responses of primary endings of cat muscle spindles. J Physiol 1984;356:465-77.

125. Grice AS. Muscle tonus change following manipulation. JCCA 1974;18(4):29-31.

126. Shambaugh P. Changes in electrical activity in muscles resulting from chiropractic adjustment: a pilot study. J Manipulative Physiol Ther 1987;10:300-4.

127. Johnston WL, Elkiss ML, Marino RV, Blum GA. Passive gross motion testing: Part II. A study of interexaminer agreement. J Am Osteopath Assoc 1982;81:304-8.

128. Gill K, Krag MH, Johnson GB, Haugh LD, Pope MH. Repeatability of four clinical methods for assessment of lumbar spinal motion. Spine 1988;13:50-3.

129. Zachman ZJ, Traina AD, Keating JC Jr, Bolles ST, Braun-Porter L. Interexaminer reliability and concurrent validity of two instruments for the measurement of cervical ranges of motion. J Manipulative Physiol Ther 1989;12(3)205-10.

130. Mayer TG, Tencer AF, Kristoferson S, Mooney V. Use of noninvasive techniques for quantification of spinal range-of-motion in normal subjects and chronic low-back dysfunction patients. Spine 1984;9(6):588-95.

131. Leach RA. The chiropractic theories: principles and clinical applications. 3rd ed. Baltimore: Williams & Wilkins; 1994. p. 55-87.

132. Haas M. The reliability of reliability. J Manipulative Physiol Ther 1991;14(3):199-208.

133. Keating JC. Inter-examiner reliability of motion palpation of the lumbar spine: a review of quantitative literature. Am J Chiropractic Med 1989;2(3):107-10.

134. Nansel DD, Peneff AL, Jansen RD, Cooperstein R. Interexaminer concordance in detecting joint-play asymmetries in the cervical spines of otherwise asymptomatic subjects. J Manipulative Physiol Ther 1989;12:429-33.

135. Jull G, Bogduk N, Marsland A. The accuracy of manual diagnosis for cervical zygapophyseal joint pain syndromes. Med J Aust 1988;148:233-6.

136. Byfield D. Preliminary studies with a mechanical model for the evaluation of spinal motion palpation in the lumbar spine. Proceedings of the 1990 International Conference on Spinal Manipulation. Washington, D.C.: May 11-12, 1990. p. 215-9.

137. Herzog W, Read LL, Conway PJW, Shaw LD, McEwen MC. Reliability of motion palpation procedures to detect sacroiliac joint fixations. J Manipulative Physiol Ther 1989;12:86-92.

138. Jull G, Zito G, Trott P, Potter H, Shirley D. Interexaminer reliability to detect painful upper cervical joint dysfunction. Aust J Physiother 1997;43:125-9.

139. Jull G. Manual diagnosis of C2-3 headache. Cephalalgia 1985;5 Suppl I5:308-9.

140. Jull G, Trott P, Potter H, Zito G, Niere K, Shirley D et al. A randomized controlled trial of exercise and manipulative therapy for cervicogenic headache. Spine 2002;27:1835-43.

141. Haas M, Groupp E, Panzer D, Partna L, Lumsden S, Aickin M. Efficacy of cervical endplay assessment as an indicator for spinal manipulation. Spine 2003;28:1091-6.

142. Mennell JM. Joint pain: diagnosis and treatment using manipulative techniques. Boston: Little Brown; 1964.

143. Triano JJ. The subluxation complex: outcome measure of chiropractic diagnosis and treatment. Chiro Tech 1990;2(3):114-20.

144. Fischer AA. Pressure tolerance over muscles and bones in normal subjects. Arch Phys Med Rehabil 1986;67:406-9.

145. Fischer AA. Pressure threshold meter: its use for quantification of tender spots. Arch Phys Med Rehabil 1986;67:836-8.

146. Vernon H, Cote P, Beauchemin D, Bonnoyer B. A correlative study of myofascial tender points and joint fixations in the lumbar-pelvic spine in low back pain. Proceedings of the 1990 International Conference on Spinal Manipulation. Washington, D.C.: May 11-12, 1990. p. 236-40.

147. Vernon HT, Aker P, Burns S, Viljakaanen S, Short L. Pressure pain threshold evaluation of the effect of spinal manipulation in the treatment of chronic neck pain: a pilot study. J Manipulative Physiol Ther 1990;13:13-6.

148. Enebo B. Conservative management of chronic low back pain utilizing mobilization: a single subject descriptive case study. Chiropractic Technique 1998;10(2):68-74.

149. Keating JC, Bergmann TF, Jacobs GE, Finer BA, Larson K. Interexaminer reliability of eight evaluative dimensions of lumbar segmental abnormality. J Manipulative Physiol Ther 1990;13:463-70.

150. Vernon H. An assessment of the intra- and inter-reliability of the posturometer. J Manipulative Physiol Ther 1983;62(2):57-60.

151. DeBoer KF, Harmon RO Jr, Savoie S, Tuttle CD. Inter- and intra-examiner reliability of leg length differential measurement: a preliminary study. J Manipulative Physiol Ther 1983;6(2):61-6.

152. Fuhr AW, Osterbauer PJ. Interexaminer reliability of relative leg length evaluation in prone, extended position. J Chiro Tech 1989;1(1):13-8.

153. Rhudy TR, Burk JM. Inter-examiner reliability of functional leg-length assessment. Am J Chiro Med 1990;3(2):95.

154. Johnson WL, Vorro J. Biomechanical measurements of changes in cervical muscle function following osteopathic manipulative treatment. J Am Osteopath Assoc 1983; 83:131.

155. Vorro J, Johnston WL, Hubbard R. Biomechanical analysis of symmetric and asymmetric cervical function. J Am Osteopath Assoc 1982;82:140-1.

156. Frobin W, Leivseth G, Biggemann M, Brinckmann P. Sagittal plane segmental motion of the cervical spine. A new precision measurement protocol and normal motion data of healthy adults. Clin Biomech 2002;17(1):21-31.

157. Nansel DD, Cremata E, Carlson J, Szlazk M. Effect of unilateral spinal adjustments on goniometrically assessed cervicolateral-flexion end-range asymmetries in otherwise asymptomatic subjects. J Manipulative Physiol Ther 1989;12(6):419-27.

158. Nansel D, Peneff A, Cremata E, Carlson J. Time course considerations for the effects of unilateral lower cervical adjustments with respect to the amelioration of cervical lateral-flexion passive end-range asymmetry. J Manipulative Physiol Ther 1990;13:297-304.

159. Enebo BA. The effect of cervical spine manipulation on motor control in healthy individuals: a pilot study. Chiropractic J Australia 2003;33(3):93-7.

160. Gal J, Herzog W, Kawchuk G, Conway P, Zhang Y. Biomechanical studies of spinal manipulative therapy (SMT): quantifying the movements of vertebral bodies during SMT. JCCA 1994;38(1):11-24.

161. Cramer GD, Gregerson DM, Knudsen JT, Hubbard BB, Ustas LM, Cantu JA. The effects of side-posture positioning and spinal adjusting on the lumbar Z joints: a randomized controlled trial with sixty-four subjects. Spine 2002;27:2459-66.

162. Cramer GD, Tuck NR Jr, Knudsen JT, Fonda SD, Schliesser JS, Fournier JT et al. Effects of side-posture positioning and side-posture adjusting on the lumbar zygapophyseal joints as evaluated by magnetic resonance imaging: a before and after study with randomization. J Manipulative Physiol Ther 2000;23:380-94.

163. Keller TS, Colloca CJ, Gunzburg R. Neuromechanical characterization of in vivo lumbar spinal manipulation. Part I. Vertebral motion. J Manipulative Physiol Ther 2003;26:567-78.

164. Colloca CJ, Keller TS, Gunzburg R. Biomechanical and neurophysiological responses to spinal manipulation in patients with lumbar radiculopathy. J Manipulative Physiol Ther 2004;27(1):1-15.

165. Herzog W, Nigg BM, Robinson RO, Read LJ. Quantifying the effects of spinal manipulation on gait using patients with low back pain: a pilot study. J Manipulative Physiol Ther 1987;10:295-9.

166. Herzog W, Nigg BM, Read LJ. Quantifying the effects of spinal manipulations on gait using patients with low back pain. J Manipulative Physiol Ther 1988;11(3):151-7.

167. Manga R, Angus D, Papadopoulos C, Swan W. The effectiveness and cost-effectiveness of chiropractic management of low-back pain. Richmond Hill, Ontario: Kenilworth; 1993.

168. Cassidy JD, Quon JA, Lafrance LJ, Yong-Hing K. The effect of manipulation on pain and range of motion in the cervical spine: a pilot study. J Manipulative Physiol Ther 1992;15:495-500.

169. Cassidy JD, Lopes AA, Yong-Hing K. The immediate effect of manipulation versus mobilization on pain and range of motion in the cervical spine: a randomized controlled trial. J Manipulative Physiol Ther 1992;15(9):570-5.

170. Enebo B. Outcome measures for low back pain: pain inventories and functional disability questionnaires. Chiropractic Technique 1998;10(1):27-33.

171. Vernon H. Static and dynamic roentgenography in the diagnosis of degenerative disc disease: a review and comparative assessment. J Manipulative Physiol Ther 1982;5:163-9.

172. Hall MC. Luschka's joint. Springfield, IL: Charles C Thomas; 1965. p. 44.

173. Kirkaldy-Willis W, editor. The three phases of the spectrum of degenerative disease. In: Managing low back pain. 2nd ed. New York: Churchill Livingstone; 1988. p. 117-32.

174. Sandoz R. The natural history of a spinal degenerative lesion. Ann Swiss Chiro Assoc 1989;9:149-92.

175. McNab I. Cervical spondylosis. Clin Orthop 1975;109:69-77.

176. Iida T, Abumi K, Kotani Y, Kaneda K. Effects of aging and spinal degeneration on mechanical properties of lumbar supraspinous and interspinous ligaments. Spine J 2002;2(2):95-100.

177. Borenstein D. Does osteoarthritis of the lumbar spine cause chronic low back pain? Curr Rheumatol Rep 2004;6(1):14-9.

178. Triano JJ. Biomechanics of spinal manipulative therapy. Spine J 2001;1:121-30.

179. Grieve GP. Common vertebral joint problems. New York: Churchill Livingstone; 1981. p. 5-38.

180. Salter RB. Textbook of disorders and injuries of the musculoskeletal system. Baltimore: Williams & Wilkins; 1970.

181. Levin S. Early mobilization speeds recovery. Physicians Sports Med 1993;7(1):70-4.

182. Eck JC, Humphreys SC, Lim TH, Jeong ST, Kim JG, Hodges SD et al. Biomechanical study on the effect of cervical spine fusion on adjacent-level intradiscal pressure and segmental motion. Spine 2002;27:2431-4.

183. Chou WY, Hsu CJ, Chang WN, Wong CY. Adjacent segment degeneration after lumbar spinal posterolateral fusion with instrumentation in elderly patient. Arch Orthop Trauma Surg 2002;122(1):39-43.

184. Woo SL, Matthews JV, Akeson WH, Amiel D, Convery FR. Connective tissue response to immobility: correlative study. Biomechanical measurements of normal in immobilized rabbit knees. Arthritis Rheum 1975;18:257-64.

185. Cramer GD, Fournier JT, Henderson CNR. Degenerative changes of the articular processes following spinal fixation [abstract]. J Chiropr Ed 2002;16(1):7.

12

Buckling: A Biomedical Model of Subluxation

John J. Triano

Key Words   Motion segment buckling, load, creep shear, bend

After reading this chapter you should be able to answer the following questions:

Question 1   What are the characteristics of spinal motion segment buckling?

Question 2   What factors precipitate spinal motion segment buckling?

Question 3   What factors are required to resolve buckling behavior?

For over 100 years, the notion of vertebral subluxation has provided a conceptual basis for the chiropractic profession. Throughout that history, there has been little change in the reasoning underpinning the theory of subluxation. Parallel hypotheses have evolved as justifications for treatment by osteopathic and manipulative manual medicine practitioners[1] under the terms *osteopathic lesion* and *joint dysfunction,* respectively. Acceptance of the subluxation lesion by the broader health care community and health policy makers has been hindered primarily by the absence of tangible evidence of its existence or its mechanism. It has been essentially a heuristic theory explained only by empirical observation and thought experiments. For the profession, the subluxation denotes structural failure altering body function.

Chiropractic today is similar in its stage of theory development to that behind the treatment of diabetes mellitus in the mid-1930s. At that time, the clinical description of diabetic patients was well understood. Patients with polyphagia, polydipsia, polyuria, and sweet smelling body fluids often could be treated successfully with dietary modifications. While the mechanism of altered sugar metabolism was known, the Islets of Langerhans cells and their functional pathophysiology were unknown. Symptoms of patients that appear responsive to spinal manipulation, similarly, are known but there exist neither adequate tests nor means to objectively visualize and measure the lesion.

Good theory should reliably account for clinical observations. Classical explanations of subluxation do not. Like most advances in health care, breakthroughs are triggered by the accumulation of observations that are not explained within the theory. Early efforts to resolve these apparent conflicts gave rise to the notion of the subluxation complex.[2,3] This modification of the traditional theory sought to develop subcategories of mechanisms explaining different symptom subsets but with limited success. Within the past two decades, specific evidence has accumulated to explain the subluxation mechanism with a more complete,

biomechanically based theory able to account for clinical observations. This chapter will first review the theoretical inconsistencies followed by more recent evidence that helps to reconcile them.

The notion that the subluxation hypothesis or theory may be flawed is often met with strong condemnation from members of the profession, principally because the history of chiropractic has been to hold so tenaciously to it that some feel a loss of identity and purpose should there be any doubt. A lesson can be taken from Galen Price, D.C., who was both a tradition and part of the heritage of the Palmer University system as a professor teaching chiropractic philosophy. As early as 1969, he stated the following:

> If science proved tomorrow, that our theory of subluxation was incorrect, it would not alter what I do...I would simply find another theory.[4]

Dr. Price observed that the value of his clinical work might be independent of the hypothetical explanation available at the time. His comments perhaps were prescient because scientific evidence now shows a significant benefit from use of chiropractic methods while simultaneously demonstrating error in the underlying hypothetical framework of the lesion being treated.

Inconsistencies of Chiropractic Theory

The fundamental basis of the subluxation hypothesis was set out by Palmer[5] and specifies a cascade of events. They are (1) displacement or relative malposition between two vertebra, (2) irritation of the intervertebral spinal nerve, (3) interference of the nerve function, and (4) functional or pathological abnormality in the end organ innervated by the nerve. A direct examination of the first two tenets of the cascade demonstrates inconsistency with clinical and experimental observation.

Strong clinical and biomechanical evidence exists that make clear that there is no normal position between vertebrae in the context of the Palmer subluxation hypothesis. The body of evidence as a whole is beyond the space available for review here. However, two examples, one clinical and one biomechanical, illustrate the problems.

The clinical observation that fails to be explained by the Palmer cascade is the fact that no reliable relationship has been found between vertebral position and any health disorder, including spine pain. Figure 12-1 shows two patients, one evaluated with a history of repeated episodes of spine pain and one with no spine symptoms. Both were otherwise healthy. It is the patient with the normal appearing spine that has all of the symptoms. Indeed, this observation is a basis for two different schools of thought within the chiropractic discipline. The Logan approach, historically, would be to make every effort to straighten a curvature of the spine simply because it is present. The Palmer approach has been to assert that the spine developed in this manner and for this individual is normal and there should be no intervention to correct the curve.

The work of Frymoyer et al.[6] illustrates the dilemma of intervertebral position as a chiropractic premise. Their study was directly targeted to test for such a relationship. Radiographs of the lumbar spine were obtained for various clinical reasons. Each was distributed to both medical and chiropractic radiologists with instructions to identify two features: first, all of the clinically relevant findings, and second, the radiographs of patients with back pain. While the chiropractic participants were much more consistent than the medical providers in identifying factors they believed were

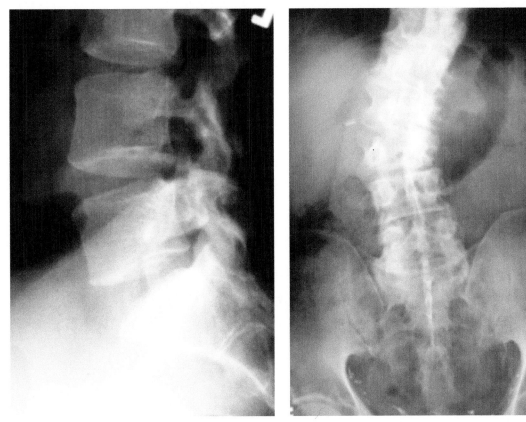

Figure 12-1   The radiograph on the left represents a "normal" lumbar spine with good lordotic curvature and relative positioning between the vertebrae. This patient had a history of recurrent episodes of severe, disabling lower back pain. On the right is an adult patient whose curvature was monitored periodically for progression. The patient had no history of back pain or any evidence of abdominal, pelvic, or lower extremity disorders.

clinically important, neither group was any more successful in correctly identifying the patients with spine complaints.

A second problem for the bone position tenet of subluxation comes with modern knowledge of spine biomechanics. However, the influence of biomechanical function on observations could be seen in clinical studies as early as 1982. Schram[7] attempted to quantify the change in position of the atlas following treatment. Figure 12-2 shows the typical type of radiographic measure used clinically for position. The location of osseous landmarks is used to determine the orientation of a vertebra with respect to some "normal" position or with respect to an earlier position. The result of treatment was a random orientation of C1 with respect to C2. There was no relationship between the position after treatment either to the pre-treatment condition or to any presumed normal position. In fact, the result appeared to be completely random and could be replicated by computer simulation.

A normal biomechanical phenomenon of vertebral joint function is now known that makes Schram's results perfectly reasonable. It is the normal presence of the articular neutral zone (Figure 12-3). The neutral zone is a region in which the vertebra will come to rest following a movement. Another description of the neutral zone is that it is a central region where there is almost no resistance from the ligamentous or discal attachments to applied loads. Disproportionately large movements occur within this neighborhood in response to spinal loads compared to outside the region where the resistance from ligaments is engaged. The neutral zone of the atlas is one of the largest of all spinal segments. Under normal circumstances, return of the head to midline following a rotation could leave the atlas rotated to one side or it may overshoot to the other. Such behavior is completely consistent with Schram's findings of random orientation following manipulation.

After positional abnormality, the Palmer cascade calls for nerve irritation with altered nerve expression. Other than the appearance of pain, itself an ambiguous symptom, rarely is there clinical evidence of direct nerve root involvement. Similarly, electrodiagnostic studies have been found to show sensitive or specific changes in nerve function at the intervertebral foramina unless pathoanatomical disease is present. The most common diseases that produce such changes include chemical neuritis associated with internal disc derangement, stenosis, and disc protrusion. Indeed, imaging studies may show significant

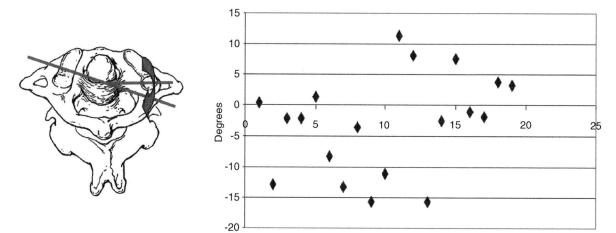

Figure 12-2   Schematic representation of a clinical measure of atlantoaxial rotation is defined by the relative position of a line drawn between landmarks on the atlas transverse processes. The graph to the right is a simulation of results that replicates the random positioning following treatment.

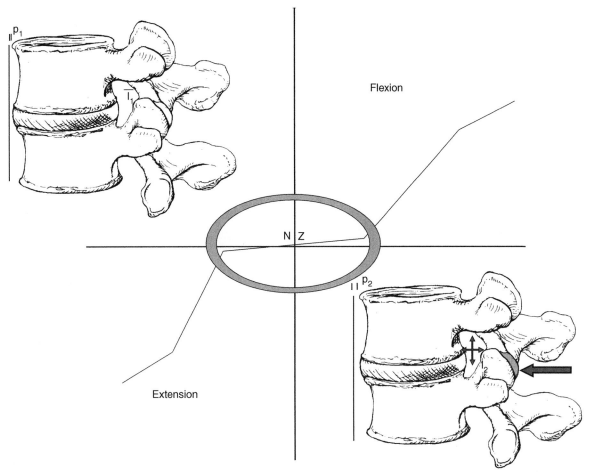

Figure 12-3   The neutral zone *(ellipse)* is plotted with displacement on the horizontal axis and load on the vertical axis. A movement from the starting position (top left) may return at completion to the bottom right. Note that the horizontal position *(p₁)* with respect to a vertical reference line is increased *(p₂)* and the shape of the intervertebral foramina will also change proportionately.

effacement of the dura or deformity of the nerve root without any reliable change in nerve amplitude, conduction velocity, or reflex response (Figure 12-4).

In the absence of consistent evidence for nerve root involvement, supplemental theories have been developed to offer mechanisms of altered proprioception and reflex changes as a basis for the claim of nerve irritation. Some evidence exists to support these ideas; however, they fail to represent mechanisms of true nerve irritation. Rather, they are normal physiological responses to altered

mechanical joint behavior as with changes in proprioceptor firing rates. Whether such changes, if they occur, are persistent or accommodate with time are unknown. Reflex responses may also vary,[8-12] but they represent secondary mechanisms that are not consistently found in patients.

Various alternative explanations have been proposed that attempt to describe the different clinical presentations that patients have. (See Chapter 10.) They include such factors as entrapped synovial tags or joint menisci and local muscle spasm. Both accounts might explain pain

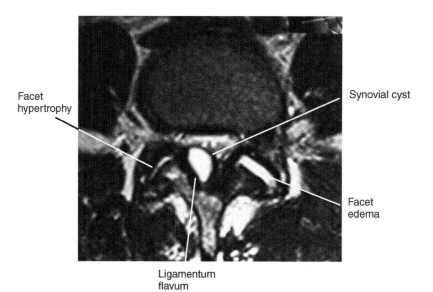

Facet hypertrophy

Synovial cyst

Facet edema

Ligamentum flavum

Figure 12-4   Pathological elements that pose increased risk for central or exiting neural element irritation or compression. A transactional image of the L3 vertebra with a synovial cyst crowding the thecal sac and compressing the nerve roots. While this patient experienced radiating, nonradicular leg pain, there were no abnormalities of nerve function measured by electromyography evaluation and nerve conduction studies.

and are intended to give a basis for how the lesion persists. Menisci are hypothesized to create a blockage of the joint, and local spasm restricts motion. Joint adhesions may develop to chronically block motion or cause it to be asymmetrical. Inconsistencies, however, remain. Menisci do exist.[13] However, because motion opens and closes the joint depending on the direction, it is not clear why an entrapped meniscus is not released with an alternate movement. Local muscle tension may exist for some; however, it has not been shown to occur uniformly. Moreover, muscles fatigue. What keeps the tension and prohibits motion then? Inflammatory conditions do cause adhesions in and around connective tissue. However, the organization of granulation tissue that yields adhesions takes time. What process retains the necessary conditions long enough?

Lantz[2,3,14] and Mootz[15,16] contributed to alternative reasoning, adding to the structured picture entitled the subluxation complex. (See Chapter 9.) This portrayal is useful since it collects the symptomatology and purported mechanisms frequently encountered into common manifestations involving muscle (myopathology), swelling, redness and inflammation (vascular pathology), scar formation (connective tissue pathology), and neural changes (neuropathology). The consolidation, however, fails to explain the underlying mechanism of the lesion or the wide variation in the clinical presentations observed in practice. Moreover, neither the traditional subluxation theory nor the revised subluxation complex account for the clinical experience of patients with known organic pathology[17,18] (Box 12-1) who may respond to spinal manipulation or adjustment.

In summary, evidence now exists that there is no normal position between vertebrae in the sense of the historical subluxation argument. Nerve irritation, although feasible, is not universal in patients who respond favorably to spinal manipulation or adjustment and the elements of subluxation complex are unable to explain how the lesion persists. The traditional theory of subluxation is incommensurate with the observations of clinical practice and scientific evidence. The gap between theoretical foundation and observation requires rethinking of our concepts of the subluxation.

BOX 12-1 ■ Examples of Pathoanatomical Disorders in Which Spinal Manipulation Is Thought to Be Helpful

Degenerative spondylosis
Discogenic pain
  • Disruption
  • Protrusion
Intermittent spinal stenosis
Painful facet arthrosis
Radicular pain syndromes
  • Compressive brachial neuropathy
  • Compressive sciatic neuropathy
Spondylolisthesis

Questioning fundamental tenets of clinical practice always raises strong debate and, for some, apprehension. However, it is the hallmark of scientific and professional maturity to identify and resolve disparity between theory and observation. A simple consolidation of clinical observations represents the common features of patients who respond to treatment with manipulation and are often classified with a diagnosis of subluxation (Figure 12-5). Modern clinical evidence supports the tenet of a mechanical lesion amenable to mechanical treatment in the form of manipulation or adjustment.

The subluxation may be static in the sense of being associated with persistent abnormal function. On the other hand, it may be dynamic,

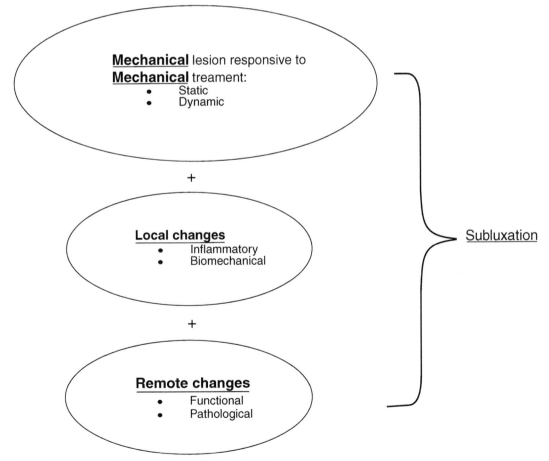

Figure 12-5 Summary elements of the subluxation lesion.

evident only within the midrange or extreme of motion. The effects may be local, remote, or both local and remote. Local changes result in altered biomechanical function that can result in proprioceptive signaling of joint behavior out of phase with the overall postural demand or task in which the patient is engaged. Such responses represent normal neurologic communication of joint function. In theory, joint receptors may accommodate with time and adjust to the new joint conditions. While the thresholds of joint activation may be inferred from physiological studies, the true behavior associated with subluxation has not yet been studied. Sufficiently altered mechanical behavior in a joint will tend to result in increased local tissue strain and foster inflammatory response.

Remote effects may arise as functional or pathological consequences of the local lesion effects. For example, if altered proprioceptive activity persists, they may contribute to the central sensitization observed in many chronic pain sufferers. Other mechanisms may include sclerotomal pain referral to an extremity, the abdomen, or the thorax. Pathologic responses may arise by separate mechanisms. Inflammatory swelling of the joint capsule may narrow the neural canal. If other pathology coexists (Box 12-2 and Figure 12-5), the thecal sac about the cord or the exiting nerve roots may be deformed, with or without nerve irritation or damage. Should disc material be torn, breakdown products of the deteriorating collagen matrix (e.g., phospholipase A2) may be released, inducing a chemical neuritis. All of these factors can result in peripheral symptoms determined by the identity and extent of the neural fibers affected.

All of the elements described in Figure 12-5 form feasible hypotheses. The implied cascade is not an all-or-nothing effect. For example, some patients have only local symptoms of spinal pain, loss of motion and muscle spasm. The sequence may be incomplete resulting in variable symptom patterns. Others have these symptoms as well as peripheral pain with or without signs of radiculopathy. While the clinical experience supports the logic of local and remote effects of subluxation, it still fails to supply a testable theoretical underpinning of the concept. The evidence surrounding the mechanical behavior of motion segment buckling describes the mechanism of subluxation.

Structural Stability and Motion Segment Buckling

The failure of any structure can be described as occurring in one of two ways, either by separation or by unacceptable deformation. That is, deformation is sufficient to result in excessive tissue strain or structural malfunction but insufficient to result in structural separation. Tissues are traumatized from a singular overload or by repetitive strains where individual components are strained beyond a threshold. The boundary for failure within a tissue is dependent both on the rate and the amount of loading. The meaning of failure by separation is obvious, constituting injuries that include fracture and structural tearing. Failure by deformation, however, may be subtler. For example, deformation of neuronal membranes at the microscopic level alters the axonal sodium transport system and impulse conduction, resulting in functional failure. Patients with rheumatoid arthritis may develop pathologic ulnar deviation of the metacarpophalangeal joints until even minimal prehensile function of the hand fails.

BOX 12-2 ■ Pathologic Changes within the Spine That Promote Chemical Neuritis or Stenosis Centrally and within the Intervertebral Canal

Congenital narrowing with degeneration
Disc protrusion
Hypertrophic elements
  • Articular pillar/facet
  • Ligamentum flavum
Internal disc derangement
Osteophytosis
Synovial cyst

Functionally, both examples represent unacceptable deformation leading to functional failure. In one case, that of acute pressure on neuronal membranes, there is no pathologic change while destructive process and pannus formation is required to deform the rheumatoid hand.

Mechanically, the spine structurally represents a multiarticular, multiligamentous, and multimuscular stability problem. It has two functional stabilizing systems. One consists of the local segmental stabilizing muscles (e.g., multifidus, rotators, intertransversarii) and the second is composed of the broad regional muscles (e.g., abdominals, quadratus lumborum, longissimus, intercostalis). These systems coordinate with each other to simultaneously meet both local and regional postural priorities. There is disagreement on the best way to represent how the body optimizes its performance, achieving extremes of motion while minimizing the risk to local tissues. It is clear, however, that the combination of joint position and load must avoid local stress concentration sufficient to reach injury threshold. Figure 12-6 models the dual control system of the lumbar spine after the seminal work of Bergmark.[19]

The lumbar spine is designed as a linkage mechanism that permits the upper and lower body segments to achieve a wide variety of postures as different tasks are performed. The large regional stabilizing muscles induce positional control and motions. The intervening spinal segments and intrinsic muscles serve as interconnected links. Each link has a limited flexibility that, cumulatively, gives rise to the range and versatility of motion. The intersegmental joint sustains the compressive, shear, and moment loads of the various activities in which the individual is engaged. Tasks from sedentary to heavy weight lifting rely on stability within both the regional and local stabilizing systems. Stability is maintained by keeping the vertebral joints as stiff as necessary to support the activity without overstressing any single tissue.

Stiffness of the spine is maintained through passive and active systems. The passive system is made up of the respective tissue properties, primarily, of the bone, disc, and ligaments. The active

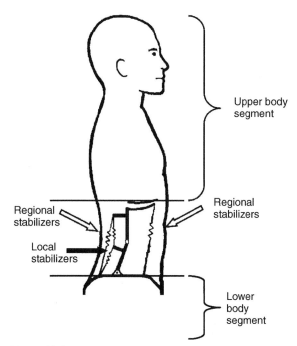

Figure 12-6　The lumbar spine, modeled as a single vertebral motion segment with hinge joint for simplicity, links the upper and lower body segments and controls their relative posture and overall stability through the regional stabilizers. Local stabilizing muscles control local motion and stability.

system is maintained by the muscular attachments (Figure 12-7). The properties of the bone and disc tolerate peak loads in compression and shear at different rates of speed. Bending moments, however, are offset by the intrinsic muscles with ligaments as range limiters. Failure of effective coordination between the regional and local muscles can lead to a local buckling event[1,20] (Figure 12-8).

Buckling is a local failure by deformation within the multisegmented structure of the spinal column. Detailed discussion of spinal buckling and its evidence can be reviewed in Triano[1] and McGill.[20] Figure 12-8 portrays the fundamental elements of the deformation itself. Under normal functional conditions, load applied to the spine results in movement that is proportional to the local balance between the applied forces, or

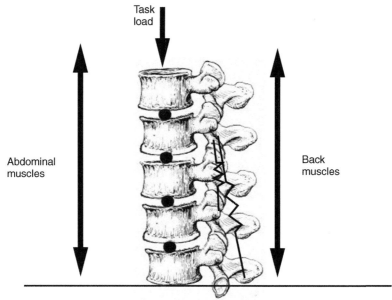

Figure 12-7   Loads from tasks attempt to compress, shear, and bend the spine. The disc is represented as a spherical ball since it can withstand compression and shear but has little stiffness against bending, which is resisted by intrinsic muscle shown here as spring elements.

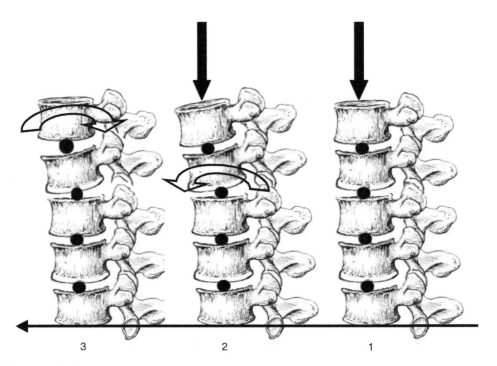

Figure 12-8   Spine load reaching its critical value *(1)* leads to a local segment undergoing a disproportionate displacement *(2)* which does not elastically recover when the load is reduced *(3)*.

moments, and the structural stiffness supplied by the spine architecture and muscle control systems. Stability will be maintained provided that the load does not exceed a critical value, which itself is dependent on five elements: load direction, speed of peak load development, spinal configuration/posture, fitness of or damage to the local tissues, and the timing of muscular response. When load exceeds the critical level or, conversely, muscle fails to create appropriate and timely stiffness consistent with the intended activity, a sudden local and disproportionate displacement occurs, leading to a concentration of local tissue stress. If sufficiently large, subcatastrophic or even catastrophic tissue damage will result in pain and inflammation. The symptom patterns that manifest are dependent on which tissue or tissues are involved (facet, nerve, disc, ligament, or muscle).

Several characteristics of buckling behavior are known (Box 12-3 and Table 12-1). Box 12-3 lists the factors that potentiate spinal buckling. An obvious causative factor is a single overload event that exceeds critical load for the conditions. For less severe tasks, the process is more complex. Normal creep deformity occurs with prolonged static posture. Creep alters the constitutive properties of the tissue and the relative critical load. Under the right conditions, even a small additional load will cause the joint to buckle.

BOX 12-3 ■ Triggering Factors Associated with Subluxation/Buckling Events

- Single overload events
- Prolonged static posture followed by an incremental load
- Loading rate higher than 500 Lb/sec
- Vibration

Table 12-1

Mechanistic Behavioral Criteria Defining the Subluxation

Mechanical phase	Characteristics
Prebuckling (normal) behavior	• Intersegmental motion is controlled by appropriate joint stiffness and is proportional to the loads applied. • Intersegmental postures are consistent with the intended tasks. • Joint and associated tissue loads remain below injury threshold.
Buckling event	• Precipitated by factors listed in Box 12-3. • Intersegmental motions are disproportionate (lower/higher) than applied loads predict. • The buckled configuration remains within the extremes of normal ranges of motion. • Intersegmental postures are inconsistent with one or more intended tasks and involve disproportionate tissue component stresses.
Postbuckling behavior	• Resembles prebuckling behavior but initiated from the buckling configuration. • One or more tasks increases tissue component stresses near to or past injury threshold. • Symptoms depend on the identity of the tissue that surpasses injury threshold. • Resolving buckling behavior requires the application of external force/moment that may be in the form of appropriate movement/exercise or manipulation/adjustment.

Rapidly applied loads also are associated with buckling and vibration reduces the threshold necessary to achieve it. Finally, tissues that are damaged, as in discopathy, may buckle sooner and reach maximum displacement (deformation) under lower peak loads than do healthy tissues.

The similarity between functional features of buckled structures and clinical observations is worth noting. Patients experience subluxation and find that the symptoms may express themselves intermittently and under specific circumstances, implying that the lesioned segment can function and sustain effort. Similarly, buckled structures often are distorted but remain functional. Data by Wilder[21,22] show that a vertebral motion segment (see Figure 12-8) functions essentially the same after buckling, but under a configuration of significantly higher mechanical stress. Moreover, patients have no measurable signs of abnormality in joint position within the precision of current clinical tests. Measures of displacement during spinal buckling demonstrate that even at the buckled extremes, the total angulation or translation remains at or within the normal ranges. The displacement, however, is disproportionate for the task and load being undertaken. The buckled site undergoes stress concentration, which for biological tissues invokes symptoms that will be typical to the tissue involved.

Summary

Patients who seem to respond to spinal manipulation span a wide spectrum of clinical descriptions. The traditional theories of the subluxation mechanism are inadequate to explain the variety of presentations and the inconsistencies in clinical and basic science evidence. Spinal buckling is a biomechanical phenomenon that occurs under defined circumstances. The characteristics of buckled spinal segments (see Table 12-1) are consistent with the findings in clinical practice and can be partitioned into prebuckling (normal), buckling, and postbuckling phases. Patients may have symptoms with or without local inflammation. Remote symptoms may occur as a result of referred pain, reflex responses, or direct neural irritation/inflammation.

The observation of subluxation no longer needs to be viewed with mystery and belief. Scientific evidence has accumulated to establish a theoretical foundation. Solid theory can be used to explore more effective methods of prevention, treatment, and rehabilitation efforts for future patients.

References

1. Triano J. The mechanics of spinal manipulation. In: Herzog W, editor. Clinical biomechanics of spinal manipulation. New York: Churchill Livingstone; 2000. p. 92-190.
2. Lantz CA. The vertebral subluxation complex. Part I: an introduction to the model and kinesiologic component. Chiro Res J 1989;1(3):1-10.
3. Lantz C. A review of the evolution of chiropractic concepts of subluxation. Topics Clin Chiro 1995;2(2):1-10.
4. Price G. Course Notes—Chiropractic Philosophy. Chiropractic Students, editor. Personal communication: 1969.
5. Boone WR, Dobson GJ. A proposed vertebral subluxation model reflecting traditional concepts and recent advances in health and science. J Vertebral Subluxation Research 1996;1:19-30.
6. Frymoyer JW, Phillips RB, Newberg AH, MacPherson BV. A comparative analysis of the interpretations of lumbar spinal radiographs by chiropractors and medical doctors. Spine 1986;11:1020-3.
7. Schram S. Error limitations in x-ray kinematics of the spine. J Manipulative Physiol Ther 1982;5(1):5-10.
8. Cramer GD, Humphreys CR, Hondras MA, McGregor M, Triano JJ. The Hmax/Mmax ratio as an outcome measure for acute low back pain. J Manipulative Physiol Ther 1993;16(1):7-13.
9. Murphy BA, Dawson NJ, Slack JR. Sacroiliac joint manipulation decreases the H-reflex. Electromyogr Clin Neurophysiol 1995;35:87-94.
10. Floman Y, Liram N, Gilai AN. Spinal manipulation results in immediate H-reflex changes in patients with unilateral disc herniation. Eur Spine J 1997;6:398-401.
11. Dishman JD, Burke J. Spinal reflex excitability changes after cervical and lumbar spinal manipulation: a comparative study. Spine 2003;3(3):204-12.
12. Dishman JD, Bulbulian R. Spinal reflex attenuation associated with spinal manipulation. Spine 2000;25(19):2519-24.
13. Giles LGF, Day RE. Intra-articular synovial folds of thoracolumbar junction zygapophyseal joints. Anatomical Record 1990;226(2):147-52.
14. Lantz CA. The vertebral subluxation complex. In: Gatterman MI, editor. Foundations of chiropractic: subluxation. St. Louis: Mosby; 1995. p. 149-74.
15. Mootz RD. Chiropractic theories: current understanding of vertebral subluxation and manipulable spinal lesions. In: Sweere JJ, editor. Chiropractic family practice. Volume I. Gaithersburg, MD: Aspen; 1992.

16. Mootz RD. Theoretical models of chiropractic subluxation. In: Gatterman MI, editor. Foundations of chiropractic: subluxation. St. Louis: Mosby; 1995. p. 176-89.

17. Cassidy JD, Kirkaldy-Willis WH, McGregor M. Spinal manipulation for the treatment of chronic low-back and leg pain: an observational study. In: Buerger AA, Greenman PE, editors. Empirical approaches to the validation of spinal manipulation. Springfield, IL: Charles C Thomas; 1985. p. 119-50.

18. Triano JJ, Bougie JD, Rogers CM, Scaringe JG, Sorrels K, Skogsbergh DR et al. Procedural skills in spinal manipulation: do prerequisites matter? Spine J 2004;4:557-63.

19. Bergmark A. Mechanical stability of the human lumbar spine [Dissertation]. Lund, Sweden: Lund Institute of Technology; 1987.

20. McGill SM. Low back disorders. In: Evidence-based prevention and rehabilitation. Champaign, IL: Human Kinetics; 2002.

21. Wilder DG, Pope MH, Seroussi RE, Dimnet J, Krag MH. The balance point of the intervertebral motion segment: an experimental study. Bull Hosp Jt Dis Orthop Inst 1989;49(2):155-69.

22. Wilder DG, Pope MH, Frymoyer JW. The biomechanics of lumbar disc herniation and the effect of overload and instability. J Spinal Disord 1988;1:16-32.

13

Three Neurophysiologic Theories on the Chiropractic Subluxation

Charles N.R. Henderson

Key Words   Chiropractic theory, subluxation, intervertebral foramen encroachment, joint receptors, proprioception, spinal cord traction, dentate ligaments

After reading this chapter you should be able to answer the following questions:

Question 1   Are the neural contents of the intervertebral foramen (nerve roots and dorsal root ganglion) equally sensitive to compression?

Question 2   By what neurologic mechanism may nonvertebral joints such as the sacroiliac, ankle, or temporomandibular joint produce long-term influences on the central nervous system?

Question 3   What are two ways in which traction through the dentate ligaments may influence neural impulses within the spinal cord?

This chapter reviews three theories that are incorporated into our neurophysiologic model of the chiropractic subluxation. The name of each of these theories tells something of the mechanism by which we think the subluxation affects the nervous system:

1. Intervertebral encroachment
2. Altered somatic afferent input
3. Dentate ligament, cord distortion

Before reviewing these three theories, it is helpful to establish our perspective by stating a few fundamental points concerning theories and models, especially those related to the subluxation. Theories should be plausible and scientifically acceptable. They are often described and examined in scientific studies by using models that help us visualize the abstract principles involved. Our models allow us to operate in a world in which the very complexity or size of reality makes it unmanageable in its full essence. The utility of a model, then, is in its manageable size and complexity. We simplify the complex, shrink the enormous, and magnify the minute until we feel comfortable. However, the very ease or comfort we feel with our models may lead us to forget that they are only models, not the full essence of reality. This is an important point. Our failure to appreciate the limits of our models leads to untold problems in our lives and our sciences. Most simply put: We think with models but we live with reality. The reader should keep this caution in mind while reading this and other chapters of this text.

Defining the term *subluxation* is necessary, even if a bit difficult. Chapter 1 on terminology introduced us to the scope of the problem. Chiropractic educators, legislators, philosophers, scientists, and practitioners hold tenaciously to a wide range of definitions. Here is a small but influential sample:

A vertebral subluxation is any vertebra out of normal alignment, out of apposition to its co-respondents above and below, wherein it does occlude a foramen, either spinal or intervertebral, which does produce pressures upon nerves, thereby interfering

and interrupting the normal quantity flow of mental impulse supply between brain and body and thus becomes THE CAUSE of all disease. A vertebral subluxation IS a vertebral subluxation whenever it IS what is stated above, ALL elements being present. It is NOT a subluxation unless the interference to transmission is present. There can be no pressure upon nerves unless the size, shape, diameter, or circumference of the foramen is changed. There can be no change in the normal size, shape, diameter, or circumference of the foramen unless one vertebra is subluxated between its co-respondents above and below [emphasis by Palmer].[1]

Subluxation is an aberrant relationship between two adjacent articular structures that may have functional or pathological sequelae, causing an alteration in the biomechanical and/or neurophysiologic reflections of these articular structures, their proximal structures, and/or body systems that may be directly or indirectly affected by them.[2]

...interference with nerve transmission and expression, due to pressure, strain or tension upon the spinal cord, spinal nerves, or peripheral nerves as a result of a displacement of the spinal segments or other skeletal structures.[3]

Intervertebral Encroachment Theory

A common theme in all of these definitions is that a chiropractic subluxation exerts a significant influence on the nervous system. In the chiropractic profession, the most popular explanation for the subluxation's impact on the nervous system is clearly the intervertebral encroachment theory. A number of other explanations have been offered, but these other explanations lack the simple appeal of the intervertebral encroachment theory. Both doctor and patient can readily understand that pressure on the neural contents of the intervertebral foramen may disrupt the normal ingress and egress of nerve impulses.

It is now well established in the clinical literature that encroachment of neural structures within the intervertebral foramen (IVF) may produce pain and paresthesias, as well as changes in muscle tone and autonomic activity. The working assumptions are that pressure on the contents of the IVF either increases or decreases neural activity. Increased neural activity produces paresthesias, pain, hypertonic muscles, vasoconstriction, and sweating. Decreased neural activity produces numbness, muscle weakness/paralysis, vasodilation, and dry skin.

It is reasonable to ask, "Just how sensitive are the contents of the IVF?" We have learned that normal dorsal root ganglia (DRG), but not the spinal roots, may be stimulated by encroachment of the IVF. In small animal studies, compressive forces rapidly applied to normal dorsal roots (10 mg) produced only brief bursts (one to two seconds) of activity.[4,5] Moreover, slowly increased pressure eventually produced a conduction block, but it did not evoke an active response within the root fibers. By contrast, DRG responded to small, slowly applied compressive forces (100 mg) with prolonged repetitive firing. Most ganglia neurons fired for at least 4 to 7 minutes; a few fired for 25 minutes.

Chronically injured dorsal nerve roots behave very differently.[5] Injured roots may respond vigorously to mechanical pressure. Rapidly applied forces produce long bursts of activity (15 to 30 seconds), and even very slowly applied 10-mg pressures fire nerve root fibers. In addition, chronic peripheral nerve injury produces spontaneous discharges within DRG. Wall and Devor[5] suggest that radiating limb pain reported during a Lasegue straight leg test could be caused by shifting the DRG to a position of increased mechanical stress. These investigators suggest that DRG discharges associated with peripheral nerve injury may explain phantom limb sensation and pain. They also comment:

> ...there are a number of therapeutic schools which claim that pain is increased or decreased by minor shifts in position of vertebrae and structures close to the vertebral column. It appears conceivable that the afferent barrage is being affected by manipulation of the dorsal root ganglia.

These small animal studies are consistent with clinical experience.[6,7] Slowly applied compression to a normal peripheral nerve (for example, the

peroneal nerve is compressed by crossing legs) produces no pain but does produce numbness, paresthesias, and muscle weakness. By contrast, rapidly applied compression to an inflamed nerve produces pain and paresthesias (Tinel's sign). At surgery, mechanical compression of normal spinal nerve roots produces sensory and motor impairment without pain. However, even minimal mechanical deformation of inflamed nerve roots produces radiating limb pain.

Recent studies demonstrate that small-caliber afferent nerve fibers do more than simply conduct impulses to the central nervous system. Stimulation of these primary afferents promotes the release of histologically potent neuropeptides such as substance P (SP) and vasoactive intestinal peptide (VIP) at their peripheral terminals.[8,9] This observation has striking implications. It suggests that the peripheral origins of sensory fibers are important sites for neurologically mediated effects. We will consider the possible consequence of such a mechanism on back pain. As shown in Figure 13-1, the posterior anular fibers of the intervertebral disc are innervated by the recurrent meningeal (sinuvertebral) branch of the spinal nerve.[10,11] Figure 13-2 demonstrates that the zygapophyseal joints are richly innervated by the medial branch of the posterior primary ramus of the spinal nerve.[12] Therefore irritation of the DRG caused by intervertebral encroachment may cause release of neuropeptides within the intervertebral disc and the zygapophyseal joints. Earlier studies showed that SP and VIP stimulated breakdown of structural proteins.[13,14] Over time, these neuropeptides may produce pathologic changes in the intervertebral disc and zygapophyseal joints.

The plausibility of IVF encroachment as a contributor to discogenic low back pain is under investigation by scientists at the University of Iowa.[14] These researchers have developed an animal model of disc degeneration caused by IVF encroachment (Figure 13-3). In this model, structural disc proteins are broken down when substance P and VIP are released by sensory nerves in the posterior anular fibers of the disc. These investigators applied low-frequency

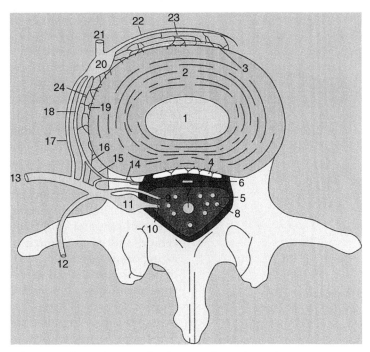

Figure 13-1   Schematic diagram of anterior spinal column and spinal canal innervation. *1,* Nucleus pulposus; *2,* anulus fibrosus; *3,* anterior longitudinal ligament/periosteum; *4,* posterior longitudinal ligament/periosteum; *5,* leptomeninges; *6,* epidural vasculature; *7,* filum terminale; *8,* intrathecal lumbosacral nerve root; *9,* ventral root; *10,* dorsal root; *11,* dorsal root ganglion; *12,* dorsal ramus of spinal nerve; *13,* ventral ramus of spinal nerve; *14,* recurrent meningeal nerve (sinuvertebral nerve of Luschka); *15,* sympathetic branch to the recurrent meningeal nerve; *16,* somatic branch to the recurrent meningeal nerve; *17,* white ramus communicans; *18,* gray ramus communicans; *19,* lateral sympathetic efferent branches projecting from gray ramus communicans; *20,* paraspinal sympathetic ganglion; *21,* paraspinal sympathetic chain; *22,* anterior paraspinal afferent sympathetic ramus; *23,* anterior paraspinal efferent sympathetic branches; *24,* lateral paraspinal afferent sympathetic ramus. Note: Afferent and efferent paraspinal sympathetic rami may be combined. *(Reprinted with permission from Jinkins JR, Whittemore AR, Bradley WG. AJR 1989;152:1277-89.)*

vibration (approximately 4 Hz) to rabbits with experimentally reduced IVFs and to control animals with normal IVFs. They observed that mechanical stimuli are more effectively transmitted to the DRG when the IVF dimension is experimentally decreased. Chronic mechanical stimulation of DRG caused small-caliber afferents in the superficial anular regions of the segmental disc to release substance P and VIP. These proteolytic neuropeptides caused degeneration of the disc. A progressive degenerative cycle developed wherein disc degeneration produced further IVF encroachment that increased the DRG stimulation. This resulted in further release of substance P and VIP and, subsequently, further degeneration of the intervertebral disc.

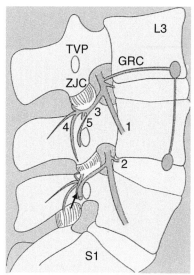

Figure 13-2   Part of the lower spinal innervation
(lateral view). *1*, Anterior primary ramus of the spinal
nerve; *2*, anterior primary ramus branch to the
intervertebral disc; *3*, posterior primary ramus of the
spinal nerve; *4*, medial branch of the posterior primary
ramus with an adjacent zygapophyseal joint capsule
(articular) branch, and a descending branch to the
zygapophyseal joint capsule (articular branch) one
joint lower; *5*, lateral branch of the posterior primary
ramus; *GRC*, gray ramus communicans; *TVP*,
transverse process; *ZJC*, zygapophyseal joint capsule;
arrow, mamiloaccessory ligament. *(Reprinted with
permission from Giles LGF. Anatomical basis of
low-back pain. Baltimore: Williams & Wilkins; 1989.)*

Altered Somatic Afferent Input Theory

Chiropractors find the IVF encroachment theory
to be very useful, and it is well supported by
clinical and research literature. But what about
upper cervical adjustments? The IVF encroachment theory cannot apply to joints lacking intervertebral foramens such as Occ-C1 or C1-C2. Do
sacroiliac or extremity joints subluxate? If so, how
is the nervous system affected? Clinical experience
suggests that chiropractic adjustments often bring
clinical improvement in the absence of demonstrable encroachment within the intervertebral

foramen. Directionally nonspecific "mobiliza-
tions" of vertebral joints are sometimes effective
in resolving the neurologic dysfunction of a subluxation. In addition, it has been suggested
by numerous clinical investigators that altered
afferent input from spinal structures such as the
zygapophyseal joints could produce signs and
symptoms previously attributed to intervertebral
encroachment.[15-20] These investigators reported
significant somatic sensory and motor responses
to altered articular afferent input. Responses consisted of changes in nociceptive and kinesthetic
sensibilities, muscle tone, deep tendon reflexes,
joint mobility, and sympathetic activity. Therefore
clinical and basic research investigations suggest
an important alternative mechanism for the effects
of a chiropractic adjustment. A chiropractic
adjustment may "normalize" articular afferent
input to the central nervous system. It is proposed
that normalized articular sensory input reestab-
lishes normal nociceptive and kinesthetic reflex
thresholds, with subsequent recovery of muscle
tone, joint mobility, and sympathetic activity.

In a study of 20 subjects, Mooney and
Robertson[17] injected hypertonic saline into the
L4-L5 or L5-S1 facet joints. They used arthro-
scopic guidance to ensure proper needle placement. These injections produced low back pain
and radiating leg pain. The entire ipsilateral lower
limb and the foot were involved in some patients.
When larger volumes of hypertonic saline were
injected, or when subjects had preexistent lumbar
facet disease, the pain radiated further down the
limb. These investigators noted marked myoelectric activity in the ipsilateral hamstring muscles
with diminished straight leg raising (by 70%). A
subsequent intracapsular injection of the local
anesthetic Xylocaine abolished all of these responses.
Several subjects with preexistent facet disease had
decreased straight leg raise (below 70 degrees) or
depressed deep tendon reflexes before saline injection. It was particularly interesting that each of
these subjects demonstrated a normal straight
leg raise and normal deep tendon reflexes within
five minutes after an intracapsular injection of
Xylocaine. The authors commented, "Based on
this preliminary experience, we no longer consider

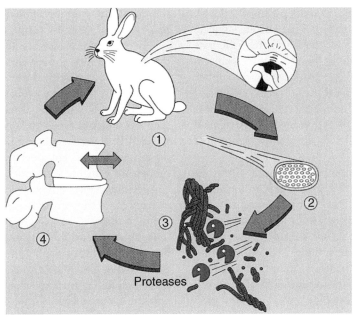

Figure 13-3   Proposed working model of dorsal root ganglia-neuropeptides-mediated degeneration of the spinal motion segment. *1,* Environmental or structural factors (for example, vibration/spinal instability) stimulate the synthesis or transport of neuropeptides of dorsal root ganglia *(2),* which in turn promote the synthesis of degradative enzymes and inflammatory agents *(3),* causing progressive degradation of the spinal motion segment *(4).* The resulting abnormal spinal motion segment renders the dorsal root ganglia more susceptible to mechanical stimuli, thereby creating a self-perpetuating, progressive, chronic condition. *(Reprinted with permission from Pedrini-Mille A, Weinstein JN, Found EM, Chung CB, Goel VK. Spine 1990;15:1252-6.)*

diminished straight leg raising or reflex changes to necessarily implicate nerve root pressure by disk protrusion."

Thabe[18] examined the segmentally related muscles of 20 upper cervical and 20 sacroiliac joints with restricted motion. Using needle probe electromyography (EMG), he observed marked spontaneous myoelectric activity in these muscles. Normal muscle does not demonstrate spontaneous EMG activity at rest. Within two minutes after injection of Xylocaine into the involved joints, there was marked reduction in spontaneous EMG activity. Spontaneous EMG activity was also reduced after gentle mobilization (nonthrust "muscle energy" technique) applied to the involved joints. It was an interesting contrast that manipulation (high-velocity thrust techniques) of the involved joints produced immediate and complete

abatement of spontaneous myoelectric activity. Thabe concluded that manipulation of the fixated joints produced a potent normalizing influence on the central nervous system, putatively caused by modified afferent input from joint receptors.

In a series of related studies, Korr et al.[16] investigated decreased electrical skin resistance (ESR) as an indicator of increased sympathetic motor activity after a variety of biomechanical stresses. In one study, they observed referred pain accompanied by segmental patterns of decreased ESR after injections of hypertonic saline into deep paraspinal tissues, deep interspinous ligaments, or paravertebral muscles. More superficial injections (skin, superficial interspinous ligaments, periosteum of spinous processes) produced only local pain and locally decreased ESR, or no pain and no changes in ESR. These investigators also reported

ESR changes in response to acute postural stresses. In this study, the pelvises of nine seated subjects were laterally tilted 15 degrees and the ESR was evaluated over a two-hour period. Other subjects received a heel lift ($\frac{1}{4}$- to $\frac{1}{8}$-inch hard rubber wedges) in one shoe. Heel lift subjects performed normal daily activities and were evaluated for ESR over one or more days. All subjects experienced reversible decreases in ESR after these acute postural stresses.

Biguer et al.[19] demonstrated that a vibratory stimulus (100 Hz) applied to the left suboccipital triangle region of normal subjects modifies the visual location and movement of a target in body-centered visual space. This stimulus apparently acts through the muscle spindles, which are especially dense in the cervical region.[21-23] In a review of causes and treatments for the "dizzy patient," Brown[20] noted the following:

> Intervertebral joint receptors from the upper cervical spine also play an important role in providing balance information and possibly control of eye movements. ... Some patients with cervical arthritis, whiplash, or other neck injury complain of persistent symptoms of light-headedness or imbalance for months to years after their incident.... Treatment modalities include vestibular suppressants, deafferentation, neck manipulation, and visual correction.

Our understanding of the basic neural processes that underlie clinical observations such as those just related has evolved from a number of animal studies. Freeman and Wyke[24] demonstrated that low-threshold mechanoreceptors in the articular capsule of the cat's ankle joint facilitate and reciprocally inhibit muscles that move the joint. In their experiments, stimulation of articular nociceptors simultaneously increased the activity of both flexor and extensor muscle groups in the ipsilateral limb as well as affecting motor activity in the contralateral limb. Joint lesions can therefore produce morbid changes in the tone of muscles that cross the joint or disrupt coordination of joint motion. In addition, these investigators reported that reflex changes in muscle tone or coordination were temporarily abolished by intraarticular injection of a local anesthetic. Electrocoagulation of

the joint capsule permanently abolished reflex responses to noxious stimuli applied to the joint.

The studies discussed to this point demonstrate the influence of relatively short-term noxious afferent input on central nervous system function. Few investigations have examined the impact of chronic noxious sensory input. However, patients seen in chiropractic and medical offices have frequently experienced chronic pain lasting months or years. The recent development of an animal model for chronic pain and rheumatoid arthritis has permitted the study of chronic, noxious articular influences on the central nervous system.[25-27] In this model a mineral oil suspension of Mycobacterium butyricum (Freund's adjuvant) is injected into the base of the rat's tail. The ensuing reversible arthritis has pathologic and biochemical features that resemble human rheumatic disease and appears to produce chronic pain. Mantyh et al.[28] examined changes within the superficial region of the dorsal horn of the spinal cord. They observed a reduction of specific neuropeptide receptors in adjuvant arthritic rats. These receptors respond to input from primary afferent nociceptors. This study demonstrated an anatomic change within the central nervous system in response to chronic altered sensory information from joints. Clinical chiropractic experience indicates that a similar effect may be produced by joint subluxation. Patients frequently experience chronic pain and neurologic dysfunction long after the site of peripheral injury achieves an apparent full recovery.

Dentate Ligament, Cord Distortion Theory

We now turn our attention to the third and final theory for our consideration. The "dentate ligament, cord distortion" theory is especially interesting to those chiropractors who limit their adjustments to the upper cervical region. With the publication of his book, *The Subluxation Specific: The Adjustment Specific,* B.J. Palmer[1] firmly stated:

> No vertebral subluxation CAN exist below axis; therefore no adjustment with any DIRECT INTENTION OR DESIGN could be given below an axis, to get sick people well [emphasis by Palmer].

B.J. Palmer ascribed the influence of subluxation to compression of the spinal cord. For approximately 20 years he adamantly denied the need to adjust below the axis. In later years he relented, admitting some value to adjustments below the axis, but asserting that these were "minor" subluxations. He maintained that only occiput/atlas/axis subluxations constituted "major" subluxations.

Little has been published on the dentate ligament, cord distortion theory. A paper by Grostic[29] relates two mechanisms by which the dentate ligaments may adversely influence the conduction of neural impulses within the spinal cord: direct mechanical irritation through dentate ligament traction; and venous occlusion and resultant local blood stasis and ischemia of the upper cervical cord, also produced by dentate ligament traction. Grostic observes that the strength of the dentate ligaments in the upper cervical region and the dynamics of cervical spine lengthening on flexion contribute to the possibility of spinal cord distress with upper cervical misalignments. Referring to the work of Breig,[30] he notes that there is an approximately 30-mm change in cervical spinal canal length from full extension to full flexion. Dural attachments to the foramen magnum and possibly to the axis and atlas are also noted. He estimates that an average lateral misalignment between the skull and atlas of 3 degrees produces an approximately 3-mm lateral displacement of the atlas. This 3-mm lateral displacement is approximately 23% of the total width of the spinal cord in the upper cervical region (approximately 13 mm).

A recent study corroborates the argument that cord distraction could produce a conduction block. Jarzem et al.[31] reported decreased spinal cord blood flow and concurrent interruption of somatosensory evoked potentials after experimental cord distraction. A study by Emery[32] underscores the mechanical strength and immobilizing character of the upper cervical dentate ligaments. Emery relates numerous cases of perinatal necropsy that demonstrated fatal kinking of the medulla-spinal cord junction in hydrocephalic children because of the interaction of a freely movable brainstem and a fixed upper cervical cord (fixed through strong dentate ligament attachments).

We have reviewed three theories that are incorporated into our current neurophysiologic model of the chiropractic subluxation. It is probable that elements of all three theories are active during a subluxation, in addition to numerous other mechanisms not covered in this presentation. We trust that further scientific research and development of our working models will enable the training of more effective chiropractic researchers, educators, and clinical practitioners.

References

1. Palmer BJ. The subluxation specific: the adjustment specific. Davenport, IA: Palmer School of Chiropractic; 1934.
2. American Chiropractic Association. Indexed synopsis of ACA policies on public health and related matters. Arlington, VA: American Chiropractic Association; 1992.
3. International Chiropractors Association. Policy handbook and code of ethics. 2nd ed. Arlington, VA: International Chiropractors Association; 1991.
4. Howe JF, Loeser JD, Calvin WH. Mechanosensitivity of dorsal root ganglia and chronically injured axons: a physiological basis for the radicular pain of nerve root compression. Pain 1977;3:25-41.
5. Wall PD, Devor M. Sensory afferent impulses originate from dorsal root ganglia as well as from the periphery in normal and nerve injured rats. Pain 1983;17:321-39.
6. Macnab I. The mechanism of spondylogenic pain. In: Hirsch C, Zotterman Y, editors. Cervical pain. New York: Pergamon Press; 1972. p. 89-95.
7. Greenbarg PE, Brown MD, Pallares VS, Tompkins JS, Mann NH. Epidural anesthesia for lumbar spine surgery. Spinal Dis 1988;1:139-43.
8. Levine JD, Clark R, Devor M, Helms C, Moskowitz MA, Basbaum AI. Intraneuronal substance P contributes to the severity of experimental arthritis. Science 1984;226:547-9.
9. Kidd BL, Mapp PI, Gibson SJ, Polak JM, O'Higgins F, Buckland-Wright JC et al. A neurogenic mechanism for symmetrical arthritis. Lancet 1989;11:1128-30.
10. Edgar MA, Ghadially JA. Innervation of the lumbar spine. Clin Orthop 1976;115:35-41.
11. Jinkins JR, Whittemore AR, Bradley WG. The anatomic basis of vertebrogenic pain and the autonomic syndrome associated with lumbar disc extrusion. AJR 1989;152:1277-89.
12. Bogduk N. The innervation of the lumbar spine. Spine 1983;8(3):286-93.
13. Lotz M, Carson DA, Vaughan JH. Substance P activation of rheumatoid synoviocytes: neural pathway in pathogenesis of arthritis. Science 1987;235:893-5.
14. Pedrini-Mille A, Weinstein JN, Found EM, Chung CB, Goel VK. Stimulation of dorsal root ganglia and degradation of rabbit annulus fibrosus. Spine 1990;15:1252-6.

15. Korr IM, Wright HM, Chace JA. Cutaneous patterns of sympathetic activity in clinical abnormalities of the musculoskeletal system. J Neur Transm 1964;25:589-606.
16. Korr IM, Wright HM, Thomas PE. Effects of experimental myofascial insults on cutaneous patterns of sympathetic activity in man. J Neur Trans 1962;23:330-55.
17. Mooney V, Robertson J. The facet syndrome. Clin Orthop 1976;115:149-56.
18. Thabe H. Electromyography as a tool to document diagnostic findings and therapeutic results associated with somatic dysfunctions in the upper cervical spinal joints and sacroiliac joints. Manual Med 1986;2:53-8.
19. Biguer B, Donaldson IML, Hein A, Jeannerod M. Neck muscle vibration modifies the representation of visual motion and direction in man. Brain 1988;111:1405-24.
20. Brown JJ. A systematic approach to the dizzy patient. Diagn Neurotology 1990;8(2):209-24.
21. Cooper S, Daniel PM. Muscles spindles in man, their morphology in the lumbricals and the deep muscles of the neck. Brain 1963;86:563-94.
22. Abrahams VC. The physiology of neck muscles: their role in head movement and maintenance of posture. Can J Physiol Pharmacol 1977;55:332-8.
23. Abrahams VC. Sensory and motor specialization in some muscles of the neck. Trends Neurosci 1981;4:24-7.
24. Freeman MAR, Wyke B. Articular reflexes at the ankle joint: an electromyographic study of normal and abnormal influences of ankle joint mechanoreceptors upon reflex activity in the leg muscles. Br J Surg 1967;54:990-1001.
25. De Castro Costa M, De Sutrer P, Gybels J, Van Hees J. Adjuvant-induced arthritis in rats: a possible animal model of chronic pain. Pain 1981;10:173-85.
26. Colpaert FC. Evidence that adjuvant arthritis in the rat is associated with chronic pain. Pain 1987;28:201-22.
27. Besson JM, Guilbaud G, editors. The arthritic rat as a model of clinical pain? New York: Elsevier; 1988.
28. Mantyh CR, Gates T, Zimmerman RP, Kruger L, Maggio JE, Vigna SR et al. Alterations in the density of receptor binding sites for sensory neuropeptides in the spinal cord of arthritic rats. In: Besson JM, Guilbaud G, editors. The arthritic rat as a model of clinical pain? New York: Elsevier; 1988. p. 139-52.
29. Grostic JD. Dentate ligament-cord distortion hypothesis. Chiro Res J 1988; 1:47-55.
30. Breig A. Adverse mechanical tension in the central nervous system. Stockholm: Almqvist and Wiksell International; 1978.
31. Jarzem PF, Quance DR, Doyle DJ, Begin LR, Kostuik JP. Spinal cord tissue pressure during spinal cord distraction in dogs. Spine 1992;17(85):S227-34.
32. Emery JL. Kinking of the medulla in children with acute cerebral oedema and hydrocephalus and its relationship to the dentate ligaments. J Neurol Neurosurg Psychiatry 1967;30:267-75.

14

T he subluxation is the greatest single factor in perpetuating any imbalance that may exist between the sympathetic and the parasympathetic nervous systems.

Muller, 1954

Vertebral Subluxation and the Anatomic Relationships of the Autonomic Nervous System

Peter Cauwenbergs

Key Words   Autonomic, preganglionic, postganglionic, splanchnic, somatic, visceral efferent, visceral afferent, sympathetic, parasympathetic, enteric, somatovisceral reflex, viscerosomatic reflex

After reading this chapter you should be able to answer the following questions:

Question 1   How are the three components of the autonomic nervous system differentiated?

Question 2   How does the location of preganglionic axons differ between the sympathetic and parasympathetic nervous systems?

Question 3   How do the functions of the sympathetic and parasympathetic nervous systems differ?

Question 4   On what basis can the treatment of visceral disorders be included in the scope of chiropractic practice?

The structure of the nervous system is commonly divided into the central nervous system (CNS), which consists of the brain, brainstem, and spinal cord, and the peripheral nervous system (PNS), which includes all neuronal processes outside of the CNS such as cranial nerves and spinal nerves, as well as ganglia associated with these nerves. Beyond pure anatomic description, however, such subdivisions are inconsequential because functional components of the nervous system extend beyond these artificial structural limits. Numerous examples can be identified in which single neurons extend axonal processes either centrally or peripherally into or out of the CNS, crossing the anatomic barrier between the CNS and PNS to form an integrated, functional system. The student of neuroanatomy should strive to understand both structural and functional relationships within the nervous system because this integrated knowledge of neuroscience is not only much more interesting and meaningful but also abundantly more useful in the clinical setting. At the same time, students should realize that we are now only beginning to understand the mechanisms whereby the nervous system monitors and modulates functional activities throughout body systems and, conversely, how stimuli remote from the CNS may be integrated into neuronal functions within the brain and spinal cord.

The autonomic nervous system (ANS) is defined traditionally as the self-regulating visceral motor (efferent) portion of the nervous system, although it is now recognized that the ANS has a major visceral afferent component. The ANS is an excellent example of structural and functional integration, encompassing the CNS, PNS, and numerous other body systems. The term *self-regulating* refers to the fact that in many ways the ANS functions independently of conscious control. *Visceral motor* (efferent) identifies the ANS as that part of the nervous system that functions largely to activate or regulate organ systems, including the heart, smooth muscle (e.g., respiratory, vascular, gastrointestinal), and glandular (exocrine and endocrine) tissues. The ANS functions to a large extent in response to environmental stimuli that may originate either outside the body or from within a specific organ or tissue. These sensory signals are carried to the CNS by afferent neuronal connections where they are integrated with other somatic or visceral sensations. An appropriate regulatory efferent response is then transmitted through the ANS to effect an alteration of visceral function if necessary. Therefore external or internal sensations such as pain, temperature, proprioception, touch, pressure, vibration, and stretch may act reflexive to elicit an autonomic response that functions to achieve and maintain homeostasis. Numerous examples of the effects of somatic or visceral sensations on visceral functions that are mediated and regulated through the ANS can be cited; they will become apparent in this chapter as the various functional systems are described. However, in many instances the neurophysiologic mechanisms involved remain poorly understood, primarily because the interneuronal connections that constitute the relevant neuronal pathways have not been described adequately.

It now appears that a more comprehensive definition of the ANS should include conscious control of external factors, such as somatic sensations, which influence the regulatory activity of the ANS. The ANS, although predominantly self-regulatory, is not limited to self-regulation. This is of particular clinical significance because therapeutic intervention that alters somatic or visceral function may have effects in body systems apparently remote from the site of applied therapy. A growing body of evidence suggests that there exists a close correlation between somatic (sensory and motor) functions and visceral (sensory and motor) functions. It appears that somatic and visceral functions are coordinated closely through somatovisceral and viscerosomatic reflex mechanisms involving the ANS, PNS, and CNS. Therefore therapeutic interventions such as vertebral manipulation, ingestion of analgesic or antiinflammatory agents, and even surgery, to name a few, can alter somatic sensations (proprioception, for example) in such a way that visceral functions may become altered. However, as stated previously, the underlying neuronal mechanisms require further elucidation through scientific investigation to understand the complexity of factors that interact to regulate organ function.[1]

The purpose of this chapter is to provide a clear, up-to-date description of the structural and functional anatomy of the ANS. The relevant neuroanatomy is discussed in some detail, focusing on neuronal centers involved with autonomic function within the PNS and CNS as they are currently understood. Throughout this chapter an integrated functional approach is employed in an effort to clarify the complex functional interactions that occur. It is hoped that a sound understanding of the ANS will stimulate students and practitioners to pursue scientific research into this basic and as yet poorly understood area of neuroscience, and that this chapter will provide a firm foundation for future research in chiropractic.

Overview of the Autonomic Nervous System

The autonomic nervous system (ANS) can be subdivided into three components: the sympathetic, parasympathetic, and enteric (intestinal) nervous systems. Each division of the ANS is composed of distinct neuronal populations interconnected by axonal processes that form an integrated functional unit. Neuron pools that make up the sympathetic and parasympathetic divisions are localized either within well-defined nuclei of the brainstem and spinal cord or within ganglia located in the periphery, whereas neurons of the enteric division are isolated in the wall of the gastrointestinal tract. Higher neuronal centers located in the hypothalamus, thalamus, hippocampus, and other areas of the cerebrum function to integrate ascending afferent stimuli from all regions of the body and are the source of descending efferent impulses that function to control and modulate autonomic activity. Like the nerve pathways of somatic portions of the nervous system, the ANS consists of visceral sensory axons that enter the CNS, ascending visceral sensory tracts within the brainstem and spinal cord, visceral reflex arcs, and descending visceral motor tracts that influence neural activity of the sympathetic, parasympathetic, and enteric divisions of the ANS.

The sympathetic and parasympathetic divisions are similar structurally, whereas the enteric division, modulated by other autonomic centers, is distinct structurally and functionally from other components of the nervous system. Sympathetic and parasympathetic divisions both originate from preganglionic neurons located within the CNS that extend thinly myelinated axonal processes that synapse with dendrites of postganglionic neurons located mostly in peripheral ganglia. All preganglionic neurons are similar functionally because, regardless of their location or which autonomic division they are part of, these neurons are cholinergic (Figure 14-1). In contrast, postganglionic neurons extend unmyelinated axonal processes that innervate specific viscera directly. In addition, unlike preganglionic neurons, which secrete the neurotransmitter acetylcholine, postganglionic neurons vary in the transmitters they synthesize and secrete. Sympathetic postganglionic neurons are largely catecholaminergic (those that innervate sweat glands are cholinergic), and parasympathetic postganglionic neurons are entirely cholinergic. Sympathetic postganglionic neurons are further subdivided functionally into α- and β-catecholaminergic neurons, which exert different influences on target tissues. Generally α-catecholaminergic innervation is excitatory to smooth muscle, and β-catecholaminergic stimulation is inhibitory.

The two-neuron chain (pre-postganglionic) pattern of innervation is unique to the ANS and is fundamentally different from the single-neuron innervation pattern that is characteristic of somatic neuronal systems. An anatomic feature that may assist in distinguishing conceptually between the sympathetic and parasympathetic divisions is the characteristic location of the ganglia, which contain postganglionic neurons. Sympathetic ganglia are localized near the CNS, indicating that sympathetic preganglionic axons are mostly short. Axons of parasympathetic preganglionic neurons are long because parasympathetic ganglia are located

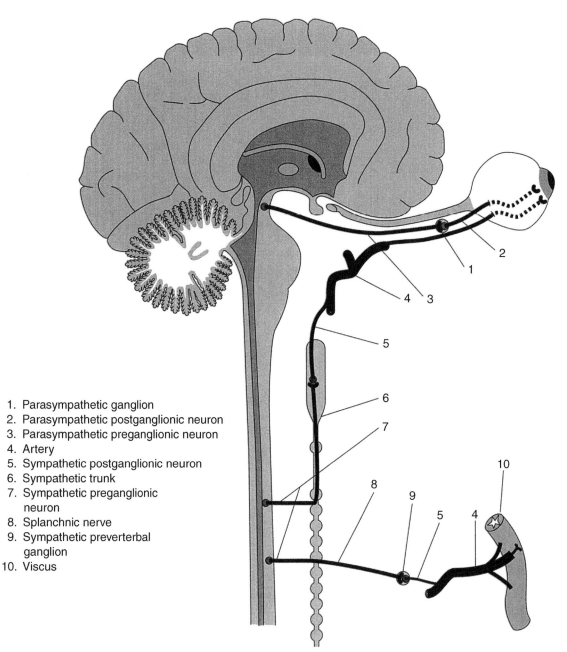

1. Parasympathetic ganglion
2. Parasympathetic postganglionic neuron
3. Parasympathetic preganglionic neuron
4. Artery
5. Sympathetic postganglionic neuron
6. Sympathetic trunk
7. Sympathetic preganglionic
   neuron
8. Splanchnic nerve
9. Sympathetic preverterbal
   ganglion
10. Viscus

Figure 14-1   Schematic diagram illustrating the general structural pattern of peripheral components of the autonomic nervous system. Note that the somata of preganglionic neurons are located within the CNS (brain and spinal cord), whereas postganglionic neuronal somata are in the peripheral ganglia. Generally, sympathetic postganglionic axons are long and course along arteries to reach target viscera (e.g., the eye), and parasympathetic postganglionic axons are short. Also note that all preganglionic neurons are cholinergic *(red)* as are parasympathetic postganglionic neurons, while sympathetic postganglionic neurons are catecholaminergic *(blue)*.

some distance away from the CNS near the viscus they innervate. (See Figure 14-1.)

The sympathetic and parasympathetic divisions of the ANS function to regulate and maintain the internal body environment. At times of emergency when there is a sudden change in external or internal body conditions such as during an argument, an examination, an athletic competition, or a drastic temperature change, the sympathetic division allows the body to cope with these stresses. The sympathetic response to external or internal stress has been referred to as the fight-or-flight reaction. This reaction, which is initiated by autonomic neuronal centers in the hypothalamus, results in increased cardiac output (rate and stroke volume), increased blood supply to appendicular muscles, increased blood glucose levels, and activation of sweat glands, erector pili muscles, and dilator pupillae. In this way, sympathetic activity is protective because it allows for a rapid response to potentially dangerous external factors.

In contrast, the parasympathetic division of the ANS serves a major role to store, conserve, and replenish body energy and can be said to be the vegetative component of the nervous system, functioning primarily at times of rest and digestion. Activation of parasympathetic neuronal centers causes increased secretion of saliva, mucus, and digestive enzymes into the gastrointestinal tract and functions to maintain basal cardiac, respiratory, and metabolic rates. Gut motility is initiated primarily through mechanical reflex activation of the enteric division of the ANS and is modulated by parasympathetic and sympathetic neuronal influences.

Although the functions of the ANS are extremely important for the maintenance of homeostasis and at times for the survival of the individual, hyperactive or hypoactive autonomics caused by pathology, trauma, aberrant physiology, or altered biomechanics can be detrimental and may give rise to characteristic symptomatology. To understand and accurately diagnose clinical presentations of abnormal autonomic function, a sound knowledge of the peripheral and central components of the ANS is necessary.

Peripheral Components of the Autonomic Nervous System

Sympathetic Division

The peripheral components of the sympathetic division, as described by Warwick and Williams,[2] include gray and white communicating rami, two bilaterally symmetric and ganglionated sympathetic trunks that house postganglionic neurons; clusters of prevertebral ganglia, which also house postganglionic neurons; splanchnic nerves, which innervate prevertebral ganglia; and vascular nerve plexuses, which conduct postganglionic axons to target viscera. In fact, most sympathetic postganglionic axons course along arterial vessels to reach viscera that they innervate. Many sympathetic axons within these vascular nerve plexuses penetrate the arterial or arteriolar wall along which they pass to supply smooth muscle in that wall and serve to regulate blood flow and blood pressure. Also in these vascular nerve plexuses are large numbers of parasympathetic axons that innervate viscera and numerous visceral afferent nerve fibers, which are sensory to the viscera and pass back to the CNS by autonomic nerves. In addition, vast numbers of sympathetic postganglionic axons course together with somatic nerve fibers within spinal nerves and their branches to reach target structures in the body wall and limbs. Still other postganglionic axons innervate viscera such as the heart and lungs as direct branches from the sympathetic trunks. The sympathetic division, which is the largest division of the ANS, therefore innervates all regions of the body by three different routes: (1) by arterial nerve plexuses, (2) as a component of somatic nerves, and (3) by direct nerve branches from the sympathetic trunks.

Spinal Origin and Peripheral Distribution of Sympathetic Preganglionic Axons

The sympathetic division is commonly referred to as the thoracolumbar portion of the ANS because all sympathetic preganglionic neurons are localized in the thoracic and upper lumbar (T1-L3) spinal cord segments. Within these cord segments, preganglionic neurons form a well-defined column of cells that is called the intermediolateral cell column because of its intermediate and lateral position between the posterior and anterior horns of gray matter. Axons of sympathetic preganglionic neurons, which are thinly myelinated, exit the spinal cord along with axons of somatic motoneurons through anterior roots of spinal nerves at the same spinal level as their soma of origin. On exiting the intervertebral foramen, preganglionic axons branch from the spinal nerve as a white communicating ramus (white because these axons are myelinated), which joins the paravertebral sympathetic trunk. Large numbers of preganglionic axons end by synapsing with dendritic branches of postganglionic neurons, the cell bodies of which are located in these ganglia. Many preganglionic axons innervate postganglionic cells in trunk ganglia located at the same vertebral level as the intervertebral foramen through which they emerge. Alternatively, numerous preganglionic axons or their collateral branches course along the length of the sympathetic trunk to innervate postganglionic neurons in trunk ganglia located more cranially or caudally than their spinal level of preganglionic origin. (See Figure 14-1.) Although all sympathetic axons enter the sympathetic trunk through white communicating rami, indicating that white rami are evident only at spinal nerve levels T1 through L3, not all of these axons terminate in sympathetic trunk ganglia as just described. Many preganglionic axons branch from the sympathetic trunk without having synapsed and course as splanchnic nerves that end in prevertebral ganglia, where additional postganglionic neuronal cell bodies are located. (See Figure 14-1.)

In summary, preganglionic axons terminate by synapsing with dendrites of postganglionic neurons located in one of two ganglionated structures, either ganglia of the sympathetic trunk or prevertebral ganglia. (Note: One exception to this general scheme that is described later is the medulla of suprarenal glands.) It is also important to realize that each preganglionic neuron normally innervates up to 20 postganglionic cells either within a single ganglion or distributed among a number of paravertebral or prevertebral ganglia. In one early study it was found that the ratio of preganglionic to postganglionic neurons in the superior cervical ganglion (described further) may be as high as 1 to 196.[3] Functionally this innervation pattern allows for divergence of sympathetic activation and coordination of postganglionic response at several spinal levels.[4] For this and other reasons that will become apparent, sympathetic activation results in a mass response, such as generalized constriction of cutaneous arteries, as compared with the more localized parasympathetic response.

Peripheral Distribution of Sympathetic Postganglionic Axons

The peripheral distribution of sympathetic postganglionic axons can be divided into two groups on the basis of the location of postganglionic somata. The first group consists of postganglionic neurons located in ganglia of the paravertebral sympathetic trunk. Postganglionic cells in these ganglia are concerned generally with innervation of viscera in the head, neck, and thorax, including lacrimal and salivary glands, pupillary dilator, heart, and lungs. These neurons also supply superficial structures in the head, neck, body wall, and limbs, including sweat glands, erector pili muscles, and smooth muscle in the walls of arteries and arterioles. The second group consists of postganglionic neurons located in abdominal and pelvic prevertebral ganglia. These postganglionic cells innervate organs associated with the gastrointestinal and urogenital systems, including the stomach, small and large intestines, pancreas, liver, gallbladder, kidneys, urinary bladder, and external genitalia. The following is a detailed description of the origin, course, and anatomic relationships of sympathetic postganglionic axons. The discussion focuses first on branches of the sympathetic trunk and subsequently on the distribution from prevertebral ganglia. A sound knowledge of the postganglionic distribution pattern is crucial to the understanding of autonomic function and clinical conditions that occur when this function is disturbed.

Relationships of the Sympathetic Trunk

The paired sympathetic trunks and their ganglia extend the length of the vertebral column (paravertebral) and are closely related to the anterolateral aspect of vertebral bodies and intervertebral discs throughout their course. For this reason, conditions such as abnormal biomechanics, subluxations, bony spurs, and other pathologies at intervertebral and costovertebral joints, which are commonly seen in chiropractic offices, as well as more severe conditions such as ankylosing spondylitis and severe osteoporosis, may have a profound influence on sympathetic functions.[5] The trunk courses through the cervical region posterior to the carotid sheath, where it is related closely to prevertebral muscles and fascia (Figure 14-2). In the thoracic region the trunk passes along the necks of upper ribs and is related directly to the fibrous capsules of costovertebral joints in the lower thoracic region (Figure 14-3). The sympathetic trunk continues into the abdominal cavity by coursing between the medial arcuate ligament of the diaphragm (anteriorly) and the psoas major muscle (posteriorly). As the trunk

descends through the abdomen, it lies adjacent to lumbar vertebral bodies and intervertebral discs anterior to the psoas major muscle and posterior to the inferior vena cava (on the right) or posterolateral to the abdominal aorta (on the left; Figure 14-4). Near its caudal termination the trunk courses posterior to the common iliac vein, descends anterior to the ala of the sacrum just medial to the anterior sacral foramina, where it lies related directly to the origin of piriformis and terminates finally by joining the trunk of the opposite side anterior to the coccyx and coccygeus muscle as the single ganglion impar (Figure 14-5).

The Cervical Sympathetic Trunk and Its Branches

In the neck extensive fusion of sympathetic trunk ganglia takes place during embryonic development,[2] resulting in three (superior, middle, and inferior) cervical ganglia that are joined by the cervical continuation of the sympathetic trunk. (See Figure 14-2.) The largest is the superior cervical ganglion, which is believed to have developed from the coalescence of the upper four cervical

1. Superior cervical ganglion
2. Right vagus nerve
3. Cervical sympathetic trunk
4. Scalenus anterior
5. Middle cervical ganglion
6. Inferior thyroid artery
7. Phrenic nerve
8. Longus capitis
9. Longus cervicis
10. Subclavian artery (note abnormal position)
11. Trachea
12. Esophagus
13. Recurrent laryngeal nerve
14. Common carotid artery

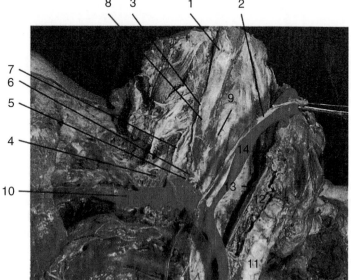

Figure 14-2   Cervical sympathetic trunk within the retropharyngeal space. The prevertebral fascia has been removed and the common carotid artery and vagus nerve are shown reflected to the left with the trachea and pharynx.

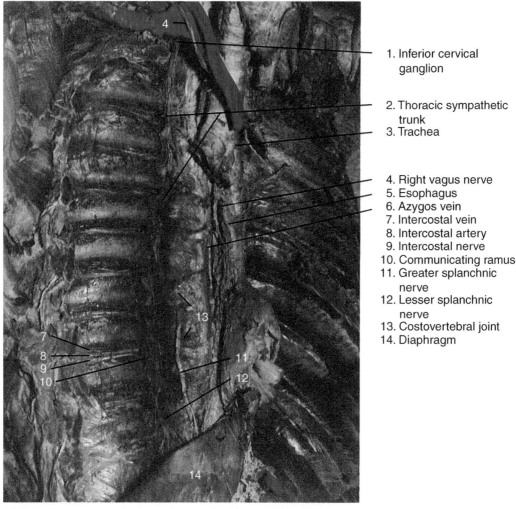

1. Inferior cervical ganglion
2. Thoracic sympathetic trunk
3. Trachea
4. Right vagus nerve
5. Esophagus
6. Azygos vein
7. Intercostal vein
8. Intercostal artery
9. Intercostal nerve
10. Communicating ramus
11. Greater splanchnic nerve
12. Lesser splanchnic nerve
13. Costovertebral joint
14. Diaphragm

Figure 14-3   Thoracic sympathetic trunk related to thoracic vertebral bodies, intervertebral discs, and costovertebral joints.

ganglia.[2] This ganglion lies at the level of C1-C3 vertebrae interposed between the carotid sheath anteriorly and the longus capitis posteriorly and, like the lower cervical sympathetic trunk, is enveloped by prevertebral fascia. Preganglionic innervation of the superior cervical ganglion, as in the middle and inferior cervical ganglia, is derived from neurons in the upper three thoracic spinal cord segments.

Postganglionic axons of neurons in the superior cervical ganglion are distributed to target struc-

tures along branches of the internal carotid artery or through a number of direct nerve branches from the ganglion. In addition, the first four cervical spinal nerves, like all spinal nerves, receive gray communicating rami composed of unmyelinated axons of postganglionic neurons from the superior ganglion and its caudal connection with the middle ganglion. These postganglionic axons are distributed to blood vessels, erector pili muscles, and sweat glands in the territory of each of these spinal nerves. Extending from the superior limit of

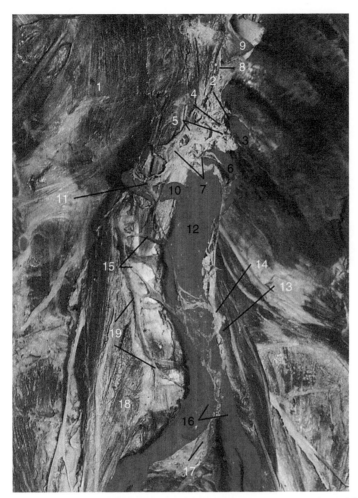

1. Diaphragm
2. Hepatic artery
3. Splenic artery
4. Celiac trunk
5. Celiac ganglion
   plexus
6. Superior mesenteric
   artery
7. Superior mesenteric
   ganglion and plexus
8. Vagal trunk
9. Esophagus
10. Renal artery
11. Aorticorenal ganglion
    and plexus
12. Abdominal aorta
13. Inferior mesenteric
    artery
14. Inferior mesenteric
    ganglion
15. Lumbar splanchnic
    nerves
16. Common iliac arteries
17. Superior hypogastric
    plexus and ganglion
18. Psoas major muscle
19. Lumbar sympathetic
    trunk

Figure 14-4   Lumbar sympathetic trunk related to psoas major muscle and lumbar vertebral column. Also shown are sympathetic prevertebral ganglia dispersed along major branches of the abdominal aorta.

the superior cervical ganglion, the internal carotid nerve conducts postganglionic axons to the internal carotid artery, which lies immediately anterior to the ganglion within the carotid sheath. The internal carotid nerve in this way forms the internal carotid plexus, which supplies the artery and its branches to regulate cerebral blood flow, although this is now thought to be only a minor role of the sympathetic division. The internal carotid plexus enters the cranial cavity along the surface of the internal carotid artery as it passes through the carotid canal and provides the clinically important sympathetic innervation to

arteries that supply the cerebrum, meninges of the anterior and middle cranial fossae, hypophysis, orbital contents, and the upper parts of the face and scalp. It is this portion of the sympathetic division that may be involved in the cause of migraine headache. As the internal carotid artery passes through the cavernous sinus, the nerve plexus on its surface extends branches that join the oculomotor, trochlear, abducens, and ophthalmic nerves through which sympathetic postganglionic axons are distributed. Thrombosis of the cavernous sinus, as may occur with infections of the orbit, nasal cavity, paranasal sinuses, and tympanic

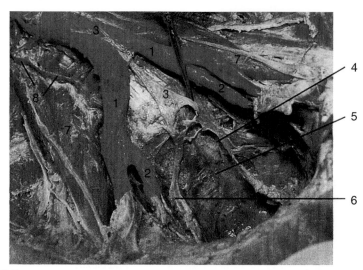

1. Common iliac artery
2. Internal iliac artery
3. Superior hypogastric plexus
4. Pelvic sympathetic trunk
5. Median sacral artery
6. Inferior hypogastric plexus
7. Psoas major muscle
8. Lumbar sympathetic trunk

Figure 14-5   Pelvic sympathetic trunk and hypogastric plexuses.

cavity, may therefore impinge on these cranial nerves, leading to characteristic cranial nerve signs and symptoms, including those associated with sympathetic blockage, as observed in a classic Horner's syndrome. The signs associated with sympathetic nerve blockage at this site include ptosis caused by the loss of sympathetic innervation to the levator palpebrae superius through the oculomotor nerve and miosis caused by unopposed parasympathetic activation of the sphincter pupillae. Sympathetic postganglionic axons reach the eye to supply the dilator pupillae and arterial vessels of the eyeball along two routes. Some axons branch from the oculomotor nerve, pass through the ciliary ganglion without synapsing, and enter the eye with parasympathetic fibers in short ciliary nerves. Other postganglionic fibers continue along the nasociliary branch of the ophthalmic nerve (CNVI) to enter the eyeball as long ciliary branches.

The internal carotid plexus also supplies sympathetic innervation to arteries and mucous glands in the tympanic cavity through the caroticotympanic nerve, which joins the tympanic branch of the glossopharyngeal nerve (CNIX) to enter the tympanic plexus. In addition, arteries and mucous glands in the nasal cavity, nasopharynx, hard palate, and soft palate receive sympathetic innervation by way of the deep petrosal branch of the

internal carotid plexus, which joins the greater petrosal nerve in the foramen lacerum.

The greater petrosal nerve traverses the pterygoid canal to reach the pterygopalatine ganglion through which sympathetic axons pass without synapsing and enters the infraorbital and nasopalatine branches of the maxillary nerve (CNV₂). These sympathetic postganglionic axons supply the lacrimal gland and mucosa of the nasal cavity, paranasal sinuses, nasopharynx, hard palate, and soft palate.

In addition to the internal carotid plexus, other nerve branches of the superior cervical ganglion innervate structures within the posterior cranial fossa, oral cavity, neck, and thorax. Small branches from the lateral aspect of the ganglion join the vagus (CNX) and hypoglossal (CNXII) nerves in the carotid sheath and are distributed with these two cranial nerves to blood vessels and mucous glands in the mucosa of the oral cavity, oropharynx, pharynx, larynx, trachea, and esophagus, as well as the submandibular, sublingual, and intralingual salivary glands.

The jugular nerve branches from the superior cervical ganglion to connect with the glossopharyngeal (CNIX) and vagus (CNX) nerves to also innervate the oral cavity and oropharynx. In addition, the meninges in the posterior cranial fossa receive sympathetic innervation through a plexus of postganglionic axons that originate in the superior cervical ganglion and join the internal jugular vein to enter the cranial cavity by way of the jugular foramen.

The cervical sympathetic trunk also contributes to the cardiac plexus through cardiac branches that arise bilaterally from all three cervical ganglia. The cardiac branch of the superior cervical ganglion courses inferiorly along the anterior aspect of the longus cervicis muscle (see Figure 14-2) partly enveloped by prevertebral fascia, where it may be influenced by damage or increased tonicity of this muscle. On the right the cardiac branch passes most commonly posterior to the subclavian artery, where it is related directly to the cupula of parietal pleura and may be affected by pathology in the apical region of the lung. The nerve continues into the thorax on the posterolateral aspect of the brachiocephalic trunk to enter the cardiac plexus posterior to the arch of the aorta, although some axons may contribute to the anterior cardiac plexus. In contrast, the left cardiac branch of the superior cervical ganglion enters the thorax most commonly along the anterior aspect of the common carotid artery to reach the anterior portion of the cardiac plexus anterolateral to the arch of the aorta. Like the right cardiac branch, the left nerve may contribute to the posterior cardiac plexus as well. En route, both the right and left cardiac branches of the superior cervical ganglia commonly receive communications from the external laryngeal, recurrent laryngeal, and cardiac branches of the vagus (CNX) nerve, indicating that, on reaching the cardiac plexus, the cardiac nerves are mixed, having both sympathetic and parasympathetic components. In addition, cardiac nerve branches of the middle and inferior cervical ganglia commonly have communicating branches with that of the superior cervical ganglion.

The cardiac plexus also receives direct cardiac branches from the upper four or five thoracic sympathetic trunk ganglia (described further) and is divided into anterior (superficial) and posterior (deep) plexuses. The anterior cardiac plexus is dispersed along the anterior aspect of the right pulmonary artery inferior to the arch of the aorta.

The posterior cardiac plexus receives input from the anterior plexus and is located near the bifurcation of the pulmonary trunk posterior to the arch of the aorta. Scattered amongst the nerve fibers of the cardiac plexus are small ganglia that contain parasympathetic postganglionic neurons that innervate the heart. (See the following discussion.) Sympathetic postganglionic axons course through the cardiac plexus along the right and left coronary arteries and their branches, which they innervate. They then penetrate the atrial and ventricular walls to supply cardiac muscle directly. Whereas the anterior cardiac plexus supplies some input to the right coronary and left pulmonary plexuses, most cardiac innervation reaches the heart by way of the posterior (deep) cardiac plexus, which can be divided into right and left halves. The right half of the posterior cardiac plexus supplies the right coronary plexus, right atrium and ventricle, and right pulmonary plexus and helps to form the left coronary plexus. The left half of the posterior cardiac plexus receives some input from the anterior (superficial) cardiac plexus and innervates the left atrium and ventricle, the left coronary plexus, and the left pulmonary plexus.

Most sympathetic postganglionic neurons are catecholaminergic including those that innervate the heart and coronary vessels, and their activation causes the release of norepinephrine (β-catecholaminergic). Interestingly, this neurotransmitter performs a dual role to control and regulate cardiac function. Cardiac myofibers are stimulated by norepinephrine to contract more forcefully and more rapidly. Concomitantly, smooth muscle in the walls of coronary arteries is inhibited, causing dilation of these vessels and increased blood flow to the heart, although Berne and Levy[6] suggest that the coronary circulation responds primarily to the metabolic needs of the myocardium and is predominantly under nonneuronal control. In fact, the sympathetic division may serve its greatest regulatory role of cardiac function indirectly by affecting the release of norepinephrine and epinephrine into the bloodstream from medullary cells of the suprarenal glands.

In addition to sympathetic postganglionic axons, visceral sensory (afferent) axons are also present in all cardiac branches of the sympathetic trunk, except those arising from the superior cervical ganglia. Cardiac pain is transmitted through these sympathetic cardiac nerves to upper thoracic spinal cord segments and for this reason may be referred to the medial aspect of the arm and adjacent thoracic wall. These neuronal pathways also may provide a viscerosomatic reflex mechanism whereby cardiac pain provokes increased tonus and even spasm of muscles innervated by upper thoracic spinal cord segments, as observed in angina pectoris and cardiac arrest.

From the superior cervical ganglion the sympathetic trunk courses inferiorly along the anterior aspect of the longus capitis and longus cervicis muscles to connect with the middle cervical ganglion at the level of the sixth cervical vertebra. (See Figure 14-2.) Occasionally this ganglion is poorly defined or absent, in which case the postganglionic neurons normally present in the middle ganglion are dispersed along the length of the cervical sympathetic trunk. The middle cervical ganglion is formed most commonly by the coalescence of the fifth and sixth cervical ganglia and is related to the inferior thyroid artery, which is innervated by a sympathetic plexus derived from this ganglion. Sympathetic postganglionic axons are distributed to branches of this artery that supply deep posterior neck muscles, prevertebral muscles, and the external vertebral arterial plexus as well as the thyroid and parathyroid glands. Postganglionic axons derived from neurons predominantly in the middle and inferior cervical ganglia form a nerve plexus on the external carotid artery. This external carotid nerve plexus supplies the artery and follows its branches to innervate structures supplied by the artery in the neck and face.

Postganglionic axons from the middle ganglion commonly enter the fifth and sixth (occasionally the fourth and seventh as well) cervical spinal nerves by gray communicating rami and are distributed to the periphery through these nerves and their branches to innervate sweat glands, erector pili muscles, and cutaneous and muscular arteries in the shoulder and upper limb regions. Because of the cervical origin of postganglionic axons that control and regulate blood flow to the upper limb,

any condition that interferes with this autonomic function, including trauma, pathology, spastic neck musculature, and abnormal somatovisceral reflexes, may compromise this blood supply and lead to numbness, tingling, and pain the upper limb, a condition commonly associated with thoracic outlet syndrome.

The cardiac plexus also receives a large cardiac branch from the middle cervical ganglion, which courses along the lateral border of the longus cervicis muscle. On the right, this cardiac nerve passes posterior to the common carotid artery; it is related directly to the trachea and enters the right half of the posterior cardiac plexus. The cardiac branch of the left middle cervical ganglion follows a similar course into the thorax but passes between the left common carotid and subclavian arteries to enter the left half of the posterior cardiac plexus.

A number of nerve cords that form the inferior continuation of the sympathetic trunk join the middle cervical ganglion to the inferior cervical (cervicothoracic) ganglion. Some nerve fibers of the cervical sympathetic trunk pass posterior and anterior to the vertebral artery to reach the inferior ganglion and may contribute to the nerve plexus around this vessel. A large nerve cord called the ansa subclavia passes inferiorly and anteriorly to the origin of the subclavian artery, loops around this vessel just medial to the internal thoracic artery, and joins the inferior cervical ganglion posterior to the subclavian artery, The ansa subclavia commonly contributes to the nerve plexuses surrounding both the subclavian and internal thoracic arteries. (See Figure 14-2.) The inferior cervical ganglion is considerably larger than the middle ganglion and is formed by the coalescence of the C7, C8, and T1 ganglia. Other names given to the inferior ganglion are the cervicothoracic ganglion, because of its embryonic origin, and the stellate ganglion, because of its shape. The inferior cervical ganglion is positioned anterior to the C7 transverse process. It extends inferiorly to the neck of the first rib just posterolateral to the origin of the vertebral artery. (See Figure 14-2.) The ganglion is also related directly to the cupula of parietal pleura and the lower vertebral attachment of the scalenus medius muscle. In some individuals the lateral border of the longus cervicis muscle is also related to the medial aspect of the inferior ganglion.

Postganglionic axons from neurons in the inferior cervical ganglion join the C7, C8, and T1 spinal nerves through gray communicating rami; they are distributed by these nerves to the periphery including cutaneous and muscular arteries of the forearm and hand. Other nerve branches of the inferior cervical ganglion are a cardiac branch, which joins the posterior cardiac plexus along with the cardiac branch from the middle cervical ganglion, and vascular branches, which form plexuses on the subclavian and vertebral arteries as well as on the thyrocervical and costocervical trunks. The subclavian plexus extends into the axilla along the first part of the axillary artery and its superior thoracic branch, but it rarely reaches arteries in the upper limb because these appendicular vessels receive direct sympathetic innervation from nerves of the brachial plexus. The large vertebral branch of the inferior cervical ganglion courses along the vertebral artery through foramina transversarii to form a vertebral nerve plexus, which supplies arteries to the cervical spinal cord, external and internal vertebral arterial plexuses, and deep muscles of the neck. The vertebral nerve plexus enters the cranial cavity with the vertebral arteries through the foramen magnum and courses along the length of the basilar artery and its branches as far as the posterior cerebral arteries. In this way postganglionic axons derived from the inferior cervical ganglion primarily supply sympathetic innervation that functions to regulate blood flow to occipital and temporal lobes of the cerebrum and cerebellum as well as vital neuronal centers in the brainstem and cervical spinal cord. It has been suggested recently, however, that neural control of cerebral blood flow may not be as important as once thought. Rather, it may be that the flow rate of blood in cerebral arterioles is regulated primarily by regional metabolic needs.[6] Near the posterior portion of the circulus arteriosus, the vertebral sympathetic plexus meets that of the internal carotid plexus. If sympathetic function in the inferior cervical ganglion is compromised, as

may happen in a variety of clinical conditions (for example, cervical rib; abnormal biomechanics of the lower cervical and upper thoracic spine), a number of signs and symptoms associated with the syndrome referred to as vertebrobasilar insufficiency are observed. Upper limb symptoms may be present, resulting in a classic thoracic outlet syndrome. Hyperactive sympathetics may give rise to tinnitus, hearing loss, dizziness, facial nerve (CNVII) palsy, blurred vision, nausea, and vomiting, as well as cardiac and respiratory arrhythmia,[7] which result from insufficient blood flow to the brainstem and cerebellum. Migraine-type headache also has been reported to occur after whiplash injury to the cervical spine[8] and may be the result of trauma or pressure on the cervical sympathetic trunks.

The Thoracic Sympathetic Trunk and Its Branches

The thoracic sympathetic trunk consists of a series of small ganglia that vary somewhat in number. Generally there is one ganglion for each thoracic spinal nerve, although the first thoracic ganglion is most commonly fused with the inferior cervical ganglion. As the sympathetic trunk descends through the thorax, the ganglia come to lie in direct contact with the fibrous capsules of costovertebral joints, except in the lower thorax, where they lie more medially adjacent to T10-11 and T11-12 intervertebral discs. (See Figure 14-3.)

Numerous nerve branches arise from the thoracic sympathetic trunk, some of which are composed of postganglionic axons of neurons in thoracic trunk ganglia, and other branches that consist of preganglionic axons of neurons located in the thoracic spinal cord. The nerves composed of preganglionic axons that innervate postganglionic cells in prevertebral ganglia are referred to as splanchnic (visceral) nerves and are described after the following description of the distribution of postganglionic nerve branches of the thoracic trunk.

Each thoracic spinal nerve receives both white and gray communicating rami from the sympathetic trunk and its ganglia, with the white ramus joining the spinal nerve slightly more distal than the gray ramus. (See Figure 14-3.) Occasionally, the white communicating rami are fused and only one mixed white and gray ramus is present. Each spinal nerve conducts these postganglionic axons to sweat glands and erector pili muscles, as well as cutaneous and muscular arteries within the thoracic and abdominal walls. Of particular clinical importance is the sympathetic nerve plexus formed by postganglionic branches of the thoracic sympathetic trunk on the aorta and its intercostal, esophageal, and bronchial branches. Segmental arteries that originate from intercostal arteries carry sympathetic innervation to the external and internal vertebral arterial plexuses and its radicular branches. By this route the autonomic nervous system can function to regulate blood flow to bones, joints, and ligaments of the thoracic vertebral column and structures within the spinal canal, including the spinal cord, spinal nerve roots, and meninges.

The pulmonary plexus receives direct input of sympathetic postganglionic axons from branches of upper thoracic (T2-T5) sympathetic trunk ganglia as well as indirect input from the anterior and posterior cardiac plexuses. As mentioned previously, the posterior cardiac plexus is formed in part by sympathetic postganglionic axons that enter the plexus directly from upper thoracic (T2-T5) trunk ganglia. From the pulmonary and cardiac plexuses, a small network of sympathetic postganglionic axons branch away to supply the mucosa of the trachea and esophagus. Within the root of the lung bilaterally, sympathetic axons from the pulmonary plexus form a delicate nerve plexus along the surfaces of pulmonary and bronchial arteries as well as on the bronchial tree to supply smooth muscle in the walls of these structures. Activation of the sympathetic division causes release of norepinephrine, which is inhibitory to bronchial smooth muscle and results in bronchodilation. It is excitatory to arterial smooth muscle, causing constriction of pulmonary and bronchial arteries. However, neuronal control of bronchial smooth muscle has been shown to be relatively insignificant when compared with the bronchiolar response to local tissue factors.[8] For example, circulating levels of norepinephrine and epinephrine secreted into the bloodstream by suprarenal glands during sympathetic activation act as potent β-catecholaminergic receptor stimulants that elicit rapid dilation of the bronchial tree.[9,10] In contrast, other local factors such as histamine and the slow reactive substance of anaphylaxis that are released from mast cells into lung tissues after exposure to allergens act as bronchoconstrictors.[11] It appears that local physiologic needs of the tissues serve as the primary regulatory control of pulmonary function, whereas direct ANS influences are limited.

Similarly, the ANS is believed to have little control over the pulmonary circulation during normal daily activity. Pulmonary vascular resistance, which is a measure of the freedom with which arterial blood flows through the pulmonary circulation, is known to be inversely proportional to cardiac output.[12,13] That is, pulmonary and bronchiolar arteries expand or collapse passively in response to an increase or decrease, respectively, in blood pressure.[14] However, a clinically significant role of the sympathetic division in the regulation of pulmonary circulation has been suggested by Fishman,[15] who indicated that pulmonary obstruction may reflexly stimulate sympathetic vasomotor activity to cause generalized constriction of pulmonary vessels and increased arterial pressure in the lung. It is also thought that constriction of larger pulmonary veins in response to sympathetic stimulation may be the primary mechanism whereby blood is shunted from the pulmonary to the systemic circulation when needed. In summary, the principal mechanism whereby the sympathetic division regulates pulmonary function is humeral because, as in the control of cardiac function, it has its greatest influence through activation of the suprarenal glands.

As mentioned previously, there are three pairs of bilaterally symmetric splanchnic (visceral) nerves, called the greater, lesser, and least (lowest) splanchnic nerves, that arise from the thoracic sympathetic trunks. The splanchnic nerves are composed of preganglionic axons of neurons located in the intermediolateral cell column of the thoracolumbar spinal cord and do not synapse within sympathetic trunk ganglia. Instead, these axons pass through the sympathetic trunk, branch medially away as splanchnic nerves, and terminate finally by synapsing with dendrites of postganglionic neurons in prevertebral sympathetic ganglia. (See Figures 14-1 and 14-3.) The prevertebral ganglia are located anterior to the lumbar spine and sacrum in association with major branches of the abdominal aorta. The largest splanchnic nerve branch of the thoracic sympathetic trunk is the greater splanchnic nerve, which is formed by five roots arising from the fifth through ninth (sometimes tenth) thoracic trunk ganglia. (See Figure 14-3.) Most preganglionic axons within the roots of the greater splanchnic nerve originate in the thoracic spinal cord segments adjacent to these ganglia. However, a small proportion of preganglionic neurons in upper thoracic spinal segments also may contribute to this nerve. The lesser splanchnic nerve is somewhat smaller, having only two roots of origin normally from the ninth and tenth (sometimes tenth and eleventh) thoracic trunk ganglia. The least (lowest) splanchnic nerve is the smallest, arising singly from the last thoracic trunk ganglion. All three splanchnic nerves course anteromedially and inferiorly along vertebral bodies and intervertebral discs to reach the diaphragm. The greater and lesser splanchnic nerves normally gain access to the abdominal cavity by piercing the crus of the diaphragm, and the least splanchnic nerve enters the abdomen with the sympathetic trunk by passing between the medial arcuate ligament of the diaphragm and the psoas major muscle. Often an enlargement of the greater splanchnic nerve called the splanchnic ganglion is present just before the nerve pierces the diaphragm.

Although the innervation of prevertebral ganglia by splanchnic nerves is somewhat variable, a general pattern can be described. The greater splanchnic nerve terminates primarily by innervating postganglionic neurons in the celiac ganglion. This large prevertebral ganglion is located anterior to the crus of the diaphragm just lateral to the origin of the celiac trunk, a large branch of the abdominal aorta at the level of the twelfth thoracic vertebral body. To a lesser degree the greater splanchnic nerve also innervates the aorticorenal ganglion, a relatively large cluster of post-

ganglionic neurons that is dispersed along the abdominal aorta near the origins of the superior mesenteric and renal arteries. The greater splanchnic nerve also innervates the suprarenal gland (described later). The lesser splanchnic nerve, which courses with the greater splanchnic nerve, supplies the celiac ganglion minimally and sends most of its axons to innervate the aorticorenal and renal ganglia. The innervation pattern of the least (lowest) splanchnic nerve is to small clusters of postganglionic neurons scattered along the renal artery and in the hilum of the kidney. For this reason the least (lowest) splanchnic nerve is often referred to as the renal nerve. The distribution of postganglionic axons of neurons in the prevertebral ganglia is described after consideration of the suprarenal glands.

The suprarenal glands are discussed in some detail because of the important functional role these glands play in the sympathetic division of the ANS. These glands are supplied by the greater splanchnic nerve, an innervation pattern that may appear unusual in that preganglionic axons innervate medullary cells of the gland directly. However, when one considers the embryonic origin of the gland, this innervation pattern can be better understood. Histologically the gland is composed of a layered cortex that develops from mesodermal cells near the developing dorsal mesentery of the embryo and a central medulla derived from neuroepithelial cells of the neural crest.[16] The medullary cells of the gland in this way develop from the same primordium as all sympathetic postganglionic neurons and may be considered to be homologous to postganglionic neurons. Like most sympathetic postganglionic neurons, medullary cells synthesize and secrete the hormones (neurotransmitters) epinephrine and norepinephrine, which when released into the bloodstream evoke a generalized sympathetic (fight-or-flight) response.

The suprarenal nerve plexus is composed of axons of the greater splanchnic nerve, which reach the plexus on the anterior aspect of the crus of the diaphragm by passing through the celiac ganglion and plexus without synapsing. The suprarenal glands, located just lateral to the crus of the diaphragm adjacent to the superomedial pole of each kidney, are said to have the largest sympathetic innervation relative to size when compared with other organs. This is understandable considering the important role this gland serves during sympathetic activation. Preganglionic axons enter the gland and terminate on two types of medullary cells called chromaffin and ganglion cells. (Note: Cortical layers of the gland that function to synthesize and secrete glucocorticoid, mineralocorticoid, and corticosteroid hormones are not innervated.) The chromaffin cells, innervated by synapse-like junctions, synthesize the catecholamines epinephrine and norepinephrine. These products then are stored in separate cytoplasmic granules recognized at the electron microscopic level to be distinct for one specific hormone. On stimulation of chromaffin cells by preganglionic axons, the granules bind with the plasmalemma and release their contents into adjacent blood vessels. The second medullary cell type innervated by preganglionic axons is a multipolar neuron-like cell referred to as a ganglion cell. However, the axons of ganglion cells and their terminations have not been studied definitively. It is possible that ganglion cells may serve to magnify incoming excitatory sympathetic stimuli and disseminate the signals to chromaffin cells. After release into the bloodstream, these hormones circulate throughout the body and act to elicit the characteristic sympathetic response to stressful conditions that the individual may be facing.

The distribution of postganglionic axons from neurons in prevertebral ganglia follows a characteristic pattern; the axons course through delicate nerve plexuses formed on the external surfaces of large branches of the abdominal aorta near the ganglion in which they originate. Each arterial nerve plexus supplies smooth muscle in the wall of the vessels along which it passes and terminates by innervating viscera supplied by the vessel. Axons of neurons in the celiac ganglion are distributed along branches of the celiac trunk, which come off the aorta at the level of the twelfth thoracic vertebra near the aortic hiatus of the diaphragm. The right and left celiac ganglia are interconnected by a massive nerve plexus called the celiac plexus that extends inferiorly to the level of the first lumbar

vertebra and surrounds both the celiac trunk and origin of the superior mesenteric artery. (See Figure 14-4.) Entering the plexus from each side are the greater and lesser splanchnic nerves and parasympathetic axons from the vagus (CNX) nerve (discussed further). Exiting the celiac plexus are sympathetic preganglionic axons, which supply the suprarenal glands, parasympathetic (vagal) axons, and sympathetic postganglionic axons that enter subsidiary plexuses to be distributed to abdominal viscera. These secondary nerve plexuses include the phrenic plexus, the left gastric, splenic, and hepatic plexuses, which course along branches of the celiac trunk, and the renal, gonadal, superior mesenteric, and inferior mesenteric plexuses, which follow lower branches of the abdominal aorta.

The phrenic plexus is small and sends nerve axons along the inferior phrenic arteries to the diaphragm and suprarenal glands. This sparse plexus contains some preganglionic axons that have traversed the celiac plexus without synapsing to aid in the innervation of the suprarenal glands. Also contained in the phrenic plexus are some postganglionic axons, which innervate smooth muscle in the inferior vena cava and then join the much larger hepatic nerve plexus. Axons that are sensory to the gallbladder also enter the hepatic plexus as branches from the phrenic nerve (a mixed somatic and visceral nerve).

Sympathetic postganglionic axons in the hepatic plexus reach the liver along branches of the hepatic artery and portal vein. The innervation that reaches the liver by this route is believed to function only to regulate blood flow to that organ because the characteristic glycogenolytic response of the liver to sympathetic activation is a result of increased circulating levels of epinephrine and norepinephrine derived from suprarenal glands. A small cystic plexus originating from the hepatic plexus contains sympathetic postganglionic axons that are inhibitory to smooth muscle in the wall of the gallbladder but excitatory to the sphincter of the common bile duct. The hepatic plexus also contributes to the nerve plexus surrounding the gastroduodenal branch of the hepatic artery to innervate the right side of the stomach, duodenum, head of the pancreas, and the most distal portion of the common bile duct. (Note: Sympathetic innervation of the gastrointestinal tract functions to inhibit neuronal activity in the enteric division of the ANS, described subsequently.)

Also extending from the celiac plexus are the left gastric and splenic plexuses, which follow the arteries of the same name and terminate by innervating the left side of the stomach, tail of the pancreas, and the spleen. The sympathetic innervation of the spleen is excitatory to smooth muscle in the capsule of this organ and causes expulsion of the relatively large reservoir of blood into the general circulation at times of need, such as during exercise or serious blood loss caused by injury. More importantly, sympathetic influences on the spleen and other lymphoid organs function to regulate the immune system.[17] The immunoregulatory role of the sympathetic nervous system is elaborated in the final section of this chapter.

The renal plexus is derived from the more inferior portion of the celiac plexus as well as the aorticorenal and renal ganglia, thus receiving input from the lesser and least (lowest) splanchnic nerves. Ganglia within the renal plexus give rise to postganglionic axons, which follow and supply branches of the renal artery and innervate glomeruli and convoluted tubules in the renal cortex. Both afferent and efferent arterioles of the glomeruli are innervated; however, the influence of sympathetic innervation on the glomerular filtration rate is only minor because neuronal control is superseded by renal autoregulatory mechanisms.[18,19] From the renal plexus, the upper part of the ureter and gonadal (testicular/ovarian) arteries also receive sympathetic innervation, which is excitatory to smooth muscle in their walls.

Finally, the superior and inferior mesenteric plexuses are located on the anterior aspect of the abdominal aorta surrounding the origin of the corresponding artery. The two plexuses contain postganglionic neurons in small ganglia dispersed along the first part of each vessel. Although some postganglionic axons from the celiac and aorticorenal ganglia enter the superior mesenteric plexus, its principle input is from the lesser splanchnic nerve, which terminates in ganglia within the plexus. Postganglionic axons from

superior mesenteric ganglia follow all the branches of the superior mesenteric artery to supply inhibitory input to the enteric division of the ANS within the jejunum, ileum, vermiform appendix, cecum, ascending colon, and most of the transverse colon. However, sympathetic innervation of the ileocecal sphincter, which reaches this site by the same route, is excitatory. The inferior mesenteric ganglia, which receives only a minor innervation from the celiac plexus, as well as lesser and least splanchnic nerves are supplied primarily by lumbar splanchnic nerves and are described with these nerves in the next section of this chapter.

The Lumbosacral Sympathetic Trunk and Its Branches

The lumbar portion of the sympathetic trunk, a continuation of the thoracic trunk, courses along the anterolateral aspect of the lumbar vertebral column within the connective tissue of the extraperitoneal space. (See Figures 14-4 and 14-5.) The lumbar trunk and its four ganglia lie in contact with medial fibers of the psoas major muscle and pass posterior to the common iliac vessels to gain access to the pelvis. Throughout their course in the abdomen the right trunk is related to the posterior aspect of the inferior vena cava, and the left trunk passes posterolaterally to the abdominal aorta. Both right and left trunks are surrounded by abdominal lymphatics, lumbar arteries, and veins, as well as connective tissues of the region. On entering the pelvis, the trunks lie anterior to the upper fibers of the anterior sacroiliac ligament and medial fibers of the iliacus muscle. (See Figure 14-5.) At this point the sacral sympathetic trunks course inferomedially just posterior to the internal iliac vessels and anterior to fibers of the piriformis muscle. The right and left trunks end anterior to the coccygeal attachment of coccygeus muscle by forming a small, unpaired ganglion impar.

Only the first two or three lumbar spinal nerves emit white communicating rami to connect with the lumbar sympathetic trunks. It should be recalled that the reason for this is that the intermediolateral cell column is present in the spinal cord down to segments L2 or L3 only. Gray communicating rami, however, are present throughout the lumbosacral region. These gray rami consist of axons of postganglionic neurons within lumbosacral trunk ganglia, which join somatic nerves of the lumbosacral plexus to supply sympathetic innervation to cutaneous and muscular arteries, erector pili muscles, and sweat glands in the lower abdominal wall, buttock, perineum, and lower limb. The gray rami in the lumbar region are relatively long when compared with those in the cervical, thoracic, and sacral regions, because to reach the lumbosacral plexus they course with lumbar arteries (which are innervated) around lumbar vertebral bodies and pass medial to the fibrous attachments of the psoas major muscle.

As in the thoracic region, many preganglionic axons that enter the lumbar sympathetic trunk do not synapse in ganglia of the trunk; instead they branch from the trunk as four lumbar splanchnic nerves to terminate in prevertebral ganglia. Of these, the first and second lumbar splanchnic nerves, which originate from the superior two or three lumbar ganglia, course posterior to the inferior vena cava and onto the anterior surface of the abdominal aorta, where they end primarily in inferior mesenteric ganglia. In most individuals the first lumbar splanchnic nerve also contributes in a minor way to the innervation of the celiac, aorticorenal, and renal ganglia. Postganglionic neurons scattered along the origin of the inferior mesenteric artery within the inferior mesenteric plexus give rise to axons that follow the artery and its branches to supply sympathetic input to the enteric nervous system in the left half of the transverse colon, descending colon, sigmoid colon, and superior part of the rectum.

The third and fourth lumbar splanchnic nerves are branches of the third and fourth lumbar trunk ganglia, which terminate by synapsing in small ganglia within the superior hypogastric (prelumbar) plexus. The third lumbar splanchnic nerve courses anteriorly to the abdominal aorta and common iliac artery, and the fourth lumbar splanchnic nerve passes posteriorly to the common iliac vessels medial to the sympathetic trunk to reach the superior hypogastric plexus. The superior hypogastric plexus is located somewhat to the

left of the median plane anterior to the bifurcation of the abdominal aorta at the level of the fourth lumbar vertebral body. (See Figure 14-5.) It extends inferiorly anterior to the left common iliac artery, median sacral artery, fifth lumbar vertebral body, and sacral promontory. In this position the plexus is related to the medial end of the sigmoid mesocolon and superior rectal vessels, which may receive nerve fibers from this plexus. The superior hypogastric plexus is continuous inferiorly with the right and left inferior hypogastric plexuses through the right and left hypogastric nerves. (See Figure 14-5.) Preganglionic axons of the third and fourth lumbar splanchnic nerves terminate by synapsing with postganglionic neurons scattered mostly amongst the nerve fibers of the superior hypogastric plexus and, to a much lesser degree, the inferior hypogastric plexus. Axons of these postganglionic cells innervate the inferior half of the ureter and contribute to nerve plexuses on gonadal (testicular/ovarian) arteries. Many axons from postganglionic neurons in the superior hypogastric plexus exit the plexus inferiorly as the right and left hypogastric nerves. These sympathetic axons pass through the inferior hypogastric plexus without synapsing for the most part to innervate pelvic viscera either as direct nerve branches to the specific organ or indirectly by passing along branches of the internal iliac artery.

In males, the inferior hypogastric plexus lies in contact with the lateral aspect of the rectum and posterior aspect of the urinary bladder, seminal vesicle, and prostate gland. In females, this plexus is similarly related to the rectum and urinary bladder and lies adjacent to the cervix of the uterus, fornix of the vagina, and the inferior portion of the uterine broad ligament. The inferior hypogastric plexus also contains small clusters of postganglionic neurons, but these are predominantly parasympathetic (described later). In summary, the sympathetic preganglionic supply for pelvic viscera originates in lower thoracic and upper lumbar (T10-L2 or L3) spinal cord segments, branches from the lumbar sympathetic trunk as lumbar splanchnic nerves, and terminates in small prevertebral ganglia, mostly in the superior hypogastric plexus. A small number of sympathetic preganglionic axons pass through both superior and inferior hypogastric plexuses to innervate postganglionic neurons in the wall of the urinary bladder.

Sympathetic postganglionic axons, mainly from cells in the superior hypogastric plexus, innervate pelvic viscera as components of three delicate nerve plexuses, namely the middle rectal, vesical, and prostatic (male) or uterovaginal (female) plexuses. The lower rectum and anal canal receive sympathetic innervation through direct colic branches of the inferior hypogastric plexus and through the middle rectal plexus, which courses along the artery of the same name. Functionally this innervation is inhibitory to the enteric nervous system of the rectum and anal canal and is excitatory to the internal anal sphincter. Activation of this portion of the sympathetic division therefore causes relaxation of expulsory musculature and contraction of the internal anal sphincter. (Note: The inferior rectal nerve, a branch of the pudendal nerve, supplies the external anal sphincter and inferior anal canal, which are under voluntary somatic sensory and motor control.)

Sympathetic innervation of the urinary bladder, seminal vesicles, and ductus deferens reaches these structures through the vesical plexus. This plexus consists of delicate branches from the anterior portion of the inferior hypogastric plexus, which contain both postganglionic axons from cells in the hypogastric plexuses and sympathetic preganglionic axons from neurons in T11-L2 or L3 spinal cord segments, which synapse with postganglionic neurons in the muscular wall of the urinary bladder. The role of the sympathetic division in the control of bladder function is somewhat controversial. Whereas some authors contend that sympathetic stimulation acts only to regulate blood flow to the urinary bladder,[9] others indicate that micturition is controlled by complex spinal reflex interactions between sympathetic, parasympathetic, and somatic components of the nervous system.[3,6] Visceral sensations from stretch and pain receptors in the wall of the bladder reach the spinal cord by passing back along both sympathetic and parasympathetic nerves that innervate the organ and act to reflexively stimulate both

spinal autonomic centers. Low-threshold receptors stimulated during filling of the bladder are thought to elicit sympathetic activity in the upper lumbar spinal cord. This activity stimulates concomitantly β-catecholaminergic receptors on fibers of the detrusor muscle, causing it to relax, and α-catecholaminergic receptors on the internal urethral sphincter, causing it to contract together with parasympathetic inhibition. Conversely, high-threshold receptors in the wall of the bladder are stimulated when the bladder is full and activate reflexly the parasympathetic division. This causes the release of acetylcholine, which binds to muscarinic receptors on fibers of the detrusor muscle and elicits contraction of this muscle to empty the bladder. In addition, somatic motoneurons located in the anterior horn of the sacral spinal cord reach the external urethral sphincter through the pudendal nerve. These somatic motoneurons are also stimulated reflexly by low-threshold receptors during bladder filling, causing contraction of the external sphincter. At times of greater distension, supraspinal neuronal centers inhibit both sympathetic preganglionic and somatic motor neurons, producing relaxation of both the internal and external urethral sphincters, contraction of the detrusor muscle, and urine flow.

In the male, the prostatic plexus provides an extensive autonomic innervation to the prostate gland, seminal vesicles, bulbourethral glands, ejaculatory ducts, and erectile tissue of the penis, as well as the prostatic, membranous, and penile portions of the urethra. Activation of the sympathetic division causes simultaneous contraction of seminal vesicles, internal urethral sphincter, and ejaculatory ducts during ejaculation, as well as subsequent constriction of arteries supplying erectile tissue of the corpora cavernosa and corpus spongiosum.

In the female, the uterovaginal plexus is formed by nerve branches from the inferior portion of the inferior hypogastric plexus, which course into the base of the broad ligament of the uterus. Sympathetic preganglionic axons pass through the uterovaginal plexus to either innervate the uterine cervix directly or course along vaginal and uterine arteries to supply the vagina, body of the uterus, uterine tubes, and ovaries. Because of extensive hormonal control of uterine function, the role of sympathetic and parasympathetic innervation is obscured. It is believed, however, that sympathetic activity produces generalized vasoconstriction in the female urogenital system, and parasympathetic activity causes vasodilation.

Parasympathetic Division

Peripheral components of the parasympathetic division of the ANS include long myelinated axons of preganglionic neurons located in the brainstem and sacral spinal cord segments S2, S3, and S4, peripheral ganglia that contain postganglionic neurons located near the viscus they innervate, and short unmyelinated axons of postganglionic neurons that reach specific target viscera. The term *craniosacral* is often applied to the parasympathetic division because of the location of parasympathetic preganglionic nuclei in cranial (brainstem) and sacral regions of the CNS.

In contrast to the sympathetic division, most parasympathetic axons reach target organs as components of cranial nerves or sacral spinal nerves, although some parts of the gastrointestinal tract receive parasympathetic innervation by way of vascular nerve plexuses similar to the sympathetic innervation. Cranial nerves with parasympathetic components are the oculomotor (CNIII), facial (CNVII), glossopharyngeal (CNIX), and vagus (CNX) nerves. The parasympathetic division therefore innervates target viscera by three principal routes—as a component of specific cranial nerves, as a component of sacral spinal nerves, and by arterial nerve plexuses. A general structural pattern that may assist the reader in understanding the ANS more clearly is related to the fact that the parasympathetic division functions to regulate visceral activity in the head, neck, thorax, abdomen, and pelvis only. For this reason, unlike the sympathetic division, parasympathetic nerves do not extend into the body wall or limbs. It should be recalled that, functionally, all parasympathetic neurons (preganglionic and postganglionic) are cholinergic, and stimulation of these cells generally acts to counterbalance sympathetic activity. Whereas sympathetic activation elicits, for

example, accelerated heart rate, increased blood pressure, and decreased gut motility to mobilize body energy reserves, parasympathetic activity decreases the heart rate and blood pressure and increases gastrointestinal peristalsis so as to conserve and replenish energy stores.

Parasympathetic Cranial Nuclei and Their Peripheral Distribution

The cranial origin of the parasympathetic division is localized in bilaterally symmetric brainstem nuclei composed of preganglionic neurons. These parasympathetic nuclei (also referred to as general visceral efferent nuclei) are centered near other nuclei of specific cranial nerves. The cranial nerves distribute these autonomic preganglionic nerve fibers to peripheral ganglia and postganglionic axons from the ganglia to target viscera. The most superior of these is the Edinger-Westphal (accessory oculomotor) nucleus, which is located in the periaqueductal gray of the midbrain at the level of the superior colliculus. The Edinger-Westphal nucleus is therefore positioned adjacent, posterior, and superior to the main oculomotor (somatic motor) nuclear complex. Parasympathetic preganglionic axons originating from neurons in the Edinger-Westphal nucleus join somatic motor axons of the oculomotor (CNIII) nerve and course anteriorly through the red nucleus and tegmentum of the midbrain. These parasympathetic nerve fibers continue as a component of the third cranial nerve as it emerges from the cerebral peduncle in the interpeduncular fossa. The oculomotor nerve courses through the subarachnoid space and passes between the posterior cerebral and superior cerebellar arteries near their origin from the basilar artery. This is a clinically important relationship because pathology of these vessels, such as a berry aneurism, may impinge the oculomotor (CNIII) nerve at this site, producing a classic progressive ophthalmoplegia with loss of the pupillary light reflex. The oculomotor (CNIII) nerve pierces the dura mater just lateral to the posterior clinoid process at the apex of the petrous ridge of the temporal bone to enter the cavernous sinus. The nerve passes through this venous sinus, where it may be affected by infective thrombosis of the sinus together with the trochlear (CNIV), abducens (CNVI), ophthalmic (CNV$_1$), and maxillary (CNV$_2$) nerves, as well as the terminal part of the internal carotid artery. Before exiting the middle cranial fossa through the superior orbital fissure, the oculomotor nerve may receive some sympathetic preganglionic axons from the internal carotid nerve plexus and conduct these into the orbit. Parasympathetic preganglionic axons course in the oculomotor (CNIII) nerve as it passes through the common tendinous ring of extraocular muscles and finally branch away from the inferior division of the oculomotor (CNIII) nerve to terminate in the ciliary ganglion. This small ganglion, which is located posteriorly in the orbit between the proximal attachment of the lateral rectus muscle (laterally) and the optic nerve (medially), contains parasympathetic axons. Postganglionic axons emerge from the ciliary ganglion as short ciliary nerves and enter the posterior aspect of the eyeball by piercing the sclera, run anteriorly through the perichoroidal space, and innervate the pupillary sphincter (constrictor) and ciliary muscle. This parasympathetic pathway balances the sympathetic system, which, as described above, supplies the pupillary dilator muscle. Thus the sympathetic and parasympathetic divisions are complementary functionally to regulate the amount of light entering the eye through the pupil by the pupillary light reflex. A bright light entering the eye stimulates reflexly the Edinger-Westphal nucleus, which causes contraction of circular smooth muscle in the sphincter pupillae, in this way narrowing the pupillary aperture and reducing the amount of light entering the eye. Conversely, in reduced light levels the parasympathetic division is quiescent, and sympathetic activity causes contraction of the dilator pupillae.

Parasympathetic innervation of the ciliary muscle in the eye is activated reflexly during near vision in the accommodation reflex. Contraction of the ciliary muscle slackens the suspensory ligaments of the lens. This gives the lens a thicker shape and allows the individual to focus better on near objects in the visual field.

The facial (CNVII) nerve also conducts parasympathetic axons to supply visceral motor innervation to lacrimal and salivary glands. Parasympathetic preganglionic axons are conducted by the facial (CNVII) nerve to two peripheral ganglia called the pterygopalatine and submandibular ganglia. These preganglionic axons originate in the caudal pons region of the brainstem from the salivatory nucleus. This nucleus is located adjacent caudally to the branchial motor nucleus of the facial (CNVII) nerve, immediately superior to the dorsal motor nucleus of the vagus (CNX) nerve. The superior portion of the salivatory nucleus (often referred to as the superior salivatory nucleus) contains preganglionic neurons, which are components of the facial (CNVII) nerve, whereas the more inferior part of the nucleus (inferior salivatory nucleus) contributes to the glossopharyngeal (CNIX) nerve. Parasympathetic preganglionic axons in the glossopharyngeal (CNIX) nerve terminate by synapsing on preganglionic neurons in the otic ganglion.

Preganglionic axons from neurons in the superior salivatory nucleus course inferolaterally through the tegmentum of the pons, along with branchial motor axons of the facial (CNVII) nerve. These parasympathetic axons continue with this cranial nerve as it emerges from the brainstem at the border between the pons and medulla, courses through the subarachnoid space and exits the posterior cranial fossa together with the vestibulocochlear (CNVIII) nerve, through the internal acoustic meatus. The facial nerve courses laterally to reach the floor of the tympanic cavity, where it diverts posteriorly and inferiorly to enter the facial canal and emerge on the external surface of the skull through the stylomastoid foramen. At the point where the nerve bends posteriorly, called the geniculum, the nerve is slightly enlarged into the geniculate ganglion. This ganglion is the site where sensory neurons, predominantly of the facial (CNVII) nerve, are located. Parasympathetic preganglionic axons traverse this ganglion without synapsing, and many branch away from the seventh cranial nerve at this point to enter the tympanic plexus of nerves on the floor of the tympanic cavity. Other parasympathetic axons continue further along the facial nerve to form the chorda tympani nerve, which branches more distally. (See following discussion.) Most axons that enter the tympanic plexus from the facial (CNVII) nerve and some from the glossopharyngeal (CNIX) nerve (discussed later) coalesce anteriorly in the tympanic cavity to form the greater petrosal nerve. This nerve emerges from the tympanic cavity onto the anterolateral aspect of the petrous temporal bone through a small, unnamed fissure and courses anteromedially to reach the foramen lacerum on the lateral aspect of the internal carotid artery as this vessel enters the middle cranial fossa from the carotid canal. At this point sympathetic axons of the deep petrosal nerve join the greater petrosal nerve to form the nerve of the pterygoid canal. This last nerve conducts the parasympathetic preganglionic axons along with sympathetic and taste fibers to the pterygopalatine ganglion, which is located deep in the pterygopalatine fossa against the sphenoid bone, where it lies between the openings of the pterygoid canal (medially) and the foramen rotundum (laterally). Only parasympathetic axons terminate in the pterygopalatine ganglion by synapsing with dendrites of parasympathetic postganglionic neurons. Axons of these postganglionic neurons branch away from the ganglion and course in two directions. One group of parasympathetic nerve fibers joins the maxillary (CNV$_2$) nerve, which enters the pterygopalatine fossa through the foramen rotundum and courses through the inferior orbital fissure and anteriorly along the floor of the orbit with the infraorbital branch of the maxillary nerve. The parasympathetic fibers then join the zygomatic nerve, which travels laterally and superiorly along the zygomatic bone to finally reach the lacrimal gland. It is thought that some parasympathetic axons reach the lacrimal gland more directly from the pterygopalatine ganglion by coursing separately into the orbit through the inferior orbital fissure, along the posterolateral wall of the orbit in the retroorbital plexus and into the lacrimal gland. Activation of this pathway produces secretion of serous fluid from the gland, which is important for the maintenance of the ocular conjunctiva. For this reason the physician must be concerned with possible desiccation and ulceration of the conjunctiva in a patient with a facial (CNVII) nerve palsy. The

second group of parasympathetic preganglionic axons emerges from the pterygopalatine ganglion and joins nasal and palatine branches of the maxillary (CNV$_2$) nerve to innervate mucous glands in the nasal cavity, nasopharynx, hard palate, and soft palate. Parasympathetic activity in this pathway causes mucous secretion in these regions.

In addition to the parasympathetic contribution of the facial (CNVII) nerve to the tympanic plexus, many preganglionic axons from the superior salivatory nucleus continue past the geniculum of the facial (CNVII) nerve. These axons, along with taste fibers, branch away from the nerve as the chorda tympani within the facial canal and course in the reverse direction back into the tympanic cavity through a small bony channel called the posterior canaliculus for the chorda tympani. The chorda tympani enters the tympanic cavity at the posterior edge of the tympanic membrane near the handle of the malleus and crosses the medial surface of the tympanic membrane and handle of the malleus near its superior end to reach the anterior canaliculus of the chorda tympani through which it passes to exit the tympanic cavity.

The chorda tympani emerges on the external aspect of the skull through the petrotympanic fissure, grooves the medial aspect of the spine of the sphenoid bone, and comes to lie on the medial aspect of the lateral pterygoid muscle as it traverses the infratemporal fossa. Near the inferior border of the lateral pterygoid muscle, the chorda tympani joins the lingual branch of the mandibular (CNV$_3$) nerve. The lingual nerve conducts these parasympathetic preganglionic axons into the floor of the mouth, where they branch from this nerve to terminate in the submandibular ganglion located on the superolateral aspect of the hyoglossus muscle. Postganglionic axons from neurons in the submandibular ganglion either branch directly into the submandibular salivary gland, which lies adjacent to the ganglion, or rejoin the lingual nerve to supply the sublingual and intralingual salivary glands. Release of acetylcholine at postganglionic axonal terminals within these glands initiates rapid dilation of arterioles within the glands and secretion of saliva into the floor of the oral cavity.

The glossopharyngeal (CNIX) nerve also conducts parasympathetic preganglionic axons from the salivatory nucleus. Axons of neurons in the more inferior portion of the nucleus join branchial motor axons from neurons in the nucleus ambiguus to enter the ninth cranial nerve. This nerve stems from the medulla oblongata through several tiny rootlets at the superior limit of the groove between the olive and the pyramid. The glossopharyngeal (CNIX) nerve has a short anterolateral course through the subarachnoid space and exits the posterior cranial fossa, along with the vagus (CNX) and accessory (CNXI) nerves and first part of the internal jugular vein, through the jugular foramen. As the ninth cranial nerve passes through the jugular foramen, it has two enlargements called the superior and inferior glossopharyngeal ganglia that house sensory neurons. Parasympathetic preganglionic axons of the glossopharyngeal (CNIX) nerve pass through the superior glossopharyngeal ganglion and branch away from the nerve at the level of the inferior ganglion to form the tympanic nerve. This tympanic nerve conducts the parasympathetic axons through the tympanic canaliculus, a small tunnel near the anterior margin of the jugular foramen, into the more anterior part of the tympanic plexus on the floor of the middle ear cavity. Within the plexus some autonomic fibers from the glossopharyngeal (CNIX) nerve may join the greater petrosal branch of the facial (CNVII) nerve, but most axons from the inferior salivatory nucleus, together with a small number from the superior salivatory nucleus (facial nerve), form the lesser petrosal nerve. The lesser petrosal nerve exits the tympanic cavity through the same opening as the greater petrosal nerve and has a short anteromedial course in the middle cranial fossa to reach the foramen ovale through which it exits the cranial cavity most commonly. The lesser petrosal nerve conducts the parasympathetic preganglionic axons to the otic ganglion, which is attached to the medial aspect of the mandibular (CNV$_3$) nerve near the roof of the infratemporal fossa. Within the otic ganglion, the preganglionic axons relay to parasympathetic postganglionic neurons, the axons of which branch from the ganglion and join

the auriculotemporal nerve, and a small branch from the ganglion also joins the chorda tympani inferiorly. As a component of the auriculotemporal nerve, postganglionic axons reach the parotid gland, which is stimulated to synthesize and secrete saliva into the vestibule of the mouth when this portion of the parasympathetic division is activated.

The fourth and final cranial nerve that has a parasympathetic (general visceral efferent) component is the vagus (CNX) nerve. Although this nerve has an extensive distribution to the gastrointestinal system, respiratory system, and heart, the density of parasympathetic preganglionic axons within the nerve relative to that of other cranial nerves having a parasympathetic component is low. In fact, most axons in the vagus (CNX) nerve are sensory (visceral afferent), which conduct sensations from the viscera to the brainstem. It may be that, as suggested by Gershon,[20] excitatory stimuli that reach the gut are magnified greatly in the enteric division of the ANS (described under Enteric Division).

Parasympathetic preganglionic neurons associated with the vagus (CNX) nerve are localized in the dorsal motor nucleus of this nerve located in floor of the fourth ventricle near the midline of the medulla oblongata. Axons of these neurons traverse the tegmentum of the medulla oblongata anterolaterally and emerge from the brainstem as a series of rootlets in the groove between the olive and the pyramid just inferior to the rootlets of the ninth cranial nerve. The vagus (CNX) nerve exits the posterior cranial fossa through the jugular foramen, where, like the glossopharyngeal (CNIX) nerve, the tenth cranial nerve has two enlargements called superior and inferior vagal ganglia, which contain sensory neurons. The vagus (CNX) nerve courses inferiorly through the neck, where it lies within the carotid sheath in the posterior groove between the internal jugular vein (laterally) and the internal carotid artery (medially). Inferior to the superior border of the thyroid cartilage, the nerve maintains a similar relationship with the common carotid artery into the root of the neck. Because of structural asymmetry between the right and left sides in the superior mediastinum, the course of the right vagus (CNX) nerve in the thorax differs from that of the left side.

The right vagus (CNX) nerve enters the thorax posterior to the terminal portion of the internal jugular vein and crosses the first part of the subclavian artery anteriorly to reach the posteromedial aspect of the brachiocephalic vein, where it gains access to the lateral aspect of the trachea. The nerve passes medial to the azygos vein and posterior to the right primary bronchus, where vagal axons are joined by sympathetic postganglionic axons from the second, third, and fourth thoracic sympathetic trunk ganglia to form the right posterior pulmonary plexus. Several vagal branches from the posterior pulmonary plexus descend further and, together with a contribution from the left vagus (CNX) nerve, form the posterior esophageal plexus. Near the inferior end of the esophagus the posterior esophageal plexus coalesces into a single posterior vagal trunk, which enters the abdomen through the esophageal aperture of the diaphragm.

On the left side, the vagus (CNX) nerve enters the superior mediastinum posterior to the left brachiocephalic vein in the groove between the common carotid and subclavian arteries. The nerve reaches the posterior aspect of the left primary bronchus by coursing lateral to the arch of the aorta, where it is crossed by the left superior intercostal vein and left phrenic nerve. In the left posterior pulmonary plexus the left vagus (CNX) nerve, like the right nerve, is joined by sympathetic postganglionic axons from T2-4 sympathetic trunk ganglia. Two or three vagal branches descend from the left posterior pulmonary plexus and are joined by a small number of axons from the right posterior pulmonary plexus to continue down the esophagus as the anterior esophageal plexus. As is the case with the posterior esophageal plexus, an anterior vagal trunk is formed inferiorly from axons of the anterior esophageal plexus, and this trunk is transmitted into the abdomen with the esophagus.

Within the abdomen, the anterior and posterior vagal trunks are distributed to abdominal viscera by two principal routes. The posterior vagal trunk, which originated primarily in the right

dorsal motor nucleus, provides a small gastric branch to the posterior aspect of the stomach and a large celiac branch that distributes parasympathetic preganglionic axons through the celiac, splenic, hepatic, suprarenal, renal, and superior mesenteric plexuses. These axons terminate by synapsing with postganglionic neurons located in or near the viscera they supply. By traversing the celiac and superior mesenteric plexuses, these vagal axons innervate the myenteric and submucosal plexuses in the walls of the duodenum, jejunum, ileum, vermiform appendix, ascending colon, and transverse colon to a point near the left colic flexure. The second route from the anterior vagal trunk supplies most of the stomach and, by branches that traverse the lesser omentum, innervates the pylorus, liver, superior and descending segments of the duodenum, the head of the pancreas, and sphincter of the common bile and pancreatic ducts.

By activation of the parasympathetic innervation, abdominal viscera are mobilized to replenish nutrient and energy stores of the body. Through pharyngeal, superior laryngeal, and recurrent laryngeal branches of both right and left vagus (CNX) nerves, mucous glands in the pharynx, larynx, and trachea receive excitatory parasympathetic stimulation. In addition, two or three cardiac branches arising from the vagus nerves as they course through the neck and superior mediastinum terminate by synapsing with postganglionic neurons dispersed primarily in the posterior cardiac plexus. Axons of these parasympathetic postganglionic neurons innervate cardiac muscle in the walls of the right and left atria by passing through the subepicardial tissue. Numerous parasympathetic axons also course through the atrioventricular bundle to innervate ventricular muscle fibers. In addition, smaller arteriolar branches of coronary arteries receive parasympathetic postganglionic innervation. Excitation of this portion of the parasympathetic division at times of rest elicits slowing of the heart and constriction of coronary arterioles in response to the release of acetylcholine. At the same time, the respiratory rate is also slowed by activation of postganglionic neurons in the pulmonary plexuses, which innervate circular smooth muscle in the bronchial tree to cause bronchoconstriction.

Clinically, the function of the vagus (CNX) nerve can be affected either by direct effects on its neurons of origin in the cranial end of the medulla oblongata and along their peripheral course or by reflex mechanisms that may modulate the activity of vagal preganglionic neurons. For example, if the arterial blood supply to the brainstem is compromised, as in vertebrobasilar insufficiency, symptoms such as nausea, vomiting, cardiac arrhythmia, slowing of respiration, and a sense of suffocation may be observed. Somatic and visceral afferent stimuli entering the CNS through the vagus (CNX) nerve or other cranial and spinal nerves can affect the function of vagal preganglionic neurons and produce similar symptoms. A good example is how a persistent feeling of nausea and vomiting may be caused by excessive earwax in the external acoustic meatus, which stimulates the auricular (somatic sensory) branch of the vagus nerve. In addition, it has been suggested[7] that aberrant vagal activity may be caused by abnormal somatic sensations entering the cervical spinal cord as a result of a cervical vertebral subluxation. (See following discussion.)

Parasympathetic Sacral Nuclei and Their Peripheral Distributions

Clusters of parasympathetic preganglionic neurons are also present in sacral spinal cord segments (S2, S3, and S4). Like sympathetic preganglionic neurons in the thoracolumbar spinal cord, these parasympathetic neurons are in the intermediate lateral area of spinal gray matter. However, unlike sympathetic preganglionics, these neurons do not form a continuous column of cells; instead, they are organized into intermittent nuclei that cannot be called a true intermediolateral cell column. Although the axonal course from neurons in sacral preganglionic spinal nuclei is strikingly similar to that of sympathetic preganglionic axons, axons of parasympathetic neurons exit the sacral spinal cord as components of anterior roots of S2, S3, and S4 spinal nerves and have a long course through the subarachnoid space within the cauda equina. On exiting through anterior sacral foramens

within the anterior primary rami of these sacral spinal nerves, parasympathetic axons branch away to form pelvic splanchnic nerves. These nerves therefore can be compared with thoracic and abdominal sympathetic splanchnic nerves, which also are composed of preganglionic axons. The pelvic splanchnic nerves enter the inferior hypogastric plexus, where many parasympathetic preganglionic axons end by synapsing with postganglionic neurons dispersed throughout the plexus. (See Figure 14-5.) A large number of parasympathetic preganglionic axons pass through the inferior hypogastric plexus and continue as pelvic splanchnic nerves to supply postganglionic neurons within the specific viscus they innervate.

Pelvic splanchnic nerves can be traced superiorly to the left of the superior hypogastric plexus (some pass through this plexus without synapsing) to enter the sigmoid mesocolon and the mesentery of the descending colon. By this route parasympathetic preganglionic axons cross branches of the inferior mesenteric artery, which may conduct some parasympathetic axons to the colon. Most of these pelvic splanchnic nerve branches continue directly to the colon and end by supplying postganglionic neurons in the myenteric and submucosal plexuses of the transverse colon (near the splenic flexure), descending colon, sigmoid colon, and rectum. The rectum is also innervated by parasympathetic preganglionic axons, which join the nerve plexus on the middle rectal artery, as well as by the inferior rectal nerves, which are branches of the pudendal nerve (S2, S3, and S4). Parasympathetic preganglionic axons within the pudendal nerve, which is predominantly a somatic motor and sensory nerve, are axons that did not branch into the inferior hypogastric plexus. The pudendal nerve also may conduct parasympathetic preganglionic axons to the external genitalia, although the presence of postganglionic neurons in these tissues has not been demonstrated. Finally, pelvic splanchnic nerves also conduct preganglionic axons from the inferior hypogastric plexus to parasympathetic postganglionic neurons in the wall of the urinary bladder.

Other pelvic viscera are innervated by parasympathetic postganglionic axons that emanate from the inferior hypogastric plexus together with sympathetic axons passing through the plexus. For example, the testicular or ovarian plexuses, which originate predominantly from the sympathetic aorticorenal, renal, and superior hypogastric plexuses (see the Thoracic Sympathetic Trunk and Its Branches), receive parasympathetic postganglionic axons that are vasodilatory to the epididymis and ductus deferens (male) or ovary and uterine tube (female). Axons of postganglionic neurons in the inferior hypogastric plexus also enter the prostatic (male) or uterovaginal (female) plexus to provide parasympathetic innervation to arterioles, which supply erectile tissues in the corpora cavernosa and corpus spongiosum of the penis or clitoris. Activation of this portion of the parasympathetic division during erotic stimulation elicits vasodilation of these vessels and engorgement of erectile tissues.

Sexual function or dysfunction is a good example of how central processing in supraspinal and spinal neuronal centers can influence peripheral autonomic activity. Integration of neuronal activity in various cerebral and spinal systems, including olfactory, limbic, somatic, and visceral sensory, as well as visual and auditory systems, can govern autonomic regulation of sexual function. The fact that impotence is determined primarily by psychological factors points to the strong role of cerebral neuronal centers in the control of autonomic function. Of particular interest to the chiropractor and other primary health care practitioners is the profound influence that somatic and visceral sensations have on autonomic regulation of both visceral and somatic functioning. (See discussion in Central Processing in the Control of Autonomic Function.)

Enteric Division

Until recently the ANS has been described as having only two divisions: sympathetic and parasympathetic. As early as 1889, however, it was recognized that enteric function appeared to be controlled autonomously by reflex mechanical stimulation of neuronal elements within the wall of the gastrointestinal system.[21] Gershon,[20] a renowned authority on the enteric nervous system,

stated that the enteric nervous system was classified as a distinct division of the ANS in the early 1920s, but this notion was not accepted generally until the last decade. In his review paper, Gershon[20] presents convincing evidence favoring an enteric division of the ANS, and other authors have now adopted this view.[3,6] The human myenteric and submucosal plexuses within the wall of the gut are estimated to contain 10^8 neurons, which is comparable to the number of neurons in the spinal cord.[22] The vagus nerves are known to conduct fewer than 2000 parasympathetic preganglionic axons to innervate the gastrointestinal system. This huge disparity of neuron numbers suggests that many, if not most, neurons in the gut are not innervated directly by the CNS. Furthermore, the enteric nervous system can function in vitro independent of CNS influences and responds to stimuli to produce peristaltic contractions. This evidence suggests that the myenteric and submucosal plexuses contain sensory receptors, intrinsic primary afferent neurons, interneurons, and motor neurons.[20] From examination of congenitally aganglionic sections of the gastrointestinal tract, such as occurs in Hirschsprung's disease, which are known to have preganglionic innervation,[23] it appears that in the absence of intrinsic enteric neurons, local coordination and integration of smooth muscle activity are lost.[24] These researchers concluded that the enteric division of the ANS can function independent of CNS influences and is essential for the control of motor activity in the gastrointestinal system. It appears that sympathetic and parasympathetic innervation of the gut serves to regulate neuronal activity within the enteric division but is not necessary for initiation of motor activity in the gut.

The enteric division of the ANS therefore consists of sensory (visceral afferent) neurons in the wall of the gastrointestinal tract that are sensitive to mechanical stretching and chemical changes that occur in the wall. The enteric nervous system also contains motoneurons that innervate longitudinal and circular smooth muscle fibers, arteriolar networks, and secretory cells within the gut wall. These motoneurons have connections with visceral afferent neurons within the wall, either through direct collateral axonal branches from the sensory neurons or through interneurons interposed between visceral afferent and enteric motoneurons. Visceral afferent neurons are also known to have axonal processes that course back along arterial nerve plexuses like those of primary sensory neurons within posterior root ganglia of spinal nerves. However, the axons of enteric visceral afferent neurons (in the gut wall) innervate sympathetic postganglionic neurons in prevertebral ganglia. They are believed to be able to influence reflexly the neuronal activity in the enteric nervous system.

The neurons of the enteric division and their interconnecting axons are localized between the layers of the gut wall within the myenteric and submucosal plexuses.[22] The myenteric plexus is located between the external longitudinal and circular smooth muscle layers and is distinct structurally from all other parts of the peripheral nervous system. In many ways the myenteric plexus resembles structurally the CNS[25-27] and is described as having a blood barrier similar to the blood-brain barrier present in the brain and spinal cord.[28] The submucosal plexus is located between the circular smooth muscle layers and the intestinal mucosa and contains numerous pseudo-unipolar or bipolar neurons, which resemble primary sensory neurons in posterior root ganglia of spinal nerves and sensory ganglia of cranial nerves.[29]

It is believed that only a relatively small number of motoneurons within the myenteric and submucosal plexuses are in direct synaptic contact with incoming parasympathetic preganglionic axons of either the vagus (CNX) nerve or pelvic splanchnic (S2, S3, and S4) nerves.[20] For this reason, and because of the structure of the myenteric plexus, which, like the CNS, appears to be isolated from other tissues, the enteric nervous system can function autonomously. Reflex activation of parasympathetic and sympathetic preganglionic centers in the CNS by afferent (sensory) stimuli, however, plays a strong role in the regulation of activity in the enteric division. This becomes obvious at times of emergency or stress when parasympathetic or sympathetic activity within the CNS may supersede intrinsic control of the enteric nervous system. The normal function of the enteric nervous system is important for the maintenance of homeostasis through its regulation of alimentary blood supply, intestinal motility, gastric and intestinal secretions, and fluid transport. In times of stress, sympathicotonia will override the enteric nervous system and shut down normal gastrointestinal functions.

Central Processing in the Control of Autonomic Function

Hypothalamic Control or Autonomic Function

The principal central control of autonomic function originates in the hypothalamus, which regulates autonomic activity either through descending neuronal pathways to nuclei in the brainstem reticular formation and spinal cord or through the pituitary gland to influence autonomic function hormonally. Primary hypothalamic nuclei concerned with autonomic regulation are the posterior, lateral, preoptic, and mammillary nuclei, although it is now thought that the mammillary nucleus may be more concerned with the process of memory storage.[17,30,31] Axons of neurons in these nuclei project primarily to the brainstem reticular formation, dorsal motor nucleus of the vagus (CNX) nerve, and autonomic preganglionic neurons in the spinal cord. There are four main tracts that conduct descending autonomic information from the hypothalamus (Figure 14-6). First, the dorsal longitudinal fasciculus, which originates predominantly in the posterior nucleus and to a lesser degree in the preoptic nucleus, courses into the tegmentum of the midbrain to innervate midbrain reticular formation and through the central tegmental tract, the dorsal motor nucleus of the vagus (CNX) nerve, and spinal cord nuclei. Second, the medial forebrain bundle contains large numbers of descending axons from neurons in the lateral and preoptic nuclei and forms a major descending pathway to innervate the reticular formation, dorsal motor nucleus of the vagus (CNX) nerve, nucleus solitarius, and spinal cord nuclei. In addition, the medial forebrain bundle is a major route whereby

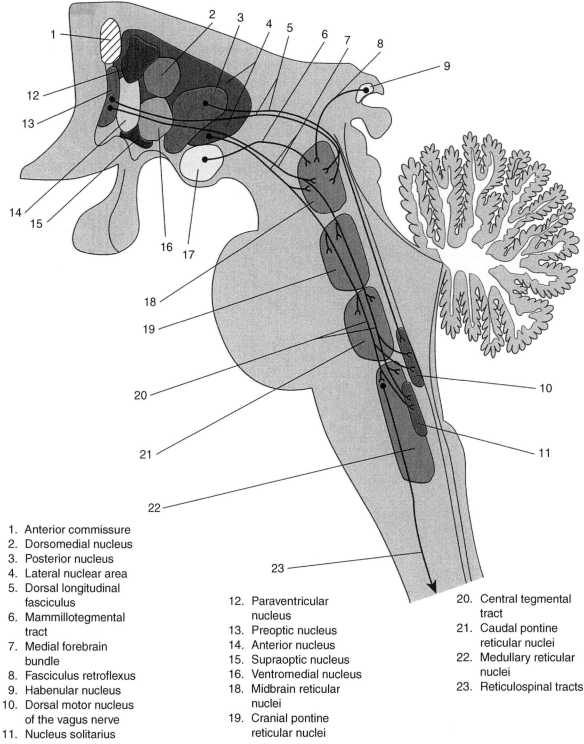

1. Anterior commissure
2. Dorsomedial nucleus
3. Posterior nucleus
4. Lateral nuclear area
5. Dorsal longitudinal fasciculus
6. Mammillotegmental tract
7. Medial forebrain bundle
8. Fasciculus retroflexus
9. Habenular nucleus
10. Dorsal motor nucleus of the vagus nerve
11. Nucleus solitarius

12. Paraventricular nucleus
13. Preoptic nucleus
14. Anterior nucleus
15. Supraoptic nucleus
16. Ventromedial nucleus
18. Midbrain reticular nuclei
19. Cranial pontine reticular nuclei

20. Central tegmental tract
21. Caudal pontine reticular nuclei
22. Medullary reticular nuclei
23. Reticulospinal tracts

Figure 14-6   Schematic diagram illustrating hypothalamic nuclei and the principal descending neuronal pathways from the hypothalamus, which regulate autonomic activity in the brainstem and spinal cord.

ascending sensory information reaches the hypothalamus and deep cortical centers in the cerebrum. Finally, the mammillotegmental tract and the fasciculus retroflexus are descending pathways that originate in the mamillary and habenular nuclei, respectively, and innervate the brainstem reticular formation.

Afferent (sensory) stimuli entering the CNS through spinal and cranial nerves reach the hypothalamus by relaying in the nucleus solitarius and reticular formation of the brainstem. The nucleus solitarius, located in the superior part of the medulla oblongata, receives visceral afferent stimuli from most organs of the body and integrates this information to modulate autonomic activity in two ways. First, neurons in the nucleus project to lower brainstem nuclei in the reticular formation, which in turn send reticulospinal axons to autonomic preganglionic neurons in the spinal cord. By this pathway, sympathetic and parasympathetic preganglionic neurons are regulated reflexively. Second, neurons in the nucleus solitarius project to higher brain nuclei, such as the paraventricular nucleus of the hypothalamus, which further integrates information from still higher cortical centers and relays back to the nucleus solitarius to regulate more complex autonomic activity. By this sophisticated interneuronal network the nucleus solitarius receives information from the highest cortical levels as well as from afferent sensory pathways and can coordinate gastrointestinal functions through direct and indirect projections to the dorsal motor nucleus of the vagus (CNX) nerve and spinal autonomic preganglionic neurons.

In summary, the hypothalamus is the major CNS center that coordinates and regulates autonomic neuronal activity. Various hypothalamic nuclei function to integrate sensory stimuli ascending from the spinal cord and brainstem with information derived from cortical and subcortical nuclei of the cerebrum and diencephalon. Outflow from the hypothalamus relays in the brainstem reticular formation and nucleus solitarius and reaches autonomic preganglionic neurons in the brainstem and spinal cord to modulate neuronal activity in peripheral components of the ANS.

Reflex Regulation of Autonomic Activity

The importance of sensory information in the control of autonomic function cannot be overstated. In fact, the primary CNS mechanism whereby autonomic neuronal activity is regulated originates in visceral and somatic sensations and is reflexogenic. Today the term *autonomic nervous system* incorporates both visceral efferent and visceral afferent (also referred to as autonomic afferent) components, even though the original definition of the ANS was restricted to visceral efferent components exclusively. Under normal conditions, impulses of visceral sensation reach the CNS along peripheral processes of primary sensory neurons like those of somatic sensation and provoke reflex responses in the organs. When an organ functions abnormally because of a pathologic condition or injury, visceral afferent neurons may conduct pain sensations to the spinal cord segments that supply the involved organ. Often these painful sensations are referred to a region of the body wall or limbs innervated by the same spinal cord segments as those that supply the painful viscus. Because visceral sensory neurons are localized in sensory ganglia of cranial nerves and posterior root ganglia of spinal nerves and their peripheral processes are distributed with autonomic preganglionic and postganglionic axons to reach the viscera, it becomes important to have a good understanding of the spinal segmental pattern of autonomic innervation to the viscera (described in Peripheral Components of the Autonomic Nervous System) to differentiate somatic pain from referred pain of visceral origin.

Autonomic afferents are divided into two types, both of which exert profound influences on autonomic activity. These are the special visceral afferent (olfactory, gustatory) and general visceral afferent (stretch, pain) sensations. These visceral sensations function at an unconscious level, for the most part, to provoke reflex responses in the viscera. However, visceral sensations also lead to conscious awareness of a feeling of fullness in hollow organs such as the stomach, intestine, or urinary bladder and also contribute to the feeling of well-being or malaise.[32]

Generally, the somata of autonomic afferent neurons are localized in sensory ganglia of the vagus (CNX) and glossopharyngeal (CNIX) nerves, as well as in posterior root ganglia of thoracic and upper lumbar (T1-T2 or T3) or midsacral (S2, S3, and S4) spinal nerves. Peripheral processes of general visceral afferent neurons are distributed to thoracic and abdominal viscera through white communicating rami of thoracic and upper lumbar (T1-T2 or T3) spinal nerves and follow sympathetic preganglionic and postganglionic axons without synapsing in peripheral autonomic ganglia to terminate in the wall of the viscus. For sensations from pelvic viscera, the visceral afferent nerve fibers course with pelvic splanchnic nerves to reach the lower gastrointestinal tract and other pelvic organs.

It is important to realize that, although general visceral afferent stimuli play a significant reflexogenic regulatory role at an unconscious level in the ANS, somatic sensations also control autonomic activity by reflex pathways. In fact, at times when sympathetic activation is required, somatic sensations involving special senses (visual, auditory, olfactory, vestibular) or general sensations (touch, vibration, pain, temperature, pressure) most often initiate the autonomic response. Elevation of blood pressure and pupillary dilation are well-known somatovisceral reflex sympathetic responses to painful sensations. For example, relaxation of skeletal muscle with soft tissue therapy such as massage, although largely caused by proprioceptive mechanisms, may be caused in part by reflex activation of parasympathetics or inactivation of sympathetics. Viscerosomatic reflexes are also recognized. For example, visceral pain is known to cause increased tonus and even spasm of skeletal muscle. Although these reflex responses have been recognized for some time, little research has been undertaken to elucidate the mechanisms of somatovisceral or viscerosomatic interactions.

Autonomics in Chiropractic

During the initial history of chiropractic, autonomics were held in high regard and treatment of visceral disorders by manipulative therapy in chiropractic offices was common. The reason for this is simple: Early chiropractic practitioners observed that spinal manipulative therapy ameliorates specific visceral disorders. Indeed, chiropractors today continue to report such observations.[33] However, the chiropractic profession has received much criticism, primarily from allopathic medical practitioners, throughout most of this century because of the lack of scientific evidence supporting this contention. For this reason, spinal manipulative treatment of visceral problems reached the point where few if any chiropractors performed such therapy or would admit to doing so.

It now appears that visceral disorders may once again be included in the scope of chiropractic practice, and again the frequency of reported successful treatments is increasing exponentially. The reason for this trend once again is obvious. It appears that reports from early chiropractors, although based on empirical observation alone, are now beginning to find some foundation in basic science.[34]

In his synopsis of the role of autonomics in chiropractic, Muller[35] recognized the need for a more scientific approach but failed in his effort because of paucity of valid research at the time. Since then, scientific evidence supporting the role of chiropractic manipulative therapy is mounting. Sato et al.[36,37] demonstrated a visceral response (decreased gastric motility) to somatic stimulation (skin pinch), a necessary first step toward elucidating the mechanism whereby spinal manipulative therapy may affect visceral function. More recent studies from Sato's laboratory[38,39] and others[40,41] support this early evidence and suggest that the mechanism of this somatovisceral response may involve reflex activation of the autonomic nervous system. Since these initial studies, there has been an explosion of reports that describe relief of symptoms in various visceral disorders after spinal manipulative therapy at specific vertebral motion segments. Varying degrees of benefit have been reported after chiropractic manipulation of the vertebral column in such diverse visceral problems as headache,[42,43] cardiovascular dysfunction,[44,45] asthma,[46] and dysmenorrhea.[47] However, nearly all studies to date focus on the therapeutic benefits of spinal manipulative therapy and fail to investigate the cellular mechanisms that underlie the observed effects of manipulation.[48]

One exception is the reports from Brennan's laboratory that indicate an increased respiratory burst of immunologically competent cells (neutrophils and monocytes) after chiropractic manipulation of the thoracic spine.[48,49] Effects of spinal manipulative therapy that enhance the immune response have far-reaching implications for the chiropractic profession. A large body of evidence is accumulating rapidly in the scientific literature[50] that indicates that the nervous system exerts a profound regulatory influence on immune activity and that this effect may be manifested through activation of the autonomic nervous system.[51] The challenge for investigators in the field of chiropractic is to establish the links between spinal manipulative therapy, autonomic function, and the positive therapeutic effects of manipulation in patients with visceral disorders.

References

1. Jamison JR. Chiropractic adjustment in the management of visceral conditions: a critical appraisal. J Manipulative Physiol Ther 1992;15(3):171-80.
2. Warwick R, Williams PL, editors. Gray's anatomy. 35th ed. Philadelphia: WB Saunders; 1978. p. 1065-83.
3. Ebbesson SOE. Quantitative studies of superior cervical sympathetic ganglia in a variety of primates including man. 1. The ratio of preganglionic fibres to ganglionic neurons. J Morph 1968;124:117-32.
4. Dodd J, Role LW. The autonomic nervous system. In: Kandell ER, Schwartz JH, Jessel TM, editors. Principles of neural science. 3rd ed. East Norwalk, CT: Appleton and Lange; 1991. p. 761-75.
5. Lipschitz M, Bernstein-Lipschitz L, Nathan H. Thoracic sympathetic trunk compression by osteophytes associated with arthritis of the costovertebral joint. Acta Anat 1988;132:48-54.
6. Berne RM, Levy MN. Physiology. 2nd ed. St. Louis: Mosby; 1988. p. 543-4, 553-4.
7. Dhami MSI, DeBoer KF. Systemic effects of spinal lesions. In: Haldeman S, editor. Principles and practice of chiropractic. East Norwalk, CT: Appleton and Lange; 1992. p. 115-35.
8. Winston KR. Whiplash and its relationship to migraine. Headache 1987;27:452-7.
9. Guyton AC. Textbook of medical physiology. 3rd ed. Toronto: WB Saunders; 1991. p. 410-2, 415-8.
10. Sant' Ambrogio G, Mathew OP. Control of upper airway muscles. New Physiol Sci 1988;3:167.
11. Forster RE II. Introduction to respiratory physiology. Annu Rev Physiol 1987;49:555.
12. Harada RN, Repine JE. Pulmonary host defense mechanisms. Chest 1985;87:147.
13. Mark AL, Mancia G. Cardiopulmonary baroreflexes in humans. In: Shepherd JT, Abbout FM, editors. Handbook of physiology. Sec. 2, Vol 3. Bethesda, MD: American Physiological Society; 1983.
14. Piene H. Pulmonary arterial impedance and right ventricular function. Physiol Rev 1986;66:606.
15. Fishman AP. Vasomotor regulation of the pulmonary circulation. Annu Rev Physiol 1980;42:211.
16. Moore KL, Persaud TVN. The developing human: clinically oriented embryology. 5th ed. Philadelphia: WB Saunders; 1993. p. 279-80.
17. Loewy AD, Spyer KM. Central regulation of autonomic functions. New York: Oxford University Press; 1990.
18. Edwards RM. Direct assessment of glomerular arteriole reactivity. News Physiol Sci 1988;3:216.
19. Morel F, Doucet A. Hormonal control of kidney functions at the cellular level. Physiol Rev 1986;66:377.
20. Gershon MD. The enteric nervous system. Annu Rev Neurosci 1981;4:227-72.
21. Bayliss WM, Starling EH. The movements and innervation of the small intestine. J Physiol Lond 1889;24:99-143.
22. Furness JB, Costa M. Types of nerves in the enteric nervous system. Neuroscience 1980;5:1-20.
23. Penninckx F, Kerremans R. Pharmacological characteristics of the ganglionic and aganglionic colon in Hirschsprung's disease. Life Sci 1975;17:1387-94.
24. Rogawski MA, Goodrich JT, Gershon MD, Touloukian RJ. Hirschsprung's disease: absence of serotonergic neurons in the aganglionic colon. J Pediatr Surg 1978; 13:608-15.
25. Gabella G. Fine structure of the myenteric plexus in the guinea pig ileum. J Anat 1972;111:69-97.
26. Cook RD, Burstock G. The ultrastructure of Auerbach's plexus in the guinea pig. Part I. Neuronal elements. J Neurocytol 1976;5:171-94.
27. Cook RD, Burstock G. The ultrastructure of Auerbach's plexus in the guinea pig. II. Non-neuronal elements. J Neurocytol 1976;5:195-206.
28. Gershon MD, Bursztajn S. Properties of the enteric nervous system: limitation of access of intravascular macromolecules to the myenteric plexus and muscularis externa. J Comp Neurol 1978;180:467-88.
29. Schofield GC. Anatomy of muscular and neural tissues in the alimentary canal. In: Code CF, editor. Handbook of physiology. Section 6, Alimentary canal. Vol. 4: Washington, DC: American Physiological Society; 1968. p. 1903-60.
30. Kupfermann I. Hypothalamus and limbic system: peptidergic neurons, homeostasis, and emotional behavior. In: Kandel ER, Schwartz JH, Jessel TM, editors. Principles of neural science. 3rd ed. East Norwalk, CT: Appleton and Lange; 1991. p. 735-49.

31. Ciriello J, Calaaresu FR, Renaud LP, Polosa C, editors. Organization of the autonomic nervous system: central and peripheral mechanisms. New York: Liss; 1987.

32. Barr ML, Kiernan JA. Visceral innervation. In: The human nervous system: an anatomical viewpoint. 6th ed. Philadelphia: JB Lippincott; 1988. p. 364-76.

33. Wiles MR. Visceral disorders related to the spine. In: Gatterman MI, editor. Chiropractic management of spine related disorders. Baltimore: Williams and Wilkins; 1990. p. 379-96.

34. Mootz RD. Chiropractic models: current understanding of vertebral subluxation and manipulable spinal lesions. In: Sweere JJ, editor. Chiropractic family practice: a clinical manual. Gaithersburg, MD: Aspen; 1992.

35. Muller RD. Autonomics in chiropractic: the control of autonomic imbalance. Toronto: The Chiro Publishing Co; 1954.

36. Sato A, Schmidt RF. Somato-sympathetic reflexes: afferent fibers, central pathways, discharge characteristics. Physiol Rev 1973;53:916-47.

37. Sato A, Sato Y, Shimado F, Torigata Y. Change in gastric motility produced by nociceptive stimulation of the skin in rats. Brain Res 1975;87:151-9.

38. Sato A, Swenson R. Sympathetic nervous system response to mechanical stress of spinal columns in rats. J Manipulative Physiol Ther 1984;7:141-8.

39. Sato A. Physiological studies of the somato-autonomic reflexes. In: Haldeman S, editor. Modern developments in the principles and practice of chiropractic. New York: Appleton-Century-Crofts; 1980; p. 93-106.

40. Leach RA. The chiropractic theories: a synopsis of scientific research. Baltimore: Williams and Wilkins; 1980;133-42.

41. Coote JH. Central organization of somatosympathetic reflexes. In: Haldeman S, editor. Modern developments in the principles and practice of chiropractic. New York: Appleton-Century-Crofts; 1980. p. 107-16.

42. Vernon HT. Spinal manipulation and headaches of cervical origin: reviews of the literature. J Manipulative Physiol Ther 1989;12(6):455-68.

43. Vernon H. Spinal manipulation and headaches of cervical origin: a review of literature and presentation of cases. Manual Med 1991;6:73-9.

44. Tilley RM. The role of palpatory diagnosis and manipulation therapy in heart disease. Osteopathic Ann 1976;4:272-7.

45. Crawford J, Hickson G, Wiles MR. The management of hypertensive disease: a review of spinal manipulation and the efficacy of conservative therapeusis. J Manipulative Physiol Ther 1986;9:27-31.

46. Monti RL. Mechanisms and chiropractic management of bronchial asthma. Dig Chiro Econ 1981;26:48-51.

47. Kokjohn K, Schmid DM, Triano JJ, Brennan PC. The effect of spinal manipulation on pain and prostaglandin levels in women with primary dysmenorrhea. J Manipulative Physiol Ther 1992;15(5):279-85.

48. Brennan PC, Kokjohn K, Kaltinger CJ, Lohr GE, Glendening C, Hondras MA et al. Enhanced phagocytic cell respiratory burst induced by spinal manipulation: potential role of substance P. J Manipulative Physiol Ther 1991;14:399-408.

49. Brennan PC, Triano JJ McGregor M, Kokjohn K, Hondras MA, Brennan DC. Enhanced neutrophil respiratory burst as a biological marker for manipulation forces: duration of the effect and association with substance P and tumor necrosis factor. J Manipulative Physiol Ther 1992; 15(2):83-9.

50. Fabris N, Jankovic BD, Markovic BM, Spector NH, editors. Ontogenetic and phylogenetic mechanisms of neuroimmunomodulation: from molecular biology to psychosocial sciences. Ann N Y Acad Sci 1992;650.

51. Pantic VS, Pantic SM. Opposite actions of alpha-androgenic vs beta-androgenic influences on humeral immune response in guinea pigs. In: Fabris, Jankovic, Markovic, and Spector, editors. Ontogenetic and phylogenetic mechanisms of neuroimmunomodulation: from molecular biology to psychosocial sciences. Ann N Y Acad Sci 1992; 650:165-9.

15

Review of the Systemic Effects of Spinal Manipulation

Patricia C. Brennan

Key Words   Viscerosomatic effects, polymorphonuclear neutrophils (PMN), natural killer (NK) cells, respiratory burst, heat shock proteins (HSP), tumor necrosis factor (TNF), substance P (SP)

After reading this chapter you should be able to answer the following questions:

Question 1   Is there a response in vitro to polymorphonuclear neutrophils challenge after spinal manipulation?

Question 2   Has a change in tumor necrosis factor (TNF) been demonstrated after manipulation?

urrently it is not possible to determine whether there are identifiable systemic consequences, including immunologic consequences, of vertebral subluxation as defined in this text. The demonstration of such cause and effect relationships requires that stringent criteria are satisfied.[1] These criteria include the relative strength of the study designs used to determine causality, the consistency of the association, the temporal sequence of exposure (subluxation) and outcome (systemic effect), and freedom from bias of the diagnosis of a subluxation and the appearance of the presumed outcome (Box 15-1). We have no convincing evidence that a vertebral subluxation causes a systemic effect. What we do know is that spinal manipulation used by chiropractors to treat subluxation elicits some very specific effects on both cells and the concentrations of some soluble factors found in the body that are quantifiable by well-defined techniques. These cells and soluble factors are involved in immune responses, but they play other physiologic roles as well.

That spinal manipulation elicits viscerosomatic effects is a concept common to both chiropractic and osteopathy.[2-7] Convincing evidence for such effects comes from animal model systems, notably the work of Sato and Swenson,[8] who showed that experimental mechanical stimulation of rat spinal cord afferents decreased blood pressure and both adrenal and renal nerve activity. More recently, DeBoer et al.[9] demonstrated an inhibition of gastrointestinal myoelectric activity (EMG) in con-

scious rabbits by experimental manipulation of the thoracic spine, and Deloof et al.[10] showed that stimulation of afferents in the central end of the cut vagus nerve inhibited gastric EMG for up to six minutes. In contrast, efforts to demonstrate viscerosomatic effects in humans after spinal manipulation have produced conflicting results. Vernon et al.[11] reported a slight but significant increase in β-endorphin levels after spinal manipulation; however, Christian et al.[12] were unable to demonstrate differences in the plasma levels of adrenocorticotropic hormone (ACTH), β-endorphin, or cortisol between sham-treated or manipulated subjects before or after treatment. Although it has also been hypothesized that spinal manipulation affects cells of the immune system,[4,13,14] until recently little experimental or clinical evidence supported this hypothesis. Vora and Bates's preliminary report[15] that spinal manipulation twice a week for four weeks increased the absolute numbers of B lymphocytes in five of eight patients with documented neuromuscoloskeletal disorders has never been repeated.

We have approached the question of systemic responses to spinal manipulation in a number of ways. First, we studied the ability of polymorphonuclear neutrophils (PMN) from both healthy subjects and patients with low back pain to respond in vitro to a particulate challenge after spinal manipulation.[16-18] Further, in the healthy patients we explored the plasma concentration of the neuroimmunomodulator substance P (SP), and we investigated the in vitro production of tumor necrosis factor (TNF) by mononuclear cells, primarily lymphocytes.[16,17] Second, we applied forces similar to those associated with manipulation to PMN in vitro and measured the production of stress proteins. Stress proteins, also known as heat shock proteins (HSP), are believed to be protective against a variety of stressors. They are highly conserved genetically and are produced by every eukaryotic and prokaryotic organism studied.[19] Third, in a small pilot study, we explored the hypothesis that spinal manipulation reduced both pain and plasma levels of prostaglandins, specifically prostaglandin $PGF_{2\alpha}$ in women suffering from primary dysmenorrhea.[20] $PGF_{2\alpha}$ is believed to be the putative cause of primary dysmenorrhea.

BOX 15-1 ■ Criteria to Determine Cause and Effect of the Subluxation

The relative strength of the study designs used to determine causality

The consistency of the association

The temporal sequence of exposure (subluxation) and outcome (systemic effect)

Freedom from bias of the diagnosis of a subluxation and the appearance of the presumed outcome

To study cells responsible for the adaptive immune response, we determined the number and function of natural killer (NK) cells and other lymphocyte subpopulations in asymptomatic subjects with a variety of complaints who presented to the National College Chiropractic Center (National University of Health Sciences), our main clinic.[21,22] Finally, we examined, as a secondary outcome, lymphocyte subpopulations in patients enrolled in a randomized clinical trial of manipulative therapy for low back pain of mechanical origin.[23]

Methods

Setting

All treatment interventions were administered at the National College Chiropractic Clinic, a private outpatient chiropractic teaching clinic in the suburban Chicago, Illinois, area.

Interventions

Treatment interventions were performed by licensed chiropractic physicians. For the studies involving the thoracic spine, manipulation was delivered to the clinically relevant segment between T1 and T6 and consisted of a high-velocity, short-lever, low-amplitude thrust sufficient to produce an auditory release or palpable joint movement. Sham manipulation consisted of a low-velocity, light-force thrust to the selected segment. In the primary dysmenorrhea study, the interventions were delivered with the subject placed in a side-lying position with the bottom leg straight and the top leg flexed at the knee and hip. Subjects who received manipulation received a high-velocity, short-lever, low-amplitude thrust to all clinically relevant vertebral levels within T10 and L5-S1 and the sacroiliac joints. Subjects who received a sham manipulation in this study were placed in a side-lying position with both hips and knees flexed. The manipulation consisted of a thrust to the midline base of the sacrum. In the randomized clinical trial of manipulative therapy for chronic low back pain of mechanical origin, patients were randomly assigned to one of three intervention groups: (1) a high-force, high-velocity, low-amplitude manipulation procedure delivered to all levels of the spine between T12 and S1 and including the sacroiliac joints that were clinically relevant for that patient; (2) a low-force, high-velocity, low-amplitude procedure (LFP ["sham"]) delivered to a single level of the lumbar spine; or (3) a series of educational lectures regarding lower back pain, with no physical contact between physician and patient or exercise recommendations provided.

Measurement of Manipulation Forces

The procedures used to measure the forces delivered to the thoracic spine have been described in detail elsewhere.[16,24] Briefly, subjects were positioned on a specially constructed force table and were then treated up to six times each with spinal manipulation, using intended force magnitudes ranging from 0% to 100% in increments of 20%. Each manipulation was performed on separate days, with the magnitude delivered on any particular day assigned randomly.

Outcome Measures

In those studies involving the collection of blood, the blood samples were collected by venipuncture in ethylenediaminetetra-acetic acid (EDTA) Vacutainer tubes (Becton Dickinson, Rutherford, N.J.). The blood was collected 15 minutes before treatment and 15 minutes after treatment in the PMN, SP, and TNF studies. In the primary dysmenorrhea study, the postintervention blood sample was collected 60 minutes after treatment because it takes that long for preexisting $PGF_{2\alpha}$ to clear the circulation. Isolation of cells was performed within 30 minutes of collection over a modified Ficoll-Hypaque gradient as previously described.[16] Plasma was separated by centrifugation and stored frozen at either $-20°$ C or $-70°$ C until assayed for the analyte of interest. Both SP and $PGF_{2\alpha}$ are stable for at least a year when stored frozen. We analyzed all samples within a month of collection. In the randomized clinical trial, blood was collected at the initial visit, at the twelfth visit, and again after a two-week no-treatment follow-up period. Lymphocyte profiles were determined within 1 hour of collection of the blood sample.

Perceived abdominal and back pain were measured in the women with primary dysmenorrhea with a visual analogue scale, and the effect of menstrual distress on the activities of daily living was measured with the menstrual distress questionnaire.[20] The respiratory burst (RB) of PMN was measured using the chemiluminescent (CL) response to an in vitro challenge with a standardized suspension of opsonized zymosan. Endotoxin-stimulated TNF production by cultured mononuclear cells was determined in the culture supernatant solutions by a standard cytotoxicity assay using actinomycin D-treated 1929 mouse fibroblasts.[6] Enumeration of lymphocyte subpopulations was performed using cell surface-specific monoclonal antibodies labeled with fluorescent dyes and either conventional fluorescence microscopy or flow cytometry.[22,25] Functional assessment of NK cell activity was made with a standard ^{51}Cr release cytotoxicity assay.[25]

The soluble factors measured in the plasma of subjects in these studies were the neuroimmunomodulator SP and the prostaglandin $PGF_{2\alpha}$ metabolite, 15-keto-13, 14-dihydro-prostaglandin $F_{2\alpha}$ ($KDPGF_{2\alpha}$). Substance P was determined by radioimmunoassay (RIA) using commercially available reagents after a petroleum ether extraction.[16,26] $KDPGF_{2\alpha}$ was determined in the women enrolled in the dysmenorrhea study by RIA as previously described.[20]

The in vitro production of HSP by PMN in response to manipulation forces was determined by Western blot analysis after exposure of the cells to a static pressure of approximately 200 pounds/square inch, which is equivalent to 1379 Kilo-Pascals. For the Western blot procedure, 10 µl previously frozen PMN samples were loaded onto an 8% polyacrylamide mini-gel and subjected to electrophoresis. The proteins were then transferred to 0.45-µm nitrocellulose paper and incubated with a primary antibody specific for 70-kD HSP. This incubation was followed with a secondary biotinylated antibody. Bound antibody was detected using an avidin-horseradish-peroxidase stain.

Results and Discussion

Polymorphonuclear cells isolated from apparently healthy subjects or from patients with diagnosed

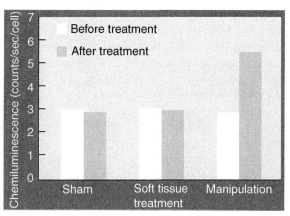

Figure 15-1 Peak chemiluminescent response of polymorphonuclear neutrophils isolated from peripheral blood obtained 15 minutes before and 15 minutes after each treatment. Shown is the mean peak response of all subjects ±2 standard error of the mean (SEM). *(From Brennan PC, Kokjohn K, Kaltinger CJ, Lohr GE, Glendening C, Hondras MA et al. J Manipulative Physiol Ther 1991;14:399.)*

low back pain of mechanical origin who receive a single spinal manipulation to the thoracic or the lumbar region of the spine are primed to respond to a particulate zymosan challenge with an enhanced RB as measured by CL. Results from a typical series of patients are shown in Figure 15-1. The mean before- versus after-treatment peak counts/second/cell difference in response for cells from subjects receiving a thoracic spine manipulation ranged from 2.2 to 2.9, depending on the study.[16-18,27] The magnitude of the after- versus before-treatment enhancement of the RB was similar in PMN isolated from subjects who received a manipulation to the lumbar spine, ranging from 2.15 to 3.2 peak counts/second/cell.[25,27] The *P* values for these data, based on paired students' *t*-tests, were consistently less than .001. The force threshold for this response was found to lie somewhere between 450 and 500 N for the thoracic spine.[24] Representative manipulation force magnitudes for the manipulative versus the sham procedure are shown in Figure 15-2. The force threshold for this biologic response delivered to the lumbar spine is estimated at approximately 400 N (Triano, unpublished). When we examined the in vitro endotoxin-stimulated production of TNF by mononuclear cells isolated from subjects who had received a thoracic spine manipulation (Table 15-1), we found that there was approximately twice as much endotoxin-stimulated TNF produced by cells isolated after manipulation compared with the production by cells isolated before manipulation.[17] Similarly, manipulation of the thoracic spine resulted in approximately a twofold increase in the concentration of plasma SP.

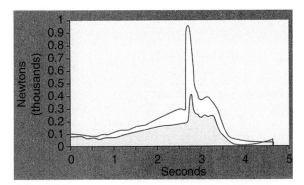

Figure 15-2   Representative manipulation force magnitudes of the manipulation procedure *(upper curve)* and sham procedure *(lower curve)* are shown. For comparison, the time has been shifted so both the sham and the manipulation procedure are aligned. *(From Brennan PC, Kokjohn K, Kaltinger CJ, Lohr GE, Glendening C, Hondras MA et al. J Manipulative Physiol Ther 1991;14:399.)*

(See Table 15-1.) These results strongly suggest that spinal manipulation results in at least short-term priming of PMN for an enhanced RB and also a short-term priming of mononuclear cells for enhanced production of the cytokine TNF. The fact that these priming effects are accompanied by modest but significantly increased plasma levels of the undecapeptide SP suggests that SP is functioning as a regulatory molecule in our subjects as opposed to a mediator of pain. Whether SP or TNF is the proximate priming agent for the enhanced RB of PMN is unclear. However, we suggest that there is a positive feedback loop between TNF, SP, and probably other cytokines as well.

In a preliminary nonrandom trial to examine the number and percentage of T cells, B cells, and NK cells using conventional fluorescence microscopy, there was no statistically significant difference between patients and asymptomatic control subjects in percentage of lymphocytes or in percentage of T and B cells.[22] Neither was there a difference in the absolute numbers of these cells. However, the mean percentage of NK cells in patients was significantly less than the percentage of NK cells in controls (unpaired t = 4.35; P = .000). The absolute number of NK cells was also significantly lower in patients than in asymptomatic subjects (unpaired t = 2.62; P = .011). Using sensitive flow cytometric techniques, we verified these findings.[21] Table 15-2 shows flow cytometric results from this study.

Table 15-1

SP, TNF, and CL 15 Minutes before and 15 Minutes after Spinal Manipulation

Time	SP (n = 21) (pmol/l plasma)	TNF (n = 26) (pg/ml/10⁶ cells)	CL (n = 26) (count/sec/cell)
Before treatment	29.8 ± 15.3	810.6 ± 595.5	2.8 ± 1.2
After treatment	52.0 ± 42.0*	1309.4 ± 766.8†	5.0 ± 1.8‡

From Brennan PC, Kokjohn K, Kaltinger CJ, Lohr GE, Glendening C, Hondras MA et al. J Manipulative Physiol Ther 1991;14:399.
Values are the mean ± SD (standard deviation).
SP, Substance P; *TNF,* tumor necrosis factor; *CL,* chemiluminescent.
*Paired students t before versus after = 2.913; P = .009.
†Paired students t before versus after = 3.615; P = .001.
‡Paired students t before versus after = 5.715; P = .000.

Table 15-2

Flow Cytometric Analysis of Lymphocyte Subpopulations in a Nonrandom Sample of Patients and Asymptomatic Control Subjects

	Percent lymphocyte subpopulation				
	Total T	Tн	Ts	NK	Total B
Asymptomatic controls	85.7 ± 1.8	47.2 ± 3.3	25.3 ± 2.5	14.9 ± 2.3	12.8 ± 3.1
Patients	83.9 ± 4.1	46.9 ± 4.1	29.2 ± 4.8	8.6 ± 1.6	13.9 ± 2.4

Shown is the mean ±2 standard error of the mean (SEM).

Table 15-3

Functional Ability of NK Cells in a Nonrandom Sample of Patients and Asymptomatic Control Subjects

	Percent NK cell cytotoxicity for K562 target cells*	
	Effector: target ratio 25:1	Effector: target ratio 6.25:1
Asymptomatic controls	66.0 ± 7.4	43.1 ± 7.6
Patients	63.8 ± 10.4	48.8 ± 9.4

*Shown is the mean ±2 standard error of the mean (SEM).

Although both the percentage and absolute numbers of NK cells were lower in patients presenting to our main clinic, the functional ability of NK cells as determined in a cytotoxicity assay did not differ between the two groups in this study (Table 15-3). In a recently completed trial of manipulation for the treatment of chronic low back pain of mechanical origin in 209 patients, the mean percentage of NK cells before any treatment was administered was 9.1 ± 0.84.[23] This compares favorably with the data presented in Table 15-2 and is less than the published minimum critical values for this lymphocyte subset in healthy adults.[28] The results of this study are the first that examine lymphocyte profiles in patients with diagnosed low back pain using flow cytometric analytic methods to quantitate cells. Table 15-4 shows the mean percentage of each lymphocyte subpopulation for each intervention at the three sample times, and Table 15-5 displays the mean absolute number of each cell type. The

appropriate method for determining whether there were treatment differences over time is the test of significant treatment-time interactions in the context of a repeated measures analysis of variance. As shown in Table 15-6, the cell types for which the interaction tests were at or near statistical significance are: Tн counts: $P = .0208$, total T cell percentage: $P = .0928$, and total T cell counts: $P = .0908$. Interaction tests for differences in either percent or absolute counts of B cells, Ts cells, NK cells, or cells bearing both the NK and Ts marker were not statistically significant. (See Table 15-6.) Thus we failed to demonstrate dramatic effects of spinal manipulation on several immune cell subsets. However, these negative results must be interpreted in the light of some methodologic issues. Lymphocyte profiles were not the primary outcomes in this trial, and medication usage was restricted only if it was intended to relieve the symptoms associated with low back pain. Detailed histories of the use of medications

Table 15-4

Mean (Standard Deviation) Percent of Lymphocyte Subpopulations in the Total Lymphocyte Pool at the Initial Visit, Final Treatment Session (Twelfth Visit), and after a Two-Week No-Treatment Interval (Follow-up)

Cell type		Treatment		
		Manipulation	LFP*	Lecture series
Total T cells	n	54	46	48
	Initial	81.4 (5.2)	82.1 (4.6)	83.0 (5.6)
	Twelfth visit	82.5 (4.9)	82.9 (4.0)	83.0 (5.5)
	Follow-up	82.0 (4.8)	83.2 (4.2)	83.0 (6.0)
TH cells	n	53	45	48
	Initial	50.6 (7.4)	50.6 (7.7)	47.8 (5.6)
	Twelfth visit	51.0 (8.8)	51.1 (7.0)	48.6 (6.0)
	Follow-up	51.3 (7.5)	50.9 (8.0)	48.4 (6.0)
Ts cells	n	53	45	48
	Initial	23.4 (5.9)	23.5 (6.3)	25.4 (5.2)
	Twelfth visit	23.2 (6.4)	23.6 (5.0)	25.1 (5.2)
	Follow-up	23.5 (6.2)	23.7 (5.4)	25.5 (5.5)
NK cells	n	53	45	48
	Initial	9.3 (5.7)	8.4 (3.5)	9.2 (5.1)
	Twelfth visit	9.4 (5.6)	8.9 (4.7)	8.6 (5.8)
	Follow-up	8.8 (4.6)	9.0 (5.2)	8.9 (5.2)
TsNK cells	n	53	44	41
	Initial	3.5 (2.7)	3.0 (1.4)	3.5 (2.0)
	Twelfth visit	3.6 (2.6)	3.2 (1.8)	3.4 (2.4)
	Follow-up	3.3 (2.4)	3.2 (2.0)	3.3 (2.2)
B cells	n	54	46	48
	Initial	15.5 (4.7)	15.1 (5.0)	16.1 (8.4)
	Twelfth visit	15.4 (5.1)	13.9 (4.3)	14.9 (6.2)
	Follow-up	15.1 (4.5)	14.0 (4.5)	14.5 (5.6)

From Brennan PC, Graham MA, Triano JJ, Hondras MA, Anderson RJ. J Manipulative Physiol Ther 1994;17:219-27.
*Low-force, high-velocity, low-amplitude procedure.

such as drugs for depression (psychoactive drugs) or drugs with cyclooxygenase-inhibiting activity (such as over-the-counter cold medications) were not obtained from these patients. Both classes of drugs can influence levels of leukotrienes and prostaglandins, and these, in turn, can either upregulate or downregulate the immune system, depending on their concentration.[29] Thus poten-tial confounding by medications cannot be assessed in this study. A second limitation may be the time frame over which the interventions were administered. All treatments were given over a two-week period, with the follow-up evaluation two weeks later. In the immune system, there is continuous renewal and selection of immunocom-petent cells and the total number of cells is under

Table 15-5

Mean (Standard Deviation) Absolute Numbers of Each Lymphocyte Subpopulation/μl in the Total Lymphocyte Pool at the Initial Visit, Final Treatment Session (Twelfth Visit), and after a Two-Week No-Treatment Interval (Follow-up)

		Treatment		
Cell type		Manipulation	LFP*	Lecture series
Total T cells	n	54	46	48
	Initial	2068 (685)	2197 (919)	2051 (640)
	Twelfth visit	1969 (724)	2173 (861)	1936 (636)
	Follow-up	2078 (1016)	1930 (554)	1890 (540)
TH cells	n	53	45	48
	Initial	1247 (379)	1351 (613)	1192 (429)
	Twelfth visit	1184 (442)	1336 (598)	1151 (442)
	Follow-up	1289 (670)	1174 (406)	1113 (374)
Ts cells	n	53	45	48
	Initial	585 (237)	620 (313)	629 (246)
	Twelfth visit	549 (266)	610 (281)	584 (224)
	Follow-up	588 (379)	545 (204)	579 (208)
NK cells	n	53	45	48
	Initial	223 (142)	211 (108)	223 (137)
	Twelfth visit	211 (132)	224 (133)	198 (133)
	Follow-up	213 (126)	205 (119)	202 (123)
TsNK cells	n	53	44	41
	Initial	85 (70)	78 (48)	84 (53)
	Twelfth visit	83 (70)	85 (57)	77 (56)
	Follow-up	82 (66)	77 (54)	77 (55)
B cells	n	54	46	48
	Initial	413 (232)	409 (224)	390 (242)
	Twelfth visit	385 (243)	365 (169)	371 (248)
	Follow-up	413 (339)	335 (161)	351 (223)

From Brennan PC, Graham MA, Triano JJ, Hondras MA, Anderson RJ. J Manipulative Physiol Ther 1994;17:219-27.
*Low-force, high-velocity, low-amplitude procedure.

strict control. Each newly produced lymphocyte can establish itself only on loss of other cells, and that new cell then has to compete with other newly produced or resident cells for survival. In such a dynamic system, it takes time to establish sufficient numbers of new cells to be detected as differences in either percentages or absolute numbers. In short, we simply may not have treated these patients over a long enough time frame or followed them long enough to detect changes in lymphocyte profiles. A third limitation of this study is that we were not able to couple our determination of lymphocyte profiles with a functional assessment of either NK cells or any other

Table 15-6

Repeated Measures Analysis of Variance Tests for Treatment-Time Interaction

Cell type	Value
Total T Cells	
Counts	0.0908
Percent	0.0928
TH Cells	
Counts	0.0208
Percent	0.9468
Ts Cells	
Counts	0.2075
Percent	0.9723
TsNK Cells	
Counts	0.7231
Percent	0.3547
B Cells	
Counts	0.1459
Percent	0.4394

From Brennan PC, Graham MA, Triano JJ, Hondras MA, Anderson RJ. J Manipulative Physiol Ther 1994;17:219-27.

lymphocyte subset. The design of the trial allowed for sporadic entry of patients into the trial. Functional assays for NK cells require target cells labeled with ^{51}Cr, and it was not economically or technically feasible to prepare such cells daily when we did not know if a new patient would be entering the trial. Similarly, assays for T or B cell function require considerable preplanning. Therefore the assessment of functional ability of T cells, B cells, and NK cells in patients with chronic low back pain awaits further studies.

In our published pilot study of women with primary dysmenorrhea treated with spinal manipulation,[20] we found that the perception of pain and the level of menstrual distress were significantly reduced by spinal manipulative therapy 60 minutes after administration of the intervention (Table 15-7). For perceived abdominal pain, there was a statistically significant difference between the preintervention and postintervention scores of the two groups, with the sham treatment group having higher postintervention scores ($F = 5.92$; $P = .019$). Similarly, there was a significant difference between groups for the menstrual distress scores. The group receiving sham treatment had higher

Table 15-7

Pretreatment and Posttreatment Means and Mean Differences in Pain and Menstrual Distress Scores

Outcome measure and intervention	Pretreatment means	Posttreatment means	Mean differences	SD
Abdominal Pain*				
SM (n = 23)	5.87	3.78	2.09	2.30
Sham (n = 21)	6.00	5.19	0.81	1.50
Back Pain*				
SM	4.83	2.96	1.87	1.94
Sham	5.21	4.43	0.78	1.57
Menstrual Distress†				
SM	44.22	25.17	19.05	15.36
Sham	47.86	37.57	10.29	11.27

Modified from Kokjohn K, Schmid DM, Triano JJ, Brennan PC. J Manipulative Physiol Ther 1992;15:279.

SD, Standard deviation; SM, spinal manipulation.

*10 cm VAS; 0 = no pain.

†MDQ; 0 = no distress.

Table 15-8

Pretreatment and Posttreatment Means and Mean Differences in Plasma KDPGF$_{2\alpha}$

Treatment	Pretreatment means	Posttreatment means	Mean differences	SD
Spinal manipulation (n = 20)	133.86	116.18	17.68	32.253
Sham manipulation (n = 19)	142.82	126.27	16.55	33.948

From Kokjohn K, Schmid DM, Triano JJ, Brennan PC. J Manipulative Physiol Ther 1992;15:279.
SD, Standard deviation.

postintervention scores ($F = 9.97$; $P = .003$). Interestingly, regardless of treatment, the plasma KDPGF$_{2\alpha}$ levels significantly declined after intervention, and overall, the differences between plasma levels of KDPGF$_{2\alpha}$ were statistically significant ($t = 3.276$; $P = .002$). However, the sham treatment group and the manipulation group were not significantly different from one another (Table 15-8). The data reported in this small pilot study suggest that spinal manipulative therapy is effective in relieving the perception of pain and menstrual distress in women with primary dysmenorrhea, at least for a short time after treatment. The data further demonstrate that this reduction in pain is accompanied by a reduction in PGF$_{2\alpha}$. The reduction in PGF$_{2\alpha}$ in the group that received sham treatment was not altogether unexpected. A similar placebo effect on prostaglandin levels has been reported in trials of pharmacologic agents for primary dysmenorrhea.[30] It is also possible that manipulation affects other mediators of the pain associated with primary dysmenorrhea such as circulating vasopressin or leukotrienes. Nevertheless, whatever the mechanisms at work in this study, it is clear that spinal manipulation and possibly the spinal mobilization used for the sham procedure affect plasma prostaglandin levels 60 minutes after treatment. A trial conducted over several menstrual cycles is in progress and is expected to resolve some of the questions raised by the pilot study.

Finally, Kokjohn[19] previously reported that PMN subjected to an in vitro pressure force similar to forces achieved during a spinal manipulation did not manifest the stress response with the production of HSP. Slight modifications resulting in improvement in the Western blot technique used in our laboratory have clearly demonstrated that PMN do produce a 70-kD HSP when subjected to a force of 680 N pressure. Heat shock (45° C water bath for 60 minutes) produces a similar 70-kD HSP. Control cells incubated at 37° C do not produce a band corresponding to the 70-kD marker protein. The extent to which HSP are produced in response to the more dynamic thrust of a spinal manipulation is unknown.

We believe that the results summarized here and reported in detail in the publications cited support the hypothesis that spinal manipulation evokes short-term systemic effects. They are a beginning, but they are only a beginning. As in most research, the questions raised by the results are more numerous than the answers the research provides. To name but a few of these questions, we know that there is a short-term reduction in perceived pain in women with primary dysmenorrhea after manipulative therapy; we do not yet know if this persists through successive menstrual cycles. We do not know if the placebo effect of sham manipulation on plasma KDPGF$_{2\alpha}$ disappears in succeeding menstrual cycles, as it does with pharmacologic placebos. We do not know if women who receive spinal manipulation experience a diminution of their pain as treatment progresses. We do not know if the function of NK cells changes with manipulative therapy. We do not know the biologic significance of HSP or if they are actually produced by circulating PMN in vivo. We have no idea about the relationship of a variety of cytokines such as TNF, or neuroimmunomodulators such as SP and the RB of PMN, in patients with musculoskeletal conditions. It is hoped that studies planned or in progress will address these issues.

Acknowledgments

The work summarized in this chapter was supported by The National College of Chiropractic, by grants from the Foundation for Chiropractic Research, and by a restricted grant to the Foundation for Chiropractic Education and Research made possible by the Foundation for the Advancement of Chiropractic Education.

I am indebted to all of my colleagues in the Research Department of The National College of Chiropractic who have been involved in the studies summarized in this chapter. Most of their names appear in the Reference section of this paper. I owe a special thanks, however, to Drs. Hondras and Kokjohn, and Ms. Graham, without whom this work would not have been possible.

References

1. Sackett DL, Haynes RB, Guyatt GH, Tugwell P. Clinical epidemiology: a basic science for clinical medicine. 2nd ed. Toronto: Little, Brown, and Company; 1991.
2. Beal MC. Viscerosomatic reflexes: a review. J Am Osteopath Assoc 1985;85:786-801.
3. Johnston RJ. Vertebrogenic autonomic dysfunction subjective symptoms: a prospective study. J Can Chiro Assoc 1981;25:51-7.
4. Korr IM. Somatic dysfunction, osteopathic manipulative treatment, and the nervous system: a few facts, some theories, many questions. J Am Osteopath Assoc 1986;86:109-14.
5. Korr IM. The spinal cord as organizer of disease processes. II. The peripheral autonomic nervous system. J Am Osteopath Assoc 1979;79:82-90.
6. Korr IM. The spinal cord as organizer of disease processes. III. Hyperactivity of sympathetic innervation as a common factor in disease. J Am Osteopath Assoc 1979;79:232-9.
7. Korr IM. The spinal cord as organizer of disease processes: some preliminary perspectives. J Am Osteopath Assoc 1976;76:35-45.
8. Sato A, Swenson RS. Sympathetic nervous system response to mechanical stress of the spinal column in rats. J Manipulative Physiol Ther 1984;7:141-7.
9. DeBoer KF, Schutz M, McKnight ME. Acute effects of spinal manipulation on gastrointestinal myoelectric activity in conscious rabbits. Manual Med 1988;3:85-94.
10. Deloof S, Bennis M, Rousseau JP. Inhibition of antral and pyloric electrical activity by vagal afferent stimulation in the rabbit. J Auton Nerv Sys 1987;19:13-20.
11. Vernon HT, Dhami MS, Howley TP, Annett R. Spinal manipulation and beta-endorphin: a controlled study of the effect of spinal manipulation on plasma beta-endorphin levels in normal males. J Manipulative Physiol Ther 1986;9:115-23.
12. Christian GF, Stanton GJ, Sissons D, How HY, Jamison J, Alder B et al. Immunoreactive ACTH, 13-endorphin and cortisol levels in plasma following spinal manipulative therapy. Spine 1988;13:1411-7.
13. Leach RA. The chiropractic theories. 2nd ed. Baltimore: Williams & Wilkins; 1986.
14. Spector NH. Anatomic and physiologic connections between the central nervous and the immune systems. In: Research forum. Davenport, IA: Palmer College of Chiropractic; 1987.
15. Vora GS, Bates HA. The effects of spinal manipulation on the immune system (a preliminary report). ACA J Chiro 1980;14:5103-5.
16. Brennan PC, Kokjohn K, Kaltinger CJ, Lohr GE, Glendening C, Hondras MA et al. Enhanced phagocytic cell respiratory burst induced by spinal manipulation: potential role of substance P. J Manipulative Physiol Ther 1991;14:399-408.
17. Brennan PC, Triano JJ, McGregor M, Kokjohn K, Hondras MA, Brennan DC. Enhanced neutrophil respiratory burst as a biological marker for manipulation forces: duration of the effect and association with substance P and tumor necrosis factor. J Manipulative Physiol Ther 1992;15:83-9.
18. Brennan PC, Hondras MA. Priming of neutrophils for enhanced respiratory burst by manipulation of the thoracic spine. In: Wolk S, editor. Proceedings of the 1989 International Conference on Spinal Manipulation. Washington, D.C., March 31-April 1, 1989. Foundation for Chiropractic Education and Research, Arlington, Virginia. p. 160-3.
19. Kokjohn K et al. In vitro stress response of PMN to manipulation forces. In: Callahan D, editor. Proceedings of the 1992 International Conference on Spinal Manipulation, May 15-17, 1992, Chicago, Illinois. Foundation for Chiropractic Education and Research, Arlington, Virginia. p. 123-4.
20. Kokjohn K, Schmid DM, Triano JJ, Brennan PC. The effect of spinal manipulation on pain and prostaglandin levels in

women with primary dysmenorrhea. J Manipulative Physiol Ther 1992;15:279-85.

21. Graham MA, Brennan PC. Functional ability of natural killer cells as an outcome measure for chiropractic treatment efficacy. In: Wolk S, editor. Proceedings of the 1991 International Conference on Spinal Manipulation, Arlington, Virginia, April 12-13, 1991. Foundation for Chiropractic Education and Research. p. 84-6.

22. Lohr GE et al. Natural killer cells as an outcome measure of chiropractic treatment efficacy. In: Wolk S, editor. Proceedings of the 1990 International Conference on Spinal Manipulation, May 11-12, 1990, Washington, D.C., Foundation for Chiropractic Education and Research; 17:109-12, 219-227.

23. Brennan PC, Graham MA, Triano JJ, Hondras MA, Anderson RJ. Lymphocyte profiles in patients with chronic low back pain enrolled in a clinical trial. J Manipulative Physiol Ther 1994;17:219-27.

24. Triano JJ, Brennan PC, McGregor M. A study of threshold response to thoracic manipulation. In: Wolk S, editor. Proceedings of the 1991 International Conference on Spinal Manipulation, Arlington, Virginia, April 12-13, 1991. Foundation for Chiropractic Education and Research, Arlington, Virginia. p. 150-2.

25. McGregor M, Brennan PC, Triano JJ. Immunologic response to manipulation of the lumbar spine. In: Wolk S, editor. Proceedings of the 1991 International Conference on Spinal Manipulation. Arlington, Virginia, April 12-13, 1991. Foundation for Chiropractic Education and Research, Arlington, Virginia. p. 153-5.

26. Brennan PC et al. Quality control in a randomized clinical trial using cellular chemiluminescence. In: Callahan D, editor. Proceedings of the 1992 International Conference on Spinal Manipulation, May 15-17, 1992, Chicago, Illinois. Foundation for Chiropractic Education and Research, Arlington, Virginia. p. 125.

27. Reichert T, DeBruyere M, Deneys V, Totterman T, Lydard P, Yuksel F et al. Lymphocyte subset reference ranges in adult Caucasians. Clin Immunol Immunopathol 1991; 60:190-208.

28. Phipps RP, Stein SH, Roper RL. A new view of prostaglandin E regulation of the immune response. Immunol Today 1991;12:349-51.

29. Fedele L, Marchini M, Acaia B, Garagiola U, Tiengo M. Dynamics and significance of placebo response in primary dysmenorrhea. Pain 1989;36:43-7.

30. Arimura A, Lundqvist G, Rothman J, Chang R, Fernandez-Durango R, Elde R et al. Radioimmunoassay of somatostatin. Metabolism 1978;27(9 Suppl 1):1139-44.

Spinal Cord Mechanisms of Referred Pain and Related Neuroplasticity

Richard G. Gillette

| Key Words | Convergence-projection, supersegmental, convergence, neuroplasticity, central sensitization, facilitated state, long-term potentiation, phasic inhibitory control, tonic inhibitory control |

After reading this chapter you should be able to answer the following questions:

Question 1 What is the contribution of central neuronal plasticity and referred pain?

Question 2 What mechanism may account for ongoing back pain independent of proprioceptive afferent input from the periphery?

Question 3 By what mechanism can spinal manipulation inhibit low back pain?

I.   Referred pain and hyperalgesia from deep tissue damage
     A. Skin versus deep tissue pain
     B. Axial versus extremity deep tissue pain
II. Clinical phenomenology of referred low back pain
     A. Clinical presentation
     B. Where is the pain coming from?
III. Neurobiologic explanations of referred pain
     A. Peripheral axon-reflex explanation
     B. Convergence-projection explanation
     C. Suprasegmental convergence explanation
IV. Neurophysiologic evidence for central convergence
     A. Single-neuron recording evidence
     B. Clinical implications
V.   The contribution of central neuroplasticity to referred back pain and hyperalgesia
     A. Pain referral and spinal plasticity
     B. Nociception-triggered "central sensitization"
     C. Clinical implications
VI. Sympathetic nervous system and low back pain
     A. Single-neuron recording evidence
     B. Clinical implications
VII. Neurophysiology of paraspinal antinociceptive mechanisms
     A. "Phasic" inhibitory controls
     B. "Tonic" inhibitory controls
     C. Clinical implications
VIII. Recapitulation and conclusions

Most clinically significant pains are triggered by damage to deep somatic and visceral tissues. For many years clinicians have observed that when tissues lying deep to the skin are injured, inflamed, or diseased, the patient reports that not only is the local area of damage painful but surrounding and sometimes distant uninjured areas are also painful; this phenomenon is called *pain referral*.[1-6] Referred pains are often felt in, or referred to, structures innervated by the same spinal cord segment as that innervating the damaged structure (isosegmental convergence); however, the painful region often expands or spreads (radiation of pain) to tissue areas served by other adjacent spinal segments.[1-4,7] This dynamic change in the perceived area of pain is usually triggered by continued or recurrent injury of the original site of deep tissue damage.[1-4]

The patient with deep tissue referred pain also has difficulty locating the source(s) of his or her pain, in contrast to a skin injury, the pain of which is seldom if ever mislocated by the patient.[1,3,4] As a general rule, the deeper and the more proximal the damaged structure, the greater the degree of pain mislocation by the patient.[2-4] Referred pain also arises rapidly and becomes maximal only a few minutes after deep somatic or visceral tissue injury and may last from hours to days in normal individuals[1,2] or for much longer periods (weeks, months, years) in symptomatic patients.[1-4]

Besides being difficult to localize, pains of deep somatic or visceral origin have a dull aching quality and are often associated with tissue tenderness that results in exaggerated painful sensation on palpatory stimulation (called *referred tenderness* or *hyperalgesia*).[1-3] This referred tenderness, felt locally in the area of injury, can be provoked also in the area of referral where the tissues are normal. Interestingly, local anesthetic injections into the referral area blocks the referred hyperalgesia but not the local tenderness, whereas injections into the area of deep injury block both the local and the referred tenderness.[2-4] These findings suggest that painful input from the damaged deep tissues is crucial for the production and elaboration of both the local and the referred hyperalgesia.

Because deep referred pains are poorly localized by the patient, it is difficult for the attending physician to diagnose the exact source and cause of the patient's problem. This is especially so when there is deep tissue damage of axial structures like the back (or head), but it is seldom a problem in the case of an extremity injury like a sprained ankle.[1,2] Because of the importance of the symptom of referred back pain and its alleviation in clinical chiropractic practice, and because of the recent appearance of uniquely new findings on the lumbar spine pain-signaling system,[8-13] this chapter focuses on the neurophysiologic correlates of lumbar spinal pain and referral.

Clinical Phenomenology of Pain Originating from the Lumbar Spine

Commonly, chiropractic physicians are asked to help patients whose primary complaint is back pain and, more specifically, low back pain (Figure 16-1).[14] The crucial initial clinical question for determining diagnosis and subsequent treatment is "Where is the pain coming from?" Traditionally, the back pain is assumed in most instances to arise from previous or ongoing injury or disease of lumbar "motion-segment structures" such as facet (zygapophyseal) joints, muscles, ligaments, intervertebral discs, bone or periosteum, meninges (dura), and associated vascular elements.[1-23] (See Chapter 2.) Indeed, numerous clinical investigations have shown that all of these spinal tissues, when appropriately stimulated, can give rise to generalized low back and referred leg pain (called *referred* or *nonradicular pain*) in normal or symptomatic individuals, and local anesthetic blockage of these same structures or their neural innervations can eliminate such pain.* Typically, the pain arising from these structures is poorly localized to the low back and hip region bilaterally and is reported as having an aching quality felt deep to the skin surface (Figure 16-1, *A*). In addition, associated abnormal skin sensations are sometimes reported, including hyperalgesia to mechanical and thermal stimuli.[2,25,26]

In addition to these features, the low back pain patient frequently reports that the pain spreads (radiates) from the back into the hip and leg as the condition continues to worsen (Figure 16-1, *B*).† The radiating leg pain is often called *sciatica*[2,19,22,23] and should be clinically distinguished from the superficially localized "electric shock-like" leg and foot pain arising from segmental nerve root compression (called *true radicular pain*).[19,23] Radicular and nonradicular (referred) leg pain are currently believed to arise from quite different pathophysiologic processes.[1,2,19,23]

Explanatory Hypotheses

Neurobiologic explanations of referred pain have historically rested on some anatomic feature of the peripheral innervation, an organizational feature of the spinal cord, or some process occurring in the brain (Figure 16-2). The clearest formulation of a peripheral explanatory hypothesis of pain referral was that of Sinclair et al.[6] published some decades ago (Figure 16-2, *A*). They speculated that

> ...the factor in the production of referred pain is the existence of branching among the sensory pathways conveying the sensation of pain. This branching is of such a type that one limb of a branched axon passes to the site of origin of the disturbance and the other passes to the sites to which the pain is referred (axon reflex). This mechanism works in two ways: first by leading to a misinterpretation by the central nervous system of the true origin of the pain impulses and secondly by the liberation of metabolites at the terminals in the region where the referred pain is experienced, thus giving rise to secondary pain impulses actually having origin at the periphery.[6]

Evidence suggests that this explanation is inadequate for pain referral in general and referred lumbar pain in particular for at least three reasons. First, the patient's report of the location of the back pain usually involves widespread areas of the back, hip, and legs that are served by completely separate and non-overlapping peripheral neural innervations.[16,18,19,23] Second, the peripheral branching of somatosensory pain afferents with one branch in back tissues and the other branch innervating the hip or leg is yet to be confirmed experimentally.[1,27] Third, and most important, this type of "static" anatomic explanation cannot account for the consistent clinical observation that these pains are "dynamic," that the painful area grows in size and spreads into uninjured tissue regions (for example, hip and leg) served by other spinal segments as the condition worsens or is exacerbated by reinjury (Figure 16-1, *B*).* All of these considerations argue against the peripheral

---

*References 2, 4, 15, 17, 20, 22, 24, 25.
†References 2, 15, 17, 19, 21, 24.

---

*References 2, 7, 15, 17, 22, 23.

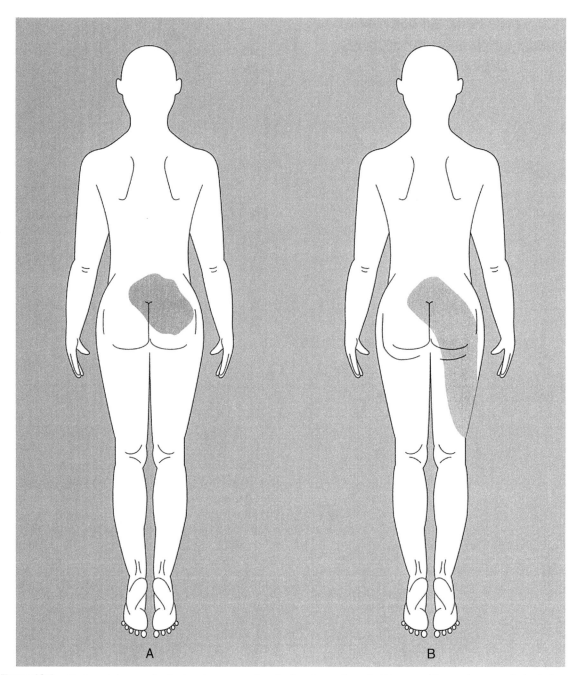

Figure 16-1   Referred (nonradicular) pain pattern for the lumbar spine. **A,** Diagram illustrating area (stippled region) of perceived low back pain resulting from low back "motion-segment" tissue (for example, facet joint or disc) damage. **B,** Same patient some days later, showing enlargement of pain area and "radiation" of pain into the hip and proximal thigh caused by reinjury of the back. Both depictions are derived from numerous clinical studies in humans.

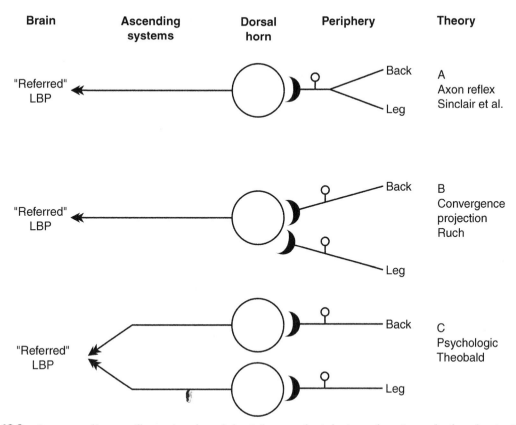

Brain	Ascending systems	Dorsal horn	Periphery	Theory

Figure 16-2 Summary diagram illustrating three "classic" neurophysiologic explanations of referred pain. See text for details.

axon reflex mechanism as an explanation for referred deep tissue pains in general and low back pain in particular.

If peripheral innervation is unable to explain the clinical symptomology, then where do we go to find a more satisfactory explanation? An obvious place to look is within the central nervous system itself. Because of the uniformity of the pain pattern produced by provocative stimulation of lumbar paraspinal structures, Livingston[4] and later Kellgren[19] suggested that there must be an underlying population of pain-signaling neurons that receive convergent input from all of the clinically relevant deep spinal sources. Moreover, they argued that when these neurons are driven to

activity by painful (nociceptive) injury messages coming from any injured spinal tissue, the brain interprets the projected impulse activity of these cells to mean that pain is originating from all of the tissue areas having potential connections with these neurons, and so the pain is "referred" to a much larger region than the actual area of injury. This idea, called the *convergence-projection theory of pain referral* (see Figure 16-2, *B*), had originally been suggested by Ruch[5] to explain pain referral of visceral disease to somatic tissues of the body. Even though ample neurophysiologic evidence supporting somatovisceral convergence-projection at the spinal cord level has appeared in recent years,[1,7,28] a search for somatosomatic convergence in pain-signaling neurons serving the vertebral column has never been attempted until recently. A consideration of these issues prompted experiments in animals (rats and cats) to see if spinal cord neurons could be found that show convergence of nociceptive input from the low back, hip, and leg region, as originally suggested by Kellgren[19] and others.[2,4,18,22] This evidence is discussed in detail in the next sections of this chapter.

Finally, Theobald[29] many years ago postulated that deep tissue pain and referral might result from the processing of neuronal impulse traffic from the damaged and referral territories only at psychological (that is, suprasegmental) levels (Figure 16-2, C). This possibility has received only limited experimental analysis, yet there is no question now that single nerve cells in the somatosensory thalamus and neocortex show the requisite evidence of interaction of peripheral inputs. However, the available evidence relates only to somatic tissues of the extremities.[30] Because nothing is known about how suprasegmental regions of the somatosensory pathway process pain input from the vertebral column, our appraisal of the neurobiologic evidence related to referred low back pain is restricted to that obtained at the spinal cord level.

Neurophysiologic Evidence for Central Convergence-Projection

In our initial experiments, we have recorded from individual somatosensory neurons within the spinal cord that respond to tissue damage in the low back region, neurons likely to mediate low back pain.[8,10,11] We found that most of these "low back" pain-signaling neurons, located exclusively in the lateral dorsal horn of the lumbar cord (Figure 16-3), were responsive to noxious, damaging stimuli applied to many different tissues of the low back, hip, and proximal leg; that is, within the "receptive field" of the cell. Recall that a neuron's receptive field is that area of tissue within which peripheral stimulation causes the neuron to

generate an action potential, that is, the neuron receives information from that tissue.[1,7] Because of the remarkable input convergence to these cells from multiple back and hind limb tissues, we now refer to these neurons as "hyperconvergent" low back pain neurons (hereafter, "low back neurons").

Individual low back neurons were found to be either responsive to noxious and nonnoxious stimulation (multireceptive or wide-dynamic range [WDR] neurons, 77%) or noxious stimulation only (high-threshold or nociceptive-specific [NS] neurons, 23%) of paraspinal muscles, ligaments, discs, periosteum, facet joints, dura, and skin, as well as tissues of the hip and leg (Figures 16-3 and 16-4). Evidence strongly suggests that WDR neurons are responsible for the generation of subjective pain in humans and NS units appear not to contribute to this sensation.[7] In addition, all of the WDR and NS neurons that we examined were found to be more powerfully activated by nociceptive input from deep tissues than from skin, which we believe may explain why back pain is felt to originate from deep rather than superficial tissues. We have also established that some of the recorded neurons (for example, units shown in Figures 16-3, 16-4, 16-8, and 16-10) project axons into well-recognized ascending pain pathways (for example, the spinothalamic, spinoreticular, and spinocervical tracts).[8]

The low back neurons we examined also had very large hyperconvergent receptive fields in the low back and proximal leg that included both skin and deep somatic tissues innervated through both the dorsal (back/hip) and ventral (leg/ventral spine) primary rami. (See Figure 16-3.) The finding that low back neurons respond to damage of many paraspinal structures implies that damage to any deep lumbar tissue probably produces the same or similar pain and may partially explain why it is often difficult to identify a specific cause of low back pain.* It had been shown in earlier studies that analogous spinal neurons serving the

---

*References 15, 19, 20, 21, 23, 25.

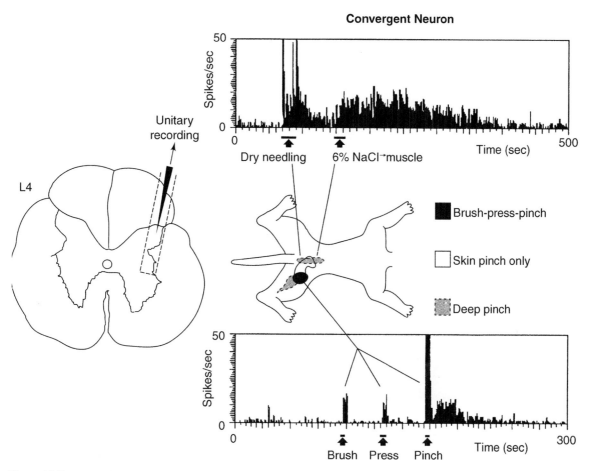

Figure 16-3 Recordings from a representative "hyperconvergent" (WDR) low back neuron located in laminae II of the lateral dorsal horn of the L4 spinal cord (spinal cross-section at left). Response histograms reflect number of action potentials/unit of time. Stippled areas show locations of deep receptive fields; the shaded area denotes the cutaneous receptive field. Note that the unit was modestly responsive (lower histogram) to innocuous *(brush, press)* mechanical stimulation but more responsive to noxious *(pinch)* stimulation of skin receptive field—the "classic WDR response." Neuron was maximally responsive (upper histogram) to noxious mechanical *(dry needling)* and chemical (hypertonic 6% NaCl solution) stimulation within the deep paraspinal receptive field. *(From Gillette, Kramis, and Roberts, unpublished data.)*

limbs are responsive to sensory inputs from fewer individual tissues over very small areas, often just from skin,[1,7,11,31] making diagnosis of an origin of pain in a limb much easier than for the low back.

Finally, these neuronal response properties, especially the "hyperconvergence" from multiple back and leg tissues (Figure 16-5), match the requisite features of the convergence-projection explanation of pain referral originally proposed by Ruch[5] and Kellgren.[19] We discuss in the following section whether central convergence is sufficient to account for referred low back pain and hyperalgesia.

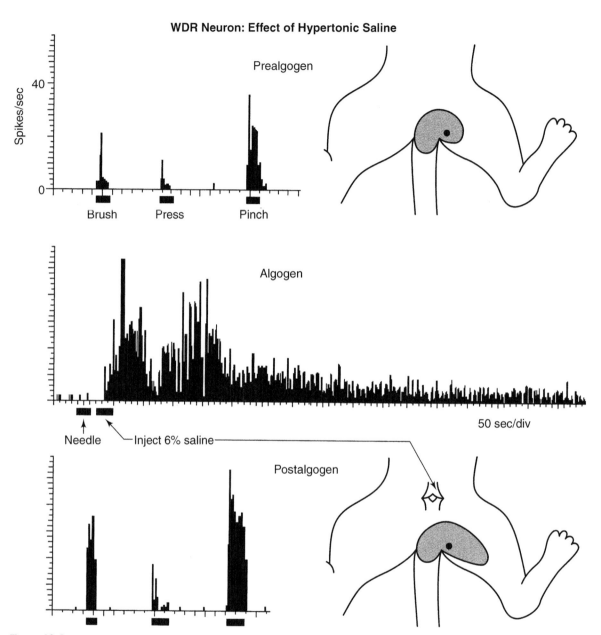

Figure 16-4   Neuroplastic changes in a low back neuron after noxious stimulus-induced central sensitization. Top *(prealgogen)* histogram illustrates baseline response to innocuous brush, press, and noxious pinch stimulation applied at dot location in the unit's receptive field shown at right. Middle histogram shows neuronal response to injection of noxious, hypertonic (6%) saline into a lumbar facet joint *(arrow)* that produces long-lasting ongoing discharge in the unit and sensitization of the cell to subsequent mechanical stimulation (lower postalgogen histogram) while enlarging the receptive field (compare upper and lower RFs). *(From Gillette, Kramis, and Roberts, unpublished data.)*

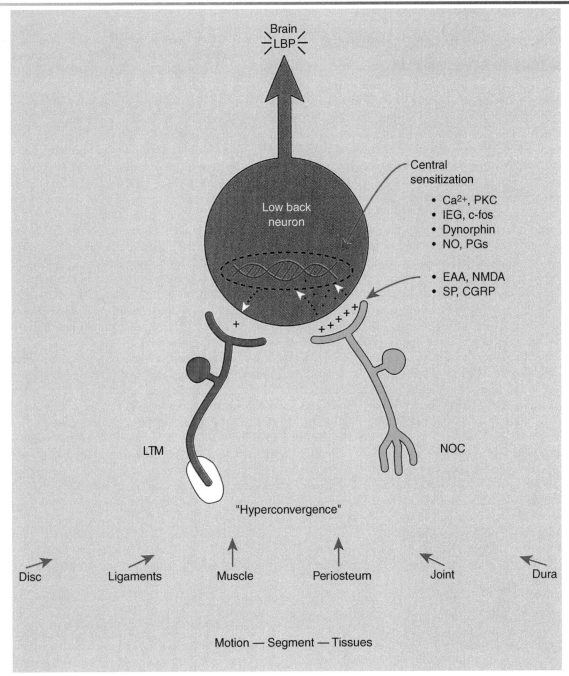

Figure 16-5 Schematic diagram illustrating some of the cellular mechanisms thought to be involved in central sensitization of low back neurons. Paravertebral motion-segment tissue damage causes release of excitatory amino acid (*EAA;* for example, glutamate) and neuropeptide transmitters *(SP, CGRP)* from converging nociceptive *(NOC)* afferents that "sensitize" spinal low back neurons through changes in second-messenger *(Ca²⁺, PKC)* cascades and postsynaptic (for example, glutaminergic\NMDA) receptors. As central sensitization progresses *(open arrowheads)*, genes are induced to transcribe through IEGs (for example, *c-fos*) new pronociceptive proteins (for example, *dynorphin*) to further enhance neuronal excitability and effectiveness of nociceptive *(NOC)* and nonnociceptive *(LTM)* input *(open arrowheads)*. "+" denotes excitatory synaptic actions.

The Contribution of Central Neuronal Plasticity to Referred Pain

On several occasions since the publication of Theobald's original hypothesis,[29] investigators have been drawn again to a central psychogenic explanation to account for some of the more perplexing characteristics of referred back pain that cannot be explained by convergence-projection alone.[32,33] Four features of low back pain in particular appear to be troublesome: (1) its dynamic spread or radiation to involve tissues served by multiple spinal segments; (2) its occurrence in response to normally nonnoxious stimulation like minor movements, deep pressure, and touch; (3) its occurrence and persistence in many patients in the absence of identifiable peripheral tissue pathology; and sometimes, (4) its relief by treatment with a placebo. However, an appeal to suprasegmental processes to explain these issues is not needed because changes in the response properties of spinal low back neurons now appear to be sufficient.[11] Based on the neurophysiologic evidence discussed later, features 1, 2, and 3 may be interpreted as being caused by enduring excitability changes in these spinal neurons, changes that render these units excessively responsive to a variety of inputs after painful paraspinal damage.[8,10-12,34] Evidence is also presented to show that these same neurons are under the influence of powerful inhibitory controls that may operate in a variety of clinical settings to alleviate pain (feature 4).

To examine these issues more closely, we review the results of our recent animal experiments designed to explore neuroplastic processes in relation to the neurophysiology of the low back.[8,11-13] We have found, for example, that not only are low back neurons activated by noxious mechanical and chemical (algesic) stimulation of the lumbar region, they are also "sensitized" by this input (68% of 37 units examined), meaning that they become hyperresponsive to all subsequent stimuli delivered to their receptive fields. (See Figure 16-4; compare top and bottom histograms.) These neurons also showed dramatic expansion of their superficial and deep receptive fields after noxious

stimulation of paravertebral tissues (see Figure 16-4) and often showed ongoing or background discharge independent of any further peripheral stimulation.[8,10,11]

These dynamic neurophysiologic changes, called activity-dependent "central sensitization,"[11,12,28,35-37] may explain why tenderness develops over a wide area after a localized back injury and why the pain seems to expand and radiate to the hip and out into the proximal leg (features 1 and 2). Similar dynamic neuronal processes were described some years ago by Korr[38] (the "facilitated state") and more recently by Patterson and Steinmetz[39] ("spinal fixation") to explain spinally mediated autonomic and motor pathophysiology. Although these concepts were not proposed as explanations for clinical pain symptomology, it still appears quite likely that what Korr and Patterson and Steinmetz have described is very much like what we call central sensitization.

With regard to the modern view of the cellular mechanisms underlying neuroplastic changes, our findings[8,10-13] and those of others[28,35-37,40] indicate that central sensitization is caused at least in part by changes in the intrinsic characteristics of the spinal neurons involved rather than by changes in the damaged peripheral tissues. (See Figure 16-5.) This process, however, is importantly dependent on an initial activation of nociceptive (NOC) afferents and the subsequent corelease of excitatory amino acids (EAAs; for example, glutamate and aspartate) and neuropeptides (for example, substance P [SP] and calcitonin gene-related peptide [CGRP]) from their central axon terminals.[28,35-37,40] These substances in turn bind to postsynaptic glutamate[37,40] (for example, the N-methyl-D-aspartate, or NMDA) and neuropeptide receptors[35,36,40,41] on spinal nociceptive neurons, where they trigger a cascade of cellular changes including increases in ion channel-mediated electrical activity as well as alterations in intracellular enzyme cascades. (See Figure 16-5.) The biochemical cascades use various second-messenger systems (for example, Ca^{2+} and protein kinase C, or PKC) to trigger phosphorylation of membrane receptors (for example, glutamate and neuropeptide types) and ion channels (both ligand- and voltage-gated) that ultimately leads to enduring increases in neuronal excitability.[11,28,35-37,40,41]

The excitability change is reflected in a dramatic increased responsiveness to both nociceptive (NOC) and nonnociceptive, low-threshold mechanoreceptive (LTM) afferent input (see Figures 16-4 and 16-5) from the neuron's receptive field and a tendency for the cell to generate ongoing discharges on its own.[8,10-12] (See Figures 16-3 and 16-4.) Interestingly, this persistent increase in neuronal responsiveness shows many of the features of a form of synaptic learning or plasticity, called "long-term potentiation," or LTP, wherein temporally coincident synaptic inputs are strengthened, a process that appears to be widespread in many parts of the brain[28,34-36] and spinal cord.[42,43]

Finally, nociceptor afferent input to spinal neurons,[28,35,40,41] including low back neurons,[11,13] also leads to alterations in gene transcription (through immediate early genes [IEGs] like c-fos and c-jun) and the associated production and release of pain-promoting neuroactive peptides like dynorphin and diffusible messengers like nitric oxide (NO) and prostaglandins.[28,35,40,41] (See Figure 16-5.)

One might speculate that, through these mechanisms, a positive feedback cycle of pronociceptive excitability is triggered, refreshed, and maintained for varying lengths of time within individual pain-signaling neurons of the low back sensory system by periodic nociceptive and nonnociceptive paraspinal inputs.[11,34] (See Figure 16-5.)

It is also important to consider how the spread of excitability across populations of pain-signaling neurons in adjacent spinal segments might occur during the elaboration and radiation of low back pain (feature 1).[2,7,19,20,22] Recent evidence suggests that there are a number of processes involved, including activation of increasing numbers of paraspinal nociceptive afferents with widely divergent central terminations along the rostrocaudal axis of the spinal cord.[9,11] Increased activity in these afferents is believed to "unmask" latent excitatory synapses[34,44] that contact low back neurons so that progressively more nerve cells are recruited into the active (impulse-generating) population as

nociception continues. Furthermore, there is some limited evidence to suggest that this spread of excitability is in part mediated by the local release and diffusion of neuroactive peptides like SP and CGRP from these afferents[27] as well as the local release of pronociceptive substances like dynorphin and NO from targeted spinal neurons.[35,41] (See Figure 16-5.) All of these mechanisms appear to be able to operate in concert to produce increases in neuronal excitability across populations of spinal nociceptive neurons, including those serving the low back.[11-13]

One could further speculate that if sensitization of these spinal neurons continues for a long time because of persistent or refreshed nociceptor activation, the back pain may become self sustaining (that is, chronic) and independent of nociceptive afferent input from the periphery.[11,34] This may explain why patients suffering from chronic low back pain seldom show evidence of peripheral tissue pathology[32] (feature 3); that is, the peripheral tissues have healed but the central nervous system is still abnormal.[8,41]

Finally, some recent experimental findings suggest that the development of central sensitization and persistent pain may be promoted and maintained by the progressive loss of inhibitory controls that normally play on spinal nociceptive neurons to prevent hyperexcitability.[28,35] It is believed that the small inhibitory neurons operating within the pain system are particularly vulnerable to "excitotoxic effects" of excessive and prolonged NMDA receptor activation by the nociceptive EAA transmitter, glutamate.[28,35,41] This also might occur in the low back pain signaling system; however, there is no evidence available to assist in the verification of this suggestion.

Sympathetic Nervous System Involvement in Low Back Pain

Because persistent low back pain is often found to exist in the absence of any detectable, ongoing injury or disease,[32] and because other types of chronic pain have been found to be dependent on activity in the sympathetic division of the autonomic nervous system,[31] we have also tested to determine whether low back neurons respond to electrical stimulation of the lumbar sympathetic trunk, located just outside the spinal column.[10]

We found that most (70%) spinal neurons serving the low back region were indeed activated by applying electrical pulses to visceral and somatic afferent and sympathetic efferent axons within the sympathetic trunk, suggesting that activity in these nerve fibers may contribute to low back pain.[10,11] This finding in animals is consistent with reports from clinical studies by others indicating that some chronic low back pain patients benefit from local anesthetic or ablative blocks of the sympathetic trunk.[10,31,45] This procedure of blocking the sympathetic trunk is not commonly used to diagnose or treat low back pain, partly because there has been no clear physiologic evidence to suggest that the sympathetic division of the autonomic nervous system has a direct influence on pain from this region.

Our data indicate that at least two types of nerve fibers in the lumbar sympathetic trunk contribute to the activation of these spinal neurons.[10] One type is sensory, being the parent axons of nociceptor (NOC) and mechanoreceptor (LTM) sensory afferents originating in muscles, ligaments, and other retroperitoneal (visceral) tissues near the spinal column and running in the sympathetic trunk to finally enter the spinal cord over the dorsal roots to directly affect low back neurons (Figure 16-6).[10,11,16] The convergent input to low back neurons from visceral nociceptive afferents projecting through the sympathetic chain (see Figure 16-6, VISC) could help to explain how pain from pelvic visceral disease is referred to the low back region,[9,10] a classic example of viscerosomatic convergence.[5]

The second type of activated nerve fiber appears to be sympathetic motor efferent fibers that project out to all tissues, where they act to control blood flow and other processes.[10,31] Activity in these sympathetic efferent fibers indirectly triggers activity in other sensory mechanoreceptive (LTM) and nociceptive (NOC) afferent fibers[10,11,31] that in turn project back into the spinal cord to affect low back neurons (Figure 16-7). We have also shown that this sympathetic process can be blocked by the alpha-adrenergic antagonist drug phentolamine (see Figure 16-7), which most commonly is used to control hypertension or for other diagnostic tests unrelated to pain.[10,11] We are investigating whether this drug may provide a safe and harmless means for testing whether the sympathetic nervous system contributes to low back pain in patients with chronic discomfort.[26]

The importance of these sympathetically mediated effects is in their capacity to greatly increase the excitatory synaptic drive onto already sensitized low back neurons to maintain them in a hyperexcitable state. (See Figures 16-6 and 16-7.) Conceivably, a sympathetically triggered nonnociceptive (LTM) afferent drive could eventually be sufficient to maintain the spinal low back neuron (see Figure 16-7) in a sensitized state, even after peripheral tissues have healed and related nociceptor afferent input has decreased (feature 3).[10,11]

Neurophysiology of Paraspinal Antinociceptive Systems

While studying the response properties of the low back pain-signaling neurons, we have also examined, to a limited extent, inhibitory phenomena that may be important in pain suppression as opposed to pain production. For example, a subset of the dorsal horn low back neurons from which we have recorded data (approximately 20%) show complex forms of response suppression to mechanical stimulation of paravertebral structures.[8,10,11]

These inhibitory responses fell into two groups based on the modality of triggering afferent input and the duration of the inhibitory effects produced. In some instances, brief inhibition of cellular discharge (both ongoing and stimulus-evoked) could be obtained by applying innocuous mechanical stimulation to the skin receptive field of these cells (Figure 16-8). Interestingly, the suppression of neuronal responses in these cases immediately ceased with the removal of the innocuous stimulation. (See Figure 16-8.) This short-lived ("phasic")

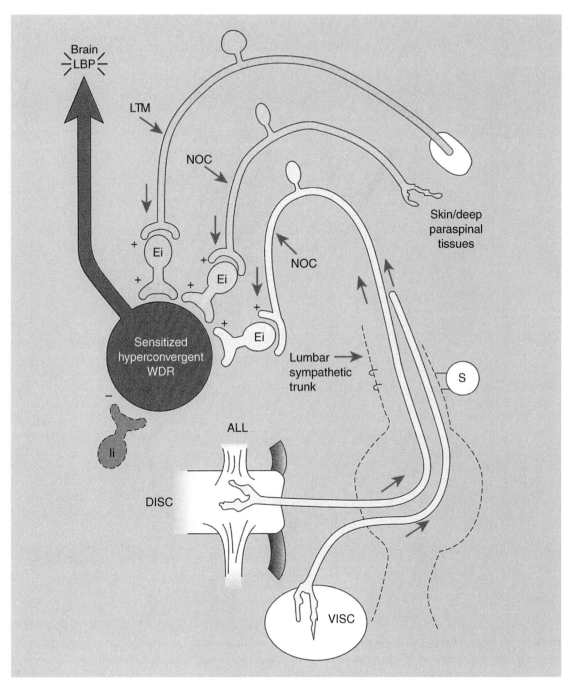

Figure 16-6 Diagram of neuronal pathway proposed to mediate responses of low back neurons to sympathetic trunk stimulation—the "direct sensory afferent loop." Electrical stimulation of sympathetic trunk *(S)* activates somatic *(DISC)* and/or visceral *(VISC)* nociceptive afferents, which act directly or via interneurons to excite and sensitize hyperconvergent *(WDR)* low back neurons. "+" denotes excitatory synaptic actions; *Ei*, excitatory interneuron; *Ii*, inhibitory interneuron.

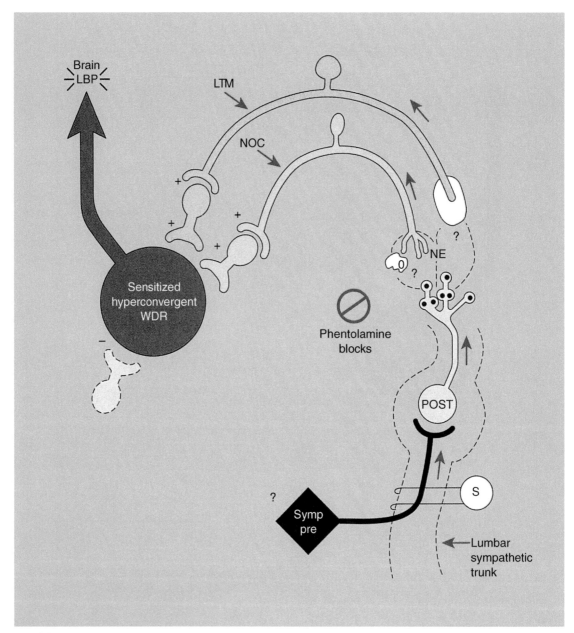

Figure 16-7   Diagram of neuronal pathway proposed to mediate responses of low back neurons to sympathetic trunk stimulation—the "indirect sympathetic efferent/sensory afferent loop." Electrical stimulation of sympathetic chain *(S)* activates preganglionic axons, which excite sympathetic postganglionic neurons. These neurons in turn excite primary *(LTM and NOC)* afferents through a sympathetic-sensory coupling to indirectly excite and sensitize hyperconvergent *(WDR)* low back neurons. Sympathetic efferent-to-afferent coupling appears to be noradrenergically *(NE)* mediated because it can be blocked by phentolamine; however, other unknown mediators *("?")* such as prostaglandins and cytokines may also contribute. "+" denotes excitatory synaptic actions.

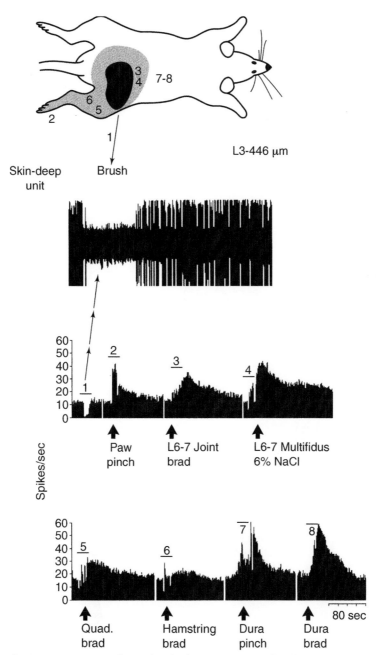

Figure 16-8 Brief "phasic" suppression of impulse discharge (top record and middle histogram at *1*) in a low back neuron by innocuous "brush" stimulation of the superficial receptive field (*black area in top figure*). This unit was vigorously excited and sensitized by skin pinch (stippled area) and by noxious mechanical and algesic stimulation of deep paraspinal (records *3, 4, 7, 8*) and hind limb (records *2, 5, 6*) structures. *Brad*, bradykinin; *6% NaCl*, hypertonic saline; *Dura*, spinal dura mater. Unit isolated in the lateral dorsal horn of spinal segment L3. *(From Gillette, Kramis, and Roberts, unpublished data.)*

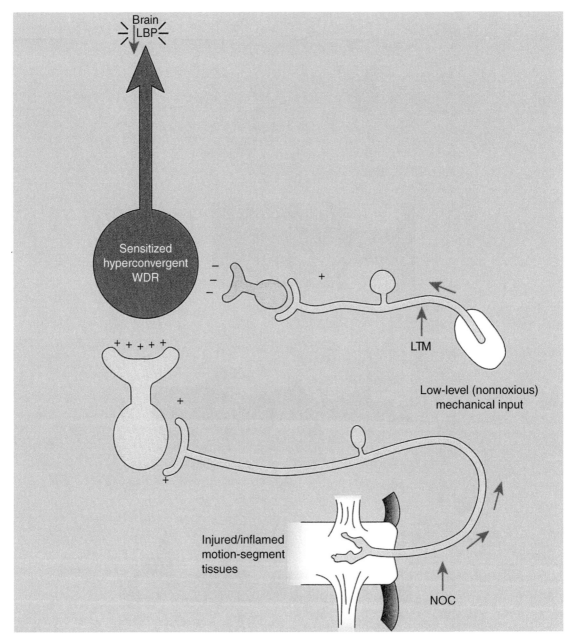

Figure 16-9 Schematic illustrating proposed neural circuitry involved in producing "phasic" antinociception or response suppression shown in Figure 16-8. In the depiction, a low back *(WDR)* neuron has been sensitized by nociceptive *(NOC)* afferent bombardment reaching the cell from damaged paravertebral structures. The diagram illustrates how activation of low-threshold mechanoreceptive afferents *(LTM)* by innocuous mechanical (for example, touch, press, brush) stimulation could activate small spinal inhibitory neurons that subsequently inhibit the hyperexcitable low back neuron resulting in a decrease in pain transmission *(↓ LBP).* "+" denotes excitatory synaptic actions; "−" denotes inhibitory synaptic actions.

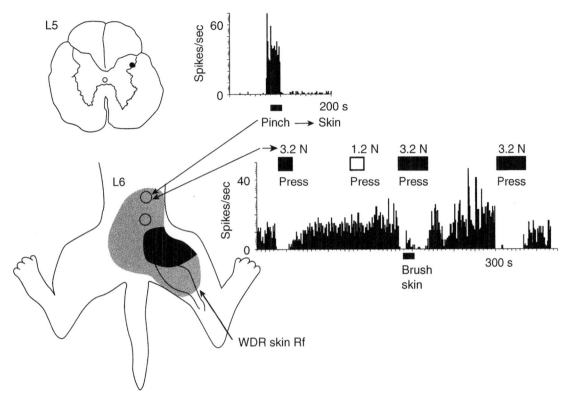

Figure 16-10   Single-unit recordings showing that high-level mechanical stimulation of paravertebral tissues can effectively suppress impulse activity in low back neurons. This neuron was initially inactive, but after pinching the skin receptive field (upper histogram) and injecting algogens (for example, Brad, 6% NaCl) into deep paraspinal tissues (responses not shown), the cell developed an ongoing discharge that was effectively inhibited during and after forceful mechanical stimulation over the L5-6 facet joint (3.2 N stimulus, *black boxes*). Although noxious *(3.2 N)* mechanical input very effectively attenuated unit discharge, less forceful probing had no effect (1.2 N stimulus, *open box*). Excitatory "breakthrough" (*Brush skin* region of histogram) during 3.2 N stimulus-induced inhibition demonstrates that the discharge suppression is neurally mediated. Unit isolated in lateral lamina II of L5 dorsal horn. *(From Gillette, Kramis, and Roberts, unpublished data.)*

response suppression is reminiscent of the spinally mediated pain-gating postulated some years ago by Melzack and Wall (Figure 16-9).[1,46]

It was also found that noxious mechanical pressure applied to deep tissues of the back and hip (Figure 16-10) produced a more marked and longer lasting ("tonic") inhibition of neuronal discharge that showed striking similarities to the segmental[47,48] and suprasegmental\descending modulatory inhibition (Figure 16-11) described originally by Le Bars et al.[49,50] and more recently

by others.[1,7,11,51,52] Evidence suggests that these inhibitory mechanisms use both GABA-ergic and opioidergic transmitter pharmacologies to suppress nocireceptive neuron excitability.[1,7,34,50,53]

These experimental findings are consistent with a speculative hypothesis published several years ago that argued that the mechanical forces produced by various forms of chiropractic manipulation (CM) were of sufficient magnitude to coactivate both low-threshold mechanoreceptive (LTM) and high-threshold nociceptive (NOC) afferents in

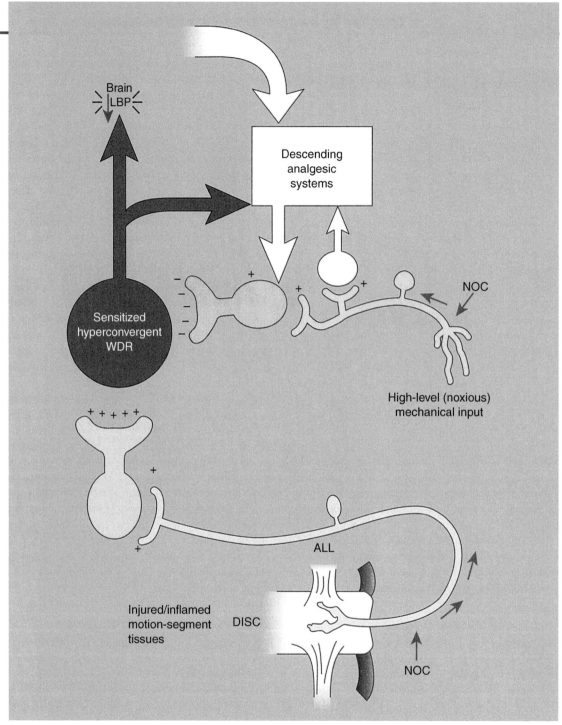

Figure 16-11 Diagram of the postulated neural circuitry believed to underlie the inhibitory phenomena shown in Figure 16-10. Brief but noxious mechanical input to paravertebral tissues activates paraspinal nociceptive afferents *(NOC)* that activate spinal inhibitory interneurons both directly (segmentally) and indirectly through a suprasegmental analgesic loop. The spinally and supraspinally activated inhibitory interneuron decreases the electrical excitability and impulse discharging of "already sensitized" low back *(WDR)* neurons, leading to a decrease in perceived low back pain *(↓ LBP)*. The descending analgesic system can also be independently activated by higher-order brain regions (top, *open arrow*) to produce "context-dependent" antinociception (for example, with placebos). "+" denotes excitatory synaptic actions, and "–" denotes inhibitory synaptic actions.

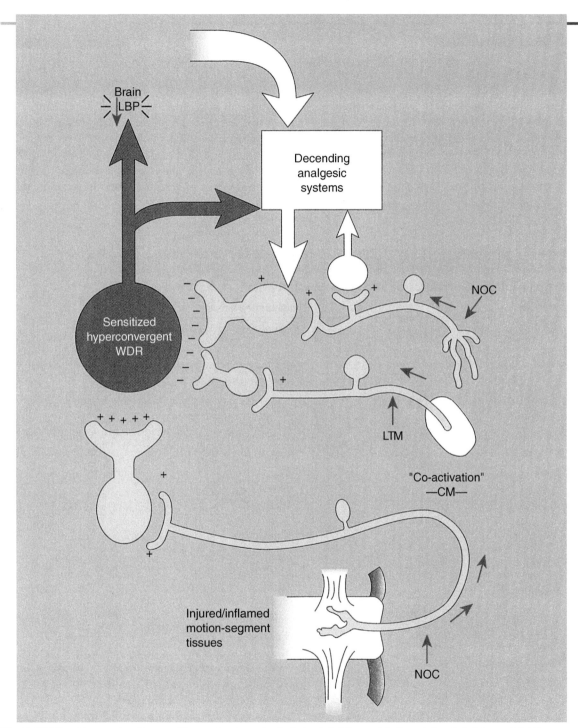

Figure 16-12 Composite diagram illustrating how both "phasic" (Figure 16-9) and "tonic" (Figure 16-11) antinociceptive circuits might be coactivated by mechanically forceful chiropractic manipulation *(CM)* and how these mechanisms could work together to reduce the hyperexcitability of "sensitized" low back pain transmission neurons. A subsequent decrease in excitability and impulsing across the majority of low back *(WDR)* neurons would lead to a subjective decrease in referred low back pain, that is, an analgesia *($\downarrow$ LBP)*. "+" denotes excitatory synaptic actions, and "−" denotes inhibitory synaptic actions.

paraspinal tissues.[47,54] It was further argued that this type of sensory input could simultaneously activate both "phasic" and "tonic" antinociceptive systems, which would act to suppress the hyperexcitability of spinal cord neurons set up by noxious input from damaged paravertebral structures (Figure 16-12).[47,54] Perhaps both of these inhibitory processes could act to decrease neuronal excitability by clamping membrane voltages at levels that favor the promotion of "long-term depression" (or LTD) of neuronal excitability rather than LTP.[34,42] Finally, these central antinociceptive systems may operate in conjunction with peripheral antinociceptive mechanisms, particularly when there is inflammation in damaged peripheral tissues.[34] Indeed, Stein[53] and associates have recently shown that a powerful, peripheral opioidergic antinociceptive system is upregulated in peripheral tissues

Table 16-1

Neurophysiologic Correlates of Referred Low Back Pain

Clinical feature	Postulated neural correlate
Poorly localized back, hip, and leg pain	Spinal neuron "hyperconvergence" and large unit receptive fields
Referred pain to arise from deep tissues	Nociceptive input to low back neurons from deep tissues more powerful than skin input
Spontaneous, ongoing low back pain	Ongoing discharge in many spinal low back neurons after central sensitization/LTP
Referred hyperalgesia (stimulus-provoked tenderness)	Increased responsiveness to mechanical (LTM and NOC) input in the receptive field after central sensitization/LTP
Radiation of pain	Unit receptive field expansion over time because of central sensitization/LTP Recruitment of additional low back neurons into the active population by: • Release and spread of pro-nociceptive neuroactive substances from afferents • "Unmasking" of latent excitatory synapses by NOC inputs and sensitization/LTP • Recruitment of additional low back neurons by sensitization/LTP and release of diffusible substances
Persistent, referred low back pain	Sensitization/LTP produces: • Sympathetically mediated increases in LTM and NOC input—refreshes and maintains neuron hyperexcitability • Increased nonnociceptive (LTM) afferent drive maintains neuron hyperexcitability • Loss of inhibitory controls promotes hyperexcitability
Pain relief (analgesia) by treatment interventions (for example, CM) and placebos	Recruitment of "tonic" and "phasic" antinociception by: • Coactivation of paraspinal NOC and LTM afferents • Central/psychogenic triggers

LTM, Mechanoreceptor; *NOC*, nociceptor; *LTP*, long-term potentiation; *CM*, chiropractic manipulation.

in the presence of deep somatic tissue inflammation and, moreover, that this system can be activated by further transient noxious stimulation. These speculations and neurophysiologic findings are consistent with recent clinical trial results showing the antinociceptive effectiveness of forceful chiropractic manipulation (CM) in low back pain patients.[55-57]

It appears that the low back nocireceptive neurons that we have investigated are subject to powerful inhibitory controls that may be activated by various location-specific mechanical interventions (for example, spinal manipulation) and location-nonspecific interventions (for example, placebos[11,26,50,55,56]) currently applied for the amelioration of lumbar spine pain (feature 4).

Recapitulation and Conclusions

Table 16-1 summarizes our current understanding of the neurophysiologic processes that underlie the sensory/symptom dimensions of referred low back pain and hyperalgesia.[8-11,34,47,54] This summary includes a number of working and speculative hypotheses concerning the neurobiologic correlates of lumbar spine pain phenomenology and should help explain some of the unique clinical features of this problem in humans, including its persistence, poor localization, deep referral, tendency to radiate, and its attenuation by placebos and other interventions.

The future holds much promise for those researchers prepared for a protracted campaign of attack on this refractory and expensive health care problem.

Acknowledgments

The experimental work described in this chapter was supported by the National Institutes of Health; R.S. Dow Neurological Sciences Center of Good Samaritan Hospital and Medical Center, Portland, Oregon; the Tarter Trust of the Medical Research Foundation of Oregon; and Western States Chiropractic College, Portland, Oregon. The author would also like to thank Professors Robert Boal, PhD, and David Peterson, DC, for critically reviewing an earlier version of this chapter.

References

1. Fields HL. Pain. New York: McGraw-Hill; 1987.
2. Hockaday JM, Whiny CWM. Patterns of referred pain in the normal subject. Brain 1967;90:481-96.
3. Lewis T. Pain. London: Macmillan; 1942.
4. Livingston WK. Pain mechanisms. London: Macmillan; 1943.
5. Ruch TC. Visceral sensation and referred pain. In: Fulton JF, editor. Howell's textbook of physiology. Vol. 15. Philadelphia: Saunders; 1946.
6. Sinclair DC, Weddell G, Feindel WH. Referred pain and associated phenomena. Brain 1948;71:184-211.
7. Price DD. Psychological and neural mechanisms of pain. New York: Raven Press; 1988.
8. Gillette RG, Kramis RC, Roberts WJ. Characterization of spinal somatosensory neurons having receptive fields in lumbar tissues of cats. Pain 1993;54:85-98.
9. Gillette RG, Kramis RC, Roberts WJ. Spinal projections of cat primary afferent fibers innervating lumbar facet joints and multifidus muscle. Neurosci Lett 1993;157:67-71.
10. Gillette RG, Kramis RC, Roberts WJ. Sympathetic activation of cat spinal neurons responsive to noxious stimulation of deep tissues in the low back. Pain 1994;56:31-42.
11. Kramis RC, Gillette RG, Roberts WJ. Neurophysiology of chronic back pain. In: White A, editor. Spinal medicine and surgery: a multidisciplinary approach. St. Louis: Mosby; 1995.
12. Roberts WJ, Gillette RG, Kramis RC. Dorsal horn plasticity relating to low back pain. Journal of the CCA 1992;36(2):108-9.
13. Roberts WJ, Gillette RG, Kramis RC, Byers MR. Bilateral c-fos expression in dorsal horn after unilateral low back capsaicin injections: enhancement by prior conditioning stimulation [Abstract]. IASP World Congress of Pain 1993;7:747.
14. Shekelle PG, Brook RH. A community-based study of the use of chiropractic services. Am J Public Health 1991;81:439-42.
15. Bogduk N. Lumbar dorsal ramus syndrome. Med J Aust 1980;2:537-41.
16. Bogduk N. The innervation of the lumbar spine. Spine 1984;8:286-93.
17. Fernstrom U. A discographic study of ruptured lumbar intervertebral discs. Acta Chir Scand Suppl 1960;258:1-60.
18. Hirsch C, Ingelmark BE, Miller M. The anatomical basis for low back pain. Acta Orthop Scand 1963;33:1-17.
19. Kellgren JH. The anatomical source of back pain. Rheumatol Rehabil 1977;16:3-12.
20. Kuslich SD, Ulstrom CL, Michael EJ. The tissue origin of low back pain and sciatica: a report of pain response to tissue stimulation during operations on the lumbar spine using local anesthesia. Orthop Clin North Am 1991;22:181-7.
21. Mooney V. Where is the pain coming from? Spine 1987;12:754-9.

22. Mooney V, Robertson J. The facet syndrome. Clin Orthop 1976;115:149-56.
23. O'Brien JP. Mechanisms of spinal pain. In: Wall PD, Melzack R, editors. Textbook of pain. London: Churchill Livingstone; 1984.
24. El Mahdi MA, Latif UA, Janko M. The spinal nerve root innervations and a new concept of the clinicopathological interrelations in back pain and sciatica. Neurochirurgia 1981;24:137-41.
25. Hansson P, Lindblom U. Quantitative evaluation of sensory disturbances accompanying focal or referred nociceptive pain. In: Vecchiet L, Albe-Fessard D, Lindblom U, editors. New trends in referred pain and hyperalgesia. London: Elsevier; 1993.
26. Fine PG, Roberts WJ, Gillette RG, Child TR. Slowly developing placebo responses confound tests of intravenous phentolamine to determine mechanisms underlying idiopathic chronic low back pain. Pain 1994;56:235-42.
27. Mense S. Referral of muscle pain: New aspects. APS Journal 1994;3:1-9.
28. Coderre TJ, Katz J, Vaccarino AL, Melzack R. Contribution of central neuroplasticity to pathological pain: Review of clinical and experimental evidence. Pain 1993;52:259-85.
29. Theobald GW. Referred pain: a new hypothesis. Colombo: Times of Ceylon; 1941.
30. Guilbaud G. Central neurophysiological processing of joint pain on the basis of studies performed in normal animals and in models of experimental arthritis. Can J Physiol Pharmacol 1991;69:637-46.
31. Roberts WJ, Kramis RC. Sympathetic nervous system influence on acute and chronic pain. In: Fields HL, editor. Pain syndromes in neurology. London: Butterworth; 1990.
32. Haldeman S. Failure of the pathology model to predict back pain. Spine 1990;15:718-24.
33. Waddell G. A new clinical model for the treatment of low back pain. Spine 1987;12:632-44.
34. Gillette RG, Boal R. Molecular neutronal plasticity, low back pain and spinal manipulative therapy. J Manipulative Physiol Ther 2004;27:314-26.
35. Dubner R, Ruda MA. Activity-dependent neuronal plasticity following tissue injury and inflammation. Trends Neurosci 1992;15:96-103.
36. McMahon SB, Lewin GR, Wall PD. Central hyperexcitability triggered by noxious inputs. Curr Opin Neurobiol 1993;3:602-10.
37. Woolf CJ, Thompson WN. The induction and maintenance of central sensitization is dependent on N-methyl, D-aspartic acid receptor activation: implications for treatment of post-injury hypersensitivity states. Pain 1991;44:293-9.
38. Korr IM. The neural basis of the osteopathic lesion. J Am Osteopath Assoc 1947;47:191-8.
39. Patterson MM, Steinmetz JE. Long-lasting alterations of spinal reflexes: a potential basis for somatic dysfunction. Manual Med 1986;2:38-42.
40. Coderre TJ. The role of excitatory amino acid receptors and intracellular messengers in persistent nociception after tissue injury. Mol Neurobiol 1994;7:229-46.
41. Zimmermann M, Herdegen T. Control of gene transcription by Jun and Fos proteins in the nervous system: beneficial or harmful molecular mechanisms of neuronal response to noxious stimulation? APS J 1994;3:33-48.
42. Randic M, Jiang MC, Cerne R. Long-term potentiation and long-term depression of primary afferent neurotransmission in the rat spinal cord. J Neurosci 1993;13:5228-41.
43. Wall PD. Neurophysiologic mechanisms of referred pain and hyperalgesia. In: Vecchiet L, Albe-Fessard D, Lindblom U, editors. New trends in referred pain and hyperalgesia. London: Elsevier; 1993.
44. Wall PD. The presence of ineffective synapses and circum stances which unmask them. Phil Trans R Soc Lond Biol 1977;278:361-72.
45. Sluijter ME. The use of radio frequency lesions for pain relief in failed back patients. International Disability Studies 1988;10:37-43.
46. Melzack R, Wall PD. Pain mechanisms: a new theory. Science 1965;150:971-9.
47. Gillette RG. Potential antinociceptive effects of high-level somatic stimulation: chiropractic manipulative therapy may coactivate both tonic and phasic analgesic systems. Trans Pac Consort Chirop Res 1986;1:A1-9.
48. Chung JM, Fang ZR, Hori Y, Lee KH, Willis WD. Prolonged inhibition of primate spinothalamic tract cells by peripheral nerve stimulation. Pain 1984;11:259-65.
49. Le Bars D, Dickenson AH, Besson JM. Diffuse noxious inhibitory controls (DNIC): Effects on dorsal horn convergent neurons in the rat. Pain 1979;6:283-304.
50. Le Bars D, Villanueva L, Bouhassira D, Wilier JC. Diffuse noxious inhibitory controls (DNIC) in animals and in man. Path Physiol Exp Ther 1992;4:55-65.
51. Basbaurn AI, Fields HL. Endogenous brain control system: brainstem spinal pathways and endorphin circuitry. Annu Rev Neurosci 1984;7:309-38.
52. Fields HL, Heinricher MM. Anatomy and physiology of a nociceptive modulation system. Phil Trans R Soc Lond Biol 1985;308:361-74.
53. Stein C. Peripheral mechanisms of opioid analgesia. Anesth Analg 1993;76:182-91.
54. Gillette RG. A speculative argument for the coactivation of diverse somatic receptor populations by forceful chiropractic adjustments. Manual Med 1987;3:1-14.
55. Postacchini F, Facchini M, Palieri P. Efficacy of various forms of conservative treatment in low back pain. Neuroorthopedics 1988;6:28-35.
56. Waagen G, Haldeman S, Cook G, Lopez D, DeBoer KF. Short-term trial of chiropractic adjustments for the relief of chronic low back pain. Manual Med 1986;2:63-7.
57. Herzog W. Biomechanical studies of spinal manipulative therapy. J CCA 1991;35:156-64.

Part THREE

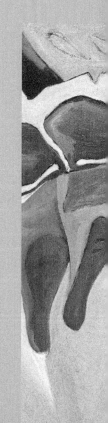

The Subluxation Syndromes

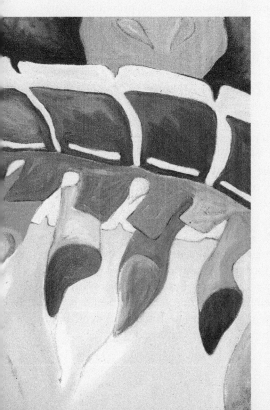

T he subluxation syndromes are the aggregate of signs and symptoms produced by subluxation of the various spinal and pelvic motion segments. Case studies along with a limited number of larger studies link the subluxation of articulations with patterns of signs and symptoms characteristic of each region of the spine and pelvis. Each subluxation syndrome is presented with pathophysiology and dysfunction typical of that region of the spine along with appropriate diagnostic and therapeutic measures employed by the chiropractic profession. In each syndrome articular subluxation is amenable to manual therapy, including manipulative and adjustive procedures.

Although the focus of this section of the text is the identification and management of subluxation syndromes, it must be emphasized that the focus of chiropractic care is the patient. Patient-centered care has been identified with the long-standing satisfaction experienced by chiropractic patients. This satisfaction has been related to chiropractors' egalitarian manner in dealing with patients, understandable explanations of the patient's condition, and holistic approaches to the care of each individual. This care includes use of the patient's belief that recovery is possible, diagnostic and therapeutic touch, and counseling aimed toward healthy lifestyle changes. Paramount in the chiropractor patient encounter is actively involving the patient in the recovery process and in health promotion. This focus on the patient as an individual and not just on subluxations or pain patterns prevents separation of the patient from the disease and is the ingredient sought by patients when seeking health care.

Chapter 17 "Cervicogenic Headache" describes the mechanisms whereby headaches result from cervical subluxations. Cervicogenic headaches are frequently classified as muscle tension headaches involving referred pain; however, through autonomic modulation, some migrainous presentations are benefited by manipulation. This chapter presents the evidence supporting the treatment of cervicogenic headaches with manipulation.

Chapter 18 "Cervicogenic Sympathetic Syndromes" relates subluxation of the cervical spine to sympathetic syndromes that show a favorable response to manipulation. Cervicogenic vertigo, Horner's syndrome, and Barré Liéou syndrome are among the sympathetic conditions that may be produced by the dysfunction caused by subluxation of the cervical spine.

Chapter 19 "The Cerebral Dysfunction Syndrome" presents a theory that explains the various manifestations of cerebral dysfunction purportedly relieved by manipulation. The proposal that decreased blood flow that inhibits normal cerebral functioning can be reversed through manipulation is supported by ophthalmologic measurement. The widespread effects of improvement in cerebral function through spinal manipulation of upper cervical vertebrae have been demonstrated.

Chapter 20 "Whiplash" discusses the ramifications of whiplash injuries. The mechanism of injury and pattern of injury are outlined. Subluxation of cervical motion segments from whiplash injuries is commonly treated by chiropractors, with supporting evidence that early manipulation of the neck after this type of injury proves beneficial to the patient.

Chapter 21 "Cervicogenic Dorsalgia" is a syndrome in which pain originating in the cervical spine is referred to the thoracic region of the spine. As in any pain pattern referred from a subluxation in another area of the spine, manipulation of the subluxation produces dramatic relief from the referred pain.

Chapter 22 "The Thoracic Outlet Syndrome: First Rib Subluxation Syndrome" can be produced by cervical and first rib subluxations that respond dramatically to manipulation. The hand and arm symptoms produced by these subluxations are often mistaken for other causes of thoracic outlet syndrome. The anatomic relationships that lead to compromise of the structures passing through the thoracic outlet are discussed in this chapter in addition to management of thoracic outlet syndromes.

Chapter 23 "Thoracic and Costovertebral Subluxation Syndromes" cause needless suffering when the sharp chest pain produced by these subluxations goes unrecognized. The mechanism, diagnosis, and management of thoracic and costovertebral subluxations is presented. Early recognition and appropriate treatment of these syndromes can prevent much needless anxiety and suffering.

Chapter 24 "Facet Subluxation Syndrome" has been shown to benefit greatly from chiropractic manipulation. Subluxation of the lumbar facet joints, which produces low back pain, has been the focus of numerous studies that have demonstrated the effectiveness of manipulation in the treatment of pain-producing subluxations in the low back.

Chapter 25 "Intervertebral Disc Syndrome" has been demonstrated in some cases to respond to chiropractic manipulation. Both flexion distraction therapy and procedures using rotation have proven beneficial. The mechanism, diagnosis, and management of intervertebral disc syndromes using manipulation are discussed.

Chapter 26 "Sacroiliac Subluxation Syndrome" has a favorable response rate of 97% to manipulation of the sacroiliac joints. Long considered the most controversial subluxation syndrome, sacroiliac subluxation as a cause of buttock and referred leg pain is recognized as responsive to manipulation. This chapter discusses the mechanism, diagnosis, and treatment of sacroiliac subluxation syndrome.

Chapter 27 "Coccygeal Subluxation Syndrome" produces coccydynia, one of the most painful conditions to respond to manipulation. Mechanisms of injury, diagnostic procedures, and therapy directed to the coccygeal subluxation syndrome are presented in the final chapter.

17

Cervicogenic Headache

Howard Vernon and
Meridel I. Gatterman

Key Words   Cervicogenic headache, tension headache, vertebrogenic migraine, convergence projection, central sensitization, central facilitation, aura

---

After reading this chapter you should be able to answer the following questions:

Question 1   What is the most common level of motion segment blockage (subluxation) found in subjects suffering "cervical headache"?

Question 2   What is the proposed neuroanatomic basis of headache referred from the neck?

Question 3   What cervical subluxogenic signs have been noted in headache sufferers?

Question 4   Can there be a cervical component in tension-type and migraine-type headaches?

Question 5   Do the results of manipulation studies automatically imply the existence of a causative cervical component to benign headaches?

Question 6   Can a subluxation associated with a headache be either the cause or the effect of the headache syndrome?

Acknowledgment of the role of the cervical spine in headache has increased since the 1990s. In 1988 a spectrum of headache subtypes that might have some kind of cervicogenic involvement was defined (Figure 17-1).[1] At that time the spectrum ranged from "tension headache with neck muscle pain" through "cervicogenic headache," defined in chiropractic terms as symptomatic head pain and cephalic dysfunction caused by subluxation of a spinal joint, to a proposed "vertebrogenic migraine." Also in 1988, the International Headache Society (IHS) published its report on the classification of headaches.[2] This classification recognized a headache subtype known as cervicogenic headache (CH). The definition of CH according to the 1988 IHS classification is shown in Box 17-1. This headache owes much of its definition to the work of Ottar Sjaastad and his colleagues,[3-6] which first appeared in print in 1983.

In a subsequent publication,[7] this very narrow definition of CH was challenged and contrasted with the characteristic headache subtypes that chiropractic, manual medicine, osteopathic, and physiotherapeutic experts had addressed in the literature spanning the greater part of the twentieth century. The IHS version of CH was also contrasted with the headache subtypes that had been included in the clinical studies of the outcome of spinal manipulation by the same array of practitioners. In these studies of both tension-type and migraine-type headaches (definitely different from the narrow

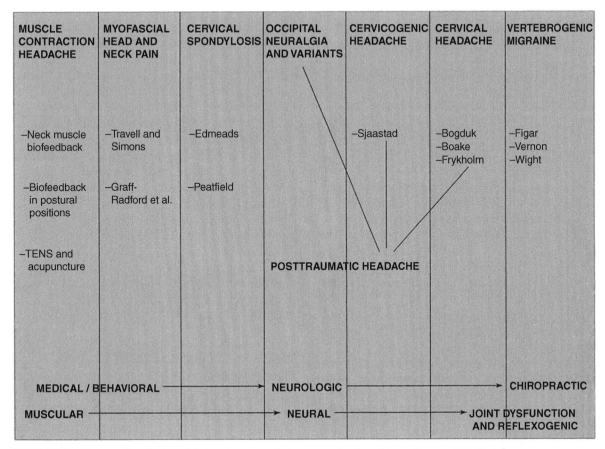

Figure 17-1   Types of headache with involvement of the cervical spine. *(From Vernon HT. Vertebrogenic headache. In: Vernon HT, editor. The upper cervical syndrome: chiropractic diagnosis and treatment. Baltimore: Williams & Wilkins; 1988. p. 152-88.)*

BOX 17-1 ■ Classification of Cervicogenic Headache Diagnostic Criteria

A. Pain localized to neck and suboccipital region. May project to forehead, orbital region, temples, vertex, or ears.
B. Pain is precipitated or aggravated by special neck movements or sustained neck postures.
C. At least one of the following occurs:
   1. Resistance or limitation of passive neck movements
   2. Changes in neck muscle contour, texture, tone, or response to passive stretching or contraction
   3. Abnormal tenderness of neck muscles
D. Radiologic examination shows at least one of the following:
   1. Movement abnormalities in flexion-extension
   2. Abnormal posture
   3. Fractures, congenital abnormalities, bone tumors, rheumatoid arthritis, or other distinct pathology (not spondylosis or osteochondrosis)

From International Headache Society. Cephalalgia 1988;8 Suppl 7:1-96.

IHS features of the CH category), the results of manipulation for (presumably) some cervical spine dysfunction range from fair to excellent.

This leaves us in a quandary asking the following questions: Is there a putative cervical component in tension-type and migraine-type headaches? Is it similar to or different from the dysfunction in CH? Do the results of manipulation studies automatically imply the existence of a causative cervical component to these forms of benign headaches?

Alternatively, is there one kind of cervical component that might contribute to, or manifest as, different forms of headache experiences and thus may be diagnostically labeled as different headache categories? This chapter explores this quandary with a clear bias toward accepting this alternate

hypothesis. This is done by first briefly reviewing the current research on pain mechanisms in CH and following with the results of clinical studies of spinal manipulation for headaches. Literature is reviewed on findings of cervicogenic dysfunction in headache groups that are clearly not IHS-CH. Finally, the argument is made for the alternative hypothesis: that subluxation/dysfunction of the spine makes a significant contribution to the cause of a number of benign forms of headache.

Mechanisms of Pain in Cervicogenic Headache

In 1988 a vertebrogenic model of headache was presented[1] that contained four categories: (1) extra-segmental, referring to the long regional myofascial structures such as the trapezius and long extensor muscles, ligamentum nuchae, and interface between the occipitofrontalis muscle and the regional cervicothoracic structures; (2) intersegmental, referring to the three-joint complexes of C2-C3-C4 and the articulations of C0-C1-C2 with their ligaments and deep intersegmental muscles; (3) infrasegmental, referring to the nerve structures in and around the intervertebral foramina and, in the cervical spine, those near the lateral portions of the vertebrae (the sympathetic trunk; the vertebral nerve; the C2 dorsal root ganglion; the greater, lesser, and third occipital nerves; and the sensory roots of C1); and (4) intrasegmental, referring to the spinal cord and medullary dorsal horn with the nucleus subcaudalis of the trigeminal nerve.

Bogduk[8] considers the possible cervical source of headache to lie in any of the structures innervated by the first three cervical nerves. Knowledge of upper cervical innervation patterns must first be considered.[9]

Innervation Patterns of the First Three Cervical Nerves

1. C1 and C2 Anterior Ramus
   • Deep anterior suboccipital muscles
   • Posterior dura
   • Posterior cranial vessels

- The C2 anterior ramus contains the sensory fibers of the hypoglossal nerve, which run in the ansa hypoglossus
2. C1 Posterior Ramus
   - The posterior ramus is very small, but its existence was demonstrated by Kerr[10]
3. C1 Anterior Ramus
   - Superior oblique muscles
4. C2 Posterior Ramus
   - The C2 posterior ramus has two branches: the medial and the lateral. The medial branch becomes the lesser occipital nerve and innervates the rectus capitus posterior major and minor and the medial C1-2 joint and ligaments. The lateral branch is the largest posterior ramus of the spine and is called the greater occipital nerve. The greater occipital nerve gives off an articular branch to the inferior oblique muscle, then courses posteriorly and superiorly to pierce between the semispinalis capitus and trapezius muscle insertions, where it becomes cutaneous, innervating the skin of the posterior skull until the midline.
5. C3 Posterior Ramus
   - The C3 posterior ramus has been referred to as the "third occipital nerve" by Bogduk.[8,11] It innervates the C2-3 zygapophyseal (Z) joint and deep muscles as well as provides the recurrent meningeal nerve that innervates the C2-3 intervertebral disc (IVD).

Localization of Somatic Tissues Innervated by the First Three Cervical Nerves

Extrasegmental

The relatively superficial, long occipitothoracic muscles in the neck include the trapezius, sternocleidomastoid, and splenius cervicis. The occipitofrontalis muscle is also an important consideration related to cranial pain. Other important extrasegmental structures include the vertebral artery (implicated in the Barré-Liéou syndrome[1] and vertebrobasilar ischemic syndrome) as well as the ascending sympathetic chain and superior cervical ganglion. Older theories implicated compression or irritation of these sympathetic structures in generating cranial pain and cranial vasomotor

dysregulation. These theories have fallen out of favor, having been supplanted by sensorimotor theories of pain.

Myofascial dysfunction results from macrotrauma, microtrauma, and postural strain. Trigger points with typical pain referral patterns have been charted by Travell and Simons.[12] Occupational stress that produces repetitive strain can produce static overload of muscles producing local and referred pain.[13]

Intersegmental

These structures include the classic spinal joints and deep spinal muscles, i.e., the semispinalis occiput and cervicalis, multifidus and suboccipital muscles (posterior, lateral, and anterior). Note that there is no intervertebral disc between the C0-1 and C1-2 spinal motion segments. The suboccipital articulations include the bilateral atlantooccipital joints, the bilateral atlantoaxial joints, the atlantodental joint, joints of Luschka, and the C2-3 intervertebral disc. The suboccipital region contains a large number of specialized ligamentous structures.[14]

Subluxation of the C0-3 spinal motion segments is thought to be a common precipitator of cervical headaches. A number of authors have mapped local and referred pain patterns in the cervical zygapophyseal joints. Dreyfuss, Michaelson, and Fletcher[15] have used provocation and anesthetic procedures to study pain patterns for the C0-1 joint. Feinstein et al.[16] and others[17-19] have similarly studied the C1-2 and C2-3 articulations. Anesthetic blockades have been used to identify the C2-3 Z-joint as the primary pain generator in more than 50% of a group of whiplash patients suffering from headaches.[20,21]

Pain patterns from trigger points in the deep intersegmental and suboccipital muscles have also been implicated.[12] Tenderness in the deep suboccipital muscles is the most commonly reported finding in clinical trials.[22] At least one tender point was found in 84% of a sample of tension-type and migraine headache sufferers with most exhibiting two or more. Others[23] found a high prevalence of paraspinal tenderness at the C3-4 level. Bouquet et al.[24] found trigger points at the C2-3 level in 24 cervicogenic headache sufferers with "enlarged C2 spinous processes," proposed to be due to rotational misalignment at that level. Misalignment and tenderness around the transverse process of C1 were reported by Jaeger[25] in a study of 11 cervicogenic headache patients.

Intrasegmental

This category involves the neural and vascular structures contained in the intervertebral environment of C1-2 and the intervertebral foramina of C2-3—specifically, the anterior and posterior rami of C1 and C2, the C2 dorsal root ganglion, as well as the C3 posterior nerve root. For an extensive review of upper cervical anatomy see Bogduk.[8,26]

Entrapment of the greater occipital nerve and its ganglion has long been purported to cause greater occipital neuralgia. Recent evidence by Bogduk[8,26] casts more doubt on this theory, because anesthetization of the greater occipital nerve would reduce pain from any of the tissues it innervates. Irritation of the sensory fibers in the anterior ramus of C2 by inflammation or osteophytes from the C1-2 lateral joint has been reported as a cause of the uncommon "neck tongue syndrome"[27] characterized by shooting pain into one side of the tongue.

Infrasegmental

Included in this category are the spinal cord and lower brainstem. Of particular importance is the spinal tract of the trigeminal nerve, which contains descending afferents from the trigeminal sensory ganglion that terminate as far caudally as C3 in the spinal nucleus of cranial nerve V. The descending tract contains three components: the pars oralis (upper), pars intermedialis, and the pars or subnucleus caudalis (lowest). These afferent fibers terminate on the same second order neurons as do the afferents from the upper three cervical roots. The second order neurons form a continuous column of cells called the "trigeminocervical nucleus" by Bogduk and Marsland[28] and the "medullary dorsal horn" by Gobel.[29] This "neural anastomosis" of converging afferents is the fundamental neuroanatomical basis by which

painful structures in the upper cervical region might generate referred pain to the cranium (Figure 17-2).

Only two direct mechanisms related to mechanical disturbances of the upper cervical cord have been identified. The first involves a mechanism reported by Hack and Koritzerin[30] in which a ligamentous connection was noted between the rectus capitus posterior minor and the dural lining at the atlantooccipital junction. In a small number of reported cases, surgical ligation of this ligament has resulted in improvement in headache patients. The second mechanism involves a herniation of the C2-3 intervertebral disc. Reported in 1950 by Eldridge and Choh-Luh,[31] this is thought to be relatively rare. Recently disc fusion surgery with the use of discogram imaging has resurrected this idea.

A significant role played by the spinal cord in cervicogenic headache lies in the previously described phenomenon of afferent convergence of the upper cervical and trigeminal systems.[32] This mechanism explains the referred pain to the cranium resulting from upper cervical deep-tissue pain. It should be remembered that the same convergence phenomenon explains why posterior intracranial pathologies result in referred upper cervical pain. This may be one of the mechanisms involved in the creation of upper cervical pain and myofascial dysfunction in migraine. Painful and inflamed posterior cranial vessels can refer pain to the suboccipital region contributing to diagnostic confusion.

Implications for Headache of Cervical Origin

Central sensitization provides a mechanism to explain the clinical phenomena seen so regularly in headache sufferers of (1) persistent somatic pain; (2) pain referred from the cervical spine or posterior occipital region into the frontoorbital regions and perceived as "headache" when it is actually referred neck pain; (3) tender hyperalgesic muscle zones ("trigger points"), which often expand as the headache pain increases; (4) muscular tension in the deep suboccipital, superficial occipital, and craniofacial muscles, which has for many years been thought to be the sole basis of muscle contraction

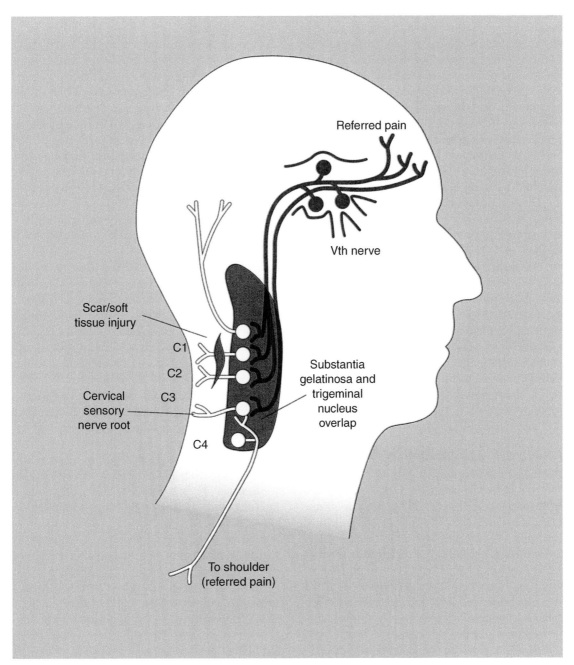

Figure 17-2   The trigeminocervical nucleus. *(From Hooshmand H. Chronic pain. London: CRC Press; 1993. p. 52.)*

or tension-type headache.[33] Conversely, the mechanism of "convergence-sensitization-projection" also serves to explain how pain arising from intracranial structures such as posterior cerebellar tumors or the intracerebral blood vessels (proposed by Moskowitz[34] in the case of migraine) may be referred to the posterior occipital and suboccipital regions, masquerading as cervical pain.

In summary, the trigeminocervical nucleus and the extensive afferent convergence from numerous craniocervical peripheral tissues onto these second-order neurons (a phenomenon called convergence-projection)[35] serves to explain the neuroanatomic basis of headache referred from the neck. The neurophysiologic basis of such pain referral, particularly from inflammatory pain arising from the posterior suboccipital muscles and joints, is explained by the phenomenon of "central sensitization" and the neuroplastic changes that these second-order neurons undergo in response to prolonged peripheral deep somatic pain. These are the mechanisms thought for many years by chiropractors to arise from the subluxation or dysfunction state of the vertebral motion segment. Certainly this is consistent with the older model of "central facilitation" proposed by Korr et al.[36] and adhered to by several generations of chiropractors.

Cervicogenic Dysfunction in Headache

A 1992 report by Vernon et al.[22] on cervicogenic dysfunction in muscle contraction (that is, "tension-type headache" [TTH]) and common migraine (that is, "migraine without aura" [MWA]) defined the components of cervicogenic dysfunction, and the literature up to 1988 was reviewed in defense of the notion of a broad, highly prevalent basis of cervicogenic dysfunction in headache. A 1991 report[7] also addressed how high prevalence of cervicogenic dysfunction in these types of headaches argued against the position adopted by the IHS (based principally on the work of Sjaastad and his colleagues[3-6]) that "cervicogenic headache" was a narrowly defined, infrequently encountered form of headache. This controversy was again addressed by Vernon in 1999.[37]

Components of cervicogenic dysfunction:

1. Hypomobility; variously termed *subluxation, joint blockage, segmental dysfunction, fixation* (See Chapter 1.)
2. Tender points in the soft tissues; local areas of hypersensitivity that produce a pain response to light pressure
3. Trigger points; palpable nodules in muscles that refer pain in consistent patterns
4. Radiographic findings of misalignment and dynamic intersegmental abnormality
5. Static segmental misalignment on palpation
6. Static malposition of the head and neck (specifically, anterior carriage of the head and low rounded shoulders)
7. Reduced regional ranges of cervical motion

Hypomobility

In 1985 and 1986, Jull[38,39] reported on both the reliability of upper cervical joint motion palpation and its use in headache subjects to determine the lesioned segment. The comparison between headache and nonheadache subjects[39] showed dysfunction at C0-1, C1-2, and C2-3 in 60%, 40%, and 55% of headache subjects, compared with 5%, 12%, and 22%, respectively, in controls. These palpatory findings were confirmed by Jull, Bogduk, and Marsland[40] and Dwyer et al.[41] using diagnostic anesthetic blocks as the gold standard.

In the 1992 report by Vernon et al.,[22] three motion palpation procedures described by Fligg[42] were used. They were A-P glide, rotation, and lateral flexion. A major blockage in any of these three procedures on either side at C0-3 was indicative of segmental fixation. It was reported that only 16% in each group had a fixation at only one level. In the tension-type group, 54% had fixations at two levels and 30% at all three; for migraine subjects these figures were 42% and 42%, respectively. In both groups, 84% had a fixation in at least two of three upper cervical segments.

In 1993 Watson and Trott[43] used multiple outcomes (others are discussed later) to assess cervical headache subjects. They reported on the reliability of posterior-to-anterior glide palpation in 12 of the subjects examined on two occasions by the same examiner. (Kappa values ranged from 0.67 to 1.0 depending on the segment.) They also included as positive signs of joint dysfunction the presence of tenderness and muscle stiffness. (See later discussion.) When all three signs—fixation, tenderness, and palpatory stiffness—were included, far more positive findings were found in headache subjects (N = 30) than in controls (N = 30). The most prevalent level was C0-1.

In 1997 Jull et al.[44] reported high rates of agreement between several pairs of examiners in their abilities to detect the presence or absence of treatable upper cervical dysfunction. Agreement levels were somewhat lower on the exact segment of dysfunction but still good at 70% overall. The highest frequency of joint dysfunction was found at the C1-2 segment. The sensitivity of motion palpation was reported by Jull et al.[44] as 100%. They also reported high levels of agreement between motion palpation findings that were obtained by examiners without pain cues and from headache subjects' subsequent reports of pain during each procedure at each cervical motion segment. This established validity of motion palpation without the subject providing pain-related feedback. Much higher levels of significant joint dysfunction were found in the upper cervical segments of cervical headache subjects versus controls in this study. Jensen, Nielson, and Vosmer[45] reported findings of hypomobility before and after treatment with manipulation compared to the use of cold packs, in a clinical trial of 19 posttraumatic headache patients. The most frequently blocked segment was C1-2. Fourteen of the subjects had at least one level of joint blockage in the upper cervical and upper thoracic region, whereas four had blockage only in the upper cervical region for a total of 18 out of 19 patients with upper cervical hypomobility.

Vernon, Steiman, and Hagino[22] found that 54% of tension-type headaches had hypomobility at two upper cervical segments, whereas 30% had all three levels affected at least unilaterally. They also found that migraine headache sufferers had 42% and 42%, respectively. At least 84% in both groups had at least two upper cervical segments exhibiting hypomobility.

In a posttraumatic headache study[46] that compared headache subjects with an age- and gender-matched control group, at least one segment in the headache group demonstrated marked hypomobility in the upper cervical spine. Much greater joint dysfunction was noted between C0-3 in the headache group as compared with the control group.

In a cervical migraine study, Stodolny and Chmeilewski[47] reported that all 31 of the headache patients had significant joint dysfunction at C0-1 on manual palpation. More than 80% of these subjects had at least two cervical motion segments demonstrating joint dysfunction, remarkably consistent with the findings of Vernon, Steiman, and Hagino[22] in their study of tension-type headaches and migraine subjects.

Craniovertebral Tender Points

Tenderness to palpation of the skin[48] and deep tissues of the craniovertebral and paraspinal region is the most commonly reported sign of headache of cervical origin. Virtually every relevant author has reported on the subject, from Lewit,[49] who reported on "pain over the posterior arch of atlas," to Sachse et al.,[50] who reported similar suboccipital and scapular tenderness, to Graff-Radford et al.[51] and Jaeger,[25] who have reported on the numerous cervical tender points that serve to perpetuate myofascial head pain, to Sjaastad et al.,[3,4] who reported the high prevalence of tenderness at C2-3.

A 1992 study[37] reported on the prevalence of six standard craniocervical tender points in these headache groups:
- Medial occipital brim
- Lateral occipital brim (near the TVP of atlas)
- Suboccipital (C1-2)
- Mid cervical (C2-3)
- Trapezius
- Levator scapulae

Table 17-1 lists the studies of manual tenderness assessment in neck pain and headaches.

In the 1992 report, the pressure algometer[37] was used to verify true tenderness in cervical tender points in tension-type and migraine-without-aura sufferers. This type of assessment has been used with great success by fibromyalgia[52] and headache[53] researchers. Table 17-2 summarizes studies of

Table 17-1

Studies of Manual Tenderness Assessment in Neck Pain and Headaches

Author(s)	Findings	Location
Lebbink, Spierings, and Messinger	Neck muscle soreness, stiffness, and prior neck injury more common in 164 headache sufferers than in 108 controls	Neck muscles
Jensen et al.	Studied 14 muscles sites bilaterally in normals; used Langemark et al. method of scoring; norms reported; older subjects had lower TTS values, females had higher TTS scores	Cranial and large neck muscles
Jensen et al.	TTS scores in TTH and migraine headache sufferers compared; TTHs had lower overall scores; TTHs with headache that day had higher TTS than matched non-HA group	Cranial and large neck muscles
Jensen, Nielsen, and Vosmar	In 19 PTHAs, 42% had tenderness at C2-C3, 89% at C3-C4, and 63% at C4-C5	Neck paraspinal muscles
Hatch et al.	HA subjects had at least one tender muscle more often than controls; TTS in HAs greater than controls; EMG findings not correlated to tenderness	Four cranial muscles Two posterior cervical muscles
Watson and Trott	PTHAs had more tenderness findings than controls, particularly in upper cervical spine	Neck paraspinal muscles
Mercer, Marcus, and Nash	HA subjects had higher values of tenderness than controls	Neck paraspinal muscles
Levoska, Keinanen-Kiukaannierni, and Bloigu	Test-retested correlation of manual palpation of scapular muscles was high; interrater reliability only fair	Scapular muscles
Levoska et al.	Neck pain sufferers had higher number of tender points than controls	Neck paraspinal muscles
Hubka and Phelan	Interrater reliability of segmental TTS scores was highly correlated (Kappa, 0.68)	Neck paraspinal muscles
Sandmark and Nisell	Cervical tenderness was most sensitive (82%) and specific (79%) for neck pain patient discrimination	Neck paraspinal muscles
Nilsson	TTS scores in neck pain patients; high interrater reliability	Neck paraspinal muscles
Sandrini et al.	Mean TTS scores higher in ETTH and CTTH subjects than controls	Trapezius
Persson and Carlsson	TTS scores higher in CH vs. controls	Suboccipital, neck paraspinal, and scapular muscles
Stolk-Hornsveld et al.	Segmental tenderness on passive motion at C1-C4 higher in CH vs. other headache types; good interrater reliability	Suboccipital and neck paraspinal muscles

From Redwood D, Cleveland CS. Fundamentals of chiropractic. St. Louis: Mosby; 2003. p. 515-6.
TTS, Total tenderness score; *TTH,* tension-type headache; *HA,* headache; *PTHA,* posttraumatic headache; *EMG,* electromyogram; *ETTH,* episodic tension-type headache; *CTTH,* chronic tension-type headache; *CH,* cervicogenic headache.

Table 17-2

Studies of Pressure Algometry in Neck Pain and Headache

Author(s)	Findings	Location
Reeves, Jaeger, and Graff-Radford	High correlation coefficients for intraexaminer and interexaminer reliability; average value for C0-C1, 3.0 kg/cm^2; for trapezius, 3.5 kg/cm^2	Occipital and suboccipital
Jensen et al.	Highly consistent values bilaterally and over 3-week interval in normals	Temporalis muscle
Drummond	High intraexaminer reliability; HA subjects had lower algometer values than normals; no difference between TH and migraine HA	Scalp and upper cervical muscles
List, Helkimo, and Falk	High intraexaminer reliability; algometry scores highly correlated to manual palpation findings; TMJ pain subjects had lower values than normals	Temporalis and suboccipital
Langemark et al.	Temporalis algometry negatively correlated to headache intensity and to TTS on manual palpation; high correlation between temporal and occipital sites	Cranial muscles
Takala	High intrarater and interrater reliability in normal subjects; women had lower algometry values than men; lower values in subgroup with minor neck pain and HA	Scapular muscles
Hogeweg et al.	Good reliability to normals; cervical points have lower algometry values than lumbar points	Spinal muscles
Bovim	Lower algometry values in cervicogenic HA group vs. migraine, TTH, and controls; CH group had lower values in posterior cranial area and on the affected side	Cranial and suboccipital muscles
Chung, Un, and Kim	Electronic pressure algometer showed good reliability and test-retest consistency in normals	TMJ and neck muscles
Jensen et al.	Algometry values lower in TTH vs. controls	Cranial muscles
Kosek, Ekholm, and Nordema	Algometry in normals showed good 1-week consistency; lower values in upper part of body	Whole body
Levoska, Keinanen-Kiukaanniemi, and Bloigu; Levoska	Reliability high in neck pain and normals; pain group had lower values	Scapular muscles
Massotta et al.	PPT values significantly lower in ETTH vs. controls	Temporalis
Sandrini et al.	PPT values significantly lower in ETTH and CTTH vs. controls	Frontalis and trapezius
Stolk-Hornsveld et al.	High levels of interrater reliability; sensitivity and specificity for CH vs. controls, 82% and 62%	Suboccipital and neck paraspinal muscles
Bendtsen et al.	Reported on an electronic finger pressure pad for palpating tenderness; high levels of interexaminer reliability	Cranial muscles

From Redwood D, Cleveland CS. Fundamentals of chiropractic. St. Louis: Mosby; 2003. p. 517.
HA, Headache; *TTH,* tension-type headache; *TMJ,* temporomandibular joint; *TTS,* total tenderness score; *CH,* cervicogenic headache; *PPT,* pressure pain threshold; *ETTH,* episodic tension-type headache; *CTTH,* chronic tension-type headache.

pressure algometry in neck pain and headache. In fact, the 1988 IHS classification[2] includes the presence or absence of pericranial tender points as part of the subclassification of tension-type headaches. (See Box 17-1.) A recent report by Kanieki[54] has found tender points in migraineurs during attacks.

The findings of Watson and Trott[43] in which detection of joint dysfunction in headache (HA) subjects and non-HA subjects included pressure palpation for tenderness were described above. Again, this procedure was found to have good intraexaminer reliability and was found to distinguish HA subjects from non-HA subjects with higher prevalence of findings in the HA subjects.

Finally, tenderness to palpation has been used as one of the cardinal signs by Jull, Bogduk, and colleagues[38-41] to locate the level of zygapophyseal joint dysfunction potentially responsible for neck pain and headache. These findings correlate very well with the signs of joint hypomobility previously discussed. This combination of tenderness and hypomobility (as with Watson and Trott[43]) correlates very highly with joint blockades used as a gold standard for diagnosis.

A finding associated with muscle tenderness is increased muscle stiffness. In 1992 Vernon and Gitelman[55] reported on a single case of bilateral tension-type headache with cervical dysfunction. Pressure algometry showed clinically significant tenderness bilaterally in the suboccipital region. Muscle stiffness of the mid-cervical paraspinal and trapezius muscles was measured using Fischer's tissue compliance meter.[56] Higher than expected values were found in both muscle sites.

Sakai et al.[57] used a computerized compliance meter in a comparison of 37 tension-type headache subjects and 63 normal individuals. In 65% of HA subjects there was significantly increased trapezius stiffness, and the overall mean values (756 + 121 versus 538 + 89) significantly distinguished headache from control subjects. An orally administered muscle relaxant greatly reduced this increased stiffness in headache subjects, implying that active tension contributed to the stiffness.

It is evident that the more recent studies of myofascial dysfunction (pain/tenderness and stiffness) employ more sophisticated methodologies and instrumentation and are being conducted in case-control design formats. The findings of these studies even more strongly substantiate the clinical and empirical experience of a high prevalence of craniocervical tenderness in headache sufferers, which is strongly associated with other signs (including misalignment and joint hypomobility) of spinal segmental subluxation. Studies that also employ manipulation or joint blockade have by the relief of symptoms obtained further implicated cervicogenic joint dysfunction in the cause of headache.

Trigger Points That Refer Pain to the Head

Trigger points have been differentiated from tender points based on the pain referral patterns.[12,13,58,59] Travell and Simons[12] have mapped consistent referral patterns that accompany trigger points associated with myofascial pain. Tender points are characterized by localized tenderness from hyperexcitability of spinal cord sensory neurons without referral patterns.[13,58,59] Tender points are characteristically found in patients with fibromyalgia syndrome.[60]

Pain referral from myofascial trigger points does not follow a simple segmental pattern. Neither does it follow familiar neurological patterns, nor the known referral pain of visceral origin. Myofascial pain frequently but not always occurs within the same dermatome, myotome, or sclerotome as that of the trigger point, but it does not involve the entire segment. Additional segments may also be involved. A dermatome is the area of the skin supplied by the afferent nerve fibers of a single posterior nerve root, a myotome is the group of muscles, and a sclerotomes is the area of bone so innervated.[12] The severity and extent of the pain referral pattern depends on the degree of trigger point irritability, not on the size of the muscle.

Pain Guide to Involved Muscles
The most common muscles that refer pain to the head have been identified by Travell and Simons[12] as follows:
Vertex Pain
- Sternocleidomastoid (sternal portion)

Back of the Head
- Trapezius
- Sternocleidomastoid (sternal and clavicular portions)

Temporal Headache
- Temporalis
- Trapezius
- Sternocleidomastoid (sternal portion)

Frontal Headache
- Sternocleidomastoid (clavicular and sternal portions)
- Frontalis
- Zygomaticus major

Eye and Eyebrow Pain
- Sternocleidomastoid (sternal)
- Temporalis
- Splenius cervicis
- Masseter
- Occipitalis
- Orbicularis oculi

Chiropractors treat trigger points and their referred pain employing sustained pressure over the painful nidus. Termed *ischemic compression* by Travell and Simons,[12] this technique was pioneered by Nimmo more than 40 years ago. This Texas chiropractor referred to it as the receptor tonus technique.[61] Specific pressure applied to the center of the trigger point to the patient's tolerance is applied for approximately 30 seconds until release is felt. Stubborn or long-standing trigger points may require a number of treatments until relief from the pain referral pattern is obtained.[13]

Radiologic Findings of Cervicogenic Misalignment and Dysfunction

Functional radiographs are practical tools for the evaluation of spinal segmental motion. Since Hviid[62] in 1963, chiropractors including Sandoz,[63] Anderson,[64] Conley,[65] West,[64] Grice,[66] and Henderson[67] have employed cervical templating techniques to determine hypomobility, hypermobility, and instability of spinal motion segments. Functional radiographs may be used to evaluate the segmental range of motion by comparing the neutral position to the end range of movement in either the sagittal or coronal planes. Medical inves-

tigators, including Penning[68] and Dvorak,[69] have established normative values for gross segmental flexion and extension without reference to the neutral lateral or AP view. However, clinical information may be lost when the information from the neutral position is not included in the assessment.

Pfaffenrath et al.[70] used a computer-aided method of analyzing segmental cervical motion on flexion-extension radiographs. They found a statistically higher incidence of restrictions at C0-C1 in cervicogenic headache subjects as compared with normal controls.

In a 1992 report[37] on tension-type and migraine headache subjects, a similar method that rated segmental movement against the normative data from Dvorak et al.[71] was used. In addition, Penning's method[72] was used for C0-1 (with Fielding's norms for flexion and extension at C0-1). The mean ±1 SD (standard deviation) for occipital flexion in both headache groups was 3.17 degrees ± 2.24 degrees; whereas for extension it was 10.6 ± 7.7 degrees. The percentage of subjects showing reductions in motion below a lower cutoff for normal (−1 SD) was 90% for flexion and 70% for extension. These results agree with those of Pfaffenrath et al. For the rest for the cervical spine, a pattern emerged of greater hypermobility at C1-2 and hypomobility at C4-5-6.

The key to accurately evaluating motion on functional spinal radiographs is precise standards of patient positioning.[73] Meticulous attention to the details of positioning cannot be overemphasized if the information obtained from the resultant radiographs is to be considered a reliable assessment of that particular patient's function. Functional radiographic studies have traditionally been performed with active movement by the patient. Dvorak et al.[74] emphasized the value of obtaining functional radiographic studies of the cervical spine both actively and passively. While they claim that many more hypermobile segments are discovered on the passive stress studies, the application of force at the end of active range of motion risks injury to the patient. These systems of functional radiographic analysis may be of clinical value to the doctor of chiropractic who provides spinal manipulation/adjustments to specific levels of segmental dysfunction. The reliability[71] and clinical validation[74] of cervical flexion extension studies have been demonstrated.

Nagasawa et al.[75] reported changes in cervical function in headache sufferers as determined by x-ray analysis. They compared 372 tension-type headache subjects with 225 normal controls. They found a statistically significant reduction of the neutral curve as measured by a "cervical spine curvature index" (14.6 ± 11.9% versus 19.4 ± 11.1%, P < .001). They also found that segmental instability was less frequent in headache subjects than in controls. Finally, they found a higher frequency of low-set (in other words, rounded) shoulders in headache sufferers (57.5%) versus controls (41.8%, P < .01, χ^2 = 16.6). These findings confirm that tension-type headache sufferers have significant cervical postural and segmental motion abnormalities, typical of subjects whose headaches could be labeled as "cervicogenic."

Static Segmental Misalignment on Palpation

Careful manual assessment can identify misalignments between upper cervical segments. Palpable misalignment of the C1 transverse processes, the C2 spinous process, and the C0-3 posterior joints are common findings. Jaeger[25] noted misalignment around the transverse process of C1 in a number of cervicogenic headache patients.

Cervical Posture, Muscular Weakness, and Range of Motion

Watson and Trott[43] studied 60 subjects, 30 with recurrent cervical headache (a combination of cervicogenic, migraine without aura, and tension-type headache and 30 controls). They studied: (1) the degree of anterior head carriage, measured photographically, (2) the isometric strength and endurance of the upper cervical flexor muscles, measured by strain gauge dynamometry, and (3) the presence of "joint dysfunction," by combining manual palpatory findings of restricted joint play, tenderness, and stiffness (as described above). They found a smaller mean angle of forward head position (FHP) in headache sufferers (that is, a straightened cervical spine). Headache sufferers had smaller strength values and smaller endurance values of upper cervical flexors. These findings correlated well with the degree of FHP. They concluded that FHP increases the load on the posterior muscles that rotate the head (occiput) backward to maintain the orthostatic horizontal position of the eyes. This in turn weakens the antagonist muscles (upper cervical flexors) and contributes to upper cervical joint and myofascial dysfunction, ultimately leading to upper cervical pain. This nociception reinforces the local muscle spasm (as found experimentally by Hu et al.[75]) and creates a vicious cycle of pain, spasm, altered mechanics, pain, etc., all leading to the potential for referred cranial pain.

Reduced Regional Ranges of Cervical Motion

Evidence for the development of regional muscular stiffness and reduced range of cervical motion comes from Kidd and Nelson's report,[77] using a very simplistic observer's evaluation of neck ROM in 64 subjects, 37 with and 37 without benign headache. The headache sufferers more frequently had a reduction of two or more ranges of motion. All of these findings combine to create a composite of cervicogenic dysfunction, much of which has been observed in tension-type headaches and migraine without aura. This profile includes regional alterations in anterior head posture, straightened cervical curve and low-set shoulders, regional muscular stiffness and reduced ROM, as well as upper cervical subluxogenic signs including misalignment, joint hypomobility, and frequent segmental myofascial tenderness. The high potential for upper cervical pain to occur, not only unilaterally, but bilaterally, creates potent opportunities for cranial pain referral.

Headache and Spinal Manipulation

Studies of the treatment of headache with manipulation generally follow three groups from the International Headache Society classification and include tension-type, cervicogenic, and migraine. Less studied is posttraumatic headache.

Tension-Type Headache

Tension-type headaches (see Box 17-1) have been described as usually unilateral and characterized by pressing, tight, vise-like pain—not throbbing and not aggravated by routine physical activity. They are generally mild to moderate and do not inhibit activity. They may last from 30 minutes to 7 days. Precipitating factors include stress, emotional conflict, and depression. Hoyt, Shaffer, Bard et al.[78] reported in 1979 on a trial that compared a combination of osteopathic manipulation and soft tissue procedures with two control interventions (palpatory exam alone and a 10-minute rest period). Treatments were administered for an isolated episode of "muscle contraction" headache associated with posterior cervical discomfort. The soft tissue procedures were described as kneading, deep pressure, and stretching over the entire axial skeleton. Manipulation was described as a high velocity, low amplitude procedure to reduce restriction. Headache severity was assessed before and immediately after treatment. Headache severity was decreased by 49% in the manipulation group but remained unchanged in both the palpatory examination and rest period control groups. This small trial (n = 22) measured the effect of a single session of treatment on acute/ongoing headache.

Boline et al.[79] in a randomized controlled trial (reported in 1990) studied parallel groups for 4 weeks pretreatment and 4 weeks posttreatment. In the group receiving spinal manipulation (n = 5), treatment was given two times a week for 4 weeks with evaluation at 4 weeks posttreatment. The amitriptyline group (n = 5) received 10 mg on day 1, 20 mg on day 2, and then 30 mg/day. No statistically significant difference between groups was found in this small pilot study. A subsequent study by Boline, Kassak, and Brontfort[80] randomized 150 patients to similar interventions. Spinal manipulation described as short lever, low amplitude, high velocity thrusts were administered in two sessions per week for 6 weeks. Amitriptyline doses were begun at 10 mg/day and increased by 10 mg/day each week up to 30 mg daily. The mean daily headache intensity at 6 weeks was lower for amitriptyline than for spinal manipulation. However, when the amitriptyline was stopped and no further manipulation was performed, posttreatment differences were statistically significant (P < 0.01) favoring the manipulation group.

In a 1998 study by Bove and Nilsson,[81] soft tissue therapy plus cervical manipulation was compared to soft issue therapy plus low-power laser light therapy to the upper cervical spine. Each group received 2 sessions/week for 4 weeks following 2 weeks pretreatment. Patients were assessed at 7 weeks and at the end of the trial. By week 7, both treatment groups experienced significant reductions in headache duration, compared with pretreatment values. Significant reductions from pretreatment levels were maintained throughout the trial. This study suggests that manipulation does not confer additional benefits on patients given massage and trigger point therapy. Equating chiropractic care solely with one treatment modality (manipulation) does a disservice to patients if reported that "chiropractic care does not help patients with tension headaches" since chiropractors commonly employ soft tissue therapy (see the following discussion on trigger point therapy).

Cervicogenic Headache

The IHS describes headaches associated with the neck as localized to the neck/occipital region that may project to the forehead, temples, vertex, ears, or orbits. The features of cervicogenic headache are outlined in Box 17-1. While the classification of cervicogenic headache is poorly recognized in medical circles, it is readily described in the chiropractic, osteopathic, physiotherapy, and manual medicine literature.[82-84]

Nilsson et al. reported in 1995[85] and 1997[86] on cervicogenic headache trials. Both studies compared manipulation with soft tissue therapy. Statistically significant improvements in headache intensity and frequency were reported in the manipulation group compared to the control group. These results are consistent with an uncontrolled study in 1995 by Martelli et al.[87] of a group of 36 cervicogenic headache sufferers who received 12 treatments within 4 weeks and whose improvements were retained after a further 4-week follow-up.

A recent clinical trial[88] examined the effect of 6 weeks of manipulative therapy, exercise therapy, combined manipulation and exercise, or a control treatment in 200 subjects with cervicogenic headache. The 12-month follow-up demonstrated significantly greater reductions in headache frequency and intensity in the manipulation and exercise groups, while the combined therapy group did not show a significantly greater improvement.

Migraine Headache

The treatment of migraine headache by chiropractors is more controversial that either cervicogenic or tension-type headaches. Evidence supporting manipulation for migraine relief, however, suggests a cervicogenic component that may act as a trigger. Other triggers that have been suggested include biochemical factors particularly from foods rich in tyramine such as chocolate, cheese, red wine, and any sort of alcohol and fermented foods; environmental factors, such as changes in barometric pressure, ambient odors, loud harsh sounds, and certain kinds of lighting; sleep deprivation, psychosocial factors, particularly those associated with stress and anxiety; and hormonal factors where menstruation may aggravate migraine and pregnancy may relieve it or make it worse.[89]

An early study that became the center of this controversy was reported in 1978 by Parker, Tupling, and Pryor.[90] In this study, 85 subjects (33 male and 52 female) were randomly allocated to three treatment groups. Of these subjects, 70% suffered common migraine (migraine without aura) while 30% suffered from classic migraine (migraine with the premonitory aura). Included in the baseline assessment were psychological tests. Following the baseline examination that included standard medical and neurological tests, the subjects were randomly assigned to one of three treatment groups: chiropractic manipulation, medical manipulation, and a purported control group that received mobilization by physical therapists. The study design included a 2-month pretreatment phase, a 2-month treatment phase, and a further 2-month follow-up phase. An average of seven treatments was given in the treatment phase. The mean improvement level for all groups was 28%. Only one hypothesis achieved an acceptable level

of statistical significance ($P < 0.01$). Pain intensity was reduced in the chiropractic manipulation group. This finding became controversial when it was suggested that the measures of treatment expectation was higher in the chiropractic manipulation group. Further, design flaws led to a follow-up published in 1980 by Parker et al.[91] It was noted that at a 20-month follow-up period, a further 19% of subjects had achieved an improved rating constituting a 47% success rate for manual therapy.

Vernon[1] has noted that data was omitted from statistical analysis which indicated 14 of the subjects achieved a complete recovery (8 in the chiropractic manipulation group, 1 in the medical manipulation group, and 5 in the mobilization group). The follow-up study attempted to correlate certain psychosocial values and only gender achieved the appropriate level of statistical significance; female patients responded more favorably than males to the forms of manual therapy studied by Parker et al.[91]

In 1989, Stodolny and Chmielewski[92] reported on 31 subjects (24 women, 7 men; average age of 48 years) with "cervical migraine." They employed tests for intersegmental blockage and found that 100% of subjects demonstrated spinal motion segment blockage at C0-1, 75% at C7-T1, and 25% between C1-2 and C3. The treatments consisted of two to three manual therapy sessions largely employing manipulative techniques. They reported results at the end of 7 days that included the following:

- Complete relief of headache in 75% of subjects
- Average increases of cervical range of motion of 9 degrees (statistically significant)
- Fixations reduced in 28 of 31 subjects
- Reports of dizziness in subjects greatly reduced

There was no further follow-up reported. Obviously, no control comparison or blinding of the assessors was included in their protocol. Results must be interpreted cautiously, all the more so because of the short treatment period.

More recently Nelson[93] reported on the efficacy of spinal manipulation, amitriptyline, and the combination of both therapies for the prophylaxis of migraine headache. Nelson used a similar design for his tension headache trial with clinical improvement noted in all three groups. Significant differences were noted over time with reduction of headaches reported on the headache index amounting to 24% for the amitriptyline group, 42% for the spinal adjustment/manipulation group, and 25% for the combined group.

In 2000 Tuchin, Pollard, and Bonello[94] presented findings of a randomized controlled trial of chiropractic spinal manipulative therapy for migraine. In comparing manipulation to detuned ultrasound, the study found significant improvements from manipulation in headache frequency, duration, disability, and level of medication use.

Posttraumatic Headache

Jenson, Nielsen, and Vosmer[95] reported on the treatment of posttraumatic headache that compared manual therapy with cold packs. Subjects were randomly assigned to one of the two parallel groups. The design included 5 pretreatment weeks followed by 2 treatments one week apart, with assessment at 7 weeks posttreatment. Outcomes were assessed using a headache diary and a headache index. A reduction of 43% in posttraumatic headache in the manual group compared to the cold therapy group was demonstrated at 2 weeks posttreatment.

Issues Surrounding the Treatment of Cervicogenic Headache by Chiropractors

An ongoing problem in the area of cervicogenic headache is the lack of clarity that exists for the etiology and definition of cervicogenic headache. By a broad definition it must involve pain referred to the head originating from structures in the cervical spine. The upper cervical spine has been particularly implicated, principally because the upper cervical spinal cord and lower brain stem share a common input of pain afferent fibers from the trigeminal and upper cervical sensory systems.[37] Also problematic is the narrow International

Headache Society definition of cervicogenic headache that leaves little room for the characteristic subtypes of headaches treated by practitioners of manual therapy. Challenged by Vernon[22] in consideration of the results of manipulation to cervical spine dysfunction that range from fair to excellent, this narrow classification does a disservice to patients suffering from headaches that form a much broader classification.

Finally, the treatment of headache by chiropractors goes beyond the use of manipulative high velocity, low amplitude thrust procedures to include a variety of adjustive and soft tissue techniques. To dismiss chiropractic treatment of muscle tension headaches as adding no additional benefit based on the solely on one procedure (manipulation) ignores the many effective therapies employed by chiropractors including trigger point therapy and myofascial release.

Conclusion

It is speculative to assert the conclusion that relief of headache by manipulation proves the hypothesis that spinal dysfunction (presumably the target of the manipulative treatment) causes or is associated with these forms of headache. This is because, although correction of the causative agent is one acceptable hypothesis to explain these results, other equally plausible explanations exist, including the strong placebo effect that is typically generated in headache patients, the natural history effect, and the selection bias. Once again, controlled studies are required for theoretical and pathophysiologic conclusions, as well as for conclusions regarding clinical efficacy.

Much has been learned about these mechanisms since 1988. The focus has centered on the pain pathways of the upper cervical cord and their convergence on cells in the nucleus subcaudalis, a mechanism called the trigeminocervical nucleus by Bogduk.[95] (See Figure 17-2.) Recent data presented by Burnstein[96] suggest that fibers from the spinal trigeminal nucleus may affect structures in the lower cervical spine as well. Upper cervical cord and trigeminal nucleus subcaudalis neurons are particularly responsive to deep nociceptive inputs that, as Hu[97,98] has said, "unmask or strengthen... central somatosensory neuronal relays of convergent afferent inputs that normally are relatively 'ineffective' ('silent') in exciting (these) neurons."

As such, deep nociceptive inputs are particularly effective in creating the most significant increase of cutaneous hypersensitivity and an increase in the receptive fields of dorsal medullary horn neurons. In clinical terms, this underlies several important features of deep tissue pain, including its poor localization (explained by multiconvergence on numerous central neurons), hyperalgesia (so-called secondary hyperalgesia), spread of hyperalgesia, and its referral to distant cutaneous regions. All of these phenomena are well-known attributes of myofascial pain and, in particular, spinal pain syndromes. These are also important components of myofascial dysfunction and pain referral likely to be operative in headache of cervical origin. Central sensitization in tension-type headaches is evidenced by widespread distribution of pain as well as a qualitative difference of pain following a peripheral noxious stimulus. The role of a central mechanism in migraine is suggested by an involvement of hypothalamus serotonin excitatory amino acids, central trigeminal pathways, and cerebral events. Nicolodi[99] examined existing data and concluded that hyperalgesia related to CNS neuropathic changes is crucial for both migraine and fibromyalgia syndrome.

Deep pain inputs activate local and, in some cases, distant muscles, presumably in some kind of early protective response. However, it can be presumed that this muscular reactivity contributes to the pain and dysfunction of clinical syndromes involving the neck and jaw articulations. There is a complex neurochemical control of these mechanisms that balances inhibitory and excitatory influences within the entire sensorimotor system involved with cephalic and facial pain. All of these mechanisms are consistent with the phenomenon of central sensitization, which has been demonstrated previously in spinal systems.[100] This phenomenon is consistent with the model of neuroplasticity proposed by Dubner and Ruda[101] in that changes in central processing of nociceptive transmission contribute to the development and prolonged maintenance of the pathophysiology associated with pain arising from deep somatic tissues.

Summary

The literature on headaches of cervical origin has been reviewed and has focused on three areas: (1) recent advances in the understanding of craniocervical pain mechanisms, (2) the results of studies employing manipulation and facet or neural anesthetic blockade, and (3) recent studies of cervicogenic dysfunction in several categories of headache, including cervicogenic, tension-type, and migraine without aura. This chapter concludes that the 1988 IHS approach to "cervicogenic headache" is too narrow and will create many false misattributions, typically in the direction of underdiagnosing the cervicogenic component of a great many more benign headache conditions. Kanieki[54] has concluded that many migraine attacks are accompanied by tension headache-like symptoms such as neck pain. Conversely, he notes that the previously defined tension-type headaches are often accompanied by migraine-like symptoms such as photophobia, phonophobia, and aggravation by activity. He concludes that the health care provider should be cognizant of these overlaps and their complications. The overlap of headache classification along with the removal of the tension-type headache category from the 2003 revised IHS criteria[102] only adds to the confusion in terminology. This classification existed under the original IHS diagnostic criteria and was removed from the updated 2003 revised criteria. The following comment was added:

> Headache attributed to disorder of neck but not fulfilling the criteria for any of *Cervicogenic headache*, *Headache attributed to retropharyngeal tendonitis* and *Headache attributed to craniocervical dystonia* are not sufficiently validated.

In conclusion, there are likely three categories of benign headache:

1. Those in whom the cervicogenic component is etiological. This group, ideally, will derive primary benefit from spinal manipulation or other treatments aimed at cervical dysfunction.
2. Those in whom the cervicogenic component is secondary but synergistic. This group ideally could derive significant benefit from spinal manipulation in conjunction with other therapeutic measures.
3. Those in whom the cervicogenic component is negligible, reactive, or fully absent. This group would derive little if any benefit from spinal manipulation.

Today as in 1988, it is still the case that only careful yet comprehensive research that takes full account of cervicogenic dysfunction will ultimately determine the validity of this model.

References

1. Vernon HT. Vertebrogenic headache. In: Vernon HT, editor. The upper cervical syndrome: chiropractic diagnosis and treatment. Baltimore: Williams & Wilkins; 1988. p.152-88.
2. International Headache Society. Classification and diagnostic criteria for headache disorders, cranial neuralgias, and facial pain. Cephalalgia 1988;8 Suppl 7:1-96.
3. Sjaastad O, Saunte C, Hovdahl H, Breivek H, Gronback E. Cervicogenic headache: an hypothesis. Cephalalgia 1983;3:249-56.
4. Sjaastad O, Fredrickson TA, Stolt-Neilsen A. Cervicogenic headache, C2 rhizopathy, and occipital neuralgia: a connection. Cephalalgia 1986;6:189-95.
5. Fredrickson TA, Hovdahl H, Sjaastad O. Cervicogenic headache: clinical manifestations. Cephalalgia 1987;7:147-60.
6. Fredrickson TA. Cervicogenic headache: the forehead-sweating pattern. Cephalalgia 1988;8:203-9.
7. Vernon HT. Spinal manipulation and headaches of cervical origin: a review of literature and presentation of cases Manual Med 1991;6:73-9.
8. Bogduk N. Cervical causes of headache and dizziness. In: Greive GP, editor. Modern manual therapy of the vertebral column. Edinburgh: Churchill Livingstone; 1986. p. 289-302.
9. Vernon H. Cervicogenic headache. In: Gatterman MI, editor. Chiropractic management of spine related disorders. 2nd ed. Philadelphia: Lippincott Williams & Wilkins; 2003. p. 282-9.
10. Kerr FW. Structural relation of the trigeminal spinal tract to upper cervical roots and the solitary nucleus in the cat. Exp Neurol 1971;4:134-48.
11. Bogduk N, Marsland A. On the concept of third occipital headache. J Neurol Neurosurg Psychiatry 1986;49:775-80.
12. Travell JG, Simons DG. Myofascial pain and trigger point manual. Baltimore: Williams and Wilkins; 1983.
13. Gatterman MI, Blunt K, Goe DR. Muscle and myofascial pain syndromes. In: Gatterman MI, editor. Chiropractic management of spine related disorders. 2nd ed. Baltimore: Lippincott Williams & Wilkins; 2003. p. 319-69.
14. Gatterman MI, Panzer DM. Disorders of the cervical spine. In: Gatterman MI, editor. Chiropractic management of spine related disorders. 2nd ed. Baltimore: Lippincott Williams & Wilkins; 2003. p. 231-2.
15. Dreyfuss P, Michaelsen M, Fletcher D. Atlanto-occipital and lateral atlanto-axial joint pain patterns. Spine 1994;19:1125-31.
16. Feinstein B, Langton JN, Jameson RM, Schiller F. Experiments on pain referred from deep somatic structures. J Bone Joint Surg Am 1954;36-A:981-97.
17. Bogduk N, Marsland A. The cervical zygapophyseal joints as a source of neck pain. Spine 1988;13:610-7.
18. Dwyer A, April C, Bogduk N. Cervical zygapophyseal joint pain patterns. I. A study in normal volunteers. Spine 1990;15:453-7.
19. April C, Dwyer A, Bogduk N. Cervical zygapophyseal joint pain patterns II. A clinical evaluation. Spine 1990;15:458-61.
20. Barnsley L, Lord SM, Wallis BJ, Bogduk N. The prevalences of chronic cervical joint pain after whiplash. Spine 1995;20:20-5.
21. Lord SM, Barnsley L, Bogduk N. The utility of comparative local anesthetic blocks vs placebo-controlled blocks for the diagnosis of cervical zygapophyseal joint pain. Clin J Pain 1995;11:208-13.
22. Vernon H, Steiman I, Hagino C. Cervicogenic dysfunction in muscle contraction and migraine headaches: a descriptive study. J Manipulative Physiol Ther 1992;15:418-29.
23. Sjaastad O, Fredreckson TA, Stolt-Neilsen A. Cervicogenic headache, C2 rhizotomy and occipital neuralgia: a connection? Cephalalgia 1986;6:189-95.
24. Boquet J, Boismare F, Payenneville G, Leclerc D, Monnier JC, Moore N. Lateralization of headache: possible role of an upper cervical trigger point. Cephalalgia 1989;9:15-24.
25. Jaeger B. Cervicogenic headache: a relationship to cervical spine dysfunction and myofascial trigger points. Cephalalgia 1987;Suppl 7:398-9.
26. Bogduk N. The clinical anatomy of the cervical dorsal rami. Spine 1982;13:26.
27. Terrett A. Neck-tongue syndrome and spinal manipulative therapy. In: Vernon HT, editor. Upper cervical syndrome: chiropractic diagnosis and treatment. Baltimore: Williams and Wilkins; 1988. p. 223-39.
28. Ad Hoc Committee on Classification of Headache. Classification of headache. Arch Neurol 1962;613:6.

29. Goebel S. An EMG analysis of the transsynaptic effects of peripheral nerve injury subsequent to tooth pulp extirpations on neurons in laminae I and H of the medullary dorsal horn. J Neurosci 1984;4:2281.

30. Hack GD, Koritzer RT. Anatomic relationship between the rectus capitus posticus minor muscle and the dura mater. Spine 1995;20:2484-6.

31. Elvidge AR, Choh-Luh L. Central protrusion of cervical intervertebral disc involving the descending trigeminal tract. Arch Neurol Psychiat 1950;63:455-66.

32. Sessle BJ, Hu JW, Yu X. Brainstem mechanisms of referred pain and hyperalgesia in the orofacial and temporomandibular joint region. In: Veccheit L, Albe-Fessard D, Lindbolm U, Giamberardino MA, editors. New trends in referred pain and hyperalgesia. Amsterdam: Elsevier; 1993.

33. Pozniak-Patewicz E. "Cephalgic" spasm of the head and neck musculature. Headache 1976;15:261-5.

34. Moskowitz M. The neurobiology of vascular head pain. Ann Neurol 1984;16:157-68.

35. Fulton JF, editor. Howell's textbook of physiology. 15th ed. Philadelphia: WB Saunders; 1947. p. 385-401.

36. Korr IM. The neural basis of the osteopathic lesion. Am Osteoph Assoc 1947;191-5.

37. Vernon HT, McDermaid CS, Hagino C. Systematic review of randomized clinical trials of complementary/alternative therapies in the treatment of tension-type and cervicogenic headache. Complementary Therapies in Medicine 1999;7:142-55.

38. Jull G. Manual diagnosis of C2-3 headache. Cephalalgia 1985;5 Suppl 5:308-9.

39. Jull GA. Headaches associated with the cervical spine: a clinical review. In: Grieve GP, editor. Modern manual therapy of the vertebral column. New York: Churchill Livingstone; 1986.

40. Jull G, Bogduk N, Marsland A. The accuracy of manual diagnosis for cervical zygapophyseal joint pain syndromes. Med J Aust 1988;148:233-6.

41. Dwyer A, Aprill C, Bogduk N. Cervical zygapophyseal joint pain patterns I: a study in normal volunteers. Spine 1990;15:453-7.

42. Fligg B. Motion palpation of the upper cervical spine. In: Vernon HT, editor. Upper cervical syndrome: chiropractic diagnosis and management. Baltimore: Williams & Wilkins; 1988. p. 113-23.

43. Watson DH, Trott PH. Cervical headache: an investigation of natural head posture and upper cervical flexor muscle performance. Cephalalgia 1993;13:272-82.

44. Jull G, Zito G, Trott P, Potter H, Shirley D. Interexaminer reliability to detect painful upper cervical joint dysfunction. Aust J Physiother 1997;43-125-9.

45. Jensen OK, Nielsen FF, Vosmer L. An open study comparing manual therapy with the use of cold packs in the treatment of post-traumatic headache. Cephalalgia 1990;10:241.

46. Trelevan J, Jull G, Atkinson L. Cervical musculoskeletal dysfunction in post-concussional headache. Cephalalgia 1994;14:273.

47. Stoldolny J, Chmieleski H. Manual therapy in the treatment of patients with cervical migraine. Man Med 1989; 4:49.

48. The Quebec Headache Study Group. Painful intervertebral dysfunction: Robert Maigne's original contribution to headache of cervical origin. Headache 1993;33:328-34.

49. Lewit K. Manipulative therapy in the rehabilitation of the locomotor system. London: Butterworth; 1991.

50. Sachse J, Eckhardt E, Lieb A. A phenomenological investigation in migraine patients. Manual Med 1982;20: 59-64.

51. Graff-Radford SB, Reeves JL, Jaeger B. Management of chronic head and neck pain: effectiveness of altering factors perpetuating myofascial pain. Headache 1987; 27:186-90.

52. Tunks E, Crook J, Norman G, Kalahen S. Tender points in fibromyalgia. Pain 1988;34:11-19.

53. Bovim G. Cervicogenic headache, migraine and tension-type headache: pressure-pain threshold measurements. Pain 1992;51:169-73.

54. Kaniecki RG. Diagnostic challenge in headache: migraine as the wolf disguised in sheep's clothing. Neurology 2002;58 Suppl 6:1-2.

55. Vernon HT, Gitelman R. Pressure algometry and tissue compliance measures in the treatment of chronic headache by spinal manipulation: a single case/single treatment report. J Can Chiro Assoc 1990;34:141-4.

56. Fischer AA. Clinical use of the tissue compliance meter for documentation of soft tissue pathology. Clin J Pain 1987;3:23-30.

57. Sakai F, Ebihiara S, Horikawa M, Akiyama M. Quantitative measurement of muscle stiffness in tension-type headache: development of a new method. Cephalalgia 1991;11 Suppl 11:115-16.

58. Baldry PE. Myofascial pain and fibromyalgia syndromes: a guide to diagnosis and management. St. Louis: Mosby; 2001.

59. Rachlin ES, Rachlin IL. Myofascial pain and fibromyalgia: Trigger point management. 2nd ed. St. Louis: Mosby; 2002.

60. Wolfe F, Smythe HA, Yunus MB, Bennett RM, Bombardier C, Goldenberg DL et al., editors. The American College of Rheumatology 1990 criteria for the classification of fibromyalgia. Report of the Multicenter Criteria Committee. Arthritis Rheum 1990;33:1863-4.

61. Nimmo R. Receptors, effectors and tonus ... a new approach. J NCA 1957;21-3, 60-4.

62. Hviid H. Functional radiography of the cervical spine. Ann Swiss Chiro Assoc 1963;3:37-65.

63. Sandoz R. Newer trends in the pathogenesis of spinal disorders. Ann Swiss Chiro Assoc 1971;5:112.

64. Swartz JB. Cervical templating. Digest of Chiro Economics 1984;March/April.

65. Conley RW. Stress evaluation of cervical mechanics. J Clin Chiro 1974;3:46-62.

66. Grice AS. Preliminary evaluation of fifty sagittal motion radiographic examinations J CCA 1977;21(1):33.

67. Henderson DJ, Dorman TM. Functional roentgeno-metric evaluation of the cervical spine in the sagittal plane. J Manipulative Physiol Ther 1985;8:219-27.

68. Penning L. Normative movements of the cervical spine. AJR 1978;130:317-26.

69. Dvorak J, Panjabi MM, Grob D, Novotny JE, Antinnes JA. Clinical validation of functional flexion/extension radiographs of the cervical spine. Spine 1993;18:120-7.

70. Pfaffenrath V, Dandekar R, Mayer E, Hermann G, Pollman W. Cervicogenic headache: results of computer based measurements of cervical spine mobility in fifteen patients. Cephalalgia 1988;8:45-8.

71. Dvorak J, Froelich D, Penning L, Baumgartner IT, Panjabi MM. Functional radiographic diagnosis of the cervical spine: flexion/extension. Spine 1988;13:748-55.

72. Penning L. Functional rontgenderzock Bij degenerative en tramatische afwijkingen der laag-cervicale beweg-ingssegmenten. Netherlands: University of Gronikge; 1960.

73. Peterson C. Chiropractic radiography. In: Gatterman MI. Chiropractic management of spine related disorders. 2nd ed. Baltimore: Lippincott Williams & Wilkins; 2003. p. 108-28.

74. Dvorak J, Panjabi MM, Grob D, Novotny JE, Antinnes JA. Clinical validation of functional flexion/extension radiographs of the cervical spine. Spine 1993;18:120-7.

75. Nagasawa A, Sakakibara T, Takahashi A. Roentgeno-graphic findings of the cervical spine in tension-type headache. Headache 1993;33:90-5.

76. Hu JW, Yu X-M, Vernon HT, Sessle BI. Excitatory effects on neck and jaw muscle activity of inflammatory irritant applied to cervical paraspinal tissues. Pain 1993;55:243-50.

77. Kidd RF, Nelson R. Musculoskeletal dysfunction of the neck in migraine and tension headache. Headache 1993;33:566-9.

78. Hoyt WH, Shaffer F, Bard DA, Benesler JS, Blankenhorn GD, Gray JH et al. Osteopathic manipulation in the treatment of muscle-contraction headache. J Am Osteo Assoc 1979;778:322-5.

79. Boline PD, Kassak K, Nelson C et al. Spinal adjustments and pharmaceutical therapy—a randomized controlled trial of treatment for muscle contraction headaches: a pilot study. Proceedings of the International Conference on Spinal Manipulation 1990;241-1.

80. Boline PD, Kassak K, Bronfort G, Nelson C, Anderson AV. Spinal manipulation vs. amitriptyline for the treat-ment of chronic tension-type headaches: a randomized clinical trial. J Manipulative Physiol Ther 1995;18:148-54.

81. Bove G, Nilsson N. Spinal manipulation in the treatment of episodic tension-type headache: a randomized con-trolled trial. JAMA 1998;280:1576-9.

82. Vernon HT. Spinal manipulation and headaches of cervical origin. J Manipulative Physiol Ther 1989;12:455.

83. Vernon HT. Spinal manipulation and headaches of cer-vical origin: a review of the literature and presentation of cases. J Man Med 1991;6:73-9.

84. Vernon H. Spinal manipulation and headaches: an update. Top Clin Chiro 1995;2:34-46.

85. Nilsson N. A randomized controlled trial of the effect of spinal manipulation in the treatment of cervicogenic headache. J Manipulative Physiol Ther 1995;18:435-40.

86. Nilsson N, Christensen HW, Hartvigsen J. The effect of spinal manipulation in the treatment of cervicogenic headache. J Manipulative Physiol Ther 1997;20:326-30.

87. Martelli P, Latour D, Giacovazzo M. A spectrum of pathophysiological disorders in cervicogenic headache and its therapeutic implications. J Musculoskel Sys 1995;3:182-7.

88. Jull G, Trott P, Potter H, Zito G, Niere K, Shirley D et al. A randomized controlled trial of exercise and manipulative therapy for cervicogenic headache. Spine 2002;27:1835-43.

89. Vernon H. Headaches. In: Redwood D, Cleveland CS. Fundamentals of chiropractic. St. Louis: Mosby; 2003. p. 497-529.

90. Parker GB, Tupling H, Pryor DS. A controlled trial of cervical manipulation for migraine. Aust NZ J Med 1978;8:589-93.

91. Parker GB, Pryor DS, Tupling H. Why does migraine improve during clinical trial? Further results from a trial of cervical manipulation for migraine. Aust NZ J Med 1980;10:192-8.

92. Stodolny I, Chmielewski H. Manual therapy in the treat-ment of patients with cervical migraine. Manual Med 1989;4:49-51.

93. Nelson CF, Bronfort G, Evans R, Boline P, Goldsmith C, Anderson AV. The efficacy of spinal manipulation, amitriptyline, and the combination of both therapies for the prophylaxis of migraine headache. J Manipulative Physiol Ther 1998;21:511-9.

94. Tuchin PJ, Pollard H, Bonello R. A randomized con-trolled trial of chiropractic spinal manipulative therapy for migraine. J Manipulative Physiol Ther 2000;23:91

95. Bogduk N. A neurological approach to neck pain. In: Glasgow EF, Twomey IV, Seall ER, Kleynhans AM, Edczak RM, editors. Aspects of manipulative therapy. 2nd ed. New York: Churchill-Livingstone; 1985. p. 136-46.

96. Yarnitsky D, Goor-Aryeh I, Bazwas ZH, Ranil BJ, Cutrer FM, Sattile A et al. Possible parasympathetic contributions to peripheral and central sensitization during migraine headaches. J Head Face Pain 2003;43:704-14.

97. Mense S. Considerations concerning the neurological basis of muscle pain. Can J Physiol Pharmacol 1991;69:610-6.

98. Hu JW, Yu M, Vernon H, Sessle BJ. Excitatory effects of on neck and jaw muscle activity of inflammatory irritant applied to cervical paraspinal tissues. Pain 1993;55:243-50.

99. Nicolodi M, Volpe AR, Sicuteri F. Fibromyalgia and headache. Failure of serotonergic analgesia and N-methyl-D-aspartate-mediated neuronal plasticity: their common clue. Cephalalgia 1998;18 Suppl 21:41-4.

100. Woolf CI, Thompson SWN. The induction and maintenance of central sensitization is dependent on N-methyl-D-aspartic acid receptor activation: implications for the treatment of post-injury pain hypersensitivity states. Pain 1991;44:293-9.

101. Dubner R, Ruda MA. Activity-dependent neuronal plasticity following tissue injury and inflammation. Trends Neurosci 1992;15:96-102.

102. Headache Classification Subcommittee of the International Headache Society. The international classification of headache disorders, 2nd ed. Cephalalgia 2004;24(Suppl 1):1-160.

18

Cervicogenic Sympathetic Syndromes

Donald Fitz-Ritson

Key Words   Cervical sympathetic ganglia, Horner's syndrome, Barré-Liéou syndrome, Meniere's disease, cervicogenic vertigo

After reading this chapter you should be able to answer the following questions:

Question 1   How does the position of the upper cervical ganglion make it vulnerable to an upper cervical subluxation?

Question 2   How can a subluxation produce cervicogenic vertigo?

Question 3   What is the role of manipulation and other forms of chiropractic adjustment in the treatment of cervicogenic sympathetic syndromes?

The extremely flexible cervical spine, the body's most complicated and mobile articular system, is located strategically between the head and body. It is designed for mobility, which significantly influences its stability. Subluxation syndromes affect both the mobility and stability of the cervical spine. The cervical spine is an anatomic complex of many crucial and sensitive tissues crowded into a small area. It is the "Times Square" of the human frame, with enormous volumes of traffic going in both directions.

Many delicate and vital structures pass through this 7-inch portion of the spine, which is made up of seven of the most fragile vertebrae. These are held together by 17 articular joints, 12 joints of Luschka (for a total of 29 joints), 6 intervertebral discs, and a musculoligamentous network that involves approximately 50 pairs of muscles. The musculoligamentous system, along with the architectural shapes of the vertebrae and joints, allows enormous maneuverability and range of motion, but also supports the head, which weighs approximately 8 to 10 pounds.

At least 70 clinically separate and distinct syndromes arise from abnormalities of the tissues of the cervical spine. Even more syndromes arise from distant structures but are associated with signs and symptoms referable to the cervical spine, head, shoulders, and upper extremities. These disorders are related to the subluxation syndrome and constitute a sizable portion of any chiropractor's practice.

Anatomy

This brief overview addresses anatomy relevant to injury of the cervical spine.

Sympathetic Nervous System

The sympathetic, or thoracolumbar, division of the autonomic nervous system has major functions in vasoconstriction of the skin and shifting of blood supply to more essential organs during periods of stress. The cervical sympathetic trunk (CST) consists of ascending preganglionic axons, which traverse the white rami communicantes. Peripherally, post-ganglionic fibers accompany sensory fibers to specific cutaneous areas that closely correspond to sensory dermatomes.

There are generally three cervical sympathetic ganglia that are formed from the fusion of the eight primordial cranial nerves. The cervicothoracic or stellate ganglion is the lowermost and is considered to be a fusion of the first thoracic and inferior cervical ganglia. The usual position of the cervicothoracic ganglion is anterior to the base of the transverse process of the seventh cervical vertebra. This ganglion supplies gray rami communicantes to the cervical spinal nerves 6, 7, and 8 and also to the first thoracic nerve. An inferior cervical cardiac nerve also arises from this ganglion.

The middle cervical ganglion is the smallest and most variable in form and position. It is commonly located in close proximity to the inferior thyroid artery and the cricoid cartilage. In addition to supplying the gray rami communicantes to cervical nerves 5 and 6, it also gives rise to the middle cervical cardiac nerve.[1]

The superior cervical ganglion is the largest of the three, sometimes extending 3 to 4 cm; it lies opposite the transverse process of C2. This ganglion has many branches, including the internal carotid nerve, which distributes nerve fibers to intracranial vascular smooth muscles. Communications also exist between the superior ganglion and the inferior ganglion of the glossopharyngeal nerve, the inferior and superior ganglia of the vagus, and the hypoglossal nerve. Pharyngeal branches join the pharyngeal plexus as well as the external carotid and superior cervical cardiac plexus. In general, these fibers accompany the named blood vessels and perform vasoconstrictor, secretory, and pilomotor functions. The external carotid nerves supply all of the major and minor glands of the head and neck.[2]

The cervical sympathetic trunk lies deep to the deep layer of the cervical fascia and rests on the longus coli and longus capitis muscles. The nerve is posterior and medial to the carotid artery and the vagus nerve and usually ascends from its origin in the root of the neck superomedially.[1]

The anatomic intimacy between the sympathetic division of the autonomic nervous system and the somatic nervous system is most appropriate, because it is one of the main functions of the sympathetic nervous systems to continually tune visceral, metabolic, and circulatory activity to the rapidly changing requirements of the skeletal musculature.

Every motor activity organized through the somatic innervation originating in the spinal cord also involves the simultaneous coordinated activity of the sympathetic nervous system and the tissues and processes regulated by it. For the sympathetic nervous system to meet its supportive responsibilities to the musculoskeletal system, it must be continually apprised of the activities and requirements of that system. Hence, integration is possible only with simultaneous afferent input both to the motoneuron and to the sympathetic preganglionic neurons in the cord, from the higher centers through descending pathways, and from countless musculoskeletal reporting stations, through the dorsal roots.[3] If there is a subluxation syndrome present at a particular level of the vertebral column, this affects the ability of the spinal cord to effectively integrate incoming and outgoing information. The rapid moment-to-moment adjustments in accordance with levels of exertion and posture—or anticipation, conscious or unconscious, of exertion—are orchestrated largely by the sympathetic nervous system.[4]

Sympathetic Effects in Healthy Tissue

If we accept that in several pathophysiologic states sympathetic efferents can produce pain and hyperalgesia, an obvious question is, to what extent can similar effects occur in normal healthy tissue?[5] We know that many peripheral targets, in addition to blood vessels, receive sympathetic supply. For instance, there is good evidence for an innervation of muscle spindles, Pacinian corpuscles, and other specialized end organs in skin.[6] We also might expect a modification of sensory inflow to occur secondary to changes in blood flow or piloerection.

It is therefore not surprising that physiologic experiments have identified some actions of sympathetic efferent in normal skin. Cold thermoreceptors can be excited by low-frequency stimulation of the sympathetic trunk.[7] Similarly,

some sensitive mechanoreceptors with unmyelinated axons are also transiently excited,[8] an effect that is probably caused by small changes in the tension in the tissues secondary to vasomotor changes.[9] A most important question is whether nociceptors are excited by sympathetic stimulation. Here all workers agree that for normal nociceptors with A, d, or C axons no direct excitation occurs.[10-12] Together, these studies suggest that in normal tissue, sympathetic activity has only modest sensory effects.[5] Would the presence of a subluxation complex change this modest sensory effect?

Sympathetically Mediated Pain

The most important conditions are those of causalgia and reflex sympathetic dystrophy. Causalgia is a condition that occasionally follows trauma to a major nerve. The term was coined by Mitchell in the middle of the nineteenth century to indicate the presence of persistent burning pain in such cases. The more general term *reflex sympathetic dystrophy* is used to categorize patients with some or all of the following symptoms: spontaneous burning pain, hyperalgesia (indicates both pain to normally innocuous events and increased sensitivity to noxious events), hyperpathia (delayed and exaggerated painful response to stimuli), disturbances of vasomotor and sudomotor control, and dystrophic changes in the peripheral tissues, such as abnormalities of hair and nail growth and osteoporosis. Although there is still much confusion in the use of these terms, *reflex sympathetic dystrophy* is generally used when the condition is not associated with obvious peripheral nerve trauma. Swelling is the most constant physical finding, which if not treated early is often followed by the rapid onset of stiffness.[13] Precipitating events include minor tissue trauma and fractures, nontraumatic nerve lesions such as those seen in diabetes, and even lesions to the central nervous system. Could a subluxation syndrome be a factor in this condition?

There are two main reasons for believing that the sympathetic nervous system may be important in the genesis of pain in these conditions. First, sympathetic function is frequently abnormal. The skin of the affected region is often initially warm and red, later pale and cold. Anhidrosis or hyperhidrosis may be present. The dystrophic changes that occur are likely secondary to changes in blood flow to the area. A second and more compelling reason for implicating the sympathetic nervous system is that maneuvers that alter sympathetic activity frequently alter the patient's pain. For instance, visual and auditory stimuli, emotional disturbance, or thermal stress all provoke sympathetic arousal and all can exacerbate the pain in these patients.[5] A final important clinical finding is that pain often radiates extensively beyond the area of damaged tissue or the innervation territory of the damaged nerve. The spread usually ignores traditional boundaries such as nerve territories or dermatomes. In extreme cases, it can spread to encompass large areas of the body surface.

Central Changes

The ability of peripheral nerve lesions or peripheral tissue injury to alter spinal somatosensory processes is becoming well recognized. The ascending spinal pathways that transmit information rostrally begin to respond more vigorously to peripheral inputs and indeed can become responsive to totally new inputs that normally do not drive them. These cells also relay aberrant activity generated from the periphery. This process can develop quite rapidly with peripheral tissue injury, and it is possible that once established it may become largely independent of the precipitating event.[14] The subluxation syndrome, if at the level of the injured peripheral nerve or tissue, affects the spinal somatosensory processing.

A second type of disturbance is seen in the response properties and patterns of reflex organization in the sympathetic nervous system. Within the dorsal horn, the representation of the body surface is very compressed, especially in the mediolateral plane. Expansion of receptive fields over quite substantial areas of the body surface is therefore possible and provides an explanation for the radiation of pain.[5]

Neck Proprioceptors

Proprioceptors provide information to the central nervous system (CNS). The receptors that send the information are specialized and located in extraspinal and spinal structures. Muscles, by their share of volume in the body, contain the most. The receptors are somewhat different and more numerous in the spinal musculature, especially in the cervical muscles. A review of the receptors, spinal muscles, and their spinal and CNS correlates has already been published.[15] The essential points and new information related to the development of symptoms after trauma to the cervical area are covered in this section.

Muscle Receptors

Most muscle contains at least four types of receptors:
1. Muscle spindles
2. Golgi tendon organs
3. Paciniform corpuscles
4. Free nerve endings

Muscle spindles and Golgi tendon organs have been thought to signal changes in muscle length or force development. However, paciniform corpuscles and free nerve endings also play a role in proprioception.

Muscle Spindles

In the cervical musculature, the spindles are arranged in elaborate configurations such as paired, parallel, and tandem (Figure 18-1). Because of their volume per gram of tissue and their configurations, these spindles signal enormous volumes of information to the spinal cord and CNS when tiny changes occur in muscle. With a subluxation syndrome in the cervical spine, the information entering the spinal cord and CNS therefore is affected.

Golgi Tendon Organ

The Golgi tendon organ (GTO) is an encapsulated receptor that lies in series with extrafusal fibers at the musculotendinous junction (Figure 18-2). Most GTOs are located in the rostral half of the large muscles. In neck muscles, spindles and GTOs are often clustered together in complicated receptor arrays. Stretching of muscle, whether tonic or dynamic, causes the GTOs to inhibit the muscles.

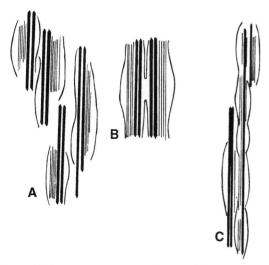

Figure 18-1 Diagrams of muscle spindles in various configurations. **A,** Four paired spindles. Note that no intrafusal fibers are shared. **B,** Parallel spindles. Note the capsule discontinuity at the equatorial regions of spindles. **C,** Spindle array in which five spindles exist in tandem sharing one common nuclear bag fiber. *(Adapted from Richmond F, Abrahams V. J Neurophysiol 1985;38:1312-21.)*

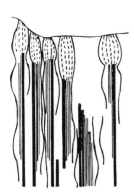

Figure 18-2 Diagram of spindle complex located in the intertransverse muscle group of the C2-C3 joint region. Tendons are shown as stippled regions. Golgi tendon organs at the ends of spindles are shown as encapsulated regions containing broken lines. *(Adapted from Bakker D, Richmond F. J Neurophysiol 1982; 48:62-74.)*

Paciniform Corpuscles

Paciniform corpuscles are small cylindrical encapsulations that ensheathe the end of a sensory nerve. In muscle, because they are located near contracting fibers, they may be signaling changes in muscle length.

Free Nerve Endings

Free nerve endings are distributed widely throughout all types of muscle and connective tissue. They respond to mechanical stimuli and muscle contraction.[16] Mechanoreceptors also provide information to the spinal cord and CNS.[15]

Biomechanics

The essential biomechanics of the cervical spine, both upper and lower, are expertly reviewed by Moroney.[17] Other pertinent information is presented here. There are five intervertebral discs (IVDs) from C2 through C7. The discs adhere above and below to hyaline articular cartilage, which covers the articular surfaces of the vertebral bodies. These five IVDs account for 25% of the total length of the cervical spine.[18]

Compared with the foraminal diameter at the neutral position, there are statistically significant reductions in foramen diameter (10% and 13% at 20 degrees and 30 degrees of extension, respectively). Conversely, in flexion there are statistically significant increases of 8% and 10% at 20 degrees and 30 degrees of flexion, respectively. A subluxation syndrome affects the spinal mechanics, causing the vertebrae above or below the affected area to move more excessively.

It has been stated that the foraminal encroachment by an uncovertebral osteophyte with narrowing of the foramen results in direct compression of the nerve root. This is thought to be a major source of pain in cervical degenerative disc disease. Anatomically, the nerve roots have a less protective epineurium as compared with the peripheral nerves, and this has been implicated in their susceptibility to compression. Therefore the understanding of the alteration in the size of the foramen with cervical motion becomes an important factor in understanding the mechanism of trauma and its management.

Also reported were greater absolute and relative changes in the foraminal size at C6 and C7 foramens compared with the C5 foramen. This may be related to the relative flexibility of these levels. The study by Yoo et al.[19] shows that the percent change of C5 foramen size was only 55% to 60% of C6 and C7 foramen size change, possibly reflecting a two-thirds decrease in flexibility. This relatively decreased motion may prevent greater excursion of the facets at the C4-5 interspace, accounting for the decrease in the alteration in the foramen size of C5.[19]

Age

In sagittal motion, there is an inverse relationship between age and range of motion; that is, as age increases, mobility decreases.[18] Hayashi et al.[20] compared three groups of healthy volunteers aged 20 to 40, 40 to 60, and 60 to 82 years. They found a 25% reduction in the maximum flexion and extension achieved when the group aged 60 to 82 was compared with that aged 20 to 40 years. Seventy-one percent of the decrease occurred at the C5-C7 motion segments. If there is a subluxation syndrome at these levels, it will further decrease the flexion-extension excursions.

Dvorak et al.[21] showed that significantly decreased motion differences were found between age groups within gender and between gender groups in corresponding decades. Results of rotation out of maximum flexion suggest and support earlier conclusions that rotation of the C1-2 segment does not decrease with age, but rather increases slightly to perhaps compensate for the overall decreased motion in the lower segments. A subluxation syndrome at C1-2 therefore affects the overall motion of the cervical spine.

Intervertebral Discs

Pertinent information regarding the disc is thoroughly covered,[22] and newer information is provided here. The major biochemical changes observed in the disc matrix with aging are similar to those described in other connective tissues. The most noticeable in the disc, however, is dehydration of nucleus pulposus (NP) and the loss of sulphated glycosaminoglycans (GAGs) accompanied by a large increase in noncollagenous proteins. The water content of the NP of the human disc decreases from 88% of dry weight at birth to 69% at 77 years. In the anulus fibrosis, water content declines from 78% at birth to 70% at 30 years, remaining relatively constant thereafter. The absolute amount of collagen also may increase with aging, but only slightly as a fraction of dry weight.

Numerous histopathologic studies of human discs at autopsy have confirmed that a high incidence of primary degenerative changes is present in individuals older than age 30, and this increases with age. However, retrospective investigations of the medical records of these individuals do not show a history of back complaints in all cases. This indicates that disc degeneration does not invariably lead to clinical symptoms of back pain. From these findings we may conclude that, with aging, biochemical changes take place within the matrix of the disc, which can reduce its ability to achieve efficient dissipation of the mechanical stresses imposed on the spine during everyday activities.[23] A subluxation syndrome limits movement at a particular motion segment; this also affects the blood supply to the disc.

The nucleus pulposus of the human, like that of the dog, starts losing notochordal cells and depositing a hyaline-like matrix within a few years of birth. Because there is evidence in dogs that the rate at which this process takes place is genetically determined, it is not illogical to hypothesize that the disc cells of humans are similarly programmed. If this is so, then the response of discs within the human spine to restricted movement may, in part, be heritable. In animal experiments, surgical methods were used to restrict spinal movement; such procedures induced profound changes in disc metabolism within six months of application. In the case of the human spine, disc changes arising from inadequate nutrition may occur for several reasons. The subluxation syndrome may be initiated by insidious or traumatic circumstances, maintenance of bad posture such as sitting, driving, flying for long periods, lack of appropriate exercise, and smoking. These extrinsic influences coupled with an aging disc cell population and the stresses of everyday activities can lead to failure, which itself contributes to degenerate discs.[24]

In human cervical discs, nerve fibers appeared to enter the disc in the posterolateral direction and course both parallel and perpendicular to the bundles of the anulus fibrosus. Nerves were seen throughout the anulus but were most numerous in the middle third of the disc. The presence of neural elements within the IVD indicates that the mechanical status of the disc is monitored by the CNS. If the nonencapsulated nerve endings in the anulus fibrosus are pain receptors, their presence may explain the occurrence of neck or shoulder pain when there is dislocation or trauma to the disc. If the nonencapsulated nerve endings in the anulus fibrosus monitor the mechanical status of the disc, a subluxation syndrome that restricts movement affects this monitoring by the CNS. Both Pacinian corpuscles and Golgi tendon organs are mechanoreceptors and are reportedly active in response to changes in tension.

Recent studies have shown that the IVD has a complex structure and mechanical properties that vary from region to region and change with age. There is evidence that the disc is capable of some regeneration. These findings plus evidence that the disc is innervated suggest that the IVD may be more than a pad that absorbs shock and maintains the spaces between the vertebral bodies. The concentration of nerves in the middle third of the disc may be sensing superoinferior compression or deformation. The circumferential arrangement of the nerve bundles about the disc and the superficial-to-deep location of the mechanoreceptors may enable the IVD to sense peripheral compression of deformation as well as alignment.[25] However, a subluxation syndrome limits normal movement and function of the disc, affecting its inherent properties.

Trauma to the Cervical Spine

Nearly 4500 years ago, an Egyptian physician described a patient with a cervical spine injury as "one having a dislocation in a vertebra of his neck while he is unconscious of his two legs and his two arms, and his urine dribbles, an ailment not to be treated."[26] Although the current outlook is not so bleak, cervical spine injury continues to be a catastrophic event. There are approximately 280 spine injuries per million population each year in the United States, and approximately 10% to 30% result in spinal cord injury.[27,28] The most common cause by far is motor vehicle accidents, with falls and sports-related injuries also being important traumatic events.[29,30]

The mortality after traumatic spinal cord injury is 47.7%, compared with 6.7% for all trauma victims. Nearly 40% of patients die before reaching a hospital and another 10% die in the hospital.[31] Injuries to the upper cervical spine account for one third of cervical spine injuries, but they are responsible for 80% of the deaths of acute cervical trauma. Of those who survive, up to 70% suffer from significant neurologic deficits.[32]

Mechanism of Injury: General

Spinal injuries may be classified according to the mechanism of injury.[33,34]

Classification of Spinal Injuries
Hyperflexion
- Anterior subluxation syndrome
- Bilateral interfacetal dislocation
- Wedge compression fracture
- Flexion teardrop fracture

Hyperflexion and Rotation
- Unilateral interfacetal dislocation

Hyperextension
- Hyperextension fracture-dislocation
- Fracture of posterior arch of atlas
- Traumatic spondylolisthesis (hangman's fracture)
- Laminar fracture
- Subluxation syndrome

Vertical Compression
- Compression fracture
- Burst fracture
- Jefferson burst fracture (C1)

Mixed Mechanism
- Atlantooccipital dislocation
- Odontoid fractures
- Total ligamentous disruption

Flexion injuries usually result from blows to the back of the head or forceful decelerations as might be experienced in motor vehicle accidents. Pure flexion trauma may result in wedge fracture of the vertebral body, without ligamentous injuries.[33] These injuries are stable and are rarely associated with neurologic injuries. With more extreme trauma, the posterior column is disrupted. In severe injuries, the anterior ligament and disc space are also disrupted and bilateral facet joint dislocation results. These injuries are unstable and are associated with a high incidence of cord damage. Flexion-rotation injuries disrupt the posterior ligamentous complex and produce unilateral facet joint dislocation. These injuries tend to be stable and are not usually associated with spinal cord injury, although cervical root injury is common. The most severe of the flexion injuries is the teardrop fracture. Both columns are disrupted, and there is bilateral facet joint subluxation. The spine is unstable, and severe cord injury is seen.

Hyperextension injuries to the cervical spine result from a blow to the anterior part of the head or from an acceleration (whiplash) injury. Extension injuries are twice as common as flexion injuries, and approximately one third involve the atlantoaxial joint. These injuries are more often than not associated with cord damage. Hyperextension appears to be the most common mechanism of injury, accounting for approximately one third of all cases of cervical spine fracture.[32] Hyperextension combined with compressive forces (for example, in diving) may result in fracture dislocations. The lateral vertebral masses, pedicles, and laminae are often fractured in this injury.[34] Because both anterior and posterior columns are disrupted, this injury is both unstable and associated with high incidence of cord dysfunction. Violent hyperextension with fracture of the pedicles of C2 and forward movement of C2 on C3 produces the "hangman's fracture." The fracture is unstable, but the degree of neurologic compromise is highly variable because the bilateral pedicular fractures serve to decompress the spinal cord at the site of injury.[35]

Burst fractures are caused by compressive loading of the vertex of the skull in the neutral position. This type of injury is converted into a flexion or extension type with only minimal angulation of the injury force; this is relatively rare as a pure entity. Compressive forces in the lower cervical spine result in the explosion of compressed disc material into the vertebral body. Depending on the magnitude of the compression loading and associated angulating forces, the resulting injury ranges from loss of vertebral body height with relatively intact margins to complete disruption of the vertebral body. Posterior displacement of comminuted fragments may result, producing cord injury. Despite the cord injury, the spine is usually stable.[34]

A considerable number of fractures are misread on initial evaluation in the emergency room.[36-38] The incidence of missed fractures ranges from 1% to 33%, with most series reporting 10% or more. The most common reasons for missed diagnoses are failure to take radiographs or misinterpretation of the radiograph.[39] Missed injuries are often unstable, and secondary neurologic lesions are 7.5 times more common in patients who are not diagnosed at initial evaluation.[37] The major factor in the development of a secondary injury is failure to immobilize the neck.[40]

Mechanism of Injury: Specific

Occupational Lifestyle Trauma to the Cervical Spine

The existing literature on back and neck pain supports two major conclusions:

1. That the prevalence of spinal pain in the United States and elsewhere is so great that it constitutes a major health problem.
2. That spinal pain is associated with identifiable activities. A style of living or a line of work can contribute to the onset or exacerbation of back and neck disease.[41]

For society at large, prevalence rates for back and neck disorders vary from one study to another. However, they are characteristically high across investigations. Put another way, the proportion of any population that is afflicted by a back or neck problem at some point in life is exceedingly large.[42] Musculoskeletal disorders of the neck and shoulders are receiving an increasing amount of attention. Earlier reports from Japan suggested that the problem was growing, and Swedish statistics on occupational injuries showed an increase in the number of reported neck and shoulder disorders during the years 1982 to 1985. Factory workers as well as office workers were mentioned as risk groups, and women workers in Sweden reported relatively more injuries in the neck, shoulders, and arms than did men.

A variety of risk factors has been suggested for neck and shoulder disorders. One example is the introduction of modern technology resulting in specialized monotonous tasks that impose static or repetitive loads. These monotonous tasks affect the muscles, which in turn contribute to the development of subluxation syndromes. Consequently, a relationship has been shown between time spent working with office machines, including visual display units, and the occurrence of musculoskeletal symptoms. Other studies have indicated that the problem is multifactorial, with mental strain, lack of control, and low job satisfaction being important elements in the development of the disorder.

A recent study of 420 medical secretaries found that 63% had experienced neck pain at some time during the previous year. Shoulder pain during the previous year had been experienced by 62%. Age and length of employment were significantly related to neck and shoulder pain. Furthermore, working with office machines five hours or more per day was associated with a significantly increased risk of neck pain, shoulder pain, and headache. Finally, a poorly experienced psychosocial work environment was significantly related to headache, neck, shoulder, and low back pain.[43]

Workplace design, posture, joint mechanical problems, subluxation syndrome, and monotonous work have been identified as important factors in the development of occupational neck and shoulder disorders. To reduce the static muscular state caused by monotonous work, the introduction of spontaneous and scheduled pauses is advocated. Pain may result in the development of stress symptoms such as sleep problems, anxiety, or feelings of depression.[44] Musculoskeletal disorders of the neck and upper limbs, including the subluxation syndrome, have frequently been reported in workers engaged in jobs involving awkward postures and high-force, high-repetitive movements. Some investigators have pointed out that after controlling for potential co-factors such as age, constitution, and disease, the length of exposure and various ergonomic factors are the major contributors to the onset of soft tissue disorders in workers performing manual tasks. Some epidemiologic data suggest that vibration may contribute to upper limb disorders as a result of repeated microtrauma on the tissues and joints of the hand-arm system. The term *cumulative trauma disorder* has recently been suggested to refer to musculoskeletal afflictions arising from chronic exposure to microtrauma. A recent study indicated that musculoskeletal impairment to the upper limbs was more severe in chainsaw operators than in the controls who did solely manual work. This suggests that vibration stress is an important contributor to the development of musculoskeletal disorders in workers using handheld vibrating tools.[45]

The increase in musculoskeletal disorders along with the recognition of a multifactorial cause has created a shift in interest from the treatment of these disorders toward their prevention. One commonly used preventive measure is the back/neck school. Although initially directed mainly toward chronic disorders, back/neck schools have become popular tools for secondary prevention. Secondary prevention refers to interventions designed to eliminate, reduce, or prevent further development of pain. A back/neck school may be described as an educational package for increasing participants' knowledge of their back problems and the relationship to environmental and individual factors. With increased knowledge, it is hoped that the patient will modify personal behavior and surroundings (for example, the workplace) to control, limit, or prevent the pain. A recent study showed that neck schools, despite good compliance, appear to be of limited clinical value for prevention of neck and shoulder disorders.[46]

The lifestyle habit of individuals carrying purses or briefcases continually on one side slowly distorts the neck-shoulder muscles on that side, contributing to altered cervical mechanics and pain. Likewise, sleeping on the stomach predisposes the cervical spine to microtrauma of the deep muscles and ligamentous and capsular structures. This not only causes subluxation syndromes to develop, but therapeutic intervention by a chiropractor is difficult or impossible unless the habit is changed.

Athletic Trauma to the Cervical Spine

Athletic injuries to the cervical spine can be serious or fatal. One reason is the vulnerability and location of the cervical spine. Another is the mechanical disadvantage the head-neck coupling has to impact traumas. Injuries have been caused by football, soccer, skiing, water sports including diving, boxing, hockey, and the use of the trampoline.[47-49]

The number of persons participating at all levels of athletic competition has increased tremendously since the 1980s. Concomitantly, there has been a proportionate increase in athletic injuries and related problems. If you become involved in the treatment of sports injuries and are responsible for the care of athletes, at some time you undoubtedly may be required to manage an injury that could be crippling or even fatal. In such a crisis, care is a matter of sound judgment and basic knowledge of emergency techniques.[50] Athletic injuries to the neck and cervical spine can involve the bony elements, IVDs, ligamentous and muscular supporting structures, elements of the brachial plexus, nerve roots, and the spinal cord itself.

Spinal cord injuries related to sports and recreation appear to be increasing in Canada. Sports and recreation moved from the third to the second leading cause of spinal injuries treated at two Toronto hospitals between 1948 and 1983. Shallow-water diving was by far the leading contributing activity. Most of the injuries were cervical, and most caused complete paralysis below the level of the injury. Of the 47 injuries caused by diving, 33 were injury to the cord, 8 to the root, and only 13 constituted a spinal injury without neurologic deficit. The mechanism was the head striking the pool or lake bottom, with fracture-dislocation the most frequent type of spinal injury.

Hockey injuries were also assessed. Most of the injuries were in the middle to lower cervical region, with fracture-dislocation the most common type of bony injury. Of the 42 injuries, 28 were spinal cord injury, 12 of which were complete injuries. The leading mechanism was a push or check into the boards, with the helmeted head striking the boards with the neck slightly flexed.[51]

Another factor that contributes to the extent of spinal cord injury is either preexisting, or development of, spinal stenosis.[52,53] In soccer players, the simple effect of heading the ball over time caused degenerative changes in the cervical spine and injuries to the brain. Repetitive small traumas over an extended period have a detrimental effect on the cervical spine and the CNS.[54]

Motor Vehicle Flexion-Extension Injuries

The mechanism of motor vehicular injuries to the individual is addressed in detail because it is so common and of immense interest to chiropractors.

Introduction

The important concept that all who deal with motor vehicle accident (MVA) injuries should understand is that our anatomy dictates a great deal of why the injuries occur. Think for a moment about your head, which weighs approximately 8 to 12 pounds and sits on top of the most flexible area of your body—your neck. The flexible neck has approximately 29 joints, 50 pairs of muscles, and a ligamentous capsular network that is very complex. The neck sits on a stable base—the upper back, or thoracic spine. We have a ball (the head), a flexible chain (the neck), and a rigid base (the upper back). Any sudden motion of the body causes the head to wobble or to be whipped around on the neck, a flexible chain of 29 joints, developing great forces and the potential for many subluxation syndromes. This is the essence of most MVA problems.

Mechanism of Injury

Eighty percent of MVAs occur at speeds of less than 25 mph. Most "whiplash accidents" occur as a result of rear-end collisions.[55]

Data from the Research Accident Investigation Center, University of Rochester, show that even at low speeds the occupants of the vehicle that was struck will sustain serious injuries.[56] Panjabi and White[56] have shown that a 10.8 mph rear-end collision with an impact duration of 0.1 seconds produces an acceleration of the lead vehicle of five times the force of gravity. The significance of this is that collisions occurring at relatively low speeds result in large forces being applied to the lead vehicle. If this causes easy acceleration of the lead vehicle (for example, on a wet/slippery surface), extensive damage to the vehicle's occupants may result.

According to the National Highway Traffic Safety Administration (NHTSA), "a ten-mile-an-hour collision is equivalent to catching a 200-pound bag of cement dropped from a second-story window. People don't understand the dynamics of crashes."[57]

McKenzie[57] has shown that the inertia of the occupant's head and neck are in unstable equilibrium. The struck vehicle reaches its peak acceleration before the occupant's head, neck, and upper back have accelerated to any significant amount. As the head, neck, and upper back try to catch up to the peak acceleration of the vehicle, they attain speeds of 2 to 2.5 times the maximum vehicle acceleration. The head relies only on the neck, through which the force of acceleration is transmitted. As a result, the force loads at the head/neck interface can be quite extreme (in excess of 100 pounds for collisions not exceeding 15 mph).[58] This shows that even a minor accident causes significant damage to the neck of the occupant of the struck vehicle.

Who Is Injured More?

Passengers in the right front seat are injured more because they are less prepared than the driver for a collision.[59]

Women sustain injuries twice as often as men. Men have greater neck muscle strength, which seems to dampen the effects of the "whipping" cervical spine.[59,60]

Other Factors That Affect the Mechanism of Injury

The age of the person is very important because preexisting traumas, the presence of degenerative joint and disc disease, smaller stature, less muscle tone, and decreased ligamentous function, in addi-

tion to decreased reaction times, all can contribute to the severity of soft tissue injury.[61] The high proportion of osteoporosis predisposes seniors to fractures of the vertebral bodies.[62] Motion of the head, such as rotation, at impact causes damage to the C2 dorsal root ganglion.[63]

Data from the University of Rochester Accident Investigation Center show that even though all cars have headrests, they are usually not properly positioned and they reduce the frequency of neck injuries by only 14%. Most car seats are designed for the average person and are weak. Because they do not fit the contours of the back properly, excessive movement occurs or the seat breaks; both can contribute to injuries of the entire vertebral column. The size of the vehicle striking the lead vehicle is very important. Seat belts, even though they are necessary in preventing the more serious head, facial, chest, and spinal injuries, contribute to more spinal and paraspinal tissue injury. Injuries to the spine occur one to three times more frequently in belted drivers.[64,65]

Road Conditions

A wet, slippery surface causes more damage to the occupants of the vehicle struck because of the magnification of acceleration.[57] In comparison, a dry or loose gravel surface may cause more damage to the car. The physical health of the individual is significant. Any previous body injury or degenerative change, especially to the vertebral column, predisposes the patient to reinjury, causing longer treatment and rehabilitation time. A young, fit, healthy person without previous injury will rehabilitate in less time than an older, unfit person.[66]

The Extension Acceleration Injury: Rear End

Macnab[60] found that patients who sustained an extension-acceleration injury suffered more problems. Because of the anatomy of the cervical spine, which includes a variety of sensitive tissues in the anterior compartment of the neck, this is understandable. The extension injury can cause some or all of the following to occur:

- Tearing of the fibers of the sternocleidomastoid muscle

- Tearing of the fibers of the scalenus anterior muscle
- Marginal fracture of the vertebral body
- Anterior protrusion of disc
- Retropharyngeal or prevertebral hematoma
- Compression of the vertebral artery at C1
- Compression of the C2 dorsal root ganglion
- Fracture of the spinous process
- Compression of the spinal nerves C5-6-7
- Posterior subluxation syndrome of C4 on C5
- Compression of the spinal cord
- Dislocation of C3, with tearing of the Sharpey's fibers
- Tearing of the longus colli muscle
- Damage to the sympathetic chain that lies anterior to the longus muscle
- Fracture of the posterior arch of C1
- Tearing of the anterior longitudinal ligament
- Temporomandibular joint pathomechanics

The Flexion Deceleration Injury: Head-on
The injuries are not as severe because of the following:
1. The victim usually anticipates the accident and tenses for it.
2. The chin stops the head by resting on the sternum.[60]

The flexion injury can cause the following:
- Tearing of the fibers of the splenius and semi-spinalis muscles
- Posterior separation and protrusion of the disc
- Tearing of the interspinous ligament
- Tearing of the posterior longitudinal ligament
- Anterior subluxation syndrome of C5 or C6
- Flexion rotatory injuries of the cervical and upper thoracic muscles caused by seat belt use.[64,65]

The lateral flexion injury will cause the following on the flexion side:
- Pathomechanics of the intervertebral joints of Luschka
- Facet jamming caused by the anatomy of the upper thoracic and lower cervical spines

On the contralateral side:
- Tearing of the fibers of the following muscles:
- Sternocleidomastoid, scalenus group, superior trapezius, and intertransversarii

- Capsules of the intervertebral joints
- Traction of the nerve roots
- Superior subluxation of the first rib

Symptoms
From the analysis of some of the tissues injured, one can understand why cervical injuries are so difficult to assess and at times take so long to resolve. Some of the major symptoms that are the result of cervical trauma are listed in Box 18-1. A few of the symptoms listed in Box 18-1 are reviewed in the following text.

BOX 18-1 ■ Symptoms of Cervical Trauma

Peripheral

Pain
Radiculitis
Thoracic outlet syndrome
Muscle spasms/strain/sprain
Limited range of movement
Cervical dorsalgia
Altered cervical mechanics
Hematoma
Sympathetic dysfunction
Headaches/sleep disorders
Vertebral artery syndrome
Vertebral subluxation syndrome

Central

Headaches
Changes in brainstem function
Disequilibrium
Lightheadedness
Depression
Syncope
Decreased concentration
Vertigo
Blurring of vision
Meniere's disease
Nystagmus
Horner's syndrome
Barré-Liéou syndrome
Neck-tongue syndrome

Horner's Syndrome

Horner's syndrome is the most common complication associated with the cervical sympathetic trunk (CST). The complex of findings includes ptosis, anhidrosis, miosis, and enophthalmos. Other effects associated with CST injury can include alterations in cerebrovascular blood flow, increased salivary viscosity, and lability of blood pressure.[1] Blurring of vision is another sign of injury to the CST. With injury, the CST can cause flattening of the lens. This causes lack of normal accommodative power of the lens.[67] Concomitant spasm of the vertebral arteries could explain in some cases the causes of tinnitus, deafness, and mild confusion. The injury to the CST may also explain voice changes, difficulty swallowing, and dryness of the mouth.[68]

Anatomic observations show the cervical sympathetic (CS) nerves are relatively immobile as compared with the vagi. The CS trunks lie embedded in the fascia of the prevertebral muscle, longus colli, anterior to the transverse processes and posterior to the carotid sheaths. The gray rami communicantes pierce the cervical muscles in their course to the cervical spinal nerves.[69] Other symptoms of injury to the cervical sympathetic trunk include throbbing headaches, tenderness of the anterior neck, and persistent supraorbital anhydrosis.[70]

Meniere's Disease

Meniere's disease is characterized by recurrent attacks of vertigo with fluctuating hearing loss, tinnitus, and fullness in one ear. Acute attacks can last up to several hours, and residual symptoms can remain for days or even longer.[71] Meniere's disease has also been given the name *endolymphatic hydrops*[72] and is characterized specifically by paroxysmal vertigo, tinnitus, and sensorineural hearing loss.[73] The cause is unknown[72]; conditions ranging from polyarteritis nodosa, syphilis,[73] and trauma to the cervical spine have been implicated.[74]

Davis[75] showed that vertigo resulted from cervical nerve root irritation, which he thought was caused by hypertrophic arthritis of the cervical spine and responded to cervical traction. Jackson, mentioned by Braaf and Rosner,[74] stated,

> Meniere's syndrome may be part of the cervical syndrome and as much as the symptoms of equilibratory disturbances are very much the same in both instances and are due to reflex stimulation of the sympathetic nerve supply to the inner ear and to the eye.

Trauma to the cervical spine causes the development of subluxation syndrome. This produces mechanical damage and irritation of the cervical nerves or intermittent compression of the vertebral artery. With damage or irritation to the cervical nerves, reflex mechanisms are set up through the sympathetic nervous system, affecting any or all cranial nerves, producing mainly sensory and vasomotor symptoms. Treatment involves cervical traction,[74] but one must be careful regarding forces on the mandible because this will affect the temporomandibular joints. Chiropractic therapy to restore biomechanical integrity by eliminating the subluxations is necessary and provides relief if not a cure.[70,76]

Barré-Liéou Syndrome

The Barré-Liéou syndrome was first described by M. Barré in 1926. He described the headache as mainly suboccipital, vertigo as mainly precipitated by turning the head and not accompanied by any other vestibular dysfunction, and tinnitus along with visual symptoms. He noted that the patients were unable to read for long periods and usually had consulted a specialist in eye disease, but there were no objective findings. Other secondary symptoms and signs include hoarseness that appears and disappears suddenly, severe fatigue, and radiographic findings localized to C4-5-6 levels. There was also an aching on one side of the face or the eye.[77] Similar symptoms have been observed in patients injured in traffic accidents, and attention has been focused on this relationship.[78] One difficulty in assessing the syndrome is that the cranial symptoms are related to excessive movement of the neck. Research has led to a variety of opinions as to the cause of Barré-Liéou syndrome. Some of the more prevalent are occlusion of the vertebral artery,[79,80] involvement of the cervical sympathetic systems,[77] and interference with neck reflexes.[81]

In his review of the neurologic aspects of the cervical spine, Stewart[77] outlined the following information: The fifth cervical root contains sympathetic fibers that join the carotid plexus, furnishing sympathetic fibers to the neck and head. The sixth cervical root contains sympathetic fibers that proceed to the subclavian and the brachial plexuses. The seventh cervical root supplies sympathetic fibers to the cardioaortic and phrenic plexuses. There are also preganglionic sympathetic centers that arise from the mediolateral gray of the cervical cord at the C5 and C8 levels and produce fibers to form the white rami communicantes. This tangled web of sympathetic fibers and small ganglionic masses from the cord follows the vertebral artery in its course in the transverse foramens of C4 to C7. Changes in the position of the vertebra can precipitate a variety of symptoms.

Tamura[78] found a lateral soft disc at the C3-4 level in patients with Barré-Liéou syndrome that exerted pressure on the C4 and especially its ventral root. Twenty of the 40 patients had surgery to remove the disc and, except for tinnitus, all symptoms had settled compared with the group that did not have surgery. The C4 nerve root communicates with the superior cervical ganglion of the sympathetic chain through a communicating branch of postganglionic fibers. Irritation by a soft disc could give sympathetic nervous symptoms that can be explained as follows:

- Headaches may result from spasm of the internal and external carotid vessels.
- Vertigo may be caused by ischemia of the brain produced by sympathetic vasoconstriction of the internal carotid artery and its intracerebral branches.
- Tinnitus may be produced by sympathetic stimulation of the corticotympanic nerve, which derives from the internal carotid plexus.
- Ocular symptoms could be explained either by the influence of the internal carotid plexus on the ciliary muscles, causing interference with their normal regulation, or by reduced blood flow in the ophthalmic artery.

- Facial pain may be related to the fact that the superior carotid ganglion has communicating branches with the facial nerve and trigeminal ganglion.
- The bilateral nature of the symptoms could be explained by the transverse branches, which connect the sympathetic trunk on one side to the other.

Clinically, a subluxation causes some or all of these signs and symptoms. Chiropractic correction of the subluxation syndrome will relieve these signs and symptoms.

Elridge and Li[82] described a case of disc herniation of C4-5 in which the corneal sensitivity and corneal reflexes were absent along with anesthesia of the cheek and tongue. Laminectomy gave relief of all symptoms on the second postoperative day.

Cervicogenic Vertigo

It is important to stress that a cervical subluxation may be present in all forms of vertigo and dizziness. In no field is manipulation more effective than in the treatment of disturbances of equilibrium.[83] Vertigo, the sensation that you or the world around you is spinning, is a common form of disequilibrium and is one of the three most common complaints after "whiplash" injury.[84] The other two are neck muscle tenderness/pain and headache.

The body's main communication center for balance or equilibrium is found in the brainstem (medulla). The brainstem contains the vestibular nuclei, which gather and process information on position and movement through the semicircular canals (central nervous system) and the spinal cord (peripheral nervous system).

Mechanisms

1. Cervical sympathetic irritation: Injury to the cervical spine may also damage the sympathetic chain. This will affect the muscles and the blood vessels directly to the eyes.[77] These factors either cause increased input to the vestibular nuclei or affect how the vestibular nuclei respond. Both cause altered function of the vestibular nuclei.

2. Abnormal neck reflex: Because the cervical musculature and joints are richly supplied with proprioceptors,[15] when injury occurs, high volumes of information enter the spinal cord/brainstem. This affects the homeostatic equilibrium of the brainstem nuclei, resulting in vertigo/disequilibrium.[85] A subluxation in the upper cervical spine also affects the homeostatic equilibrium of the brainstem nuclei. Hinoki[84] has shown that patients with cervical soft tissue injury after whiplash show abnormal electromyelographic discharges from the neck musculature and that the level of these discharges is closely related to the patient's symptoms of vertigo during a course of treatment. Suzuki[86] showed that electrical stimulation of normal cervical muscles does not cause vertigo, but when injured muscles are stimulated, they cause vertigo.

3. Mechanical compression or stenosing of the vertebral artery[79,80]: Because trauma to the cervical spine can cause (1) tissue damage, (2) subluxation, (3) muscular spasm or splinting, and (4) pain, any of these can cause further muscular spasms or splinting and contribute to stenosing of the vulnerable vertebral artery as it passes between the occiput and C1.

We therefore must consider multiple mechanisms in the causes of cervical vertigo.[87]

Richmond[88] has shown that cat spinal muscles contain a high density of proprioceptors, and she believes that humans have the same high density. When there is damage to the muscles, they provide a great deal of proprioceptive information to the spinal cord and brainstem nuclei, namely, the vestibular nuclei. Two factors, (1) overexcitement of the cervical musculature and (2) disturbance of homeostasis of the brainstem nuclei, contribute to vertigo.[84] The factors induce disequilibrium in a trigger-and-target relationship, in which the cervical proprioceptors act as triggers and the brain stem/central nervous system is their target, causing vertigo and uncoordinated movement patterns of the eye (Figure 18-3).[89,90]

Vidal et al.[91] have shown that stimulation of the rostral portion (innervated by C1-2) of the splenius capitis muscle in a cat caused nystagmus,

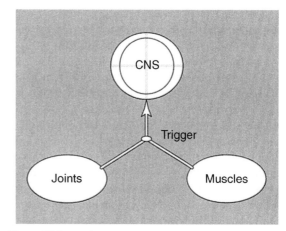

Figure 18-3   Relationship of proprioceptors to the central nervous system.

but stimulation of the caudal portion (C3-5) did not. Hildingsson et al.[92] stated that

> it seems that patients with chronic symptoms after soft-tissue injury have a localized lesion of the brain stem or an afferent proprioceptive dysfunction of the cervical spine contributing to oculomotor disturbances—one being nystagmus.

Cervicogenic vertigo is easily assessed in the clinic, and patients who have their symptoms along with upper cervical muscle and joint trauma had significant results with chiropractic therapy.[85]

Treatment

After any period of inactivity, the muscles of the neck lose tone, strength, and endurance. The joints become stiff, the ligaments become tight, and any usual activity precipitates local muscle spasm, which itself is painful.[93] Any protocol that is developed must take these factors into consideration to ensure that all injured tissues are treated effectively and that the patient does not experience increased pain.[94]

A number of researchers[95-101] have shown the beneficial effects of manipulation/mobilization of the cervical spine. The results include increased range of motion and decreased pain. Other researchers[102-105] have shown that manual therapy, including manipulation, transcutaneous electrical nerve stimulation, and traction, was not significant. The general consensus is that manipulative therapy[96,97,101] and manual therapy[95,97,99,100] have a dramatic and positive effect by decreasing cervical pain and increasing range of motion.

These studies show a treatment effect. When one considers the importance of the cervical spine with regard to its tissues, position, and the fact that it affects all parts of the body, one immediately realizes that the next level of care—rehabilitation—must be comprehensive, dealing with all the tissues in the traumatized area and with the total patient. With trauma to the cervical spine, Bogdan et al.[105] have shown that two different syndromes occur:

1. The "cervicoencephalic syndrome," characterized by headache, fatigue, dizziness, poor concentration, disturbed accommodation, and impaired adaptation to light intensity.
2. The "lower cervical spine syndrome," characterized by cervical and cervicobrachial pain. The cervicoencephalic syndrome patients had more trouble dealing with divided attention.

Trauma also contributes to injury of the intervertebral disc[106] and affects inner ear function,[107] leading to inefficient muscular control of balance and erect posture, cervical hypolordosis,[108] abnormal muscle tension,[109] postural effects through inhibition of the soleus muscle,[110] and injuries to the head, cervical muscles, and disc in the lumbar region.[111] Because cervical muscles are so important regarding control of movement and providing enormous volumes of proprioceptive information to the spinal cord/CNS,[15] it is of absolute importance to understand their response to injury and methods to effectively rehabilitate them.

Arthrogenous muscle weakness is weakness of muscles acting about an injured or inflamed joint.[112] Laboratory studies show that partial and complete muscle injuries exhibit disruption of muscle fibers near the muscle-tendon junction. Healing of partial injuries is characterized by an initial inflammatory response followed by a healing phase marked by fibrosis. Biomechanical studies show that muscle failure occurs at forces much larger than maximal isometric force, and stretch is necessary to create injury.[113] There may be up to a 20% loss of muscle strength after one week of muscle immobilization and another 20% decline in residual strength every subsequent week

of immobilization. Atrophy may occur even faster if the muscle is immobilized in a shortened position.[114] The side effects from immobilization extend beyond the muscles. If an associated joint is kept from moving, producing a subluxation syndrome, significant joint capsule, cartilage, subchondral bone, and bone-ligament changes occur.[115]

Early mobilization helps to avoid these unwanted local side effects and also promotes proper tissue healing. Collagen fiber growth and realignment can be stimulated by early tensile loading of muscle, tendon, and ligaments. The formation of adhesions between repairing tissue and adjacent structures can be limited by early motion. Proprioception is better maintained and recovers faster as well with early motion.[114] The cervical injuries for which therapeutic exercises are appropriate include acute cervical strain/sprain syndromes, brachial plexus neurapraxia, brachial plexus axonotmesis, vertebral body end plate fractures, wedge compression, and other stable fractures, along with peripheral nerve injuries.[116]

The goal is to reduce muscle tension in abnormal sensitized tissue and to develop the ability to relax such muscles when they are being maximally employed for movement and weight displacement. This may seem paradoxical, but all students of muscle physiology appreciate that fluid, efficient movement can only be achieved with a relaxed, steady, properly programmed sequence of muscle action, or muscles will fatigue, cramp, and be painful.[117]

It has been shown that progressive resistance exercises can markedly increase neck muscle strength and decrease lateral force imbalance.[118] Using the previously described protocol,[94] a preliminary study of 200 patients showed that the group receiving chiropractic treatment and performing progressive resisted exercises remained in therapy longer and had less pain and increased range of motion. Interestingly a 6-month followup found that the exercise group requested fewer chiropractic treatments and more patients maintained their overall improvement.[119]

Because the cervical muscles play a crucial role in normal cervical function, the mechanism of injury and rehabilitation and methods to enhance the efficiency of these tissues are continually being explored. Using a low-energy laser stimulates collagen synthesis and promotes more rapid healing. When the laser was combined with exercises in acute MVA victims, it produced very pronounced increases in extensor muscle strength. Also effective in rehabilitating patients with cervical injuries is the new "phasic" component system, which seems to be related to the vestibular ocular reflex. In a study addressing this component, patients with chronic cervical injuries responded significantly to new types of exercises that were "phasic," involving eye, head, neck, arm, and body movements.[120]

Conclusion

The cervical spine is truly the most complex and interesting seven inches of the human frame. One can easily understand how its injury and subluxation syndromes cause a constellation of signs and symptoms, not just localized, but referred cephalad to the head and caudal to the rest of the body. The next frontier is accurate diagnosis, effective treatment, and total rehabilitation.

References

1. Stern SJ. Cervical sympathetic trunk at the root of the neck. Head and Neck 1992;Nov/Dec:506-9.
2. Collins SL. The cervical sympathetic nerves in surgery of the neck. Otolaryngol Head Neck Surg 1991;105:544-55.
3. Korr IM. The spinal cord as organizer of disease processes: some preliminary perspectives. JAOA 1976;76:35-45.
4. Korr IM. The spinal cord as organizer of disease processes. II. The peripheral autonomic nervous system. JAOA 1979;79:57-65.
5. McMahon SB. Mechanisms of sympathetic pain. Br Med Bull 1991;47(3):585-600.
6. Akoen GN. Catecholamines, acetylcholine, and excitability of mechanoreceptors. Frog Neurobiol 1980;15:269-94.
7. Davis SN. Sympathetic stimulation causes a frequency-dependent excitation and suppression of thermoreceptive cells in the trigeminal nucleus of the rat. J Physiol 1984;350:22.
8. Roberts WJ, Ehardo SM. Sympathetic activation of unmyelinated mechanoreceptors in cat skin. Brain Res 1985;339:123-5.
9. Barasi S, Lynn B. Effects of sympathetic stimulation on mechanoreceptive and nociceptive afferent units from the rabbit pinna. Brain Res 1986;398:21-7.
10. Shea VK, Perl ER. Failure of sympathetic stimulation to affect responsiveness of rabbit polymodal nociceptors. J Neurophysiol 1985;54:513-19.
11. Sanjue H, Jun Z. Sympathetic facilitation of sustained discharges of polymodal nociceptors. Pain 1989;38:85-90.
12. Sato J, Perl ER. Sympathetic activation increases nociceptor responses after nerve injury. Soc Neurosci Abstr 1989;15:176.
13. Gellman H, Keenan MA, Stone L, Hardy SE, Waters RL, Stewart C. Reflex dystrophy in brain-injured patients. Pain 1992;51:307-11.
14. McMahon SB, Wall PD. Receptive fields of rat lamina. I. Projection cells move to incorporate a region of nearby injury. Pain 1984;19:235-47.
15. Fitz-Ritson D. Neuroanatomy and neurophysiology of the upper cervical spine. In: Vernon H, editor. Upper cervical syndrome. Baltimore: Williams & Wilkins; 1988. p. 48-85.
16. Bakker D, Richmond F. Muscle spindle complexes in muscles around upper cervical vertebrae in the cat. J Neurophysiol 1982;48:62-74.
17. Moroney SP. Biomechanics of the cervical spine. In: Haldeman S, editor. Principles and practice of chiropractic. 2nd ed. Norwalk, CT: Appleton-Century Crofts; 1992. p. 137-48.
18. Crosby ET, Lui A. The adult cervical spine: implications for airway management. Can J Anaesth 1990;37(1):77-93.
19. Yoo JU, Zou D, Edwards WT, Bayley J, Yuan HA. Effect of cervical spine motion on the neuroforaminal dimensions of human cervical spine. Spine 1992;17(10):1131-6.
20. Hayashi H, Okada K, Hamada M, Tada K, Ueno R. Etiologic factors myelopathy: a radiographic evaluation of the aging changes in the cervical spine. Clin Orthop 1987;214:200-9.
21. Dvorak J, Antinnes JA, Panjabi M, Loustalot D, Bonomo M. Age and gender related normal motion of the cervical spine. Spine 1992;17(10 Suppl):S393-8.
22. Bishop PB. Pathophysiology of the intervertebral disc. In: Haldeman S, editor. Principles and practice of chiropractic. 2nd ed. Norwalk, CT: Appleton-Century Crofts; 1992. p. 185-96.
23. Ghosh P. Basic biochemistry of the intervertebral disc and its variation with age and degeneration. Manual Med 1990;5:48-51.
24. Ghosh P. The role of mechanical and genetic factors in degeneration of the disc. Manual Med 1990;5:62-5.
25. Mendel T, Wink C, Zimny M. Neural elements in human cervical intervertebral disc. Spine 1992;17:132-5.
26. Cloward RB. Acute cervical spine injuries. Clin Symp 1980;32:3-32.
27. Connoly JF. Injuries of the cervical spine. In: Connoly JF, editor. The management of fractures and dislocations. Vol 1. Philadelphia: WB Saunders; 1981. p. 259-398.

28. Kalsbeek WD, McLaurin RL, Harris BS 3rd, Miller JD. National head and spinal cord injury: major findings. J Neurosurg 1980;Suppl:S19-31.
29. McSweeney T. Injuries of the cervical spine. Ann R Coll Surg Engl 1984;66:1-6.
30. Walter J, Doris PE, Shaffer MA. Clinical presentation of patients with acute cervical spine injuries. Ann Emerg Med 1984;13:512-5.
31. Frost E. Central nervous system trauma. Anaesthesiol Clin North Am 1987;Suppl:565-85.
32. Karbi OA, Caspari DA, Tator CH. Extrication, immobilization, and radiologic investigation of patients with cervical spine injuries. Can Med Assoc J 1988;139:617-21.
33. Babcock JL. Cervical spine injuries. Arch Surg 1976;111:646-51.
34. Whitley JE, Forsyth HF. The classification of cervical spine injuries. AJR 1960;83:633-44.
35. Pierce DS, Barr JS. Fractures and dislocations at the base of the skull and the upper cervical spine. In: The cervical spine. Cervical Spine Research Society. Philadelphia: JB Lippincott; 1983:196-232.
36. Bachulis BL, Long WB, Hynes GD, Johnson MC. Clinical indications for cervical spine radiographs in the traumatized patient. Am J Surg 1987;153:473-8.
37. Reid DC, Henderson R, Saboe L, Miller JD. Etiology and clinical course of missed spine fractures. J Trauma 1987;27:980-6.
38. Ringenberg BJ, Fisher AK, Urdaneta LF, Midthun MA. Rational ordering of cervical spine radiographs following trauma. Ann Emerg Med 1988;17:792-6.
39. Freed HA, Shields NN. Most frequently over-looked radiographically apparent fractures in a teaching hospital emergency department. Ann Emerg Med 1984;13:900-4.
40. Podolsky S, Baraff LJ, Simon RR, Hoffman JR, Larmon B, Ablon W. Efficacy of cervical spine immobilization methods. J Trauma 1983;23:461-5.
41. Anderson R. The back pain of bus drivers. Spine 1992;17(12):1481-87.
42. Kelsey JL. Epidemiology of musculo-skeletal disorders. New York: Oxford University Press; 1982.
43. Kamwendo K, Liton SJ, Moritz U. Neck and shoulder disorders in medical secretaries. Part 1. Pain prevalence and risk factors. Scand J Rehabil 1991;23:127-33.
44. Kamwendo K, Liton SJ, Moritz U. Neck and shoulder disorders in medical secretaries. Part II. Ergonomical work environment and symptom profile. Scand J Rehabil Med 1991;23:135-42.
45. Bovenzi M, Zadini A, Franzinelli A, Borgogni F. Occupational musculoskeletal disorders in the neck and upper limbs of forestry workers exposed to hand-arm vibration. Ergonomics 1991;34(Suppl):547-62.
46. Kamwendo K, Liton ST. A controlled study of the effect of neck school in medical secretaries. Scand J Rehabil Med 1991;23:141-52.
47. Alley R. Head and neck injuries in high school football. JAMA 1964;188(5):118-22.
48. Ellis WG, Green D, Holzaepfel NR, Sahs AL. The trampoline and serious neurological injuries. JAMA 1960;174(13):1673-6.
49. Funk F, Wells R. Injuries to the cervical spine in football. Clin Orthop 1972;109:50-8.
50. Haldeman S. Spinal manipulative therapy in sports medicine. Clin Sports Med 1986;5:277-93.
51. Tator C. Sports and recreation are rising cause of spinal cord injury. Physician Sports Med 1986;14:157-67.
52. Herzog RJ, Wiens JJ, Dillingham MF, Sontag MJ. Normal cervical spine morphometry and cervical spinal stenosis in asymptomatic professional football players. Spine 1991;16(6 Suppl):S178-85.
53. Denno JJ, Meadows GR. Early diagnosis of cervical spondylitic myelopathy. Spine 1991;16(12):1353-5.
54. Tysvaer AT, Locken EA. Soccer injuries to the brain. Am J Sports Med 1991;19(1):56-60.
55. Macnab I. Acceleration extension injuries of the cervical spine. In: Rothman RH, Simeone FA, editors. The spine. Vol II. Philadelphia: WB Saunders; 1975.
56. White A, Panjabi M. Clinical biomechanics of the spine. Philadelphia: JB Lippincott; 1978. p. 647-660.
57. McKenzie JA, Williams JF. The dynamic behavior of the head and cervical spine during "whiplash." J Biomech 1971;4:477-90.
58. La Rocca H. Acceleration injuries of the neck. Clin Neurosurg 1978;25:209-17.
59. Fitz-Ritson D. Unpublished data.
60. Macnab I. Acceleration injuries of the cervical spine. J Bone Joint Surg 1964;64A:1797.
61. Teasdale N, Stelmach GE, Breunig A, Meeuwsen HJ. Age differences in visual sensory integration. Exp Brain Res 1991;85:691-6.
62. Wales M. Potentially fatal asphyxia following a minor injury of the cervical spine. J Bone Joint Surg 1977;59B:93-4.
63. Keith W. "Whiplash": injury of the 2nd cervical ganglion and nerve. Can J Neurol Sci 1986;13:133-7.
64. Deans GT, Magalliard JN, Kerr M, Rutherford WH. Neck sprain: a major cause of disability following car accidents. Injury 1987;18:10-2.
65. Nygren A. Injuries to car occupants: some aspects of interior safety of cars. A study of a five-year material from an insurance company. Acta Otolaryngol Suppl 1984;395:1-64.
66. Fitz-Ritson D. Unpublished data.
67. Middleton JM. Ophthalmic aspects of whiplash injuries. Int Rec Med 1956;169:19-20.
68. Kitamura K. Brain symptoms in patients with whiplash injury. In: Itami K, editor. Whiplash injury. Tokyo: Manehara-Shuppan; 1972. p. 9-16.
69. Pick J. The autonomic nervous system. Philadelphia: JB Lippincott; 1970. p. 375-404.

70. Khurana R. Bilateral sympathetic dysfunction in post-traumatic headaches. Headache 1986;26:183-8.
71. Slater R. Vertigo. Post Grad Med 1984;5:58-67.
72. Sackett JF, Strother CM, Arenberg IK, Goldman G. The vestibular aqueduct: tomographic evaluation in Meniere's disease: a preliminary report. Head Neck Surg 1980; 2:282-6.
73. Hood NA. Diseases of the central nervous system. Br Med J 1975;15:398-400.
74. Braaf MM, Rosner S. Meniere-like syndrome following whiplash injury of the neck. J Trauma 1962;2:494-501.
75. Davis D. A common type of vertigo relieved by traction of the cervical spine. Ann Intern Med 1953;38:778-86.
76. Zerillo G, Lynch M. Importance of chiropractic in otovestibular pathology. In: Mazzarelli JR, editor. Chiropractic interprofessional research. Milan: Offset Olona; 1983. p. 69-75.
77. Stewart DY. Current concepts of the "Barré syndrome" or the "posterior cervical sympathetic syndrome." Clin Orthop 1962;24:40-8.
78. Tamura T. Cranial symptoms after cervical injury: etiology and treatment of the Barré-Liéou syndrome. J Bone Joint Surg 1989;71B(2):283-7.
79. Limousin CA. Foramen arcuale and syndrome of Barré Liéou: its surgical treatment. Int Orthop 1980;4:19-23.
80. Buna M, Coghlan W, deGruchy M, Williams D, Zmiywsky O. Ponticles of the atlas: a review and clinical perspective. J Manipulative Physiol Ther 1984;7(4):261-6.
81. Ryan G, Cope S. Cervical vertigo. Lancet 1955;ii:1355-8.
82. Elridge A, Li C. Central protrusion of the cervical intervertebral disc involving the descending trigeminal tract. Arch Neurol Psychiatry 1950;63:455-7.
83. Lewit K. Manipulative therapy and rehabilitation of the locomotor system. London: Butterworth; 1985. p. 327-9.
84. Hinoki M. Neuro-otologic studies on vertigo due to whiplash injury. Equilibrium Res Suppl 1971;1:5-29.
85. Fitz-Ritson D. Assessment of cervicogenic vertigo. J Manipulative Physiol Ther 1991;14(3):193-8.
86. Suzuki M. The effect of electricity of flowing electrode. J Physiol Soc Japan 1955;17:223-34.
87. Hinoki M. Vertigo due to whiplash injury: a neurological approach. Acta Otolaryngol (Stockh) Suppl 1985;419:9-29.
88. Richmond F. The sensorium: receptors of neck muscles and joints. In: Peterson BW, Richmond FJ, editors. Control of head movement. New York: Oxford University Press; 1988. p. 49-62.
89. Neuhuber WL, Bankoul S. The "cervical position" of the vestibular apparatus: connections between cervical receptors and vestibular nuclei. Manual Med 1992;30:53-7.
90. Bohmer A. Vertigo neuro-otologic examination procedure in the practice. Manual Med 1992;30:58-61.
91. Vidal P, Roucoux A, Berthoz A. Horizontal eye position-related activity in neck muscles of the alert cat. Exp Brain Res 1982;46:448-53.
92. Hildingsson C, Wenngren BI, Bring G, Toolanen G. Oculomotor problems after cervical spine injury. Acta Orthop Scand 1989;60:513-16.
93. Wilson PR. Chronic neck pain and cervicogenic headaches. Clin J Pain 1991;7:5-11.
94. Fitz-Ritson D. The chiropractic management and rehabilitation of cervical trauma. J Manipulative Physiol Ther 1990;13(1):17-25.
95. Brodin H. Cervical pain and mobilization. Int J Rehabil Res 1984;7:190-1.
96. Cassidy JD, Lopes AA, Yong-Hing K. The immediate effect of manipulation versus mobilization on pain and range of motion in the cervical spine: a randomized controlled trial. J Manipulative Physiol Ther 1992;9:570-5.
97. Jensen OK, Nielsen FF, Vosmar L. An open study comparing manual therapy with the use of cold packs in the treatment of post-traumatic headaches. Cephalalgia 1990;10:242-50.
98. Howe DH, Newcombe RG, Wade MT. Manipulation of the cervical spine: a pilot study. J R Coll Gen Pract 1983;33:574-9.
99. Koes BW, Bouter LM, van Mameren H, Essers AH, Verstegen GM, Hofhuizen DM et al. The effectiveness of manual therapy, physiotherapy, and treatment by the general practitioner for nonspecific back and neck complaints. A randomized clinical trial. Spine 1992;17:28-35.
100. Mealy K, Brennan H, Fenelon GC. Early mobilization of acute whiplash injuries. Br Med J 1986;22:228-32.
101. Vernon HT, Aker P, Burns S, Viljakaanen S, Short L. Pressure pain threshold evaluation of the effect of spinal manipulation in the treatment of chronic neck pain: a pilot study. J Manipulative Physiol Ther 1990; 13:13-16.
102. British Association of Physical Medicare (Brewerton DA, chairman). Pain in the neck and arm: a multicentre trial of the effects of physiotherapy. Br J Med 1966; 1:253-8.
103. Nordemar R, Thorner C. Treatment of acute cervical pain: a comparative study group. Pain 1981;10:93-101.
104. Sloop PR, Smith DS, Goldenberg E, Dore C. Manipulation of chronic neck pain: a double blind controlled study. Spine 1982;7:532-5.
105. Bogdan P, Radanov BP, Dvorak J, Valach L. Cognitive deficits in patients after soft tissue injury of the cervical spine. Spine 1992;17(2):127-31.
106. Rizzolo SJ, Piazza MR, Cotler JM, Balderston RA, Schaefer D, Flanders A. Intervertebral disc injury complicating cervical spine trauma. Spine 1991;16 (6 Suppl):S187-9.
107. Chester JB. Whiplash, postural control, and the inner ear. Spine 1991;16(7):716-20.
108. Pedersen PL. Review of cervical trauma in relation to cervical hypolordosis. Eur J Chiro 1990;38:141-7.
109. Laxton AH. Practical approaches to the normalization of muscle tension. J Manual Med 1990;5:115-20.

110. Rossi A, Mazzocchio R, Mondelli M, Scarpini C. Postural neck reflexes involving the lower limb extensor motoneuron in man. Electromyogr Clin Neurophysiol 1987;27:195-201.
111. Luo Z, Goldsmith W. Reaction of a human head/neck/torso system to shock. J Biomech 1991;24(7):499-510.
112. Stokes M, Young A. The contribution of reflex inhibition to arthrogenous muscle weakness. Clin Sci 1984;67:7-14.
113. Garrett WE Jr. Muscle strain injuries: clinical and basic aspects. Med Sci Sports Exer 1990;22(4):436-43.
114. Herring SA. Rehabilitation of muscle injuries. Med Sci Sports Exer 1990;22(4):453-6.
115. Akeson W, Woo S, Amiel D. The connective tissue response to immobility: biomechanical changes in peri-articular connective tissue of the immobilized rabbit knee. Clin Orthop 1973;93:356-359.
116. Vegso JJ, Torg E, Torg JS. Rehabilitation of cervical spine, brachial plexus, and peripheral nerve injuries. Clin Sports Med 1987;6(1):135-58.
117. Rosomoff HL, Fishbain D, Rosomoff RS. Chronic cervical pain: radiculopathy or brachialgia. Non-interventional treatment Spine 1992;17(10 Suppl): S362-6.
118. Axen K, Hans F, Schicchi J, Merrick J. Progressive resist-ance neck exercises using a compressible ball coupled with an air pressure gauge. J Orthop Sports Phys Ther 1992;16(6):275-80.
119. Fitz-Ritson D. Unpublished data.
120. Fitz-Ritson D. Phasic exercises for cervical rehabilitation after "whiplash" trauma. J Manipulative Physiol Ther 1995;18:21-4.

The Cerebral Dysfunction Syndrome

Allan G.J. Terrett

Key Words   Cerebral dysfunction, hibernation, diaschisis

After reading this chapter you should be able to answer the following questions:

Question 1   Is decreased circulation to the brain leading to loss of cell function reversible?

Question 2   Is decreased cerebral blood flow a rational explanation for previously observed effects of spinal manipulation?

After spinal manipulation, patients often comment on the relief of some other health complaint that is not apparently related to the problem for which treatment was given. This chapter gives only an overview of the concepts mentioned. The development of reversible penumbra and irreversible infarction zones appear to depend on time as well as intensity of ischemia. Some regions of the brain are more vulnerable to ischemia than others: white matter is more resistant than gray matter, and there are differences in effects of degrees of ischemia between humans, nonhuman primates (even between monkeys and baboons), and other animals (for example, cats and rats).

Over time, observant practitioners are able to recount instances in which patients mentioned improvement in vision, concentration span, learning ability, memory, or general feeling of well being, as well as decreases in tiredness, clumsiness, irritability, depression, or anxiety. Some patients return again when they feel problems with these functions. These effects cannot be explained by theories commonly put forward to explain the effects of manipulation such as the following:

- Nerve compression/irritation
- Spinal cord compression/irritation
- Somatovisceral (autonomic) reflexes
- Viscerosomatic reflexes
- Sympathetic nerve irritation
- Joint fixation (intrinsic and extrinsic)
- Vertebrobasilar ischemia
- Intraarticular meniscoid locking
- Neurodystrophic hypothesis

The cerebral dysfunction theory[1,2] was developed to explain some of the reported and observed effects of manipulation. It is proposed that manipulation can result in increased cerebral blood flow (CBF), which restores normal cerebral functioning. Therefore manipulation can have hibernocerebrosomatic, hibernocerebrocognitive, and hibernocerebropsychologic effects.

Brain Hibernation

Ischemic penumbra was a term coined in 1981[3] to describe a condition in which CBF was between normal blood flow (allowing normal functioning) and blood flow low enough to result in irreversible tissue damage (causing cell death), much like a solar eclipse in which the penumbra is an area between normal light and darkness. In this penumbra state, neurons may be paralyzed (electrocerebral silence) yet viable (ionic pump function is maintained).

CBF normally approximates 0.5 ml/g/min in human beings with cerebral oxygen consumption of about 0.035 ml/g/min. A decrease in CBF is compensated for by an increase in oxygen extraction from the bloodstream (that is, the brain has a perfusion reserve). Such compensation (to allow normal neuronal functioning) can be made down to a level of approximately 0.23 ml/g/min.[4,5] Neurophysiologic research[4-18] demonstrates that if circulation to the brain is further decreased, cells may remain alive but their function ceases. If adequate circulation is restored, neuronal function is reactivated. Therefore areas of the brain can functionally hibernate (Figure 19-1).

The relationship between cerebral electrical activity and blood flow has been amply proven in experimental studies. Differences in actual figures are related to the experimental animals being studied. Neurologic deficits begin to appear in awake monkeys when regional CBF decreases below 0.23 ml/g/min[6] and a gradual silencing of

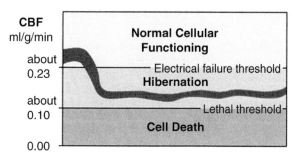

Figure 19-1   The effect of changes in cerebral blood flow (CBF) on brain function. Regional CBF above approximately 0.23 ml/g/min allows normal cell functioning. Neurologic deficits begin to appear when CBF decreases below 0.23 ml/g/min. Regional CBF below approximately 0.1 ml/g/min results in irreversible cell death.

neurons sets in. Some cells continue to fire at levels at which others have become silent,[5] with some cells still active at 0.06 ml/g/min.[7] Local CBF of approximately 0.15 ml/g/min abolishes somatosensory potential recordings in the baboon cortex.[8] Evoked potentials may be altered yet recover when flows of 0.16 ml/g/min are maintained for 14 to 60 minutes.[8] Cerebral conduction time (a function of evoked response) is affected when CBF decreases below 0.15 ml/g/min.[9] CBF below 0.18 ml/g/min in cats causes cessation of spontaneous neuronal spike activity in the cerebral cortex.[10] In humans, flattening of the electroencephalogram (EEG) occurs immediately if hemispheric flow decreases below 0.16 to 0.17 ml/g/min, as evidenced by measurements of CBF and EEG during clamping of one carotid artery in endarterectomy.[11,12] This flow level (approximately 0.23 ml/g/min) can be regarded as "critical" because electrical function in the cortex is disturbed below but is normal above this "critical" level (see Figure 19-1).

The brain uses glucose as its sole substrate. Glucose is oxidized to CO_2 and H_2O. Cell energy metabolism relies on the production of adenosine triphosphate (ATP) from adenosine diphosphate (ADP). To maintain neuronal integrity, a constant supply of ATP is required to exclude sodium ions (Na^+) from the cell and to maintain potassium ions (K^+) within the cell.

Cerebral blood flow of less than 0.10 ml/g/min results in deterioration of the energy state and ion pump failure, because in the absence of oxygen to produce ATP, anaerobic glycolysis is used. Glucose can be converted without oxygen to lactate and ATP, but the amount of energy yielded is small. This eventually leads to the accumulation of lactic acid with resultant intracellular and extracellular acidosis. When energy requirements are inadequate to maintain the normal distribution of K^+ (intracellular) and Na^+ (extracellular), membrane depolarization and ion pump failure occur with a massive efflux of K^+ from the cells. This occurs at approximately 0.08 to 0.1 ml/g/min in lightly anesthetized baboons and is most likely applicable to the human brain. (Note: The threshold of membrane and metabolic failure is higher in smaller animals.)[4,5] If such chaos persists for 5 to

10 minutes, irreversible cell damage and death occur (Figure 19-2).

Recovery of neurons suffering from a decreased blood supply is related to the duration of ischemia. Evoked potential in the baboon cortex could not recover after flow levels of 0.11 ml/g/min for 15 to 65 minutes[13]; most neurons recover from long ischemia (2 to 3 hours) only if flow levels remain above approximately 0.12 ml/g/min[6] (Figure 19-3).

Hibernation occurs between these two flow thresholds (0.12 to 0.23 ml/g/min, a difference of only 0.11 ml/g/min) and is characterized by electrical silence with normal or only slightly elevated extracellular potassium concentration. The residual perfusion (in the hibernation range) supplies

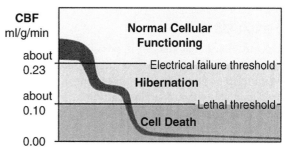

Figure 19-2   Ischemia and cell death. Further decrease in cerebral blood flow (CBF) below the lethal threshold (approximately 0.1 ml/g/min) results in brain cell death.

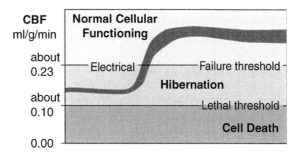

Figure 19-3   Recovery from hibernation. Most neurons recover from long ischemia only if flow levels remain above about 0.12 ml/g/min. Increase in cerebral blood flow (CBF) (from the hibernation range) to above the electrical failure threshold results in restoration of normal brain function.

sufficient oxygen to maintain a close to normal tissue concentration of ATP. Although changes in the concentrations of phosphocreatine (reduced), lactate (increased), ADP (increased), and adenosine monophosphate (AMP; increased) occur, resulting in some degree of energy failure, research suggests that this does not lead to neuronal damage.[3,4,14-16] Although electrical activity may have been lost, recovery without irreversible damage (histologic signs of structural infarction) may occur (even if the increase in blood flow is very small) only as long as the residual blood flow has been on the safe side of the threshold for energy failure and ion pump failure. There is some evidence that clinical and electrical function may turn on and off in the ischemic area of the brain.[17,18]

Diaschisis

It is proposed that diaschisis possibly occurs after hypofunctioning of one part of the brain. *Diaschisis* was a term proposed by Von Monakow in 1914[19] to describe depression of brain function at structurally intact sites remote from the brain lesion. Human and animal studies have confirmed that localized damage to one area of the brain does cause reduction of excitatory impulses to another part of the brain, resulting in depression of the distant region[20] (Figure 19-4). Neurophysiologic research of diaschisis has been done in animals and stroke victims.[21-32] These conditions represent the most severe and dramatic manifestations of diaschisis. Research has demonstrated that lesions in one hemisphere can affect functioning in the following areas:

- Contralateral cerebral hemisphere[33-36]
- Ipsilateral thalamus[34,37-39]
- Ipsilateral basal ganglia[34,37]
- Ipsilateral visual cortex; both primary and associated visual cortex[34,37,40-43]
- Contralateral cerebellar hemisphere[33,44-47]

Research has also indicated that reduction of regional CBF or metabolism in the ipsilateral frontoparietal cortex can occur in patients with lesions of the thalamus[42] and with small infarctions of the internal capsule.[34,42] Crossed cerebellar diaschisis has been reported[48,49] after hypertensive hemorrhages. Although diaschisis is proposed as part of the cerebral dysfunction theory, further research is needed to determine whether decreased brain functioning in the hibernation range has this effect and to determine the necessary severity, size, and location of the hibernating region needed to produce alterations in functioning of distant regions of the brain.

Examples of Brain Hibernation

Clinical recovery of patients with embolic transient ischemic attacks is evidence of a state of ischemic hibernation, with complete reversibility. Similarly good recovery in minor stroke patients occurring over days or weeks suggests a cortical hibernation state of longer duration.[5] Hibernation of cortical functions can occur for months or even years; when blood flow is increased, lost function returns. Cases reported in the literature tend to be the uncommon and the most severe and dramatic manifestations of this syndrome, but they are presented here to demonstrate that even in severe cases, return of adequate CBF can restore cerebral function to normal. This theory proposes that more subtle disabilities commonly occur in the brain but that they have not been considered and investigated.

1. Roski et al.[50] reported on a 50-year-old patient with a documented 7-year loss of vision (right superior homonymous hemianopia and part of the right inferior quadrants). He had an expressive dysphasia (his speech was slow and deliberate); difficulty with reading, writing, and spelling; and weakness of his right hand and a right arm drift. A computed tomography (CT) scan demonstrated a lesion in the left occipital lobe. A dynamic flow study demonstrated decreased flow in the distribution of the left middle cerebral artery. Selective arteriography demonstrated occlusion of the left internal carotid and right vertebral arteries. After an anastomosis from the left superficial temporal artery to the angular branch of the left middle cerebral artery, the visual defect immediately completely resolved. In addition, his speech was noticeably improved and his right hand grasp was normal with no arm drift.

2. Brain dysfunction associated with decreased regional CBF has been reported in cases of

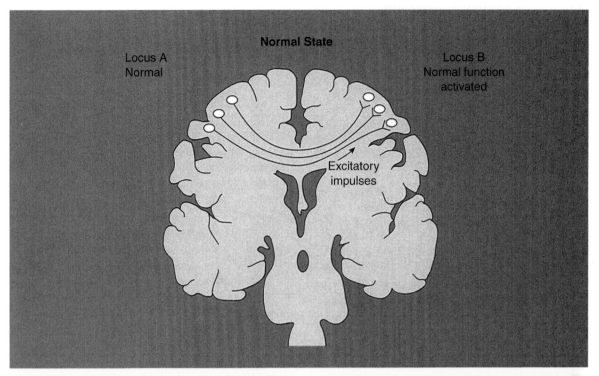

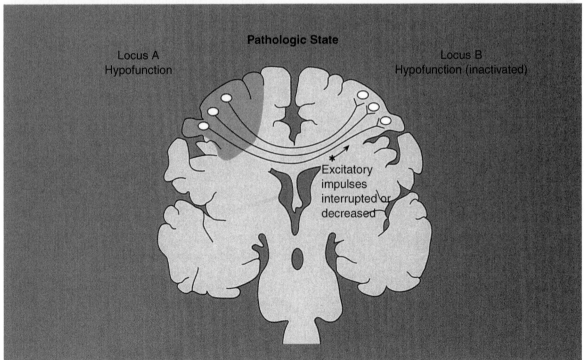

Figure 19-4   In a normal physiologic state, locus B is facilitated by stimulating impulses from neurons in locus A. If neuronal activity in locus A is decreased so that excitatory impulses from locus A are decreased, then function in locus B will be decreased. *(Adapted from Meyer JS, Hata T, Imai A. Clinical and experimental studies of diaschisis. In: Wood JH, editor. Cerebral blood flow: physiologic and clinical aspects. New York: McGraw-Hill; 1987. p. 481-502.)*

depression,[51-53] anxiety,[51,54] personality disorders,[55,56] and attention, concentration, and memory deficits.[51] Examinations of CBF in depressed patients (against control groups matched for age, sex, and handedness) showed highly reduced values for gray matter blood flow in both hemispheres when compared with controls.[51,53] The degree of depression was significantly inversely correlated with regional CBF (most manifest in the frontal regions). The authors believed that because depression is not associated with cerebral atrophy, functional hypoactivity of the neurons seems the most probable explanation for the cognitive dysfunctions (attention, concentration, and memory deficits) seen in depression. Another point relating depression to reduced CBF is that electroconvulsive therapy (ECT), which has antidepressant effects, causes cerebral blood vessel vasodilation.

Gorman[1] states the following:

It is not surprising that chiropractic manipulation lifts depression.... It is possible that chiropractic manoeuvres will become an important tool in psychiatric treatment.

3. Aphasias/dysphasias (associated with lesions of the posterior para-Sylvian association cortex) have been reversed after arterial anastomosis.[50,57,58] Jacques and Garner[57] described two patients with aphasia (one was global, the other expressive) and motor weakness (hemiparesis) that markedly regressed after superficial temporal to middle cerebral artery anastomosis (ST-MCAA).

4. Hand weakness has been reported to decrease after arterial anastomosis (increase in CBF).[50,57,58] Lee et al.[59] mention several improvements in neurologic status after an increase in CBF after ST-MCAA in patients at least three months after ischemic infarcts, so that all neurologic improvement would have occurred. They found that after ST-MCAA:
   - One patient with subjective weakness improved
   - 52% (11 of 21 patients) with mild sensory and/or motor weakness, or mild speech and/or visual impairment improved
   - 40% (two of five patients) with moderate sensory and/or motor weakness, moderate

speech and/or visual impairment, or moderate functional impairment improved
   - 71% (five of seven patients) with severe sensory and/or motor weakness, severe speech and/or visual impairment, or gross functional disturbance (but able to ambulate) improved.[59]

5. Macou and Rice[60] described the reversal of a fixed hemiplegia after ST-MCAA bypass graft.

6. Skyhoj-Olsen et al.[61] studied eight patients with completed stroke and described a clinical entity of patients with middle cerebral artery (MCA) occlusion, delayed collateral filling of the occluded vascular bed, and a deep infarct on CT, but normal overlying cortex. Patients had good recovery from the initially severe deficits, including cortical deficits like aphasia and neglect, in a matter of weeks or months. This suggests hibernation of long duration in the overlying cortex.

7. Spetzler et al.[62] studied 76 patients, who underwent extracranial-intracranial arterial bypass to increase cerebral vascularization. The researchers found that 32 presented with chronic fixed neurologic deficit (greater than three months), and that six of these demonstrated immediate improvement in neurologic examination the day after surgery (that is, after an increase in brain blood flow). Changes included improvement in hemiparesis, speech, handwriting, or combinations of these.

8. Powers et al.,[63] using positron emission tomography (PET), studied four patients with subarachnoid hemorrhage and hemiparesis caused by cerebral vasospasm. PET measurements of regional blood flows obtained early in the course of the vasospasm showed that, in the two patients who recovered, regional blood flows were 0.15 and 0.162 ml/g/min compared with 0.12 and 0.117 ml/g/min in the two who did not eventually recover (remained hemiplegic). Patient 1 also recovered from a nonfluent dysphasia.

Brain Hibernation and Spinal Manipulation

Orthodox medicine operates best when a pathologic condition is clearly definable (for example, radiographs, blood tests, cultures, biopsies).

Chiropractic usually relates to illnesses without concrete dimensions (for example, pain, aching, numbness, dizziness) but that are still disabling. Neurologists understand the effects of vascular occlusion and the resultant ischemic and stroke syndromes. The signs, symptoms, and syndromes that this theory addresses are not listed in standard neurology texts because the signs and symptoms are not so devastating as strokes, but they still cause severe health problems to the patient.

Most observant practitioners of manipulation would be able to remember patients who have described feeling better, thinking more clearly, and having clearer vision after neck adjustments. Some patients whose jobs involve complex calculations return for spinal manipulation because they believe they need it when they have difficulties with complex computations. These and other effects are commonly reported to chiropractors. It is surprising they have received very little attention in the current chiropractic literature.

The theory of brain hibernation as an explanation for many of the effects of spinal manipulation was originally proposed by two medical practitioners,[1] Eric Milne, a general medical practitioner with an interest in spinal manipulation, and Frank Gorman, an ophthalmologist with an interest in migraine. With different educational backgrounds and a patient group complaining of a much larger range of problems, they saw additional applications for and developed a different theory of the mode of action of spinal manipulation. They noted that, after spinal manipulation for headache, patients often commented that some other health complaint was relieved as well (for example, tiredness, glare distress, dizziness). After spinal manipulation in cases of interim disability, such as dizziness without the headache, the patient often mentioned the disappearance of some other health complaint. With time, the list of conditions for which spinal manipulation was indicated enlarged. The mechanism proposed to explain these postmanipulation effects was that increased CBF resulted in hibernating areas of the brain becoming functional again (Figure 19-5).

This theory proposes that arterial insufficiency to the brain resulting in decreased cerebral functioning

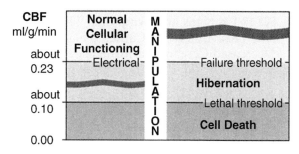

Figure 19-5 Theoretic increase of cerebral blood flow (CBF) above the electrical failure threshold following manipulation, resulting in restoration of normal brain function.

1. Is caused by constriction of the artery lumen, possibly because of
   a. Stress on the arteries in the neck caused by misaligned or malfunctioning vertebrae
   b. A sympathetic response
   c. Some mechanism still unknown.
2. Normally causes no loss of core brain functions (those that are involved in the business of existing, such as eating, walking, talking, and so on) but that it has a wide range of possible manifestations affecting sophisticated brain functions (those not essential to our existence, such as higher mathematics, concentration, "the mind," peripheral vision, mood, emotion). Box 19-1 lists signs and symptoms that are theorized to be caused by decreased cerebral functioning attributable to decreased CBF.
3. Is common and can occur without any major trauma, or after seemingly trivial trauma.
4. Causes symptoms in people who are considered "normal," and their symptoms are dismissed.
5. Has degrees of severity. As the degree of ischemia increases, the number of functioning cerebral cells decreases, and the disability becomes more severe (Table 19-1).
6. Causes people to be disabled by a mental illness of which they are unaware, which has a simple physical cause.
7. Can be relieved by spinal manipulation (by increasing CBF).

This theory proposes that it requires more "brain power" (active brain function) to be happy (not irritable), to have a good memory (not be

BOX 19-1 ■ Signs and Symptoms That Are Theorized to Be Caused by Decreased Cerebral Performance

- Giddiness/dizziness
- Lethargy/excessive tiredness
- Difficulty sleeping/insomnia
- Depression
- Nervousness
- Restlessness/anxiety
- Miserable/irritable
- Disoriented
- Personality change
- Hyperkinesias in children
- Whining child syndrome
- Tantrums
- Headache
- Problems with memory
- Learning disability
- Poor concentration
- Difficulty thinking
- Clumsiness
- Changes in visual acuity
- Visual disorders
- Auditory difficulty
- Mixing up words
- Losing track of conversations while talking
- Loss of interest in sex

forgetful), to perform complicated physical tasks (not be uncoordinated), to be bright and alive (not tired), to be articulate when speaking (not mixing words, stuttering, or losing track), to perform complicated mental tasks, to have full visual fields, and to be headache free. A child may be criticized and ridiculed with respect to intelligence or ability when in fact he or she has the potential but the cerebral dysfunction does not allow the child to use his or her assets.

Many people suffering from these complaints may be
- Given a psychologic label (and often medication)
- Told they are growing old
- Called a hypochondriac
- Labeled hysterical

and so their disability is largely ignored because
- They do not show any measurable parameters
- They do not respond to usual methods of treatment
- The absent functions are highly sophisticated and are not important to the basic business of existing (which is a poor substitute for the possibilities when the brain is fully operational).

The patient can still go about his or her day-to-day activities, but everything may be an effort, or the application of more willpower may be necessary even for quite moderate achievements, or he or she suffers excessive tiredness or irritability. An observer would not necessarily be aware of these handicaps, and because a doctor cannot detect the disabilities on radiographs, CT scans, blood or laboratory tests, or other diagnostic means, the disabilities are usually dismissed by the examiner. These disabilities are important to the patient, who may begin to assume they are normal conditions.

Gorman[64] reported on patients who underwent spinal manipulation for visual disorders. He used four ophthalmologists, independent of the author and of each other, who were asked to examine patients before and after treatment, using standard ophthalmologic assessment methods. In all cases vision improved (either the visual field and/or visual acuity). Comments by the ophthalmologists in their reports on the nonvisual field or acuity disabilities that improved after spinal manipulation included the following:
- Decreased depression
- Decreased anxiety
- Feels more positive
- Feels happier
- Feels more outgoing
- Does not wake up every morning feeling tired
- Loss of dizziness
- Loss of slurred speech
- Loss of headaches
- Improved arm movement
- Feels the light is brighter in her eyes
- Loss of sore eyes, and loss of appearance that the writing moved when reading
- Loss of a scotoma in the visual field

Table 19-1

Disorders That Are Proposed to Be Produced by Progressive Decrease in Cerebral Blood Flow (CBF)

Normal CBF (Oxygen normal) All cerebral units operational	Decreased CBF (Less oxygen than normal) Not all cerebral units operational	Further decrease in CBF (Poor oxygen supply) Few cerebral units operational
No giddiness	Giddy with use of the arms, or postural changes	Giddy all or most of the time
Normal visual field	Some loss of peripheral vision	Tunnel vision
Able to read fine print	Some visual difficulty	Only able to read large print
Happy	Irritable under stress	Irritable all the time
Able to cope with calculations	Difficulty with calculations	Unable to cope with calculations
Well rested	Easily tired	Feels continually tired
Well coordinated	Problems with manual tasks under stress	Clumsy
Never or rarely suffers headaches	Headaches under stress	Commonly suffers headaches

Testing the Theory

The value of any theory is in developing methods of testing it. If spinal manipulation is a method of reactivating hibernating cerebral neurons, the implications are enormous to both patients and the future of chiropractic. If future studies indicate this possibility, then many of the remarkable anecdotes of chiropractors will be well worth the trouble of serious investigation.

One method of investigating this theory is to
1. Develop methods of quantifying the signs and symptoms listed in Box 19-1 where no quantification system exists. Where quantification systems do exist (visual acuity, visual fields, anxiety scales, depression scales, and so on), they should be used.
2. Measure CBF in subjects before and after spinal manipulation and determine if there is any difference. Methods of measuring CBF are available.[52,56,65-75]
3. Remeasure parameters listed in step 1 after spinal manipulation and determine if there are any differences and whether these correlate with changes in CBF listed in step 2.

I have found only one report in which researchers claim to have demonstrated that spinal manipulation increases CBF. Zhang et al.[76] studied "cervical visual disturbance" in 114 people (where vision also improved after spinal manipulation) and reported the following:

> Determination of blood flow by x-ray in 18 cases of our series shows that blood flow of the cerebral hemisphere greatly improves after manipulative treatment. The same is true in similar animal tests.

The method they used to determine this is not described. Zhang et al.[76] believe that this effect of manipulation is caused by irritation of sympathetic nerves in the neck, resulting in constriction of the vertebral artery. Although this is an attractive and commonly used theory[77-80] to explain symptoms and subsequent symptomatic relief, it is not supported by recent research,[81] which found that vertebral artery blood flow was profoundly unresponsive to stimulation of any component of the cervical sympathetic system and concluded that the theory of altered vertebral artery blood flow in response to irritation of cervical sympathetic nerves is untenable. However, the vascular resistance in the carotid artery did increase with stimulation of the cervical sympathetic trunk.

It is not known by what mechanism cervical manipulation may increase CBF, but before people start postulating theories as to how blood flow is increased, further research into this possibility is needed to determine if spinal manipulation does in fact have this action.

Conclusion

Cerebral dysfunction has been proposed to explain some of the observed effects of spinal manipulation. Basic science research indicates that cerebral dysfunction (hibernation) does occur. Clinical observations suggest that this may be a mode of action to explain some of the effects of spinal manipulation. Future research is needed.

If this theory is correct, there are possible implications for the following:

- Education/learning
- Psychology/psychiatry
- Performance enhancement (physical and mental)
- Bridging gaps between professions
- Increasing scope of chiropractic practice
- Widening referral sources from:
  Industry
  Educators
  General practioners
  Psychologists
  Psychiatrists
  Speech therapists
  Rehabilitation therapists
  Occupational therapists
- Providing an explanation for some of the previously unexplainable effects of chiropractic therapy

References

1. Gorman RF. Chiropractic medicine for rejuvenation of the mind. Academy of Chiropractic Medicine, 1983. Published privately. Available from: R.F. Gorman, 7-324 Marrickville Road, Marrickville, Australia, 2204.
2. Terrett AGI. Cerebral dysfunction: a theory to explain some of the effects of chiropractic manipulation. J Chiro Technique 1993;5:168-73.
3. Astrup I, Siesjo BK, Symon L. Thresholds in cerebral ischemia: the ischemic penumbra. Stroke 1981;12:723-5.
4. Jafar JJ, Cromwell RM. Focal ischemic thresholds. In: Wood JH. Cerebral blood flow: physiologic and clinical aspects. New York: McGraw-Hill; 1987. p. 449-57.
5. Lassen NA, Astrup J. Ischemic penumbra. In: Wood JH. Cerebral blood flow: physiologic and clinical aspects. New York: McGraw-Hill; 1987. p. 458-66.
6. Jones TH, Morawetz RB, Crowell RM, Marcoux FW, FitzGibbon SJ, DeGirolami U et al. Thresholds of focal cerebral ischemia in awake monkeys. J Neurosurg 1981; 54:773-82.
7. Heiss WD, Rosner G. Functional recovery of cortical neurons as related to degree and duration of ischemia. Ann Neurol 1983;14:294-301.
8. Branston NM, Symon L, Crockard HA, Pasztor E. Relationship between the cortical evoked potential and local cortical blood flow following acute middle cerebral artery occlusion in the baboon. Exp Neurol 1974;45:195-208.
9. Hargadine JR, Branston NM, Symon L. Central conduction time in primate brain ischemia: a study in baboons. Stroke 1980;11(6):637-42.
10. Heiss WD, Hayakawa T, Waltz AG. Cortical neuronal function during ischaemia. Arch Neurol 1976;33:813-20.
11. Trojaborg W, Boysen G. Relationship between EEG, regional cerebral blood flow, and internal carotid artery pressure during carotid endarterectomy. Electroencephalogy Clin Neurophysiol 1973;34:61-9.
12. Sundt TM Jr, Sharbrough FW, Anderson RE, Michenfelder JD. Cerebral blood flow measurements and electroencephalograms during carotid endarterectomy. J Neurosurg 1974;41:310-20.
13. Branston NM, Symon L, Crockard HA. Recovery of the cortical evoked response following temporary middle cerebral artery occlusion in baboons: relation to local blood flow and pO_2. Stroke 1976;7:151-7.
14. Salford LG, Plum F, Siesjo BK. Graded hypoxia-oligemia in rat brain. I. Biochemical alterations and their implications. Arch Neurol 1973;29:227-33.
15. Salford LG, Plum F, Brierley IB. Graded hypoxia-oligemia in rat brain. II. Neuropathological alterations and their implications. Arch Neurol 1973;29:234-8.
16. Morawetz RB, DeGirolami U, Ojemann RG, Marcoux FW, Crowell RM. Cerebral blood flow determined by hydrogen clearance during middle cerebral artery occlusion in unanesthetized monkeys. Stroke 1978;9:143-9.
17. Symon L. The relationship between CBF, evoked potentials and the clinical features in cerebral ischaemia. Proceedings of the 23rd Scandinavian Neurology Congress. Acta Neurol Scand 1980;62 Suppl 78:175-90.
18. Symon L, Hargadine J, Zawirski M, Branston N. Central conduction time as an index of ischaemia in subarachnoid haemorrhage. J Neurol Sci 1979;44:95-103.
19. Von Monakow C. Die Lokalisation im grosshirn und der abbau der funktion durch kortikale herde. Wiesbaden: JF Bergman; 1914. p. 26-34. (Quoted by Reference 20)
20. Meyer JS, Hata T, Imai A. Clinical and experimental studies of diaschisis. In: Wood JH. Cerebral blood flow:

physiologic and clinical aspects. New York: McGraw-Hill; 1987. p. 481-502.

21. Ackerman RH, Correia JA, Alpert NM, Baron JC, Gouliamos A, Grotta JC et al. Positron imaging in ischemic stroke disease using compounds labeled with oxygen 15. Arch Neurol 1981;38:537-43.

22. Fieschi C, Agnoli A, Battistini N, Bozzao L, Prencipe M. Derangement of regional cerebral blood flow and its regulatory mechanisms in acute cerebrovascular lesion. Neurology 1968;18:1166-79.

23. Fujishima M, Tanaka K, Takeya Y, Omae T. Bilateral reduction of hemispheric blood flow with unilateral cerebral infarction. Stroke 1974;5:648-53.

24. Levy DE, Duffy TE. Cerebral energy metabolism during transient ischemia and recovery in the gerbil. J Neurochem 1977;28:63-70.

25. Melamed E, Lavy S, Portnoy Z. Regional cerebral blood flow response to hypocapnia in the contralateral hemisphere of patients with acute cerebral infarction. Stroke 1975;6:503-8.

26. Meyer JS, Shinoara Y, Kanda T, Fukuuchi Y, Kok NK, Ericsson AD. Abnormal hemispheric blood flow and metabolism despite normal angiograms in patients with stroke. Stroke 1970;1:219-23.

27. Meyer JS, Kanda T, Fukuuchi Y, Shimazu K, Dennis EW, Ericsson AD. Clinical prognosis correlated with hemispheric blood flow in cerebral infarction. Stroke 1971;2:383-94.

28. Meyer JS, Naritomi H, Sakai F, Ishihara N, Grant P. Regional cerebral blood flow, diaschisis and steal after stroke. Neurol Res 1979;1:101-19.

29. Meyer JS, Yamamoto M, Hayman LA, Sakai F, Nakajima S, Armstrong D. Cerebral embolism: local CBF and edema measured by CTR scanning and XeS inhalation. Neurol Res 1980;2:101-26.

30. Paulson OB, Olesen J, Christensen MS. Restoration of autoregulation of cerebral blood flow by hypocapnia. Neurology 1972;22:286-93.

31. Powers WJ, Raichle ME. Positron emission tomography and its application to the study of cerebrovascular disease in man. Stroke 1985;16:361-76.

32. Slater R, Reivich M, Goldberg H, Banka R, Greenberg J. Diaschisis with cerebral infarction. Stroke 1977;8:684-90.

33. Lenzi GL, Frackowiak RS, Jones T. Cerebral oxygen metabolism and blood flow in human cerebral ischemic infarction. J Cereb Blood Flow Metab 1982;2:321-35.

34. Celesia GG, Polcyn RE, Holden JE, Nickles RJ, Koeppe RA, Gatley SJ. Determination of regional cerebral blood flow in patients with cerebral infarction. Arch Neurol 1984;41:262-7.

35. Meyer JS, Okayasu H, Tachibana H, Okabe T. Stable xenon CT CBF measurements in prevalent cerebrovascular disorders (stroke). Stroke 1984;15:80-90.

36. Hata T, Gotoh F, Ebihara S et al. Three dimensional local cerebrovascular COl responsiveness by cold xenon method. In: Meyer JS, Reivich M, Lechner H et al., editors. Cerebral vascular disease 5. Amsterdam: Excerpta Medica; 1985.

37. Kuhl DE, Phelps ME, Kowell AP, Metter EJ, Selin C, Winter J. Effects of stroke on local cerebral metabolism and perfusion: mapping by emission computed tomography of ^{18}FDG and ^{13}NH$_3$. Ann Neuro1 1980;8: 47-60.

38. Metter EJ, Wasterlain CG, Kuhl DE, Hanson WR, Phelps ME. ^{18}FDG positron emission computed tomography: a study of aphasia. Ann Neurol 1981;10:173-83.

39. Wise RJ, Bernardi S, Frackowiak RS, Legg NJ, Jones T. Serial observations on the pathophysiology of acute stroke (the transition from ischemia to infarction as reflected in regional oxygen extraction). Brain 1983;106:197-222.

40. Bosley TM, Rosenquist AC, Kushner M, Burke A, Stein A, Dann R et al. Ischemic lesions of occipital cortex and optic radiations: positron emission tomography. Neurology 1985;35:470-84.

41. Heiss WD, Vyska K, Kloster G, Traupe H, Freundlieb C, Hoeck A et al. Demonstration of decreased functional activity of visual cortex by ^{11}C methylglucose and positron emission tomography. Neuroradiology 1982;23:45-7.

42. Lassen NA, Henriksen L, Paulson OB. Regional cerebral blood flow in stroke by ^{133}Xe inhalation and emission tomography. Stroke 1981;12:284-7.

43. Phelps ME, Mazziotta JC, Kuhl DE, Nuwer M, Packwood J, Metter J et al. Tomographic mapping of human cerebral metabolism: visual stimulation and deprivation. Neurology 1981;31:517-29.

44. Baron JC, Bousser MG, Comar D et al. Crossed cerebellar diaschisis in human supratentorial brain infarction. Trans Am Neurol Assoc 1980;105:459-61.

45. Martin WRW, Raichle ME. Cerebellar blood flow and metabolism in cerebral hemispheric infarction. Ann Neurol 1983;14:168-76.

46. Meneghetti G, Vorstrup S, Mickey B, Lindewald H, Lassen NA. Crossed cerebellar diaschisis in ischemic stroke: a study of regional cerebral blood flow by ^{133}Xe inhalation and single photon emission computerized tomography. J Cereb Blood Flow Metab 1984;4:235-40.

47. Kushner M, Alavi A, Reivich M, Dann R, Burke A, Robinson G. Contralateral cerebellar hypometabolism following cerebral insults. Ann Neurol 1984;15:425-34.

48. Kanaya H, Endo H, Sugiyama T et al. Crossed cerebellar diaschisis in patients with putaminal hemorrhage. J Cereb Blood Flow Metab 1983;3 Suppl 1:527-8.

49. Kelly RE, Ackerman RH, Davis SM et al. Positron emission tomography in cerebrovascular disease, with special emphasis on the vertebrobasilar territory. In: Berguer R, Bauer RB, editors. Vertebrobasilar arterial occlusive disease. New York: Raven Press; 1984. p. 195-213.

50. Roski R, Spetzler RF, Owen M, Chandar K, Sholl JG, Nulsen FE. Reversal of seven year old visual field defect with extracranial-intracranial anastomosis. Surg Neurol 1978;10:267-8.

51. Mathew RJ, Meyer JS, Semchuk KM, Francis DJ, Mortel K, Claghorn JL. Cerebral blood flow in depression. Lancet 1980;1(8181):1308.

52. Mathew RJ, Meyer JS, Semchuk KM, Francis D, Mortel K, Claghorn JL. Regional cerebral blood flow in depression: a preliminary report. J Clin Psychiatry 1980;41(12 Pt 2): 71-2.

53. Mathew RJ, Meyer JS, Francis DJ, Semchuk KM, Mortel K, Claghorn JL. Cerebral blood flow in depression. Am J Psychiatry 1980;137(11):1449-50.

54. Mathew RJ, Wilson WH. Anxiety and cerebral blood flow. Am J Psychiatry 1990;147(7):838-49.

55. Mathew RJ, Weinmann ML, Barr DL. Personality and regional cerebral blood flow. Br J Psychiatry 1984;144: 529-32.

56. Mathew RJ, Wilson WH. Chronicity and a low antero-posterior gradient of cerebral blood flow in schizophrenia. Am J Psychiatry 1990;147(2):211-3.

57. Jacques S, Garner JT. Reversal of aphasia with superficial temporal artery to middle cerebral artery anastomosis. Surg Neurol 1976;5:143-5.

58. Ausman JI, Lee MC, Geiger JD et al. Clinical results of middle cerebral artery-superficial temporal artery anastomosis in ischemic stroke patients in internal carotid artery distribution. Presented at The American Association of Neurological Surgeons, March 1978, New Orleans, Louisiana. (Quoted by Reference 13)

59. Lee MC, Ausman JI, Geiger JD, Latchaw RE, Klassen AC, Chou SN et al. Superficial temporal to middle cerebral artery anastomosis: clinical outcome in patients with ischemia of infarction in internal carotid artery distribution. Arch Neurol 1979;36:1-4.

60. Macou JB, Rice JF. Reversal of a fixed hemiplegia due to middle cerebral artery occlusion by delayed STA-MCA artery bypass graft. In: Spetzler RF, Carker LP, Selman WR, Martin NA, editors. Cerebral revascularization for stroke. New York: Thieme-Stratton; 1985. p. 470-4.

61. Skyhoj-Olsen T, Larsen B, Herning M, Skriver EB, Lassen NA. Blood flow and vascular reactivity in collaterally perfused brain tissue: evidence of an ischemic penumbra. Stroke 1983;14:332-41.

62. Spetzler RF, Roski RA, Zabramski J. Middle cerebral artery perfusion pressure in cerebrovascular occlusive disease. Stroke 1983;14:552-5.

63. Powers WJ, Grubb RL Jr, Baker RP, Mintun MA, Raichle ME. Regional cerebral blood flow and metabolism in reversible ischemia due to vasospasm. J Neurosurg 1985; 62:539-46.

64. Gorman RF. An observer's view of the treatment of visual perception deficit by spinal manipulation: a survey of 16 patients. Sydney, Australia: 1991 (published privately).

65. Mathew RJ, Wilson WH, Tant SR. Determinants of resting regional cerebral blood flow in normal subjects. Biol Psychiatry 1986;21(10):907-14.

66. Obrist WD, Thompson HK Jr, Wang HS, Wilkinson WE. Regional cerebral blood flow estimated by ^{133}Xenon inhalation. Stroke 1975;6:245-56.

67. Jaggi JL, Obrist WD. Regional cerebral blood flow determined by ^{133}Xenon clearance. In: Wood JH, editor. Cerebral blood flow: physiologic and clinical aspects. New York: McGraw-Hill; 1987. p. 189-201.

68. Ewing JR, Robertson WM, Brown GG et al. ^{133}Xenon inhalation: accuracy in detection of ischemic cerebral regions and angiographic lesions. In: Wood JH, editor. Cerebral blood flow: physiologic and clinical aspects. New York: McGraw-Hill; 1987. p. 202-19.

69. Yonas H, Gur D, Latchaw RE et al. Xenon computed tomographic blood flow mapping. In: Wood JH, editor. Cerebral blood flow: physiologic and clinical aspects. New York: McGraw-Hill; 1987. p. 220-42.

70. Gobbel GT, Cann CE, Iwamoto HS, Fike JR. Measurement of regional cerebral blood flow in the dog using ultrafast computed tomography: experimental validation. Stroke 1991;22:772-9.

71. Holman BL, Hill TC. Perfusion imaging with single photon emission computed tomography. In: Wood JH, editor. Cerebral blood flow: physiologic and clinical aspects. New York: McGraw-Hill; 1987. p. 243-56.

72. Herscovitch P, Powers WJ. Measurement of regional cerebral blood flow by positron emission tomography. In: Wood JH, editor. Cerebral blood flow: physiologic and clinical aspects. New York: McGraw-Hill; 1987. p. 257-71.

73. Farrar JK. Hydrogen clearance technique. In: Wood JH, editor. Cerebral blood flow: physiologic and clinical aspects. New York: McGraw-Hill; 1987. p. 275-87.

74. Warner DS, Kassell NF, Boarini DJ. Microsphere cerebral blood flow determination. In: Wood JH, editor. Cerebral blood flow: physiologic and clinical aspects. New York: McGraw-Hill; 1987. p. 288-98.

75. Ginsberg MD. Autoradiographic measurement of local cerebral blood flow. In: Wood JH, editor. Cerebral blood flow: physiologic and clinical aspects. New York: McGraw-Hill; 1987. p. 299-308.

76. Zhang C, Wang Y, Lu W et al. Study on cervical visual disturbance and its manipulative treatment. J Tradit Chin Meditor 1984;4(3):205-10.

77. Neuwirth E. The vertebral nerve in the posterior cervical syndrome. NY State J Med 1955;55:1380.

78. Stewart DY. Current concepts of "Barre syndrome" or the posterior cervical sympathetic syndrome. Clin Orthop Rel Res 1962;24:40-8.

79. Maigne R. Orthopedic medicine: a new approach to vertebral manipulations. Springfield, IL: Charles C Thomas; 1972. p. 155, 169.

80. Jackson R. The cervical syndrome. 4th ed. Springfield, IL: Charles C Thomas; 1977. p. 245-6.

81. Bogduk N, Lambert G, Duckworth JW. The anatomy and physiology of the vertebral nerve in relation to cervical migraine. Cephalalgia 1981;1:1-14.

20

Whiplash

Meridel I. Gatterman and
John K. Hyland

Key Words   Whiplash, open kinetic chain, joints of Luschka, anterior strap muscles

After reading this chapter you should be able to answer the following questions:

Question 1   How do the atypical cervical motion segments differ from the typical cervical motion segments?

Question 2   Which cervical motion segments most commonly subluxate with whiplash injuries?

Question 3   Which muscles are most likely to be strained when the patient is involved in a rear-end collision?

Whiplash is not a diagnostic term but is descriptive of the mechanical action whereby the body comes to a sudden stop followed by a sudden snap of the unsupported neck and head. This chapter is focused on the ramifications of whiplash that produce subluxations in the cervical spine.

Anatomy and Kinesiology of the Cervical Spine

Two anatomically and functionally distinct areas make up this region of the spine. The wide range of motion in all planes makes this region particularly vulnerable to injury. The head weighs approximately 10% of the body's weight, and it is balanced at the end of a long lever arm. Although it has been suggested that the term *whiplash* be abandoned, it remains a thoroughly descriptive term referring to the whip-like action that is applied to the open kinetic chain characteristic of the cervical spine. In an open kinetic chain, the most distal segment ends without attachment to any other structure.

Typical Cervical Vertebra

The lower cervical spine is composed of typical spinal motion segments from C2-3 to C7-T1. Each

motion segment is made up of two adjacent vertebral bodies, two posterior spinal joints, the elements confined within the two lateral recesses, and the intervertebral foramina, plus all the connective and muscular tissues supporting and limiting intersegmental movement. The typical cervical vertebra is wider than it is high, with comparatively large vertebral foramina. Almost 40% of the height of the cervical spine from C2 to C7 is made up of intervertebral discs so it is not surprising that this is the most mobile region of the spine.[1] Each typical motion segment contributes 20 degrees flexion-extension, 14 degrees lateral flexion, and 10 to 15 degrees side-to-side axial rotation (Table 20-1). The superior surface (superior plateau) of each vertebra is raised laterally to form the uncinate processes. These projections harbor the corresponding articular facets in the lateral inferior plateau of the vertebra above forming the uncovertebral joints (joints of Luschka).[2] Like other synovial joints, they are of clinical significance because they are subject to degenerative changes. The anterior inferior surface of the body exhibits a lip that projects downward and fits together with the transversely concave superior surface of the vertebra below. This creates a "saddle" effect that limits lateral flexion and guides anteroposterior movement during flexion-extension. The pedicles project somewhat laterally as well as backward, and the laminae are angled from them in a medial

Table 20-1							
Range of Movement (in degrees) of Cervical Motion Segments							
	C0-C1	C1-C2	C2-C3	C3-C4	C5-C6	C6-C7	C7-T1
Flexion and Extension*	15§	15	12	17	21	23	21
Lateral Bending†	3§	—	14	14	14	14	14
Axial Rotation‡	—	83	6	13	13	14	11

Modified from Adams M. Biomechanics of the cervical spine. In: Gunzburg R. Szpalski M. Whiplash injuries: current concepts in prevention, diagnosis, and treatment of the cervical whiplash syndrome. Baltimore: Lippincott Williams & Wilkins; 1998. p. 13-20.
*Data from Dvořák J, Froehlich D, Penning L, Baumgartner H, Panjabi MM. Spine 1988;13:748-55.
†Data from Penning L. Am J Roengenol 1978;130:317-26.
‡Data from Dvořák J, Panjabi MM, Gerber M, Whichman W. Spine 1987;12:197-205.
§Data from Kapandji IA. The physiology of the joints. Vol 3. The trunk and the vertebral column. London: Churchill Livingstone; 1974.

direction. The spinous processes are short and frequently bifid. The articular pillars extend from the lamina-pedicle junction and support cartilage-lined facets. The superior facets are directed backward and upward, reciprocating with the inferior facets that face forward and downward.[3] These oblique articular surfaces promote a high degree of coupled motion predominantly in lateral bending and rotation.

Atypical Cervical Vertebrae

The atypical vertebrae of the cervical spine are C1 (atlas), C2 (axis), and C7 (vertebra prominens). The first cervical vertebra is called the *atlas* because it supports the "globe-like" head. It differs significantly from all other vertebrae in that it lacks a body. Its centrum fuses with the body of the axis to form a projecting pivot (the dens) around which the atlas rotates over 80 degrees. According to Kapandji,[1] flexion and extension movements of this joint involve rolling and sliding of the lateral masses similar to the movements of the femoral condyles. The curved shape of the lateral masses ensures that axial rotation is accompanied by a vertical separation of the two vertebrae, resulting in a slight helical movement rather than pure rotation. The articulations formed by the condyles of the occiput and the superior articular facets of the atlas provide for a slipping motion with a total range of flexion-extension of 15 degrees and approximately 3 degrees of lateral flexion.[1]

The seventh cervical vertebra is atypical in that the transverse foramina are small relative to the large transverse processes, and the vertebral arteries do not normally pass through these foramina as they do in the other lower cervical vertebrae. The vertebral arteries pass upward through the transverse foramina of the typical cervical vertebrae along the uncovertebral joints looping over the posterior arch of the atlas and continuing through the foramen magnum. They are vulnerable to injury throughout their course in the cervical area when significant trauma to the cervical spine occurs. Confusing symptoms can arise inasmuch as plexuses of postganglionic sympathetic nerve fibers surround the vertebral arteries on their back surfaces, at least from C4 to C7.[4]

Stability of the Cervical Spine and Whiplash injury

The wide range of motion of the cervical spine makes stability problematic.[5] When the physiologic limits of cervical structures are exceeded, anatomical disruption of the soft tissues of the neck including muscles, ligaments, and joint capsules results. This combined with the "whip-like" mechanism of action creates a situation that facilitates subluxation of the cervical articulations.

Muscles of the cervical spine offer the first line of defense from whiplash injuries. Injury results when the neck musculature is unable to compensate for the rapidity of head and torso movement caused by the acceleration forces generated at the time of impact.[6] When the cervical muscles contract rapidly in response to impact, the potential exists for muscle injury due to lengthening contraction.[7]

Structure Injured during the Four Phases of Whiplash

When a vehicle is struck from behind, the occupant's torso is accelerated while the unrestrained head and neck lag behind.[8] As the head and neck are forced into extension, the anterior cervical muscles are stretched while contracting in an effort to prevent hyperextension. Most frequently injured by this phase are the "anterior strap muscles," including the sternocleidomastoid and scalene muscles. The splenius capitus muscles are frequently injured especially if the head and neck are rotated at the time of impact. Having the head turned at time of impact increases the risk of injury.[8]

Structures injured during the second phase of whiplash from a rear-end collision are those vulnerable to shear strain. Penning[9] speculates that the primary mechanism of injury in whiplash is actually hypertranslation of the head backwards. He notes that it is the overstretching of the ligaments of the upper cervical spine, especially of the atlantoaxial segment (including the alar ligament), that leads to disorders of proprioceptive information. It is this phase during which translation occurs that most likely contributes to subluxation of the upper cervical articulations seen clinically. When ligaments and joint capsules are stretched, the axial traction permits the joints to separate and then subsequently compress with jamming and altered alignment. Ligamentous injury occurs when the cervical muscles become stretched to the point that the ligaments are called into play to stabilize the spine. When the ligaments become stretched, further injury to the discs and articular capsules can ensue. Disc injury usually consists of a disruption of the anulus fibrosus viewed on radiographs as a widening of the posterior disc space, a narrowing of the anterior disc space, and often a concomitant anterior hypermobile subluxation caused by disruption of the posterior elements.[8] (See Chapter 8.) During phase 3, acceleration is diminished with the head and torso thrown forward straining the superficial posterior cervical muscles including the upper trapezius. During phase 4, if the body is restrained by a seatbelt, the head will continue to move forward until it strikes the chest or an external object. This is the phase when the upper cervical posterior muscular and ligamentous elements of the cervical spine become injured including the suboccipital muscles. Croft[8] maintains that it is the upper cervical spine that sustains the greatest injury from whiplash because it tends to be the biomechanical pivot point.

Mechanics of Whiplash

Initially, in a rear-end impact, the torso of the victim translates backward while the head and neck remain stationary and the vehicle moves forward underneath. This is followed by the abrupt upward movement of the torso as the thoracic kyphotic curvature is straightened. This sets the head into vertical acceleration that straightens and compresses the cervical spine. This is followed by a series of abnormal distortions of the neck. First there is an initial flexion of the upper cervical spine, followed by extension of the lower cervical segments. This induces an S-shaped distortion in the entire cervical spine.[10-12] This is then followed by extension of all levels of the cervical spine.[12] Yang and King[13] also found significant posterior shear deformation present with large facet capsular stretch. They considered this to be a major source of pain. Following the extension phase, the head is cantilevered forwards into flexion with fanning of the spinous processes.

Subluxation following Whiplash

Cervical subluxation following whiplash may take the form of simple joint locking or, more likely, be accompanied by hypermobility in other motion segments. The biomechanical injuries seen clinically that result from whiplash tend to follow a characteristic pattern. The torque and lofting of the head tends to produce hypomobility and subluxation of the upper cervical and lower cervical joints with hypermobility common in the mid-cervical region.[14] Jackson[4] noted that the greatest amount of soft tissue injury occurs at the C4-5, C5-6 motion segments. Jaeger's report[15] on 11 cervicogenic headache patients related to whiplash noted that tenderness and misalignment around the transverse process of C1 was the most frequent finding. Next to upper cervical subluxations, C7-T1 and first rib subluxations are most commonly seen. Movement of spinal motion segments may be blocked anywhere in the spine with whiplash injuries,[14,16,17] but most commonly seen clinically are upper cervical subluxations followed by fixation at the C7-T1 spinal motion segment, and first costovertebral articulation.[14]

Clinical Considerations

History

It is important to obtain as much information as possible about the whiplash injury. The direction of force, position, relationship of the head and spine, and state of tension of the neck muscles all help to determine the location of stress. The position of the patient at the time of impact should be noted. Typical questions asked of whiplash-injured patients are included in Box 20-1. These questions aid in the assessment of the severity of injury, in addition to indicating which structures are involved.

The patient with whiplash most commonly gives a history of minor to moderately severe rear-end collision.[18] Other types of vehicular crashes such as a head-on or side collision or a history of a fall can produce a whiplash mechanism. A sideways

BOX 20-1 ■ Questions Aiding in the Assessment of the Severity of Injury in Addition to Indicating Which Structures Are Involved

- Was the patient looking straight ahead or positioned with the head or body turned? Was the patient driving?
- Was the arm outstretched?
- Did the head or another body part strike something? Did something loose in the vehicle strike the patient?
- Was the patient wearing a seat restraint (lap type or combined lap-shoulder harness), and what was the nature of the head support?
- Was there loss of consciousness or mental confusion? Was the patient thrown from the car?
- What were the relative sizes of the involved vehicles, make of the vehicles, and type of suspension in the injured party's vehicle?
- What was the approximate speed involved? Was the patient's foot down hard on the brake pedal or floorboard?
- Was the seat torn loose? Did the backrest break away? Had there been a previous or old neck injury?[14]

fall on the outstretched arm can produce a lateral whiplash effect on the cervical spine similar to the side impact vehicular collision. A blow such as from a swinging object[4] may also produce whiplash. A severe form of whiplash-induced injury occurs with the "shaken baby syndrome" or "whiplash–shaken infant syndrome." Injury occurs when an adult shakes an infant repeatedly in the fore and aft direction. This mechanism can cause severe injuries and can even be fatal.[8]

Symptoms of Whiplash Injury

Patients suffering from whiplash injuries complain of a large variety of symptoms typically more broad than other neck injuries. Frequently they are not aware of significant injury immediately following the accident, but after a few minutes they can develop a feeling of discomfort in the neck, associated with some degree of nausea.[19] This is typically followed by a feeling of tightness and stiffness. After several days a broad symptom complex may develop.[18] It is wise to inform the whiplash patient who is treated immediately following a whiplash injury that he or she may gradually feel worse for several days to prevent the perception that the treatment has made the condition worse. After 72 hours, a gradual decrease in symptoms can be expected. The delay in symptoms is thought to be due to the time required for traumatic edema and hemorrhage to occur in injured soft tissues.[20]

Neck pain with limited motion is the most common complaint following whiplash injury. Neck pain may occur at the back, front, and sides of the neck.[4] The pain may radiate into the shoulders and arms to the fingers. The radiation may be unilateral or bilateral. Chest and back pain may also be present. The character of pain may be described as burning, sharp, throbbing, or stabbing, or as a dull ache. A deep, aching, or dull pain is common with joint lesions. Nerve irritation produces a stabbing or lightning-like pain that radiates in specific patterns. A sharp, localized pain may indicate a fracture. Throbbing pain is indicative of vascular involvement.[8]

Headaches are a frequent complaint with cervical spine disorders. (See Chapter 19.) The pain may be at the back of the head, the top of the head, or in the temple area.[4] It may be unilateral or bilateral, intermittent or constant, localized or generalized. Muscle contraction headaches are generally associated with occipital pain, or pain radiating to the frontal area. Often referred to as tension headaches, they may be caused by spasm, injury, or inflammation to the muscles or myofascial connection to the cranial periosteum. The greater and lesser occipital nerves may be irritated by the clinically contracted muscle or by irritating substances (bradykinins, proteolytic enzymes, etc.) that accompany inflammation. Ischemia that can accompany chronic muscle spasm frequently activates a reflex whereby the pain-spasm-pain cycle becomes chronic. Vascular headaches may occur in patients with head injuries, but they represent a small fraction of those patients suffering from posttraumatic headaches as a result of whiplash. A common source of postwhiplash head pain is subluxation (jamming) of the zygapophyseal joints referred to as a cervicogenic (vertebrogenic) headache. (See Chapter 19.) Technically all headaches arising from the neck including those caused by the cervical muscles are cervicogenic in nature, and much confusion surrounding the classification of headache remains. An accurate palpatory diagnosis can determine if the cervical motion segments are involved.

Stiffness following injury usually limits motion in the direction opposite that of the muscle spasm. Weakness of the muscles of the neck, arms, and hands may be noted by the patient, and the patient often complains of difficulty balancing the head or the neck because of weakness of the neck muscles.[4] Complaints of loss of grip strength and things slipping from the hands are common. Sensory complaints include numbness and tingling, frequently without actual demonstrable hypesthesia or sensory changes. Numbness of the neck, shoulders, arm, forearm, and fingers may be the result of nerve root irritation or compression, circulatory embarrassment, or referral from trigger points in the strained muscles.[6] Visual disturbances are frequent following trauma to the neck. Blurred vision is a common complaint and usually of short duration. It may be due to damage to the vertebral arteries or may reflect damage to the cervical sympathetic chain.[21,22] Other visual complaints can include "eye strain," fatigue, diplopia, and photophobia.[4]

Occasionally symptoms of irritation of the sympathetic nerve supply in the neck occur. This can produce dilation of one pupil with irritation of the sympathetic fibers surrounding the internal carotid arteries and their branches to the eye. Horner's syndrome is occasionally seen due to sympathetic ganglion damage around the sixth cervical level.[22] Complaints of instability or dysequilibrium with a tendency to list to one side have been reported.[4] Disruption of the proprioceptive system from injury to muscles and joints of the cervical spine or vasospasm or vasodilation with edema affecting labyrinth function may result in dizziness, unsteadiness, or lightheadedness.[22]

Dysphagia (complaints of difficulty in swallowing) and other laryngeal disturbances, with compulsive clearing of the throat,[23] may be the result of swelling of the anterior neck structures or to retropharyngeal hematoma. The latter can be seen on routine lateral radiographs as forward displacement of the air shadow of the pharynx.[22]

Less common complaints include dyspnea or shortness of breath that may be the result of pain in respiratory muscles. Heart palpitations (tachycardia) from irritation of the fourth nerve root or irritation of the cardiac sympathetic supply should be investigated thoroughly. Vertebrobasilar arterial insufficiency can precipitate drop attacks or black out sensations. Nausea and vomiting, and complaints of irritability, insomnia, and lightheadedness may also be noted. Low back pain is frequently reported in cases of moderate to severe injury resulting from rear-end collisions, and occasionally a patient complains of leg symptoms. Sprain of the lumbar region may occur from acute flexion of the low back at the time of the accident.[22] It is frequently overlooked initially because of the more severe cervical complaints at the onset.

Grieve[17] stresses the vulnerability of the whiplash victim to rough handling. He describes this as a highly reactive "brittleness" during the early stages. He notes that this is quite different from the irritability of a single peripheral joint. He states,

> If the badly injured whiplash patient is handled vigorously with careless movement, the exacerbation can be very severe with headaches of hideous intensity, bizarre visual upset, psychic distress amounting to abject misery, and cervical pain of frightening viciousness.

What appears to be a minor vehicular collision may produce a varied pattern of symptoms that can be understood by careful evaluation of the structures that can be damaged. It is not possible to determine the type or extent of soft-tissue damage by estimating the cost of auto damage.[8] Fortunately, with appropriate management the prognosis for the vast majority of these patients is favorable.

Objectively, the acute signs of whiplash injury include muscle tenderness, spasm, and restricted motion.[22] A few hours to a few days after the injury, when most patients are usually seen, there is tenderness and swelling in the anterior neck region (anterior strap muscles). Palpable spasm often occurs in the trapezius muscle accompanied by variable restriction of neck motion.[4,6] Travell[24] has noted that the splenius capitis muscles are frequently strained, especially if the head and neck are somewhat rotated at the time of impact. The sternocleidomastoid muscle resists forceful backward movement and is commonly injured by hyperextension and lateral flexion injuries along with the scalene muscles.[24] Frequently overlooked are trigger points in the posterior scalene muscle at the attachment to the second rib. These trigger points are difficult to locate because they pass beneath the levator scapulae, which must be pushed aside at the point where the levator scapulae emerges from the anterior free border of the upper trapezius.[24] Superior subluxations of the first rib are commonly found in patients suffering from whiplash injuries and are frequently associated with trigger points in the anterior scalene muscles. If the thoracic lumbar paraspinal muscles are stiffened at the time of impact, the sudden acceleration or deceleration may rapidly stretch these muscles and activate trigger points. The trapezius muscle and the levator scapulae checkrein flexion and are frequently strained in accidents involving forceful hyperflexion.[24]

In the presence of cervical nerve root irritation, the upper extremity reflexes may be hyperactive immediately following an injury. After a few days they become hypoactive, provided there is no spinal cord involvement. Sensory changes may be found anywhere along the cervical nerve-root distribution. Soon after an injury, hyperesthesia may be present, which changes to hypoesthesia after a short time.[4] Pupillary dilation may be present, which indicates irritation of the sympathetic nerve supply.[4]

Irritation of the sympathetic nerve supply gives rise to vasoconstriction of the arteries that are supplied by sympathetic fibers, and it is indicated by a wide blood pressure variation between arms. A 10- to 20-point difference can be produced by cervical spine disorders.[4] Spasm in the scalene muscles may cause diminution or oblitera-

tion of the radial pulse when the head is tilted and rotated to the opposite sides. (See Chapter 22.)

Assessment of Whiplash Injuries

Palpatory Findings

Static palpation for alignment, tone, texture, and tenderness of the bony and soft tissue structures of the neck provides valuable information in the postwhiplash patient. Palpation of cervical muscle tone and texture is palpated with the patient supine to promote optimal relaxation in injured structures (Figure 20-1). Palpation for flexion, extension, or rotation alignment of C1 in relation to C2 evaluates the C1 transverse process to mandible distance (Figure 20-2, A). Lateral flexion alignment of the atlantooccipital articulation using the inferior tip of the mastoid to C1 transverse process distance (Figure 20-2, B). Rotational and lateral flexion alignment at the atlantoaxial articulation is palpated by comparing the bilateral relationship of the C1 transverse processes to the C2 articular pillars (Figure 20-3). Palpation for the alignment of the spinous processes in the lower cervical spine is conducted in the sitting position with the patient's head flexed (Figure 20-4).

Palpation for segmental motion includes evaluation of the discrete short-range movements of a joint that are independent of the action of voluntary muscles. It is determined by springing each vertebra in the neutral position (joint play), or at the limit of its passive range of movement (end

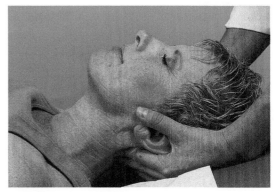

Figure 20-1   Palpation of suboccipital muscle tone and texture.

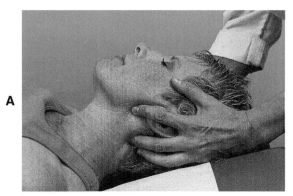
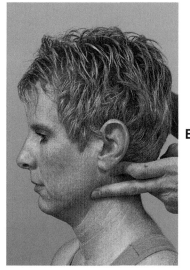

Figure 20-2   **A,** Palpation for flexion, extension, or rotation alignment of C1 on C2; evaluation of C1 transverse process to mandible distance. **B,** Lateral flexion alignment of the atlantooccipital articulation using the inferior tip of the mastoid to C1 transverse process distance.

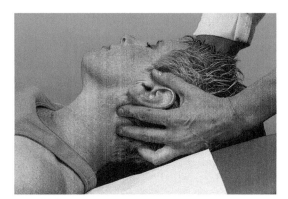

Figure 20-3   Palpation for rotation and lateral flexion alignment of the atlantooccipital articulation compares the bilateral relationship of the C1 transverse process to the C2 articular pillars.

feel), in addition to segmental range of motion. Joint play in the articulations of the cervical spine can be evaluated with the patient seated or in the supine position. In the supine position the patient's head rests on the table, which is often most comfortable for the acute patient. Joint play and posterior-to-anterior glide is assessed in the

cervical spine with the patient in the sitting position by bilaterally contacting the posterior joints with the palmar surfaces of the finger and thumb of the contact hand with the patient's forehead supported by the stabilizing hand (Figure 20-5). Each individual motion segment is evaluated for a fluid posterior-to-anterior gliding motion along the horizontal plane. With the patient in the supine position, joint play and posterior-to-anterior glide is assessed by contacting the posterior joints with the fingertips (Figure 20-6). Lateral-to-medial glide may be assessed by contacting the posterolateral surface of adjacent vertebrae with the index fingers. One hand springs the segment toward the midline as the other stabilizes. Joint play movement should be pain free and uniform on each side. Unilateral resistance or a tendency for the spine to rotate away from the midline may indicate a subluxation. A subtle gliding motion with recoil is indicative of normal joint play. Absence of this motion is indicative of joint blockage. A boggy sensation or excessive sponginess indicates possible hypermobility or instability. (See Chapter 8.) End feel is assessed by application of over pressure at the end of segmental range of motion

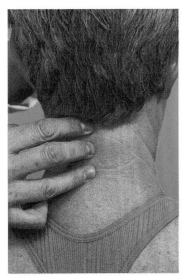

Figure 20-4   Palpation for alignment of the spinous processes in the lower cervical spine.

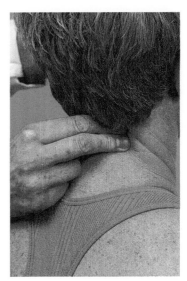

Figure 20-5   Sitting joint play assessment for posterior-to-anterior glide in the mid-cervical spine.

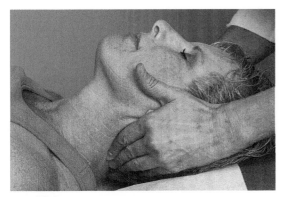

Figure 20-6   Joint play assessment for posterior-to-anterior glide in the mid-cervical spine.

testing. Atlantooccipital (C0-1) flexion and extension are evaluated by placing the tip of the index finger in the space between the mandibular ramus and the anterior tip of the atlas transverse process. This space increases during extension and decreases during flexion (Figure 20-7).

There is limited occipital rotation that occurs at the end of cervical rotation. The space between the mandibular ramus and the atlas transverse process will increase on the side opposite rotation and

decrease on the side of rotation (Figure 20-8). To assess lateral flexion at the atlantooccipital articulation, the index finger is placed between the inferior tip of the mastoid process and the atlas transverse process (Figure 20-9). The space between the mastoid and atlas transverse increases as the head is laterally flexed away from the side of contact.

Segmental range of motion at the atlantoaxial (C1-2) region is assessed by contacting the posterolateral aspect of the transverse process of the atlas and the axis with the middle and index fingers so that they bridge the C1-2 intertransverse space. With head slightly laterally flexed toward the contact, the head is passively rotated away from the side of contact (Figure 20-10). Separation of the C1-2 intertransverse space on the side opposite rotation should increase with rotation.

Segmental range of motion in the lower cervical spine from C2 to C7 can be assessed with the patient seated or supine. Contact is established on the posterior surface of the articular pillars with the index finger on the side opposite cervical rotation (Figure 20-11). The superior pillar should move forward in relation to the one below with a stair-stepping effect from the lower to the upper cervical spine on full rotation. To assess lateral

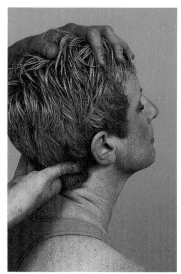

Figure 20-7   Palpation for flexion-extension movement of the right atlantooccipital articulation.

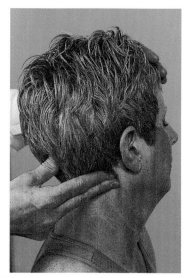

Figure 20-8   Palpation of left rotation at the atlantooccipital articulation.

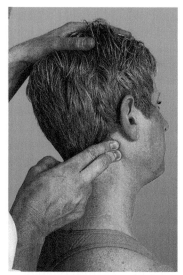

Figure 20-9   Palpation of left lateral flexion at the atlantooccipital articulation.

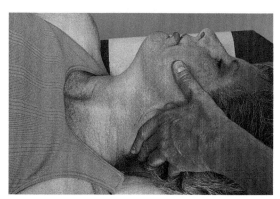

Figure 20-10   Palpation of right rotation at the atlanto-axial articulation.

flexion from C2 to C7, either a bilateral fingertip or index contact is established over the articular pillars slightly posterior to the mid-coronal plane (Figure 20-12). With the patient in a supine position, lateral flexion with a slight inferior inclination is induced and movement to each side is evaluated. To evaluate flexion and extension, contact is established bilaterally with the fingertips over the posterior articular pillars (Figure 20-13). Posterior inferior gliding of the articular pillars is palpated during extension with anterior superior gliding palpated on flexion.

Jull et al.[25-28] have demonstrated the reliability and validity of motion palpation in the detection of cervical subluxations. (See Chapter 19.) Employing diagnostic anesthetic blocks to the facet joints as the gold standard, Jull[25-28] has

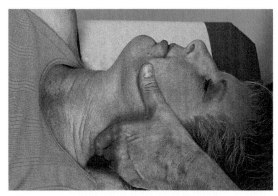

Figure 20-11   Palpation of right rotation at the C3-C4 motion segment with the patient in the supine position.

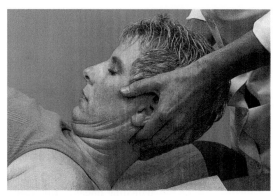

Figure 20-13   Palpation of cervical flexion with the patient in the supine position.

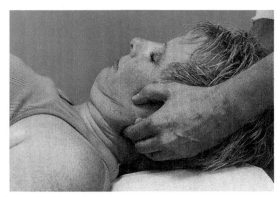

Figure 20-12   Palpation of left lateral flexion in the supine position with a fingertip contact.

reported on both noncontrolled and controlled trials. In a posttraumatic headache study[29] that compared headache subjects with an age and gender matched control group, at least one segment in the headache group demonstrated marked hypomobility in the upper cervical spine. Much greater joint dysfunction was noted between C0-3 in the headache group compared with the control group. Jensen, Nielson, and Vosmer[30] also reported findings of hypomobility in a clinical trial of 19 posttraumatic headache patients treated with manipulation.

Palpation of static segmental misalignment and tenderness can also be used to identify subluxated motion segments in patients suffering from whiplash injuries[31] (Table 20-2). Palpable misalignment of the C1 transverse processes, the C2 spinous process, and the C0-3 posterior joints are common findings. Jaeger[32] noted misalignment around the transverse process of C1 in a number of cervicogenic headache patients following whiplash injury.

Imaging Evaluation

Diagnostic imaging of the cervical spine is an important component of clinical decision making after a whiplash injury. The three-view limited cervical x-ray series (A-P, lateral, and A-P open mouth) is the recommended minimum study.[33] While these films should be carefully evaluated for the presence of fractures, dislocations, and other signs of significant damage, they are generally not sufficient to identify cervical subluxations resulting from the whiplash injury. For instance, a common finding on the lateral projection is a loss or flattening of the cervical lordosis. While this may be an indicator of subluxation, it has also been identified as a normal finding in some patients.[34,35] However, a more acute kyphotic angulation, often with a "break in George's line," is frequently associated with substantial injury to the surrounding soft tissue structures.[36] George's line, also known as the posterior vertebral line, is visualized as a smooth unbroken line extending from C2 to C7

Table 20-2

Palpatory Landmarks of the Cervical Spine

Landmark	How to locate	Clinical significance
External occipital protuberance (EOP)	*Posterior*—Midline projection of posterior aspect of skull at junction of neck	Reference landmark; adjustive contact point lateral to EOP used with occipital (C0-C1) subluxations
C2 spinous process	*Posterior*—First bony point palpated in midline inferior to EOP	Commonly used as an adjustive contact point; tender with subluxation
C6 spinous process	*Posterior*—Moves anteriorly away from palpating finger during cervical extension-easily palpated in C flexion	Commonly used as an adjustive contact point; tender with subluxation
C7 spinous process	*Posterior*—Commonly most prominent spinous process; C7 moves on T1 during C flexion and extension; palpated throughout C flexion and extension	Commonly used as an adjustive contact point; tender with subluxation
Cervical facet joints	*Posterior*—Palpated 1.5-2.0 cm lateral to spinous process	Commonly used as an adjustive contact point; soft tissues over these areas are tender with subluxation
C1 transverse process	*Lateral*—Palpated between mastoid process (prominence of temporal bone posterior to ear) and angles of the jaw	Used as an adjustive contact point; tender with subluxation

Modified from Scaringe JG, Faye LJ. Palpation: the art of manual assessment. In: Redwood D, Cleveland CS. Fundamentals of chiropractic. St. Louis: Mosby; 2003. p. 211-36.
Note: In addition to tenderness due to subluxation, vertebral fractures, infections, neoplasm sprains, and strains may also cause tenderness over the bony landmark.

along the posterior border of the vertebral bodies (Figure 20-14). Additional plain-film views are needed in some cases, and occasionally advanced imaging is indicated.

Additional X-ray Views

While the seven-view cervical study (Davis series) is commonly performed, the oblique views are often unnecessary.[37] In addition to the minimal three-view cervical series and the oblique views, flexion and extension radiographs comprise the seven view series. The exceptions are when there is a suspicion of injury to the posterior arch or of foraminal encroachment due to extensive degenerative changes; then the oblique views should be taken. Pillar views may occasionally be needed if a compression fracture of an articular pillar is suspected from the appearance on the initial views.

Dynamic (Functional) Views

The most useful x-ray views for identifying the sites and the effects of postwhiplash subluxations are the flexion and extension films.[38-40] These lateral projections are obtained at the end range of each of the movements (Figure 20-15). Because acute muscle spasm and inflammation can significantly restrict a patient's motion, these views are best deferred until the postacute stage (usually two to four weeks).[41] Once the patient is able to perform a reasonable excursion from flexion to extension, spinal levels with hypermobility (often with associated ligament damage), hypomobility, and

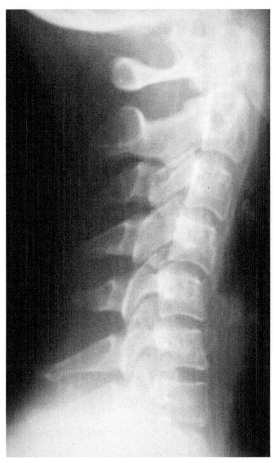

Figure 20-14   Acute kyphotic angulation with a break in George's line.

aberrant motion can be identified.[42] The templating procedure using cervical overlays demonstrates subtle areas of altered mobility by highlighting intersegmental motion.[43] (See Chapter 6.)

Advanced Imaging

When a fracture is identified or suspected from plain film evidence, a computerized tomographic (CT) evaluation should be ordered. The CT study of the cervical spine is best done with "thin-slice" (<3 mm) technique. Scintigraphy (bone scan and SPECT) is useful when there is a persistent clinical suspicion of a fracture that is not seen on plain films.[44] Magnetic resonance imaging (MRI) is most valuable for evaluating the soft tissues, especially the intervertebral discs, spinal cord, and ligaments. In addition to multiplanar anatomical morphology, MRI provides physiologic information about the tissues (fat and water content).

Management of Whiplash Injuries

People who are exposed to whiplash injuries have a greater likelihood of persistent pain, work disability, and recurrent subluxations. Because of this, timely assessment and proper care are very important. Treatments must progress from initial passive efforts to control pain and inflammation to active interventions that focus on regaining physical function and spinal stability.

Several well-designed studies have found that the risk of persistent problems after experiencing a whiplash injury is quite high. In fact, one review of the literature concluded that "between 14% and 42% of patients with whiplash injuries have chronic neck pain and...approximately 10% of this group experience constant, severe pain."[45] If patients are still symptomatic after three months, there is almost a 90% chance that they will remain so.[46] One group of investigators looked at whiplash patients an average of seven years after injury and found that such persons had two to three times greater prevalence of headaches, neck, and back pain.[47]

Comprehensive Whiplash Care

Doctors of chiropractic are well positioned to provide "multimodal treatment" to whiplash patients in order to minimize the risk of long-term problems. This has been defined as treatment that applies manual procedures (spinal manipulation, mobilization, and massage), along with physical training to improve muscle strength and endurance, including sport activities. Multimodal treatment has been found to be effective in preventing many of the persisting symptoms of "late whiplash syndrome."[23]

Spinal manipulation progressing from gentle mobilization to specific adjustments for joint fixations and subluxations should be initiated once contraindications such as fracture and instability

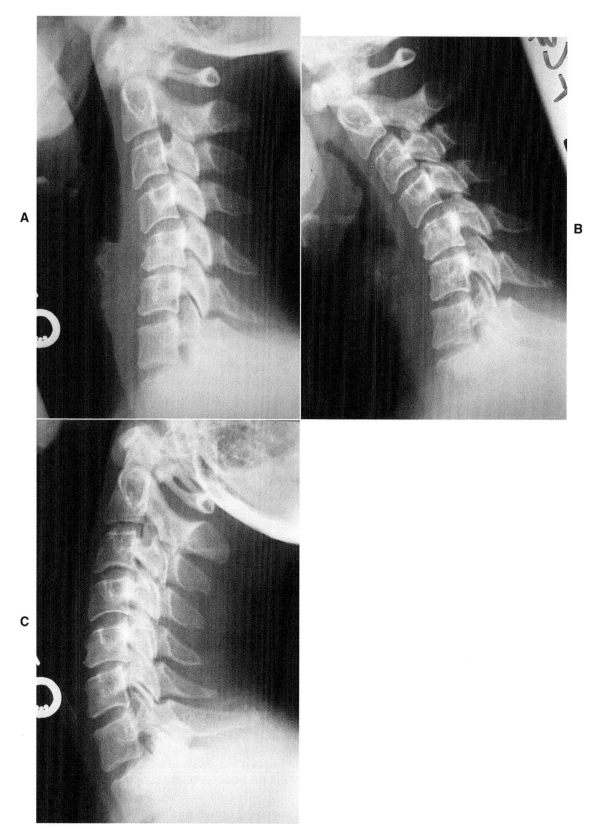

Figure 20-15 26-year-old female with hypermobility at C4-C5 and C5-C6. **A,** Neutral lateral; **B,** flexion; **C,** extension.

(see Chapter 7) have been ruled out.[48] Specific spinal adjustments have also been identified as effective treatments for patients with chronic symptoms after a whiplash injury.[49]

Studies have identified several injuries to the neurologic system that may occur after moderate whiplash injuries.[50,51] Even at low speeds, the nervous system is "jolted" during the rapid translation movement of the head and neck. A *jolt* is "a sudden, unexpected, forced stretching and/or reflex contraction of skeletal muscle induced by a barrage of impulses from receptors in muscle spindles and joint capsules."[52] This can cause a "generalized central hyperexcitability" of the nervous system, which results in muscular hyperalgesia and large referred pain areas.[53] This neurologic state is also called *central sensitization,* which has been identified as a cause of persisting disability[54,55] and is independent of psychological distress.[56] Both the biomechanical and the neurologic injuries must be taken into account when planning an effective treatment program after a whiplash injury.

Initial Postinjury Care

Protection and Support
In the first several hours (up to 72 hours), there is bleeding and effusion in the torn soft tissues (ligaments and muscles) around the spinal joints. This rapidly develops into an inflammatory response with tissue congestion. At this initial stage, activity restrictions and protection of the acutely injured area are necessary to prevent further damage. This may require the use of a soft cervical collar for one or two days. The old habit of recommending complete rest and a collar for one or two weeks has been shown to be unnecessary; in fact, this can slow the healing response.[57] It is important to keep the patient active but avoid causing further injury or aggravation of symptoms. Because additional neck trauma[58] and subsequent whiplash injuries[59] significantly increase the likelihood of prolonged disability,[60] a protective collar should be recommended any time there is injury risk, especially when in a motor vehicle.

A cervical pillow designed to support the normal curve of the cervical spine can be tremen-dously helpful throughout care. In these initial stages, the level of relaxation that is promoted helps patients to sleep through the night. Each night, the patient should relax supine on the pillow for 15 minutes before turning to the side for sleep. This procedure will help regain cervical alignment and induce muscular relaxation.

Cryotherapy
Frequent and regular cooling of the inflamed tissues not only helps to control the extent of inflammation and swelling, but also provides pain relief. A cold pack should be placed over the injured tissues every hour for ten to fifteen minutes. This can also be continued beyond the initial acute phase to provide localized cooling after each exercise session.

Active Rehabilitation
There is no doubt now that strengthening can help return injured necks to full function. Numerous studies using various exercise approaches have described the benefits of the active approach.[61,62] Dynamic exercising, using progressive resistance to stimulate the muscles and the nerves is the most useful form of active exercise.[63] Standard stretching exercises, whether at home or in the clinic, demonstrate little or questionable therapeutic value.[64] A rational approach that has withstood the test of time is to give consideration to the following[65]:
- Range of active motion of the injured spinal regions
- Strength of the related musculature
- Postural control and balance of opposing soft tissues
- General muscular power (for daily activities)
- General aerobic fitness and endurance

Loss of Support Strength
When injured, the soft tissues of the neck no longer provide adequate support for the movements and weight of the head (12 to 15 pounds). Isotonic exercise is the most efficient method to progressively stimulate these important muscles to strengthen and return to full function. During isotonic exercising, the joints move (stimulating the

mechanoreceptors) and the opposing muscles relax through reciprocal inhibition. Isotonic resistance exercise has the distinct advantage of developing neurological coordination through neuromuscular adaptation. When the cervical region is exercised in its position of function (upright), the strength and skills that are developed will transfer easily to normal daily activities. In the early phase of treatment, the amount of movement during each exercise should be limited to avoid further pain and discomfort. Persistent efforts to increase both range and strength often require verbal encouragement.

Posture and Movement Abnormalities

Many whiplash patients demonstrate an obvious anterior translation postural imbalance (forward head) (Figure 20-16). This posture is secondary to the damaging "S-curve" motion that injured the lower and upper spinal regions in very different vectors. Once in the forward head posture, a constant strain develops in the muscles of the neck and into the upper back because of the leverage of the heavy head. Without correction, this posture will develop into a chronic myofasciitis in the muscles of the upper back and shoulder girdles. This abnormal posture is also a major contributing factor to neck stiffness, since movement suffers in this position. A study of the measured difference in rotation found that in all age groups, the forward head position resulted in significant decreases in the ability to turn the head.[66] If left untreated, the patient is likely to develop a permanent limitation that affects many activities of daily living. An effective exercise to correct this postural imbalance is the posterior translation (head retraction) exercise performed against isotonic resistance in the upright weight bearing position (Figure 20-17).

Studies that have investigated the differences in movement patterns between controls and patients with neck trauma found (as expected) that individuals with a history of injury had multiple, significant limitations in their ranges of cervical motion.[67,68] In addition to sagittal plane (flexion/extension) limitations, rotation is almost always restricted and is directly associated with neck pain and headache symptoms.[69] Therefore cervical

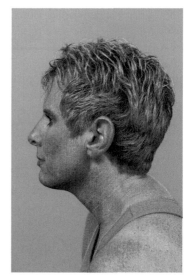

Figure 20-16   Forward head posture.

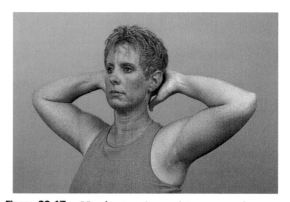

Figure 20-17   Head retraction resistance exercise.

rotation exercises against progressively increasing resistance are also frequently necessary in order to regain full, pain-free function (Figure 20-18). Whenever the head is turned during exercise, the eyes should look in the direction of rotation, leading the movement. This will help to reestablish the neurologic coupling between neck muscle activity and the ocular reflexes (the eye-head-neck interaction).[70]

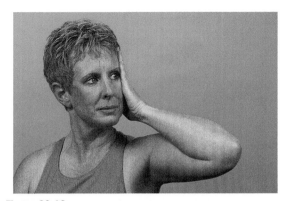

Figure 20-18   Cervical rotation against resistance.

Conclusion

Spinal adjustments for identified cervical subluxations are a necessary component of treatment after a whiplash injury. An appropriate and progressive rehabilitation program should be started early in the treatment of patients with whiplash injuries. Dynamic rehabilitation techniques for the cervical region are available that do not require expensive equipment or great time commitments. A closely monitored home exercise program allows the doctor of chiropractic to provide cost-efficient yet very effective rehabilitation care. The goals for each patient with a whiplash injury are to regain normal spinal function first and then return to full participation in daily activities. Thereafter, the doctor and patient must work together to prevent future disability and persisting symptoms.

References

1. Kapandji IA. The physiology of the joints. Vol. 3. The trunk and the vertebral column. Edinburgh: Churchill Livingstone; 1974.
2. Hall MC. Luschka's joints. Springfield, IL: Charles C Thomas; 1965.
3. Warwick W. Gray's anatomy. 35th ed. Philadelphia: WB Saunders; 1973. p. 234-236.
4. Jackson R. The cervical syndrome. 4th ed. Springfield, IL: Charles C Thomas; 1977.
5. Adams MA. Biomechanics of the cervical spine. In: Gunzburg R, Szpalski M. Whiplash injuries: current concepts in prevention, diagnosis, and treatment of the cervical whiplash syndrome. Philadelphia: Lippincott Williams & Wilkins; 1998. p. 13-20.
6. Hohl M. Soft tissue neck injuries. In: Bailey RW et al. The cervical spine. The Cervical Spine Research Society. Philadelphia: JB Lippincott; 1983.
7. Brault JR, Gunter PS, Wheeler JB. Cervical muscle response during whiplash: evidence of a lengthening muscle contraction. Clin Biomech 2000;15;426-35.
8. Foreman SM, Croft AC. Whiplash injuries: the cervical acceleration/deceleration syndrome. 3rd ed. Baltimore: Lippincott Williams & Wilkins; 2002.
9. Penning L. Backward hypertranslation of the head: participation in the whiplash injury mechanism of the cervical spine? Orthopade 1994;23:268-74.
10. Grauer JN, Panjabi MM, Cholewicki J, Nibu K, Dvorak J. Whiplash produces an S-shaped curvature of the neck with hyperextension at the lower levels. Spine 1997;22: 2489-94.
11. Kaneoka K, Ono K, Inami S, Hayashi K. Motion analysis of cervical vertebrae during whiplash loading. Spine 1999;24:763-9.
12. Panjabi MM, Cholewicki J, Nibu K, Grauer JN, Babat LB, Dvorak J. Mechanism of whiplash injury. Clin Biomech 1998;13:29-49.
13. Yang KH, King AI. Neck kinematics in rear-end impacts. Pain Res Manag 2003;8:9-85.
14. Gatterman MI, Panzer DM. Disorders of the cervical spine. In: Gatterman MI. Chiropractic management of spine-related disorders. 2nd ed. Baltimore: Lippincott Williams & Wilkins; 2003. p. 229-81.
15. Jaeger B. Cervicogenic headache: a relationship to cervical spine dysfunction and myofascial trigger points. Cephalalgia 1987;Suppl 7:398.
16. Grice AS. Pathomechanics of the upper cervical spine. In: Vernon H. Upper cervical syndromes. Baltimore: Williams & Wilkins; 1988. p. 103-12.
17. Grieve G. Common vertebral joint problems. New York: Churchill Livingstone; 1981.
18. White AA, Panjabi MM. Clinical biomechanics of the spine. Philadelphia: JB Lippincott; 1978.
19. Cailliet R. Neck and arm pain. Philadelphia: FA Davis; 1964.
20. Teasell RW, Shapiro AP. Whiplash injuries. In: Giles LGF, Singer KP, editors. Clinical management of cervical spine pain. Vol 3. Oxford: Butterworth Heinemann; 1998. p. 71-86.
21. MacNab I. Acceleration injuries of the cervical spine. J Bone Joint Surg 1964;46A:1797-9.
22. MacNab I, McCulloch J. Neck and shoulder pain. Baltimore: Williams & Wilkins; 1994.
23. Provinciali L, Baroni M, Illuminati L, Ceravolo MG. Multimodal treatment to prevent the late whiplash syndrome. Scand J Rehab Med 1996;28:105-11.
24. Travell JG, Simons DA. Myofascial pain and dysfunction: the trigger point manual. Baltimore: Williams & Wilkins; 1983.
25. Jull G. Manual diagnosis of C2-3 headache. Cephalalgia 1985;5 Suppl 5:308-9.

26. Jull GA. Headaches associated with the cervical spine: a clinical review. In: Grieve GP, editor. Modern manual therapy of the vertebral column. New York: Churchill Livingstone; 1986.

27. Jull G, Bogduk N, Marsland A. The accuracy of manual diagnosis for cervical zygapophyseal joint pain syndromes. Med J Aust 1988;148:233-6.

28. Jull G, Zito G, Trott P, Potter H, Shirley D. Interexaminer reliability to detect painful upper cervical zygapophyseal joint dysfunction. Aust J Physiother 1997;43:125-9.

29. Trelevan J, Jull G, Atkinson L. Cervical musculoskeletal dysfunction in post-concussion headache. Cephalalgia 1994;14:273.

30. Jensen OK, Nielsen FF, Vosmer L. An open study comparing manual therapy with the use of cold packs in the treatment of post-traumatic headache. Cephalalgia 1990;10:241.

31. Scaringe JG, Faye LJ. Palpation: the art of manual assessment. In: Redwood D, Cleveland C, editors. Fundamentals of chiropractic. St. Louis: Mosby; 2003. p. 211-37.

32. Jaeger B. Cervicogenic headache: a relationship to cervical spine dysfunction and myofascial trigger points. Cephalalgia 1987;Suppl 7:398-9.

33. Yochum TR, Rowe LJ. Essentials of skeletal radiology. 2nd ed. Baltimore: Williams & Wilkins; 1996. p. 692.

34. Peterson CK, Kirk RJ, Isdahl M, Humphrey BK. Prevalence of hyperplastic articular pillars in the cervical spine and relationship with cervical lordosis. J Manipulative Physiol Ther 2000;23:366-7.

35. Gore DR, Sepic SB, Gardner GM. Roentgenographic findings of the cervical spine in asymptomatic people. Spine 1986;11:521-4.

36. Green JD, Harle TS, Harris JH. Anterior subluxation of the cervical spine: hyperflexion sprain. AJNR 1981; 2:243-5.

37. Mootz RD, Hoffman LE, Hansen DT. Optimizing clinical use of radiography and minimizing radiation exposure in chiropractic practice. Top Clin Chiro 1997;4:34-44.

38. Hviid H. Functional radiography of the cervical spine. Ann Swiss Chiro Assoc 1963;3:37-65.

39. Grice AS. Preliminary evaluation of 50 sagittal cervical motion radiographic examinations. J Can Chiro Assoc 1977;21:33-4.

40. Dvorak J, Panjabi MM, Grob D, Novotny JE, Antinnes JA. Clinical validation of functional flexion/extension radiographs of the cervical spine. Spine 1993;18:120-7.

41. Wang JC, Hatch JD, Sandhu HS, Delamarter RB. Cervical flexion and extension radiographs in acutely injured patients. Clin Orthop Rel Res 1999;364:111-6.

42. Penning L. Normal movements of the cervical spine. Am J Roentgenol 1978;130:317-26.

43. Henderson DJ, Dorman TM. Functional roentgenometric evaluation of the cervical spine in the sagittal plane. J Manipulative Physiol Ther 1985;8:219-27.

44. Hildingsson C, Hietala SO, Toolanen G. Scintigraphic findings in acute whiplash injury of the cervical spine. Injury 1989;20:265-6.

45. Vendrig AA, van Akkerveeken PF, McWhorter KR. Results of a multimodal treatment program for patients with chronic symptoms after a whiplash injury of the neck. Spine 2000;25:238-44.

46. Gargan MF, Bannister GC. The rate of recovery following whiplash injury. Eur Spine J 1994;3:162-5.

47. Berglund A, Alfredsson L, Jensen I, Cassidy JD, Nygren A. The association between exposure to rear-end collision and future health complaints. J Clin Epidem 2001;54: 851-6.

48. Spitzer WO, Skovron ML, Salmi LR, Cassidy JD, Duranceau J, Suissa S et al. Scientific monograph of the Quebec task force on whiplash-associated disorders: redefining whiplash and its management. Spine 1995;20 (8 Suppl):1S-73S.

49. Woodward MN, Cook JCH, Gargan MF, Bannister GC. Chiropractic treatment of chronic whiplash injuries. Injury 1996;27:643-5.

50. Keidel M, Rieschke P, Stude P, Eisentraut R, van Schayck R, Diener H. Antinociceptive reflex alteration in acute posttraumatic headache following whiplash injury. Pain 2001;92:319-26.

51. Ide M, Ide J, Yamaga M, Takagi K. Symptoms and signs of irritation of the brachial plexus in whiplash injuries. J Bone Joint Surg [Br] 2001;83B:226-9.

52. Davis CG. Rear-end impacts: vehicle and occupant response. J Manipulative Physiol Ther 1998;21:629-39.

53. Koelbaek-Johansen M, Graven-Nielsen T, Olesen AS, Arendt-Nielsen L. Generalized muscular hyperalgesia in chronic whiplash syndrome. Pain 1999;83:229-34.

54. Hagstrom Y, Carlsson J. Prolonged functional impairments after whiplash injury. Scand J Rehab Med 1996;28: 139-46.

55. Sterling M, Treleaven J, Edwards S et al. Pressure-pain thresholds in chronic whiplash associated disorder: further evidence of altered central pain processing. J Musculoskeletal Pain 2002;10:69-81.

56. Sterling M, Jull G, Vicenzino B, Kenardy J. Characterization of acute whiplash-associated disorders. Spine 2004;29: 182-8.

57. Borchgrevink GE, Kaasa A, McDonagh D, Stiles TC, Haraldseth O, Lereim I. Acute treatment of whiplash neck sprain injuries. A randomized trial of treatment during the first 14 days after a car accident. Spine 1998;23:25-31.

58. Dolinis J. Risk factors for 'whiplash' in drivers: a cohort study of rear-end traffic crashes. Injury 1997;28:173-9.

59. Khan S, Bannister G, Gargan M, Asopa V, Edwards A. Prognosis following a second whiplash injury. Injury 2000;31:249-51.

60. Richter M, Otte D, Pohlemann T, Krettek C, Blauth M. Whiplash-type neck distortion in restrained car drivers: frequency, causes, and long-term results. Eur Spine J 2000;9:109-17.

61. Jordan A, Ostergaard K. Rehabilitation of neck/shoulder patients in primary health care clinics. J Manipulative Physiol Ther 1996;19:32-5.

62. Rosenfeld M, Seferiadis A, Carlsson J, Gunnarsson R. Active intervention in patients with whiplash-associated disorders improves long-term prognosis. Spine 2003;28: 2491-8.

63. Berg HE, Berggren G, Tesch PA. Dynamic neck strength training effect on pain and function. Arch Phys Med Rehabil 1994;75:661-5.

64. Wilkinson A. Stretching the truth: a review of the literature on muscle stretching. Aust J Physiother 1992;38: 283-91.

65. Ameis A. Cervical whiplash: considerations in the rehabilitation of cervical myofascial injury. Can Fam Phys 1986; 32:1871-7.

66. Walmsley RP, Kimber P, Culham E. The effect of initial head position on active cervical axial rotation range of motion in two age populations. Spine 1996;21:2435-42.

67. Osterbauer PJ, Long K, Ribaudo TA, Petermann EA, Fuhr AW, Bigos SJ et al. Three-dimensional head kinematics and cervical range of motion in the diagnosis of patients with neck trauma. J Manip Physiol Ther 1996;19:231-7.

68. Dall'Alba PT, Sterling MM, Treleaven JM, Edwards SL, Jull GA. Cervical range of motion discriminates between asymptomatic persons and those with whiplash. Spine 2001;26:2090-4.

69. Kasch H, Stengaard-Pedersen K, Arendt-Nielsen L, Jensen TS. Headache, neck pain, and neck mobility after acute whiplash injury. Spine 2001;26:1246-51.

70. Fitz-Ritson D. Phasic exercises for cervical rehabilitation after whiplash trauma. J Manip Physiol Ther 1995; 18:21-4.

21

Cervicogenic Dorsalgia

Glenn R. Engel and
Meridel I. Gatterman

Key Words   Cervicogenic dorsalgia, herpes zoster, anterior cervical doorbell sign

After reading this chapter you should be able to answer the following questions:

Question 1   What are the two cervical spine structures most commonly linked to production of cervicogenic dorsalgia?

Question 2   What neurologic mechanism has been proposed to account for cervicogenic dorsalgia?

Question 3   What two disorders are most often mistaken for cervicogenic dorsalgia by chiropractors?

Cervicogenic dorsalgia is pain expressed in the dorsal region and having its genesis in a disordered cervical spine. Although this descriptive phrase locates the anatomic region from which the patient's symptoms originate, the term *cervicogenic dorsalgia* is seldom an adequate diagnosis for the doctor of chiropractic. The diagnosis of cervicogenic dorsalgia serves as a rough anatomic locator and it is best accompanied by an indicator of the level of focal segmental dysfunction. If possible, the suggested pathologic nature of the lesion that gives rise to the dorsalgia, for example, subluxation of the C5-6 right posterior facet joint with right cervicogenic dorsalgia, should also be determined. An all-encompassing diagnosis such as this conjures up necessary treatment interventions instantly in the mind of the practicing clinician.

Dorsal pain of cervical origin is frequently observed in clinical practice.[1-3] The cervical spine is a freely movable and rather delicate structure sacrificing much in terms of stability for the considerable mobility it enjoys. When one compares the cervical spine possessed of its great mobility with the dorsal spine and its relatively fixed nature, it is easy to comprehend the focal action of static and dynamic stressors on such freely movable segmental structures.

One must recognize the frequency of cervical dorsalgia before embarking on an examination for dorsal (thoracic) pain of structural origin, because chronic and low-grade cases of cervicogenic dorsalgia may prove extremely difficult to elicit. It is not unusual to encounter dorsal pain of cervical origin with the patient steadfastly denying any neck pain. These cases are rarely overtly traumatic and are more commonly caused by residual static effort and postural stresses imparted to the mid to lower cervical spinal joints and their supportive soft tissue structures. The clinician must function as the ever-determined and doggedly persistent sleuth in cases of dorsalgia, gathering all essential evidence and clues both large and small to determine the condition involved and take appropriate action.

History and Examination

As in any disorder, the consulting chiropractic practitioner must explore a thorough history when investigating thoracic pain. One should diligently question the patient about viscerogenesis, being mindful of systemic signs of disease and visceral referral patterns in somatic pain syndromes. The clinician must be ever alert to the possibility of cardiac or lung pathology that gives rise to symptoms of a suspected cervicogenic dorsalgia, especially when results of testing of the relevant musculoskeletal structures are normal. Lack of reproducible symptoms on stress testing all relevant musculoskeletal structures is a definite worry to an astute clinician as is any diagnosis that relies solely on the palpation of a tender point in a soft tissue structure.

Beware the empty orthopedic examination. Radiographs of the cervicodorsal region showing degenerative change and or structural malpositions may prove misleading, especially when stress tests of the relevant structures prove negative. It has been observed that a lesioned gut, for example, a duodenal ulcer, is one of the most frequent progenitors of viscerogenic thoracic pain, with cholecystic disease a more distant second. Clinically, herpes zoster has often arisen as a nonmusculoskeletal cause of dorsalgia. Grouped vesicular lesions or a nest of small ruptured vesicles often bears witness to the herpetic origin of the dorsal pain. The greatest diagnostic difficulty arises when there is no apparent development of a herpetic dermatologic lesion or the lesions rise and pass undetected by the patient or his or her doctor. Occasionally in herpes zoster, pain precedes the vesicular eruption by a number of months even in the relatively young adult. The vesicular lesion when it does arise may be so insignificant as to be dismissed as nothing more than a small pimple.

From a historical perspective there is occasionally an obvious clue as to the cervical origin of the patient's dorsal complaint: "Doctor, when I turn my head to the left I get a stabbing pain in my left shoulder blade." or "Doctor, I have a heavy pain in my mid back and my neck is stiff and hurts to move in all directions." This type of historical comment is most often encountered when dorsal pain is of recent origin.

Much less obvious is the chronic cervicogenic dorsalgia of four to five years or more duration or the low-grade subacute case of several months duration wherein neck symptoms are entirely denied or passed off as insignificant. A methodical search of the patient's history for incidents of neck trauma, such as motor vehicle accidents, sports injuries, or ancillary symptoms such as recurrent headaches, upper extremity pain, paresthesia, or chest pain of unknown origin, may often prove rewarding! If no overt trauma is encountered in the history, often a clue may be obtained by exploring the nature of the patient's employment. In the chronic cases of cervicogenic dorsalgia, the patient is often engaged in a desk-computer type occupation or some other vocation of static effort, with the cervical spine flexed, shoulders sloped, elbows unsupported, and the suspensory apparatus of the neck and upper back unduly taxed. Often, the patient seeks relief of the painful dorsalgia by abandoning the irritating posture in favor of walking about or lying down. Most cervicogenic dorsalgia is eased by rest, although the occasional case is exacerbated by eccentric postures of the neck while sleeping.

Etiological Mechanism

Each cervical nerve innervates structures derived from the same somite (embryological origin), i.e., dermatomal (skin), myotomal (muscle), and sclerotomal (bone). The final locations of the dermatome, myotome, and sclerotome may be remote from each other. Referred pain due to cervical spine dysfunction may be perceived in any or all of the various somatic components of a nerve root.

The widespread distribution of signs and symptoms resulting from spinal muscle and joint dysfunction, including subluxation syndromes, may be explained by this mechanism. For example, pain or paresthesia perceived in the anterior or posterior chest, the shoulder, and/or down the arm may be due to irritation of the C7 zygapophyseal joint. Terrettt[3] notes that "the posterior thorax is interesting in that interposed between the thoracic

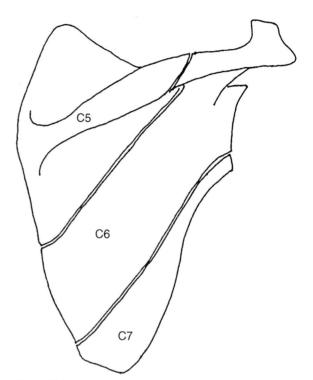

Figure 21-1   C5, C6, C7 sclerotomes of the scapula. *(From Terrett AGJ, Terrett RG. Chiro J Aust 2002;32:42-51.)*

dermatome (the skin) and the thoracic sclerotome and myotome (the ribs and intercostal muscles) lies part of the C5-C7 sclerotome (Figure 21-1) and C3-C6 myotome (Figure 21-2)."

Pain Referral Patterns

Pain referral patterns have been mapped in studies involving irritation of posterior rami innervated tissues at the C4-5, C5-6, and C6-7 levels. Figures 21-3, 21-4, and 21-5 illustrate these referral patterns. On the left of each diagram are the referral pain patterns from irritation of paravertebral muscles,[4,5] and on the right side are the referral pain patterns from irritation of the zygapophyseal joints.[6-8]

Causative mechanisms of cervicogenic dorsalgia involve a look at the most commonly involved structures seen to underlie most cervical pain syndromes, both local and referred. One causative

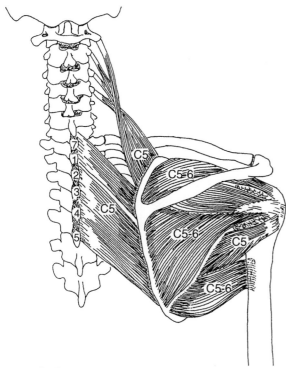

Figure 21-2   C3, C4, C5, C6 myotomes of the posterior thorax. *(From Terrett AGJ, Terrett RG. Chiro J Aust 2002;32:42-51.)*

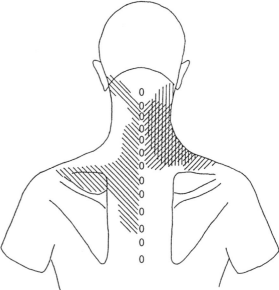

Figure 21-3   Left side: Referred pain pattern from irritation of paraspinal tissues between C4 and C5.[4,5] Right side: Referred pain pattern from irritation of zygapophyseal joints between C4 and C5 levels.[7,8] *(From Terrett AGJ, Terrett RG. Chiro J Aust 2002;32:42-51.)*

mechanism of cervicogenic dorsalgia that must be ruled out is cervical disc involvement. Discogenic nonneurogenic pain, dorsal pain emanating from disc disruption without actual nerve root compression or irritation, is often encountered clinically and frequently not recognized.

Cailliet[2] reports that in the performance of cervical discography, merely touching the anterior surface of the cervical disc with the needle caused pain in the "shoulder blade" or "interscapular region." This dorsal pain could be abolished by the injection of a small amount of local anesthetic agent through the discogram needle. Cloward[9] reported that irritation of superficial anterolateral fibers of the cervical discs produced acute pain in the ipsilateral scapular region. Irritation of the C4-5 disc produced pain at the superior-medial angle of the scapula; irritation of the C5-6 disc produced interscapular pain at the mid-scapular level; and irritation of the C6-7 level produced interscapular pain

at the inferior scapular level. The logical conclusion is that pain referred from the cervical disc caused by herniation within the disc or internal disc disruption is located in the interscapular-scapular area of referral. It has vague localization in that the superior discs refer to a superior dorsal level and lower discs refer more caudally. Dorsal pain thus expressed is often of a more diffuse nature and less spot specific.

Scapular pain on irritation of the ventral (motor) nerve roots has been noted by both Cloward[9] and Frykholm.[10] Dorsal pain of cervical origin was also recognized by Cyriax,[11] whose description of this cervicogenic dorsal pain phenomenon is one of discal-dural irritation. He perceived that when pressure is exerted on the dura mater, usually by a small displaced fragment of disc bulging out the posterior longitudinal ligament, a localized tender spot forms within the dorsal region. Cyriax notes that this lesion is very much a secondary phenomenon attributable to cervical dural irritation, although it is often mistakenly considered a

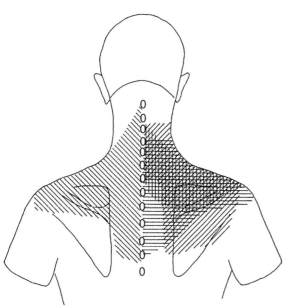

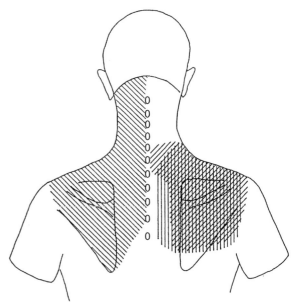

Figure 21-4   Left side: Referred pain pattern from irritation of paraspinal tissues between C5 and C6.[4,5] Right side: Referred pain pattern from irritation of zygapophyseal joints between C5 and C6 levels.[6-8] *(From Terrett AGJ, Terrett RG. Chiro J Aust 2002;32:42-51.)*

Figure 21-5   Left side: Referred pain pattern from irritation of paraspinal tissues between C6 and C7 levels.[4,5] Right side: Referred pain pattern from irritation of zygapophyseal joints between C6 and C7 levels.[7,8] *(From Terrett AGJ, Terrett RG. Chiro J Aust 2002;32:42-51.)*

primary lesion of "dorsal fibrositis," "trigger point," or "myalgic spot."

Cyriax stated that usually when a full and painless range of movement has been restored to the offending cervical segments, the dorsal pain and tenderness also eased. He also noted the amount of misdirected massage, injection, and manipulation aimed locally at this painful expression of cervical segmental pain referral.[11]

In the chiropractic profession, cervicogenic dorsalgia is most commonly misdiagnosed as a "subluxated rib" or a "trigger point" in local musculature. If a trigger point were truly to exist in local dorsal musculature, it is likely also true that this myoneural trigger point usually would lie on the course of an irritated sensory nerve from a lesioned spinal segment. "Trigger areas," according to Golding,[12] are tender spots usually on the course of a sensory nerve root from the involved spinal segment.

Subluxation of the cervical posterior facet joints is an important causative agent in the production of dorsal pain. It is also possible to have

dorsal pain emanating from both a discal source and posterior cervical facet subluxation in the same patient from interaction within the three joint complex. Lower cervical subluxation may lead to irritation of the medial branches of the dorsal primary ramus (sensory facets) or the recurrent meningeal nerve (the disc). Maigne[1] describes anastomoses between posterior branches of the lower cervical and upper dorsal nerves, especially T2. The T2 dermatome is quite extensive in the mid-dorsal region. The T2 nerve runs paravertebrally in a groove exiting close to the surface at T5 level, then laterally toward the scapula. This is thought to be the origin of the painful dorsal spot.

Thoracic pain of cervical origin may be quite simple to evoke on examination of the cervical spine, especially in the acute phase. Such is certainly not always the case for the subacute or chronic pain syndrome. Diagnosis may be as simple as having the patient actively rotate his or her head toward the acute restriction, with subjective pain noted in the dorsal region.

In the case of acute cervical disc herniation, especially when overt trauma is involved, a deep constant dorsal ache is often encountered with cervical spine ranges acutely limited in a global fashion. Radiation to one or both arms or paresthesias of the fingers of one or both hands should certainly create suspicion and concern in the mind of the clinician. Along with routine sensorimotor testing, a search for pathologic reflexes indicating upper motor neuron involvement should also be done. Many times the latter is entered into when the deep tendon reflexes (DTRs) are pathologically hyperactive. A cautiously performed Valsalva maneuver, either reinforced by having the patient's neck in the position of greatest aggravation of symptoms or maintained in neutral, may evoke dorsal pain and force consideration of a space-occupying lesion in the cervical spine such as disc prolapse or herniation. Painfully restricted forward flexion in the cervical spine, especially when other movements are largely pain free, is certainly indicative of disc involvement but is by no means exclusive. Adding bilateral nerve stretch testing while maintaining bilateral simultaneous tension on the brachial plexus further restricts an already limited flexion by causing increased tension on the spinal dura, which is already compressed by posterior migration of discal elements.

As related earlier, the subacute or chronic dorsalgia (in some cases many years) may be harder to track from the cervical spine and hence requires some diligent searching on the part of the examiner. In addition to careful motion palpation of cervical spine segments, all passive ranges must be examined with gentle overforcing in all directions to look for dorsal referral and slight limitations of end range movement. In addition to forced flexion, slight extension at the extreme of rotation may also reproduce or increase the dorsal pain.[3]

With the head supported in slight flexion the supraspinous ligament can be rubbed vigorously with the index finger of the palpating hand so that the ligament is frictioned as it courses between the spinous processes of the cervical vertebrae. Occasionally, painful radiations or paresthesia to the dorsal region or upper extremity is reported, not to mention focal selective tenderness. Symptoms thus expressed are thought to arise from irritation created by hypermobility/instability or a segmental reflex mechanism.

Posteroanterior thumb pressure can also be directed over the cervical spinous processes and should be quite forceful. The patient should be instructed to relax the neck while the forehead is supported by one of the examiner's hands in a slight attitude of flexion, allowing the posterior supportive tissues to remain slack. The patient should be assured that the procedure is necessary and painful but not in any way dangerous. An attempt can thus be made to literally "rock the vertebral segment," looking for dorsal or upper extremity radiations from facilitated joint structures. Selective deep rubbing of the facet joints with a palpating finger also may occasion the production of sought-after radiating symptoms. If necessary, forcefully deviating the spinous processes with the thumb toward and then away from the involved side also might provoke an increase in symptoms.

The "anterior cervical doorbell sign" is seen approximately 60% of the time in cervicogenic dorsalgia.[1] Moderate pressure with the index finger directed horizontally over the anterolateral portion of the lower cervical spine (the ventral emergence of the nerve root) and held for a few seconds, exploring segmental level after segmental level, may trigger the patient's dorsal pain (Figure 21-6, A and B). This phenomenon has often been dismissed as emanating from "scalene trigger points," when in fact radicular irritation is often paramount.

Skin roll is a useful procedure in which the skin and subcutaneous tissue of the dorsal region and posterior cervical spine is "pinch rolled" approximately one and one-half finger's breadth from the spine. Hyperalgesia is often seen focally in the region of T5-6 and T2, as well as C5-6 and C6-7, and corresponds to the irritated cervical segment and the entrance and emergence of the second dorsal nerve. It should be noted that this maneuver serves as a useful test in cases of fibromyalgia where the patient exhibits hypersensitivity to this procedure in addition to that experienced on palpation of the consistent pattern of tender points. If test results are equivocal for cervical dorsalgia, it

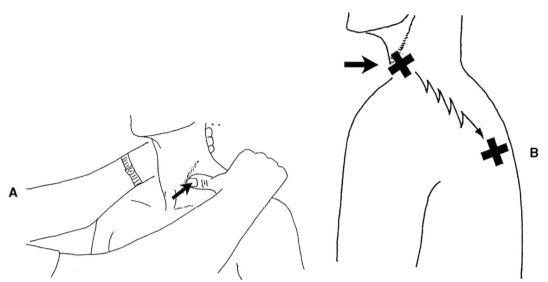

Figure 21-6   The anterior cervical doorbell sign. **A,** Pressure with the index finger is directed horizontally over the anterolateral portion of the cervical spine (the ventral emergence of the nerve root.) **B,** A positive sign is elicited when the patient's dorsal pain is reproduced. *(From Terrett AGJ, Terrett RG. Chiro J Aust 2002;32:42-51.)*

is useful to traction the brachial plexus in various positions. Tractioning the plexus through various maneuvers may serve to disclose the dorsal complaint when other more direct measures aimed at the cervical region have failed. Direct traction (stretching) of C5 and C6, C7 and C8, and T1 nerves are thus employed. It is also useful to add lateral cervical spine deviation away from the tractioned root to elicit dorsal or extremity symptoms. Occasionally, it is necessary to rotate the cervical spine globally while the roots are tractioned to produce a catch of dorsal pain. In the case of radiating upper extremity symptoms, it is frequently useful to maintain the involved arm in the position that most intensifies symptoms and then move the cervical spine through extreme ranges of motion to look for symptom escalation or amelioration.

Local palpation of the region of dorsal tenderness is necessary to assure the patient that you have found "the spot." Nowhere is the example of misleading tenderness clearer than in the case of cervicogenic dorsalgia with a clearly defined "dorsal spot." Frequently, dorsal segments in the region of the dorsal spot are "fixed" and tender to palpation. Local musculature is frequently hypertonic, evidenced by local taut and tender fibers.

The upper extremities should be examined neurologically for strength, deep tendon reflexes (DTRs), and sensory changes if present. Strength testing should be done in a repetitive challenge, comparing right with left. Triceps strength (C7) is often somewhat diminished on the side of dorsal pain even when no upper extremity symptoms are present and when DTRs are symmetric. Radiographic examination is required when the history unearths a traumatic origin to the dorsalgia, the possibility of metastatic disease, or the presence of a rheumatologic disorder such as seronegative spondyloarthropathy or rheumatoid arthritis. Such instances may require radiographic studies of both cervical and dorsal regions.

In less obvious or chronic cases, an inexperienced or hurried examiner may not exact a referral pattern from the cervical spine and may call for imaging of the dorsal region only. It is not uncommon for these dorsal radiographs to prove misleading, the cause of the patient's discomfort thought to be due to scoliosis, or dorsal degenerative changes. It is also not uncommon for radiographs of the patient's cervical spine to appear negative in a case of cervicogenic dorsalgia. This is especially true when dealing with the younger patient, frequently a young college student. Degenerative change, reversal of curve, or segmental levels of disturbed motion function may be present on the cervical radiographic study and may hint at the cervical origin of the patient's dorsal pain. It is absolutely imperative to remember that local radiographic evidence of degenerative change or structural change takes on its greatest importance only when it is consistent with the findings of a thorough examination. The obvious exception to this would be evidence of lytic disease, fracture, or rheumatic disorder of the more exotic variety. Once the diagnosis of cervicogenic dorsalgia has been established, it remains necessary to identify the pathomechanical mechanism as precisely as possible; it is on this precise diagnosis that treatment is based.

Treatment

The treatments of cervicogenic dorsalgia are varied and rely on the evocative mechanism and severity. For example, the patient with a history of going headlong into the boards during a hockey game who presents with neck stiffness, globally restricted cervical movements, an inescapable deep central dorsal ache, paresthetic hands, and equivocal long tract signs will be managed much differently than the patient with an acutely fixed neck that locked while taking a shower, who is experiencing only dorsal referred pain. In the first case, imaging with an eye to referral to a neurosurgeon would be urgently appropriate, whereas in the latter case, stabilization in a soft collar, ice therapy, soft tissue therapy, and, later, light intermittent traction therapy and specific spinal adjustment may be indicated. Fortunately, most cases encountered present with acute, subacute, or chronic unilateral subluxation with periscapular pain encountered on the ipsilateral side of restricted cervical motion.

Manipulation of the painfully restricted cervical segment in the direction of free movement often is met with a reduction in dorsal pain and a free range of cervical movement. Intermittent traction often can be successfully employed. In the chronic or subacute case of cervicogenic dorsalgia, it is often necessary to influence the zone of referred pain to bring about a more immediate response to treatment. Manipulation of subluxated thoracic segments along with treatment directed to the painful focus in the surrounding soft tissues complements manipulation of the subluxated cervical segments. The clinician may elect to employ manual compression, ultrasound, transcutaneous electrical nerve stimulation (TENS), or needle or electrical acupuncture in the treatment of painful thoracic and cervical foci.

It is often necessary to alter habitual work postures with ergometric training to reduce the stress of static postural effort on posterior cervical joints. Additional strengthening of cervical spine supportive tissues is often necessary, especially in cases of cervical discogenic segmental hypermobility. Rarely, a cervical support collar may be recommended for a period up to three weeks to abolish cervicogenic dorsalgia. This may be recommended on an intermittent basis and used when the patient must assume a habitually irritating posture. Although rarely necessary, if this method is chosen it should be combined with a program of nonirritating neck-strengthening exercises.

Conclusion

In most cases of cervicogenic dorsalgia, prolonged therapy to the area of pain produces little therapeutic benefit. Frequently, interscapular pain is not of thoracic origin, although local muscle and zygapophyseal, costovertebral, and costotransverse joint dysfunction must also be considered. Simple tests can diagnose the presence of cervicogenic dorsalgia. With treatment that includes manipulation directed to the cervical region, the thoracic pain can be relieved.

References

1. Maigne R. Orthopaedic medicine: a new approach to vertebral manipulations. Springfield, IL: Charles C Thomas; 1972. p. 261.
2. Cailliet ND. Neck and arm pain. 2nd ed. Philadelphia: F.A. Davis; 1984.

3. Terrett A, Terrett R. Referred posterior thoracic pain of cervical posterior rami origin: a cause of much misdirected treatment. Chiro J Aust 2002;32:42-51.
4. Feinstein B. Referred pain from paravertebral structures. In: Buerger AA, Tobias JS, editors. Approaches to the validation of manipulation therapy. Springfield, IL: Charles C Thomas; 1977. p. 139-74.
5. Feinstein B, Langton JNK, Jameson RM, Schiller F. Experiments on pain referral from deep somatic tissues. J Bone Joint Surg 1954;36A(5):981-7
6. Bogduk N, Marslen A. The cervical zygapophyseal joints as a source of neck pain. Spine 1988;13:610-7.
7. Dwyer A, Aprill C, Bogduk N. Cervical zygapophyseal joint pain patterns. 1. A study in normal volunteers. Spine 1990;15:453-7.
8. Fukui S, Ohseto K, Shiotani M, Ohno K, Karasawa H, Naganuma Y et al. Referred pain distribution of the cervical zygapophyseal joints and cervical dorsal rami. Pain 1996;68:79-83.
9. Cloward RB. Cervical discography. A contribution to the etiology and mechanism of neck shoulder and arm pain. Ann Surg 1959;150:1052-64.
10. Frykholm R. Deformities of dural pouches and structures of dural sheaths in cervical region producing nerve root compression: contribution to etiology and operative treatment of brachial neuralgia. J Neuro Surg 1947;4:403-13.
11. Cyriax J. Textbook of orthopaedic medicine. 8th ed, Vol. 1. Diagnosis of soft tissue lesions. London: Bailliere Tindall; 1982.
12. Golding DN. A synopsis of rheumatic diseases. 4th ed. London: Wright-PSG; 1982.

22

The Thoracic Outlet Syndrome: First Rib Subluxation Syndrome

Zoltan T. Szaraz

Key Words   Thoracic outlet syndrome, cervical ribs, interscalene triangle, trigger points, ischemic compression

After reading this chapter you should be able to answer the following questions:

Question 1   What are the anatomic boundaries of the thoracic outlet?

Question 2   What are the contents of the thoracic outlet?

Question 3   In which direction does the first rib commonly subluxate?

Question 4   Which muscle group is frequently implicated in thoracic outlet syndrome?

Significant confusion and controversy surround the thoracic outlet syndrome.[1] Historically, anatomists refer to the superior aperture of the thorax as the thoracic inlet and to the diaphragm-covered inferior aperture as the thoracic outlet.[2,3]

Sir Ashley Cooper in 1821 first described the symptom complex of the thoracic outlet syndrome.[4] Forty years later, Coote[5] excised a cervical rib with successful obliteration of symptoms. Other earlier authors considered anatomic abnormalities of the cervical spine to be the primary cause of the vascular compression and resulting neurologic symptoms as thoracic outlet syndrome (TOS).[6,7] By 1916 the presence of cervical ribs in 1% of the population had been established; however, only 10% of those were symptomatic.[8]

Further controversy and confusion stems from the fact that there are several subsets of syndromes. Adson and Coffey[9] described the scalenus anticus syndrome and their diagnostic maneuver (Adson's test) in 1927. Adson believed that intermittent vascular obstruction was pathognomonic of thoracic outlet syndrome.[10] He surmised that arterial compression meant that the brachial plexus was also irritated. However, pulse obliteration can be found in 1% to 94% of completely normal subjects.[11-13] The costoclavicular syndrome was described by Falconer and Weddell[14] in 1943. Two years later, Wright[13] identified the hyperabduction syndrome. It was Peet et al.[15] who coined the broader term *thoracic outlet compression syndromes* (TOCS). Recently, Lee et al.[16] and others[17] proposed that subluxation of the first rib may irritate neurovascular structures at the cervicothoracic area and cause radicular symptoms in the arm, hand, and neck, commonly described as thoracic outlet syndrome.

Anatomic Features

The "thoracic outlet" presents an opening bordered laterally by the first rib, medially by the vertebral column, and anteriorly by the claviculomanubrial complex. Contents of this thoracic outlet include the lower trunks of the brachial plexus and the subclavian artery (Figure 22-1). Anomalies in this region, including cervical ribs and fibrous bands, have been popularly linked to causation. The mere presence of an anatomic anomaly does not establish its causal relationship. Instead, the occurrence of neurovascular dysfunction at the thoracic outlet depends on the interplay of three conditions.[18]

The most basic factor is the anatomic fact that the neurovascular bundle comprising the subclavian artery and the lower trunk of the brachial plexus normally passes through several narrow spaces. Secondarily, a variety of physiologic and anthropomorphic factors could accentuate content-container incompatibility and lead to intermittent compression and repeated minor trauma to the bundle. Finally, space availability may be further compromised by osseous, fibromuscular, and vascular anomalies of this region that would be innocuous without the two preceding two conditions.

Narrow Passages Traversed by the Neurovascular Bundle

The subclavian vessels and brachial plexus traverse three narrow straits within the cervicoaxillary canal before reaching the arm.

Interscalene Triangle

The interscalene triangular space is bordered anteriorly by the scalene anticus muscle, posteriorly by the scalene medius muscle, and inferiorly by the medial border of the first rib. (See Figure 22-1, A.) This interscalene triangle transmits all trunks of the brachial plexus, but only the subclavian artery traverses this triangle, not the subclavian vein. The distance between the two scalenes at the base varies significantly.[19] There are therefore occasions when both the artery and the nerve trunk are clamped within this tight fibrofascial triangle.[20]

Another anatomic variation is the slope of the first rib. If the slope is unusually steep, the artery would be firmly wedged between the rib and the tendon. This obliquity seems to be more marked in women[21] and possibly in advancing age.

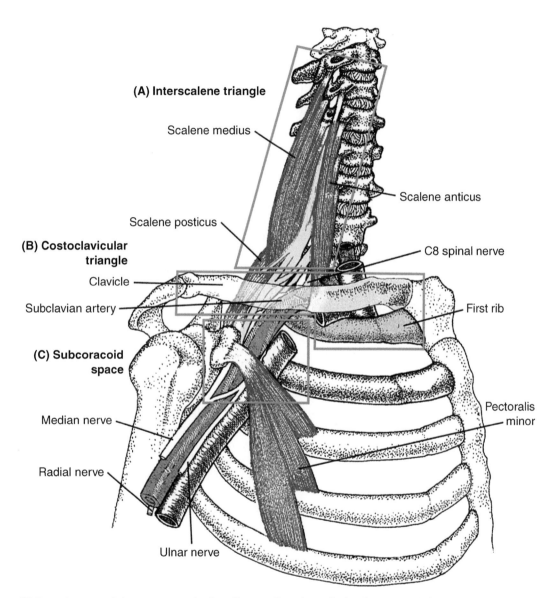

Figure 22-1   Diagram of the neurovascular bundle traveling through the three potential narrow passages. **A,** Interscalene triangle. **B,** Costoclavicular triangle. **C,** Subcoracoid space. Note that the lower branch of the brachial plexus is directly under the subclavian artery, resting on the first rib. *(Modified from Travell JG, Simons DG. Myofascial pain and dysfunction: the trigger point manual. 2nd ed. Baltimore: Lippincott Williams & Wilkins; 1999.)*

Costoclavicular Triangle

The neurovascular bundle immediately enters a second triangular space bounded anteriorly by the middle third of the clavicle, posteromedially by the anterior border of the first rib, and postero-laterally by the upper border of the scapula and the subscapularis muscle. (See Figure 22-1, B.) Both the upper and lower borders of this triangle are mobile; hence they are subject to physiologic narrowing, depending on the position of the arm and activities of the shoulder musculature.

Subcoracoid Space

The last narrow strait is provided by the insertion of the pectoralis minor tendon into the coracoid process. (See Figure 22-1, C.) During shoulder abduction, contraction of the pectoralis minor tendon may significantly narrow the subcoracoid space over the neurovascular structures.[22-24]

Physiologic Factors Compromising the Narrow Passages

Developmental Factors

In the upright position the space created between the clavicle and the first rib is chiefly determined by the inclination of the clavicle at the acromio-clavicular joint. Aging leads to progressive acromioclavicular descent, which is more marked in women.[20,24,25] This may explain the reason why women are four times more prone to develop TOS than are men.[22,23,26]

Anthropomorphic Factors

Acromioclavicular descent is also prominent in individuals with an asthenic physique, because the poorly developed shoulder muscles allow the scapula to rotate anteriorly and laterally. This is further aggravated by a long slender neck, wherein the cervical roots are even farther away from the costoclavicular passage, subjecting them to more exaggerated tension and angulation.[27-29]

Postural and Dynamic Factors

Certain body postures and arm positions may consistently produce symptoms. The most notable is hyperabduction and external rotation of the arm, such as sleeping with the arm behind the pillow. Occupations such as painting and automobile repair require the arm to be overhead for prolonged period. The anatomic mechanisms responsible for the symptoms in hyperabduction are costoclavicular compression and bowing of the axillary artery at the subcoracoid space.[13,30,31] Abduction of the arm beyond 90 degrees requires external rotation of the scapula, which brings the clavicle upward and backward at the sternoclavicular joint, closing the costoclavicular space.[13,23] Hyperabduction to 180 degrees is always accompanied by external rotation of the humerus, which tenses the costocoracoid ligament and the pectoralis minor, accentuating compression of the subclavian vein.[23,32]

Other symptom-producing factors may include wearing a heavy bag with a shoulder strap or carrying a heavy briefcase consistently with the same arm. In both situations the clavicle is brought directly or indirectly against the neurovascular bundle.[33] Water skiers, whose arms are strenuously pulled forward and downward with the body tilted backward, compress the costoclavicular space as the neurovascular bundle is dragged against the first rib and the scalene anticus tendon. Hikers carrying bulky backpacks with cross-shoulder belts suffer lower plexopathy (back palsy)[34] by the same mechanism, as do soldiers standing at attention for a prolonged period with shoulders drawn backward and chest thrust forward. These positions not only depress the clavicle but also elevate the first rib, thereby closing the costoclavicular passage.[23]

Another insidious compressive mechanism is deep inspiration, especially when forced or labored as in patients with emphysema. The first rib moves upward and forward during deep inspiration by as much as 34 mm and 22 mm, respectively, in men and by as much as 28 mm and 14 mm, respectively, in women.[35] More importantly, this is repeated approximately 33,000 times each day. In patients with emphysema, the increased functional residual lung capacity keeps the first rib in an elevated position. Added to this are the repeated strained cervical movements during forced breathing, mediated to the first rib by the scalenes. The scalenes therefore hypertrophy and can potentially narrow the interscalene passage. In emphysema patients the neurovascular bundle is repeatedly subjected to stretch, compression, and friction.[20,36]

Structural Anomalies Compromising the Narrow Passages Further

Anomalous Ribs

The association of cervical rib with TOS is well documented. Its incidence in routine nonsymptomatic patients is 0.002% to 0.5%.[9,37,38] Approximately 10% of those with cervical ribs experience symptoms. Familial occurrences with other congenital anomalies have been reported.[20,39] It is more common on the left side, although bilateral cervical ribs were found in 50% of surgical candidates.[24] It is believed that cervical ribs develop in intrauterine life more often with prefixed than with postfixed brachial plexus[20] because of the lesser resistance encountered by the small first thoracic nerve root in a prefixed plexus.[40] Rayan[41] reports numbness and tingling in the forearms of a 14-year-old girl and a 12-year-old boy brought on by athletic activities at school and caused by a cervical rib articulating with the first rib on the symptomatic side. He believes that a cervical rib more than 5.5-cm long tends to lift up and kink the subclavian artery and stretch the seventh cervical nerve root. However, it is generally considered that abnormal fibrous bands extending from the tip of an incomplete cervical rib to the first rib are the most common causes of true TOS.[1,11,20,22] Furthermore, these fibrous bands are clinically treacherous because they are invisible on x-ray films and may exist without concomitant rib anomalies.

Anomalous Muscle Insertions

Excessive and sustained scaleni muscle contraction has been thought to cause neurovascular symptoms,[11,42,43] presumably by strangling the subclavian artery and neurovascular bundle. It is now believed that such muscular actions alone are unable to produce the symptoms without some form of anomalous muscle insertions.[24,44] These anomalous muscle insertions may be a fused scalenus anticus and medius insertion that occupies an extended area over the middle third of the first rib,[24] a split tendinous insertion of the scalenus medius muscle,[33] or even a hypertrophied scalenus minimus muscle.[20]

Other Anomalies

A number of unusual causes have been reported in the literature as contributing to neurovascular compression in the costoclavicular compartment: fracture of the clavicle with subsequent pseudarthrosis,[45] malunion of a clavicular fracture,[46] unreduced dislocation of the clavicle,[47] and other rare causative factors such as osteochondroma of the clavicle and first rib.[26]

Biomechanical Considerations

Functional Cause

Because chiropractors are intimately interested in symptom-causing functional disturbances of various kinds rather than anatomic or pathologic causes, it is not unusual that we see and recognize patients with symptoms of neurovascular compression syndromes related to functional disturbances at the cervicothoracic junction. One of the major anatomic structures that may be involved in patients presenting with brachialgia, paresthesias, and pain along the ulnar nerve distribution is the first rib. Lindgren and Leino[48] reported on 22 cases of thoracic outlet syndrome-diagnosed patients who presented with a hypomobile first rib on the symptomatic side. They further reported on five additional TOS patients a year later[49] in whom the hypomobile or subluxated first rib was confirmed by cineradiographic study. These same authors also believe that normal mobility of the first rib is necessary for normal function at the cervicothoracic area and normal function at the thoracic outlet.[50]

Lewit[51] stated that there are different types of impingement syndromes. When the canal is

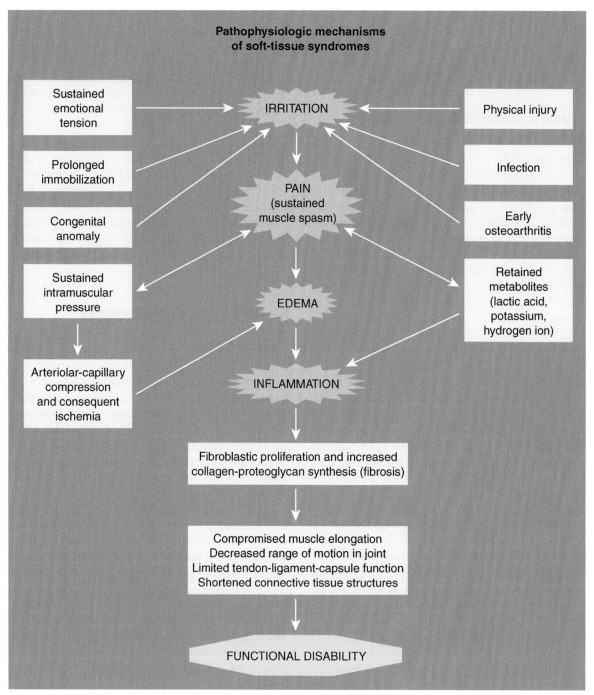

Figure 22-2 The pathophysiologic mechanism of functional disability. *(Modified from Bland JH. J Musculoskel Med 1986;3(11):23-41.)*

through a solid bone or a single groove covered by soft tissues, surgical decompression is often necessary. However, when a canal is formed by bones linked by joints capable of movement, for example, the thoracic outlet, impairment of joint mobility must be taken into consideration in pathogenesis of an entrapment syndrome. Under such conditions impaired function is the first change. If this functional loss lasts for a period, the increased strain on corresponding soft tissues, muscles, and ligaments may cause thickening of the ligament and in the end damage the nerve. This pathophysiologic mechanism is commonly shared in manual medicine (Figure 22-2).[52-56] If the offending structure is found to be a cause of functional disability as in joint dysfunction, treatment must be directed toward restoring that lost function. Lewit[51] calls this "dynamic nerve compression" or nerve compression due to impaired function. Successful treatment can be achieved by manipulation.

Impairment of function anywhere in the locomotor system involves associated structures, like a chain reaction. Patients who complain of neck, shoulder, arm, and hand pain, and who manifest poor postural habits often demonstrate lower cervical, upper thoracic, and upper rib dysfunctions. The typical restriction of movement involved with a first rib dysfunction is restriction of cervical rotation and lateral flexion.

Traumatic and Occupational Causes

Hargberg and Wegman[57] and others[58,59] evaluated the association and impact of occupational exposure and disorders of the shoulder and neck area. They found that certain tasks that are repetitive in nature or involve sustained handling of materials in primarily one direction such as is typical of assembly line workers (particularly sustained static contractions of the cervicothoracic muscles required to perform tasks at shoulder level) are clearly associated with shoulder-neck disorders.

Other commonly missed causative factors of TOS are adhesions and scarring associated with posttraumatic thoracic outlet syndrome. Dellon[60] and others[61] believe that rear end collisions cause a stretch type of injury to the brachial plexus with subsequent scarring that causes entrapment of the brachial plexus proximal to the first rib; hence such conditions are often missed in commonly used transaxillary first rib resections.

Clinical Features

From our discussion thus far, it is obvious that the clinical presentation is dependent on the underlying anatomic or functional disturbances with which patients present. In our experience, patients present with moderate symptoms with progressive deterioration, especially when symptoms are dominantly vascular. The opposite is true with neurologic dominance of symptoms. Presentations are commonly significant, especially to the patient, because they include numbness and weakness but improve gradually with conservative care (Box 22-1).

The literature appears to selectively differentiate symptoms into (1) primarily vascular causes and vascular symptoms such as swelling, cyanosis, pallor, coolness, and ischemia; and (2) primarily neurologic causes such as numbness, tingling, and paresthesia. This may have prompted a number of authors to give subclassifications to various causative factors involved. Each of these syndromes had obvious pathognomonic diagnostic tests. Adson's maneuver was specific for the scalenus anticus syndrome in which neurovascular compression occurred exclusively in the interscalene triangle. As a consequence, scalenectomy became the treatment of choice. Falconer and Weddell[14] coined the term *costoclavicular syndrome* for those patients with positive exaggerated military maneuver, which is thought to narrow the costoclavicular space. Later Wright advocated the diagnostic category of hyperabduction syndrome for patients who became symptomatic with hyperabduction of the symptomatic arm.

In practice it is more practical to associate patients with neurogenic or vascular symptoms depending on which are more dominant, as well as the degree of compression and, to a lesser extent, the lesion. This initial clinical impression often changes with treatment. Dynamic anthropomorphic factors may undergo change with lifestyle, general health, and aging.

BOX 22-1 ■ Symptoms of Thoracic Outlet Syndrome

Brachial plexus irritation

- Numbness
- Tingling (mostly ulnar side of hand, occasionally entire hand)
- Coldness
- Paresis (late manifestation)
  - Early fatigability
  - Progressive weakness
  - Dyscoordination

Venous symptoms

- Swelling
- Heaviness
- Fatigue
- Cyanosis
- Engorgement of superficial veins in supraclavicular area

Arterial symptoms

- Pallor
- Coolness
- Fatigue
- Muscle cramps from repetitive use
- Ischemic pain

Myofascial symptoms

- Catchy pain on movement of neck and shoulder(s)
- Fatigue on exertion
- Restricted and guarded cervical movements on rotation and lateral flexion
- Shoulder, arm, and hand deep, achy, constant pain

Modified from Liebenson CS. J Manipulative Physiol Ther 1988;11:493-99.

Sensory Signs and Symptoms

The most common presenting symptoms of TOS are numbness and tingling. Sanders and Pearce[62] found that 90% of TOS patients had paresthesia in the hand, 80% had arm pain, 86% had neck pain, and 69% had occipital headache. In their review of the TOS literature, Pang and Wessel[18] noted that neurologic disturbances are caused by involvement of the C8 and T1 fibers in the lower trunk of the brachial plexus and that sensory disturbances usually appear in advance of motor signs.

The pain is usually described as a dull, constant, heavy ache, and its distribution does not respect the C8-T1 dermatomal pattern. It is often diffuse in the supraclavicular and shoulder area and spreads down the arm. Paresthesia, however, is frequently segmental and mostly felt in the inner aspect of the arm and forearm, the ulnar half of the hand, and the fourth and fifth digits, including the hypothenar eminence. Constant numbness and tingling in the ulnar digits are almost pathognomonic and certainly disturbing to the patient, but occasionally a burning sensation and sharp localized pain may be experienced.[1] In some patients the pain is atypical, localized to the anterior chest wall, and may simulate angina pectoris (pseudoangina).[36]

Sensory symptoms are often precipitated by trauma to the shoulder girdle, a bout of heavy lifting or simply carrying heavy objects, or the habitual use of a heavy shoulder bag over the same shoulder. The pain is often aggravated by the use of the arm or arms because these symptoms are often bilateral.[63] Pain is worse by the end of the day, particularly in occupations involving the use of the arms overhead. Many patients are awakened during the night by arm pain and paresthesia, especially if the affected arm is raised above the pillow. Ribbe et al.[64] found that the most reliable symptoms were: (1) history of aggravation of symptoms with arm elevation, (2) history of C8-T1 paresthesia, (3) tenderness over the brachial plexus supraclavicularly, and (4) positive abduction and external rotation (AER) of the arm test. They found that three of these four tests were positive in 94% of thoracic outlet syndrome patients. This is considered the "TOS index."

Arm positions that remove traction on the brachial plexus bring relief of symptoms. Patients often find relief in sitting with elevation of the shoulder by resting the affected elbow on the arm of the chair or supporting the elbow with the opposite hand. This maneuver is effective for any brachial plexus compression syndrome, not only for TOS.

With time, objective signs of sensory denervation appear, including diminished sensation to pinprick and light touch sensation over the C8-T1 dermatome. Initially this hypesthesia is patchy over the ulnar digits, but with time it becomes evenly distributed over the entire ulnar side of the hand.[65] When this is correlated with digital tenderness over the scalene anticus and supraclavicular portion of the brachial plexus, three of the four items of the "TOS index" are satisfied and the diagnosis of TOS is certain.

Motor Signs and Symptoms

Subjective motor symptoms often accompany the onset of severe pain and paresthesia. The hands feel weak, and fine motor skills may be disturbed. Travell and Simons[66] discuss that the patient may report dropping things. Patients may complain of difficulty with buttoning their shirt or blouse in the morning. When this is accompanied by aching pain in the hand and forearm, especially in the morning, arthritic process is often suggested. Testing the individual muscles, however, shows weakness of flexors of the hand and digits, but the greatest weakness is invariably found in the intrinsic hand muscles.[20] In longstanding cases, the most characteristic pattern is severe thenar atrophy with preservation of the interossei and hypothenar muscles.[67] Within the thenar group, there is also a selective wasting of the abductor pollicis brevis and opponens pollicis with preservation of the flexor pollicis brevis, producing the characteristic guttering along the lateral aspect of the thenar pad.[18] This typical pattern of lateral thenar muscle wasting and ulnar sensory changes clinically distinguishes TOS from carpal tunnel syndrome, with its typical median nerve neuropathy.[18]

It is not unusual that carpal tunnel syndrome, especially when the patient presents with shoulder pain, is commonly confused with TOS. When a comparison of the symptom complex of the two conditions is made (Table 22-1), it is quite possible to confuse the two on symptom presentation alone. The simultaneous presentation of carpal tunnel

Table 22-1

Comparison of Positive Clinical Findings in Thoracic Outlet Syndrome (TOS) and Carpal Tunnel Syndrome (CTS)

	TOS	CTS
Symptoms		
Paresthesia	44%	79%
Pain	75%	52%
Hypesthesia	70%	0%
Weakness	41%	43%
Use numbness	0%	18%
Rest numbness	18%	18%
Shoulder-arm pain	8%	8%
Signs		
Hypertrophic scalene	3%	0%
Hypesthesia	33%	56%
Weakness	37%	20%
Atrophy	1%	42%
AER test positive	5%	0%
Pulse obliteration	37%	0%
Hyperabduction test	37%	0%
Tinel's sign	0%	63%
Phalen's sign	0%	42%
Weak pinch	1%	20%

Modified from Carroll RE, Hurst LC. Clin Orthop 1982; 164:149-53.

and thoracic outlet, however, is extremely rare.[68] Forced wrist flexion reproducing the paresthesia (Phalen's sign) and the less reliable Tinel's sign, tingling on percussion over the carpal tunnel, are good diagnostic tests.[69]

Vasomotor Disturbances and Trophic Changes

Vasomotor symptoms, blanching of the hand from exposure to cold, and purplish red discoloration of the hand and forearm when the arm is in a dependent position are usually preceded by sensory and motor complaint. These are most disturbing to the patient and, because they are often aggravated by emotional stress, usually result in diagnostic labels such as "neurotic." Unlike sensory symptoms, these vasomotor symptoms commonly occur at rest, independent of arm position, and can become very severe without concomitant pain. Sunderland[20] believes that these vasomotor disturbances always occur alongside sensory and motor changes because most of the sympathetic fibers to the upper limb course along the C8 and T1 nerve roots, converging on them as postganglionic fibers from the upper three sympathetic ganglia.[20] This may have prompted the recent advances for alternative surgical correction using dorsal sympathectomy instead of rib resection.[70]

Vascular Disturbances

Vascular symptoms are commonly divided into arterial and venous disturbances. According to Riddel and Smith,[71] venous symptoms are more common and are termed as *effort thrombosis*. Signs of venous congestion and distension are usually preceded by heavy ache in the pectoral and supraclavicular region during continual exertion of the arm. Lord and Rosati[23] believe that subclavian vein compression and subsequent thrombosis occur between the costocoracoid ligament and the first rib. Others[11,24] believe that the anterior scalene band may compress the subclavian vein against the clavicle during or after recurrent muscle contraction. In venous compression the discomfort gradually increases over several hours after exertion, and the entire arm may become swollen and cyanotic.

Arterial compression produces "ischemic-like" cramping in the hand or forearm that may lead to paresthesia during sustained exertion of the elevated arm. This is usually relieved by rest and elbow elevation (claudication). Such intermittent and position-dependent claudication may become worse in the winter months and improve in warm weather.[20] This diagnostic feature is one of the differentiating components of vascular from neurogenic TOS because neurogenic TOS is usually unaffected by climatic conditions.

Diagnosis

There are no tests or signs that are pathognomonic of TOS. The diagnosis is by elimination of other syndromes such as carpal tunnel syndrome, cervical spondylosis, cervical disc syndrome, glenohumeral dysfunction syndromes, ulnar nerve entrapment syndromes, Raynaud's disease, space-occupying diseases of the thoracic outlet such as Pancoast tumor, and cardiac pathologies (Box 22-2). Thorough and detailed case history and examination are cardinal features of diagnosis (Box 22-3). Diagnosis should include the pathomechanics of the lesion such as TOS caused by subluxation of the first rib or TOS caused by myofascial pain syndrome of the scalene muscles or as neurogenic TOS implicating cervical nerve root involvement or vascular TOS implicating involvement of the subclavian vessels.

Provocative Tests

The most reliable test according to Roos[72] and others[61,63] is the 3-minute elevated arm stress test also known in the literature as abduction and external rotation test (AER). In this test the patient's arm is abducted to 90 degrees with elbow flexed

---

BOX 22-2 ■ Differential Diagnosis of the Thoracic Outlet Syndrome

- Carpal tunnel syndrome
- Ulnar nerve entrapment at the elbow
- Cervical disc syndrome
- Cervical spondylosis
- Lower cervical facet syndrome
- Superior subluxation of the first rib
- Impingement syndrome at the shoulder
- Subacromial bursitis
- Myofascial pain syndromes of shoulder girdle muscles
- Myofascial pain syndrome of scalene muscles
- Raynaud's disease
- Pancoast tumor
- Cardiac pathology

Modified from Liebenson CS. J Manipulative Physiol Ther 1988;11:493-99.

BOX 22-3 ■ The Following Symptoms Should Be Asked for and Tests Performed

Consultation

- Distribution of pain
- Distribution of paresthesia
- Weakness or numbness in the arm and hand
- Aggravation of symptoms with arm elevated
- Aggravation of symptoms with head and neck movement
- Nocturnal symptoms

Physical Examination

- Vertebral palpation
- Ranges of active and passive mobility of the cervical spine
- Evaluation of first and second rib mobility
- Brachial plexus compression supraclavicularly
- Shoulder range of movement
- Scapular movements
- Postural assessment
  - Head position
  - Upper thoracic curve
  - Lateral spinal curves
- Elbow range of movement
- Ulnar nerve compression at the elbow
- Median nerve compression at the wrist
- Hand grip strength
- Radial and ulnar pulse tests
- "Hands-up" test (abduction-external rotation-elevation test)
- Scalene palpation
- Scalene relief test

Modified from Ribbe EB, Lindgren SHS, Norgren LEH. Manual Med 1986;2:82-5.

BOX 22-4 ■ Most Reliable Diagnostic Tests for Neurogenic TOS

Percussion pain

- Ipsilateral side of neck
- Supraclavicular, over brachial plexus
- Infraclavicular

Thumb pressure above clavicle

- Immediate pain over brachial plexus
- Gradual onset of usual symptoms in neck and arm

Weakness

- Triceps (C7)
- Interosseous hand muscles (C8, T1)
- Hand grip (C8)

Hypesthesia

- Inner forearm (C8, T1)
- Ring and small fingers, medial side of hand
- Occasional radial distribution in forearm and thumb

Elevated arm stress test (3 min)

- Premature fatigue and heaviness in involved arm
- Gradual onset of paresthesia in the fingers, spreading through hand and forearm
- Grimacing and vocal complaints
- Crescendo of distress throughout upper extremity
- Sudden, premature dropping of hand into lap
- Involved hand quite slow to recover
- Performed with arm abducted to 90 degrees elbow flexed to 90 degrees

Adapted from Liebenson after Roos DB. Vasc Surg 1979; 13:313-21.

to 90 degrees. The patient then is asked to slowly but steadily open and clinch his or her fist for a full 3 minutes. Thoracic outlet patients gradually develop symptoms of heaviness and fatigue in the involved arm and shoulders with gradual onset of numbness in the hand and have to rest the arm for relief of progressive crescendo distress that

becomes intolerable. This test is positive in both neurogenic and vascular types of TOS and, when combined with other objective signs, provides the most reliable tests for diagnosing neurogenic thoracic outlet syndrome (Box 22-4).

Adson's test is not considered a reliable test because pulse obliteration has been found in a large percentage of asymptomatic patients.[11-13] However, an increase in the symptoms with various positions of the arm is a significant component.[73]

Electrodiagnostics

Nerve conduction tests have poor reliability in the literature for definitive diagnosis.[11,63,74,75] According to Cuetter and Bartoszek,[1] nerve conduction velocities and latency values are all normal unless there is concomitant peripheral neuropathy.

Radiography

Static radiographs of the cervicothoracic region must be taken to rule out congenital anomalies, although, according to Urschel and Razzuk,[36] only 30% of thoracic outlet patients have associated congenital abnormality. Panegyres et al.[76] reported that their magnetic resonance imaging (MRI) study showed 70% sensitivity, with 87.5% specificity for deviations and distortions of nerves and blood vessels; MRI demonstrated the presence of radiographically invisible soft tissue bands in 20 TOS-suggested patients.

Functional Evaluation

Functional evaluation of biomechanical cervicothoracic lesions involves axial rotation and simultaneous lateral flexion of the cervical spine as first described by Lewit.[51] There is a typical tender spot just beneath the clavicle at the manubrium sterni[55] related to torsional stress from the subluxated first rib at the costosternal junction. Lindgren and Leino[48] describe the expiration-inspiration (E-I) test for first rib mobility (Figure 22-3) and report their study of 22 cases of TOS with 100% incidence of hypomobile first rib on the painful side. They further report a 17% recurrence of TOS as a result of subluxation of the stump of the resected first rib.[77]

When the first rib subluxates, usually in an inspiratory position, it moves cranially at the costotransverse joint. When the patient turns the head to the left, the first thoracic vertebra rotates to the left and the transverse process (TP) moves anteriorly. Restriction of cervical rotation away

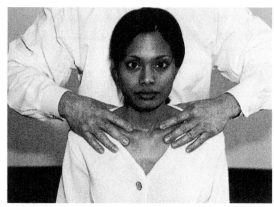

Figure 22-3   The expiration and inspiration (E-I) movement of the first rib is palpated in relation to the clavicle. The right and left sides are compared.

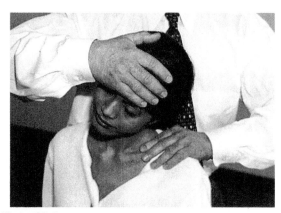

Figure 22-4   Rotation and lateral flexion of the cervical spine are restricted if the first rib is subluxated superiorly. There will be fullness and loss of inferior end joint spring of the first rib, as noted by the palpating hand.

from the side of lesion is most likely caused by the TP of the first thoracic vertebra bumping against the first rib.[50] Lateral flexion of the head toward the side of involvement is restricted because the superior position of the offending first rib; hence restriction and fullness are sensed under the palpating hand (Figure 22-4).

When superior subluxation of the first rib is suggested, all ranges of movement of the first rib should be evaluated. This includes bucket handle and caliper motion, similar to all other rib functions.[78]

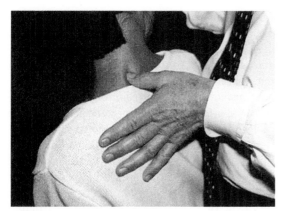

Figure 22-5 Evaluation of caliper type of motion of the first rib. When normally functioning, there will be a small range of end movement at the extreme range of cervical rotation. The head is used as a lever to magnify this small accessory joint play.

Individually and collectively, the ribs undergo these two types of motion during respiration.[79] The bucket handle motion is tested while laterally flexing the head toward the contact position over the nonarticulating tubercle of the first rib. (See Figure 22-3.) Normally the first rib depresses at the endpoint of its passive range of motion and small accessory passive joint range (joint play) motion can be elicited. Abnormal inspiratory subluxation may be attributable to scalene hypertonicity. Caliper motion is tested by using the head as a lever to magnify this small movement (Figure 22-5). The thumb is placed on the nonarticulating tubercle of the rib, and the head is rotated away from the side. The normal movement is a slight anterior springing of the transverse process and the rib (joint end feel), giving no resistance to the palpating thumb.

Management

The initial management of patients with thoracic outlet syndrome should always be conservative. Early operations should only be considered if vascular ischemia, serious embolic complication, or rapidly advancing denervations and muscle wasting are the prominent features. Surgical management

has been severely criticized in the literature, especially when large studies show that only 24% of patients with thoracic outlet syndrome actually require surgery.[63,71,73,80,81]

A well-informed patient is always a more compliant patient; hence explanation of the pathomechanical state should always be given. This alleviates the patient's often ill-defined symptom picture and provides a more receptive patient to carry out instructions. These should include postural advice, reeducation, and avoidance of carrying a heavy shoulder bag or handbag. Sleeping postures also must be evaluated and the use of a contour pillow to support the cervical curve should be considered.

Postural reeducation and correction of poor body mechanics are essential in the management of TOS. Round-shouldered or slouched postures often aggravate TOS and are the typical patient presentations. These postures not only place undue stress on the scalene and pectoralis muscles but also compromise the neural foramina and posterior zygapophyseal joints at the cervicothoracic junction. Prime concerns are correction of all associated biomechanical dysfunctions: the cervical spine, the first rib at the costovertebral and manubriocostal junctions, the sternoclavicular and acromioclavicular joints, and the shoulder complex, with special attention paid to the scapulothoracic function.

When the scalene muscles are involved, the stretching techniques advocated by Travell[66] are very effective in relieving acute spasms as well as relieving chronic painful myofascial pain syndromes. Because the sternocleidomastoid (SCM) muscle is also an important part of the myotatic unit for accessory inspiration, it likely will be involved along with the scalene. If the SCM is involved, it may be the cause of temporal and occipital headache, a TOS patient's frequent complaint. Satellite trigger points (TPs) may develop in muscles along the radiating pain pattern of the scalene. Both pectorals are often involved in radiating chest pain (pseudoangina). Satellite TPs in the long head of the triceps correspond with posterior arm pain and shoulder pain. Secondary TPs commonly develop in the brachioradialis, extensor carpi radialis, and extensor digitorum muscles, resulting in pain associated with thumb and wrist movements. The scalene-relief test identifies scalene involvement with relief of the symptoms, compared with true neurogenic TOS wherein various arm positions aggravate the symptoms (Figure 22-6). Daily passive stretching on the scalene muscles at home is critical to recovery (Figure 22-7).

Chiropractors frequently use direct pressure over trigger points (ischemic compression), first discussed by Nimmo[82] in the *Journal of the National Chiropractic Association* in 1957. He believed that pressure applied to the belly of a contracted muscle interrupts the pain-spasm-pain cycle, and relaxation of the spastic muscle follows. Ischemic compression is widely used by chiropractors as well as stretching in the treatment of trigger points.[83]

Chiropractic adjustive techniques for the cervicothoracic area, including corrections for first rib subluxations, clavicular subluxations, scapulothoracic, and glenohumeral dysfunctions, have been well described by Szaraz,[84] Kirk, Lawrence, and Valvo,[85] Gatterman and Panzer,[86] and most recently by Peterson and Bergmann.[79] Once the inferior component of the lesion is corrected, particular

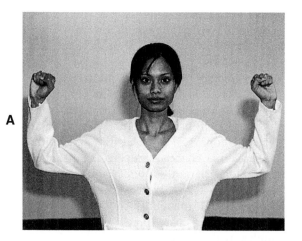

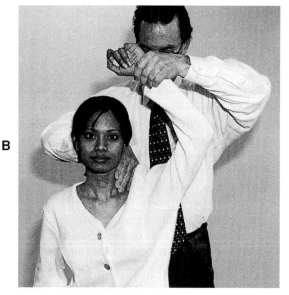

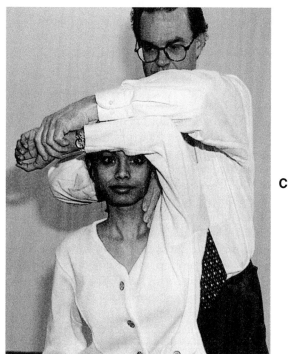

Figure 22-6   The scalene relief test helps to identify the source of referred pain from active trigger points in the scalene muscles. **A,** This is the starting position and can be combined with Roos's test. **B,** Raising the shoulder elevates the clavicle, relieving pressure on the neurovascular bundle and shortening the scalene muscles. **C,** As the shoulder is swung forward, the scapula is protracted and the clavicle moves forward and upward to fully relieve clavicular pressure on the thoracic outlet structures.

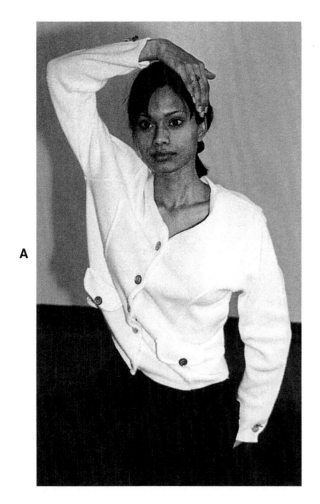

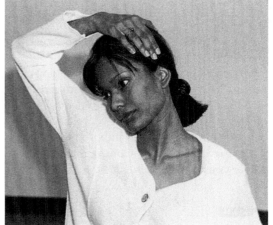

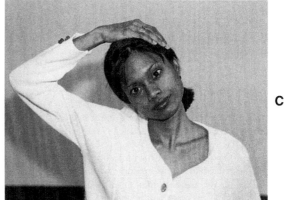

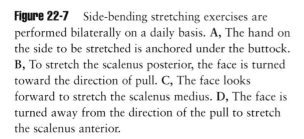

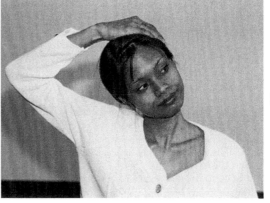

Figure 22-7   Side-bending stretching exercises are performed bilaterally on a daily basis. **A,** The hand on the side to be stretched is anchored under the buttock. **B,** To stretch the scalenus posterior, the face is turned toward the direction of pull. **C,** The face looks forward to stretch the scalenus medius. **D,** The face is turned away from the direction of the pull to stretch the scalenus anterior.

attention should also be paid to the cervical component of the lesion, especially because the scalene muscles intimately influence cervical dynamics as has been classically described by Grice.[87]

Conclusion

The thoracic outlet syndrome is a challenging clinical entity. Careful history taking and thorough physical examination, including in-depth biomechanical evaluation of the cervicothoracic area, provides the practitioner with important diagnostic clues to arrive at a solid clinical impression to undertake conservative therapeutic interventions.[88]

References

1. Cuetter AC, Bartoszek DM. The thoracic outlet syndrome: controversies, overdiagnosis, overtreatment, and recommendations for management. Muscle Nerve 1989;12:410-9.
2. Brash JC, Jarnieson EB, editors. Cunningham's textbook of anatomy. 7th ed. London: Oxford University Press; 1937.
3. Davies DV, Davies F, editors. Gray's anatomy. 33rd ed. London: Longmans; 1962.
4. Cooper A. On exostosis. In: Cooper BB, Cooper A, Travers B, editors. Surgical essays: American physician. 1st ed. Philadelphia: James Webster; 1821.
5. Coote H. Exostosis of the left transverse process of the seventh cervical vertebra surrounded by blood vessels and nerves: successful removal. Lancet 1861;1:360.
6. Todd TW. The relationship of the thoracic operculum consideration in reference to the anatomy of cervical ribs of surgical importance. J Anat Physiol 1911;45:293-304.
7. Todd TW. The vascular symptoms in 'cervical rib.' Lancet 1912;2:362-5.
8. Halstead WS. An experimental study of circumscribed dilation of an artery immediately distal to partially occluding band and its bearing on the dilation of the subclavian artery observed in certain cases of cervical rib. J Exp Med 1916;24:271.
9. Adson AW, Coffey JR. Cervical rib: a method of anterior approach for relief of symptoms by division of the scalenus anticus. Ann Surg 1927;85:839.
10. Adson AW. Surgical treatment for symptoms produced by cervical ribs and the scalenus anticus muscle. Surg Gynecol Obstet 1947;85:687-700.
11. Roos DB. Congenital anomalies associated with thoracic outlet syndrome. Am J Surg 1976;132:771.
12. Telford ED, Mottershead S. Pressure at the cervicobrachial junction: an operative and anatomical study. J Bone Joint Surg 1948;30B:249.
13. Wright IS. The neurovascular syndrome produced by hyperabduction of the arm. Am Heart J 1945;29:1.
14. Falconer MA, Weddell G. Costoclavicular compression of the subclavian artery and vein. Lancet 1943;2:539.
15. Peet RM, Hendricksen JD, Anderson TP, Martin GM. Thoracic outlet syndrome: evaluation of a therapeutic exercise program. Proc Mayo Clin 1956;31:281-7.
16. Lee R, Farquarson T, Domleo S. Subluxation und blockierung der ersten rippe: eine ursache fur das "thoracic outlet syndrome." Manuelle Medizin 1993;31:126-7.
17. Lindgren K-A, Leino E. Subluxation of the first rib: a possible thoracic outlet syndrome mechanism. Arch Phys Med Rehabil 1988;69:692-5.
18. Pang D, Wessel HB. Thoracic outlet syndrome. Neurosurgery 1988;22:105-21.
19. Daseler EH, Anson BJ. Surgical anatomy of the subclavian artery and its branches. Surg Gynecol Obstet 1959;1082:149-74.
20. Sunderland S. Disturbances of brachial plexus origin associated with unusual anatomical arrangements in the cervico-brachial region: the thoracic outlet syndrome. In: Nerves and nerve injuries. New York: Churchill Livingstone; 1978. p. 901-19.
21. Williams AF. The role of the first rib in the scalenus anterior syndrome. J Bone Joint Surg 1952;34B:200-3.
22. Brintnall ES, Lyndman OR, Van Allen MW. Costoclavicular compression associated with cervical rib. Ann Surg 1956;144:921-6.
23. Lord JW, Rosati LM. Thoracic outlet syndromes. Clin Symp 1971;23:3-32.
24. Pollack EW. Surgical anatomy of the thoracic outlet syndrome. Surg Gynecol Obstet 1980;150:97-103.
25. Todd TW. The descent of the shoulder after birth: its significance in the production of pressure-symptoms on the lower brachial trunk. Anat Anat 1912;41:385-97.
26. Nelson RM, Davis RW. Thoracic outlet compression syndrome. Ann Thorac Surg 1969;8:437-51.
27. Raaf J. Surgery for cervical rib and scalenus anticus syndrome. JAMA 1955;157:219-23.
28. Clein LJ. The droopy shoulder syndrome. Can Med Assoc 1976;114:343-4.
29. Swift TR, Nicholas FT. The droopy shoulder syndrome. Neurology 1984;34:212-4.
30. Beyer JA, Wright IS. The hyperabduction syndrome: with special reference to its relationship to Raynaud's syndrome. Circulation 1951;4:161-72.
31. Lord JW, Stone PW. Pectoralis minor tenotomy and anterior scalenotomy with special reference to the hyperabduction syndrome and "effort thrombosis" of the subclavian vein. Circulation 1956;13:537-42.
32. McCleery RS, Kesterson JE, Kirtley JA, Love RB. Subclavius and anterior scalene muscle compression as a cause of intermittent obstruction of the subclavian vein. Ann Surg 1951;133:588-602.
33. Rosati LM, Lord JW. Neurovascular compression syndromes of the shoulder girdle. New York: Grune & Stratton; 1961. p. 80-91.

34. Daube JR. Rucksack paralysis. JAMA 1969;208:2447-52.
35. Hanes RW. Movements of the first rib. J Anat 1946;80: 94-100.
36. Urschel HC Jr, Razzuk MA. Thoracic outlet syndrome. Surg Annu 1973;5:229-63.
37. Etter LE. Osseous abnormalities of the thoracic cage seen in four thousand consecutive chest photoroentgenograms. AJR 1944;51:359-63.
38. Steiner HA. Roentgenologic manifestations and clinical symptoms of rib abnormalities. Radiology 1943;40: 175-8.
39. Nguyen H, Vallee B, Person H, Nguyen HV. Anatomical bases of transaxillary resection of the first rib. Anat Clin 1984;5:221-33.
40. Turek S. Orthopedic principles and their application. 3rd ed. Philadelphia: JB Lippincott; 1977. p. 799.
41. Rayan GM. Lower trunk brachial plexus compression neuropathy due to cervical rib in young athletes. Am J Sports Med 1988;16(1):77-9.
42. Naffziger HC. The scalenus syndrome. Surg Gynecol Obstet 1937;64:119-26.
43. Oschsner A, Gage M, DeBakey M. Scalenus anticus (Naffziger) syndrome. Am J Surg 1935;28:669-95.
44. Clagetr OT. Research and prosearch. J Thorac Cardiovasc Surg 1962;44:153-66.
45. Bargar WL, Marcus RE, Ittleman FP. Late thoracic outlet syndrome secondary to pseudoarthrosis of the clavicle. J Trauma 1984;24:857-9.
46. Connolly JF, Dehne R. Delayed thoracic outlet syndrome from clavicular nonunion: management by morseling. Nebr Med J 1986;71:303-6.
47. Gangahar DM, Flogaites T. Retrosternal dislocation of the clavicle producing thoracic outlet syndrome. J Trauma 1978;18:369-72.
48. Lindgren K-A, Leino E. Subluxation of the first rib: a possible thoracic outlet syndrome mechanism. Arch Phys Med Rehabil 1988;69:692-5.
49. Lindgren K-A, Leino E, Manninen H. Cineradiography of the hypomobile first rib. Arch Phys Med Rehabil 1989; 70:408-9.
50. Lindgren K-A, Leino E, Hakola M, Hamberg J. Cervical spine rotation and lateral flexion combined motion in the examination of the thoracic outlet. Arch Phys Med Rehabil 1990;71:343-4.
51. Lewit K. Impaired joint function and entrapment syndrome. Manuelle Medizin 1978;16:45-8.
52. Bland JH. Cervical spine syndromes. J Musculoskel Med 1986;3(11):23-41.
53. Kirkaldy-Willis WH. Pathology and pathogenesis of low back pain. In: Kirkaldy-Willis WH, Burton CY, editors. Managing low back pain. 3rd ed. New York: Churchill Livingstone; 1983. p. 49-79.
54. Philips H, Grieve GP. The thoracic outlet syndrome. In: Grieve GP, editor. Modern manual therapy of the vertebral column. Edinburgh: Churchill Livingstone; 1986. p. 359-69.
55. Lewit K. Clinical aspects of disturbed function of the locomotor system. In: Lewit K. Manipulative therapy in rehabilitation of the locomotor system. 2nd ed. Oxford: Butterworth-Heinemann; 1991. p. 231-67.
56. Rashbaum RF. Multidisciplinary spinal rehabilitation: management by objectives. In: Hochschuler ST, Cotler HB, Guyer RD, editors. Rehabilitation of the spine: science and practice. St. Louis: Mosby, 1993. p. 425-33.
57. Hargberg M, Wegman DH. Prevelence rates and odds ratios of shoulder-neck diseases in different occupational groups. Br J Ind Med 1987;44(9):602-10.
58. Satow A, Taniguchi S. The development of a motor performance method for the measurement of pain. Ergonomics 1989;32(3):307-16.
59. Amano M, Umeda G, Nakajima H, Yatsuki K. Characteristics of work actions of shoe manufacturing assembly line workers, and a cross sectional factor-control study on occupational cervicobrachial disorders. Sangyo Igaku 1988;30:3-12.
60. Dellon AL. The results of supraclavicular brachial plexus neurolysis (without rib resection) in management of post-traumatic "thoracic outlet syndrome." J Reconstr Microsurg 1993;9(1):11-17.
61. Razi DM, Wassel HD. Traffic accident induced thoracic outlet syndrome; decompression without rib resection, correction of associated recurrent thoracic aneurysm. Int Surg 1993;78(1):25-7.
62. Sanders RJ, Pearce WH. The treatment of thoracic outlet syndrome: a comparison of different operations. J Vasc Surg 1989;10(6):626-34.
63. Sallstrom J, Schmidt H. Cervicobrachial disorders in certain occupations, with special reference to compression in the thoracic outlet. Am J Ind Med 1984;6:45-52.
64. Ribbe EB, Lindgren SHS, Norgren LEH. Clinical diagnosis of thoracic outlet syndrome: evaluation of patients with cervicobrachial symptoms. Manual Medicine 1986; 2:82-5.
65. Conn J. Thoracic outlet syndrome. Surg Clin North Am 1974;54:155-60.
66. Travell JG, Simons DG. Myofascial pain and dysfunction: the trigger point manual. Baltimore: Williams & Wilkins; 1983.
67. Gilliatt RW, LeQuesne PN, Logue V, Sumner AJ. Wasting of hand associated with a cervical rib or band. J Neurol Neurosurg Psychiatry 1970;33:615-26.
68. Carroll RE, Hurst LC. The relationship of thoracic outlet syndrome and carpal tunnel syndrome. Clin Orthop 1982; 164:149-53.
69. Asbury AK, Dyck PJ, Johnson AC et al. Coping with carpal tunnel syndrome. Patient Care 1985;19:76-90.
70. Urchel HC Jr. Dorsal sympathectomy and management of thoracic outlet syndrome with video-assisted thoracic surgery (VATS). Ann Thorac Surg 1993;56:717-20.
71. Riddel DH, Smith BM. Thoracic and vascular aspects of thoracic outlet syndrome. Clin Orthop 1986; 207:31-6.

72. Roos DB. New concepts of thoracic outlet syndrome that explain etiology, symptoms, diagnosis, and treatment. Vasc Surg 1979;13:313-21.

73. Stallworth JM, Horne JB. Diagnosis and management of thoracic outlet syndrome. Arch Surg 1984;119:1149-51.

74. Daube JR. Nerve conduction studies in the thoracic outlet syndrome. Neurology 1975;25:347.

75. Ryding E, Ribbe E, Rosen I, Norgren L. A neurophysiologic investigation in thoracic outlet syndrome. Acta Chir Scand 1985;151:327-31.

76. Panegyres PK, Moore N, Gibson R, Rushworth G, Donaghy M. Thoracic outlet syndrome and magnetic resonance imaging. Brain 1993;116(Pt 4):823-41.

77. Lindgren K-A, Leino E, Lepantalo M, Paukku P. Recurrent thoracic outlet syndrome after first rib resection. Arch Phys Med Rehabil 1991;72:208-10.

78. Fligg B. Spinal biomechanics. CMCC, 1989, Personal communication.

79. Peterson DH, Bergmann TF. Chiropractic technique: principles and procedures. 2nd ed. New York: Churchill Livingstone; 1993.

80. Green RM, McNamara J, Duriel K. Long-term follow-up after thoracic decompression: an analysis of factors determining outcome. J Vasc Surg 1991;14:739-45.

81. Davies AH, Walton J, Stuart E, Morris PJ. Surgical management of the thoracic outlet compression syndrome. Br J Surg 1991;78(10):1193-5.

82. Nimmo RL. Receptors, effectors, and tonus: a new approach. JNCA 1957;27:21-3.

83. Gatterman MI, Blunt K, Goe DR. Muscle and myofascial pain syndromes. In: Gatterman MI, editor. Chiropractic management of spine related disorders. 2nd ed. Baltimore: Williams & Wilkins; 1990. p. 319-69.

84. Szaraz Z. Compendium of chiropractic technique. CMCC 1984.

85. Kirk CR, Lawrence DJ, Valvo NL, editors. States manual of spinal, pelvic, and extravertebral technic. 2nd ed. Chicago: NCC; 1985.

86. Gatterman MI, Panzer DM. Disorders of the thoracic spine. In: Gatterman MI, editor. Chiropractic management of spine related disorders. 2nd ed. Baltimore: Williams & Wilkins; 2003. p. 198-228.

87. Grice AS. Scalenus anticus syndrome: diagnosis and chiropractic adjustive procedure. ICCA 1977;5:35-7.

88. Liebenson CS. Thoracic outlet syndrome: diagnosis and conservative management. J Manipulative Physiol Ther 1988;11:493-9.

Thoracic and Costovertebral Subluxation Syndromes

Adrian Grice

Key Words   Costovertebral subluxation syndromes, scoliosis, coupled motion

After reading this chapter you should be able to answer the following questions:

Question 1   Why do the traditional movement descriptions of flexion, extension, lateral flexion, and rotation need to be modified to describe segmental spinal motion?

Question 2   How does altered motion in thoracic motion segments accompanying aging lead to degenerative changes in the thoracic spine?

Question 3   What is the clinical significance of the transition area of spinous process rotation that accompanies lateral flexion?

Comparatively little is known about the neurologic, biomechanical, and physiologic relationships of this region of the spine. This is peculiar when one realizes that the thoracic spine houses the sympathetic nervous system and spinal dysfunction has been implicated in the development of somatovisceral reflex dysfunction, visceral dysfunction, and pain. What is known about thoracic physiology and biomechanics has been largely extrapolated from known functions of the cervical and lumbar spines. It would appear that our knowledge of spinal function has been driven by the need to understand the causes and treatment of spinal pain and therefore the lumbar spine. Secondarily, the cervical spine has captured most of our attention. Much of the literature relating to the thoracic spine is devoted to pathologic conditions and conditions that with a few exceptions have little to do with the clinical problems that are seen on a daily basis by the chiropractic clinician.

Clinical experience, however, demonstrates that pain syndromes and disorders of the thoracic spine and rib cage that do manifest themselves are quite frightening to the patient and produce anxiety about internal diseases that may or may not be relevant. Pain, pathology, and degenerative changes in this region of the spine have been shown to relate to postural changes, including scoliosis and kyphosis, autonomic and visceral dysfunction or pathologic condition, aberrant spinal static or dynamic function, or aberrant costovertebral function.[1-3] Aberrant static and dynamic function is related to dysfunction of the soft tissues, including ligaments, muscles, and discs. Joint function is regulated by sensorimotor reflex feedback loops.

The sensory proprioceptive system gets its main input from skin, muscles, ligaments, blood vessels, and fascia and it has been estimated to form 65% to 75% of the input; the special senses and viscera form the rest of the input. Thoracic spinal dysfunction therefore can be related to the overall neurologic regulation of the body's static and dynamic physiologic and nonphysiologic responses of viscera, including cardiovascular and respiratory systems and the locomotor system as a whole. The relationship may be through neurologic reflex changes or through direct biomechanical muscular function; for example, diaphragm contraction in respiratory change produces direct biomechanical effects on the rib cage and spine.

Diagnostic evaluation of any segment or region of the thoracic spinal or rib cage therefore should consider the following:

1. The locomotor system as a whole, as expressed in movement dynamics
2. Static body posture and our adaptation to gravity
3. The vertebral column and its function as an organ system
4. The cardiovascular and respiratory systems
5. The visceral elements and reflex responses
6. The cervical spine and its postural reflex regulation and direct muscle attachments
7. The lumbar spine, its postural regulation, and direct muscle attachments
8. The functional interaction of the thoracic spine and rib cage

Clinically Relevant Anatomy

The dorsal vertebrae are intermediate in size between the cervical and lumbar vertebrae, and they increase in size from above downward, a structural accommodation thought to relate to the increased demands of weight bearing.[4] The typical thoracic vertebra is so named because of the nature of rib attachments. The second to the eighth thoracic vertebrae are considered typical and contain two pairs of demifacets. One is located on the superior posterolateral aspect of the body and one on the inferior aspect directly below, forming the articulation with the head of the ribs on each side. Viewed from the superior aspect the typical vertebra shows a heart-shaped body with relative equal anterior-to-posterior dimensions; the spinal canal is round (Figure 23-1). The left side of the vertebral body sometimes has an impression formed by the aorta, which lies along the vertebral bodies and discs. From the lateral perspective, the vertebral body is slightly thicker on the posterior than the anterior. This vertebral shape functions in

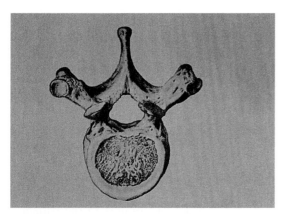

Figure 23-1   Superior view of typical thoracic vertebra. *(From Clemente C. Anatomy: a regional atlas of the human body. 4th ed. Baltimore: Lippincott Williams & Wilkins; 1997.)*

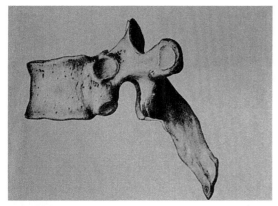

Figure 23-2   Lateral view of typical thoracic vertebra, wedge-shaped vertebral body. *(From Clemente C. Anatomy: a regional atlas of the human body. 4th ed. Baltimore: Lippincott Williams & Wilkins; 1997.)*

forming the primary normal thoracic kyphosis. The superior and inferior disc end plates should appear parallel on radiographs. The pedicles are directed backward from the body, and the inferior intervertebral notches are large and deeper than in other regions of the spine. This results in small but adequate intervertebral foramina that are circular in form (Figure 23-2).

The laminae are broad and thick, and they overlap one another like tiles on a roof. They give rise to the inferior and superior articular processes.

The superior articular processes each have an oval hyaline cartilage–covered facet that is flat and faces posteriorly, slightly superiorly, and laterally. The inferior articular processes have on the anterior surface an oval hyaline cartilage articular facet that is slightly concave transversely and faces anteriorly, inferiorly, and medially. The superior and inferior facets overlap like shingles. When viewed laterally, the joints create an angle from horizontal reported to be from 60 degrees in the upper thoracic region up to 80 to 90 degrees in the lower thoracic region.[5] (See Figure 23-2.)

The spinous processes are long, triangular, directed obliquely downward, and terminate in a bulbous extremity. The spinous tip in the mid-dorsal region is at the level of the facet of the vertebra below and produces an angle of 45 degrees up to 60 degrees or steeper in some cases. The bulbous tip of a typical thoracic vertebra is an excellent level for adjusting the intervertebral fixations/subluxations. The clinician by using an appropriate contact on the spinous process may develop an angle of force from right or left inferior to superior similar to the plane of the facet joints.

The transverse processes arise from behind the articular facets at the junction between the pedicles and the laminae. They are thick and strong, quite long, and directed obliquely backward and outward, with a clubbed extremity formed by the attachment of muscles. It is important to note that in the upper and mid-thoracic areas, the transverse processes are sometimes angled posteriorly and superiorly so that the tip is superior to the articular facet of that vertebra, a facet important in the angle to adjustive thrust. The purpose of both the spinous and transverse processes is for the attachment of muscles, and the shape of these structures is determined by the forces that act on them. The usual direction of thrust should be opposite to this direction of force. Most often a crossed bilateral is selected to facilitate the motion and not jam the facets, and the thrust delivered as torque directed from the superior is helpful. On the anterior surface, the typical thoracic transverse process contains a small concave articular facet that articulates with the tubercle of the rib.

The thorax, or chest cage, is an osseous cartilaginous structure whose principal function is to protect the principal organs of respiration and circulation. The rib cage is an important functional component of respiration, and Wyke[6] showed that by freezing the costovertebral joints the neurologic stimulus for respiration was suspended and respiration ceased. This fact may explain the benefit perceived by patients with chronic lung problems and asthma after adjustive care.

Viewed from the lateral aspect, the ribs form an angle of approximately 45 degrees as they move anteriorly and inferiorly, with a sharp superior angulation of the costal cartilages as they curve superior to attach to the sternum. The sternal costal joints of the true ribs (the first seven) unite at the sternum by hyaline cartilage. The next three or four ribs are false ribs and the hyaline cartilages connect, forming a more elastic attachment. The last two ribs have free endings without cartilaginous attachments; in some cases, the eleventh rib forms part of the false rib cartilaginous structure. The twelfth rib with the constant free distal end is sometimes called the floating rib. These costal cartilage attachments have a good deal of elasticity in the younger age-groups, but with increasing age, these cartilages become deeply yellow in color and tend to calcify and lose their elasticity. The female thorax differs from the male in that it usually has less capacity, the sternum is shorter, and the upper margin of the sternum is on the level of the lower body of the third dorsal vertebra, whereas in the male it is on the level of the lower part of the second dorsal vertebra. The upper ribs are more mobile in the female and allow greater movement of the upper thorax than in the male. These factors are important in consideration of prone adjustments in the female, particularly in the older osteoporotic or aging patient. All 12 thoracic vertebrae articulate with ribs; however, T2 through T9 have a double-rib articulation, forming a facet joint on the tip of each transverse process that articulates with the tubercle on the angle of ribs, and on the body on each side of the vertebrae as just described.

The first thoracic vertebra differs somewhat and is referred to as atypical. T1 is somewhat cervical-like, with the spinous process being thicker and proceeding posteriorly on a more horizontal plane. The vertebral body is broad transversely, with a concave superior surface slightly lipped on each side, causing the articular surfaces to be somewhat oblique. The clinician should consider the angle of the facets and the shape of the vertebral body in formulating the direction of the more effective adjustment. The concave body suggests an adjustment that includes distraction or longitudinal traction whereas a direction of thrust from superior to inferior is indicated to facilitate an adjustment with less discomfort to the patient, a factor very important in cervical adjusting as well.

The spinous process of the first thoracic vertebra is thick and may be almost as long as the vertebra prominens (spinous of C7), and during flexion of the neck, it also can appear to be quite prominent. This structure makes it an excellent contact for rotational and lateral flexion adjustments for fixations/subluxations between C7-T1 and T1-2. A thumb contact, commonly called a TM (thumb move), which is described later in this chapter, should concern itself with the thoracic vertebral shape, different patient head alignment, and thrust direction during positioning to specifically affect C7-T1 or T1-2. The head position and direction of thrust also change when we consider the holding elements involved, such as the direction of the muscle force. These factors are important for success and comfort in adjusting this region. As in all areas of the spine, the anatomy and the holding elements should be considered when applying an adjustment. This review does not deal with all the adjustments in the area; rather, special attention is drawn to areas that have been shown to produce particular difficulty for clinicians in efforts to develop efficiency, specificity, and ease of adjusting. The first thoracic vertebra is such an area. It has a complete facet for the first rib and a demifacet on the inferior of the body for the articulation of the second rib. The presence of a cervical rib may complicate pain syndromes involving the upper ribs and thoracic vertebrae but provides no particular problem for treatment and, in many cases, is present for years without symptoms. Thoracic outlet problems are common and clinically are often caused by irritation coming from the multiple pain-sensitive structures related to not only the vertebral facet joints but the rib attachments and the increased number of ligaments and muscles of this region. Muscle forces that act on these joints take their attachments from the cervical spine and occiput as well as from the thoracic spine and ribs. Correction should consider the related fixations in these regions of the spine and the interaction of the muscles. Further discussion of the cervical thoracic junction is presented in Chapter 22.

The inferior thoracic vertebrae, T9-12, are also considered atypical, particularly T11 and T12, which display characteristics of lumbar vertebrae. The ninth thoracic may or may not have an inferior demifacet, whereas the tenth usually has only one demifacet, often more laterally placed on the pedicle. The eleventh vertebra is more similar in size to a lumbar vertebra, and the articular facets for the ribs are larger and are located on the pedicle, which is also larger and stronger. The spinous process is short and nearly horizontal. The transverse processes of T11-12 are short and have no articulation with the rib. The twelfth thoracic vertebra differs from the other thoracic vertebrae in that the superior facets have a coronal facing, that of a thoracic vertebra, whereas the inferior facets have saggital facing, that of a lumbar vertebra. The biomechanical demands placed on this vertebra are unique and often necessitate special attention so that symptoms may be controlled. The thoracolumbar region exhibits the highest torsional stiffness and the highest frequency of fracture.[4] The transverse process is shorter, containing tubercles similar to mammillary or accessory processes formed by the attachments of muscles. These anatomic and biomechanical factors make this vertebra an important transitional vertebra for spinal curves and suggest that the optimal function of the spine occurs when the curves statically and dynamically make their transition at this level. Treatment should endeavor to restore or maintain this ideal function.

The presence of the anteroposterior (AP) curves in the spine gives it more resistance to weight-bearing forces, providing a springlike effect and reducing vibration. The thoracic kyphosis, unlike the lumbar spinal lordosis, ensures that in the neutral posture the facets carry little if any weight. Posture is such that when standing, we are inclined slightly forward. The result is that mild activity of posterior muscles, the erector spinae, maintains our posture. During unsupported sitting, there is slightly more activity of the posterior muscles.[7,8] This muscle also extends up the rib cage and helps posturally stabilize the spine and rib cage as a unit. During extension, the articulating facets form a close-packed system that limits motion.

The anterior compartment of the thoracic motion segment is formed by the vertebral bodies, the intervertebral disc, and longitudinal ligaments. The anterior ligament is a strong band made up of several layers, stretching from occiput to sacrum, narrower but thicker in the thoracic region, and serves to limit extension (Figure 23-3). The posterior longitudinal ligament up the posterior vertebra bodies is also thick, widens at the discal region, and narrows at the vertebral body. The axis of motion of the thoracic segment being anterior to this ligament allows it to limit flexion and translation.

The posterior compartment is formed by the vertebral arch, the transverse processes, and the zygapophyseal joints. The articular capsules are important structures in this posterior compartment because they are pain-sensitive structures and are called on to limit the movement of the thoracic motion segments in all ranges. They are attached to the lateral margins of the articular processes and are reinforced by the ligamenta flava that connect the vertebral lamina (Figure 23-4). The latter ligaments limit flexion and, to some degree, lateral flexion and rotation, and are composed largely of yellow elastic fibers. In degenerative change, the ligament may bulge and cause irritation to the nerve root.

The intrinsic elements of the thoracic spine, the discs, ligaments, and vertebral structure provide the intrinsic stability that is significant up to a few kilograms.[4] As in other areas of the spine, Nachemson[9] showed that the nucleus exerts hydrostatic pressure that acts like a coil spring,

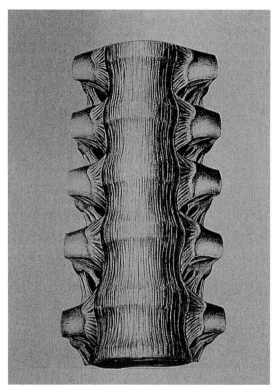

Figure 23-3   Anterior view of typical thoracic vertebra, anterior ligaments. *(From Clemente C. Anatomy: a regional atlas of the human body. 4th ed. Baltimore: Lippincott Williams & Wilkins; 1997.)*

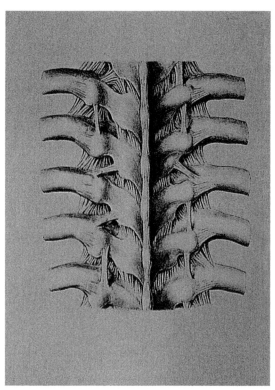

Figure 23-4   Posterior view of typical thoracic vertebra. *(From Clemente C. Anatomy: a regional atlas of the human body. 4th ed. Baltimore: Lippincott Williams & Wilkins; 1997.)*

separating the vertebrae and producing a preload stretch on the anterior and posterior compartment ligaments. Removal of the posterior ligaments, particularly the elastic ligamenta nuchae, demonstrates that the ligaments also exert compressive force or prestress on the disc, which provides for protection and enhancement of motion. As previously discussed, the rib cage also produces resistance to motion, adding to thoracic stiffness twofold and load-bearing capacity threefold (Figure 23-5).[10] All of these factors are probably why disc lesions and facet problems are less frequent in the thoracic spine. The interspinous and supraspinous ligaments limit flexion and are well developed in the thoracic region. Tenderness of the supraspinous in the mid-thorax, a common clinical finding, would seem to demonstrate that

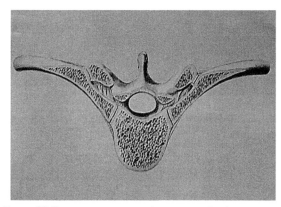

Figure 23-5   Cross-section of costovertebral connection. *(From Clemente C. Anatomy: a regional atlas of the human body. 4th ed. Baltimore: Lippincott Williams & Wilkins; 1997.)*

this region of the spine is frequently under flexion strain. Degenerative change in the anterior aspect of the dorsal vertebrae is also common, which may relate to increased compressive forces or at least to excessive anterior mobility of the body.

Biomechanics of the Thoracic Spine

Static Concepts

In general, it is often considered that the normal AP view of the thoracic spine should be relatively straight and balanced, whereas the normal lateral view should have a posterior curve. The thoracic kyphosis and the sacral curve are formed during the embryonic stage and are called the primary curves. The thoracic kyphosis, as stated previously, is attributable primarily to the wedge shape of the thoracic vertebrae, particularly characteristic in the mid-thorax. Growth changes as seen on radiograph in this normal vertebral wedging should be evaluated when an alteration in this so-called normal kyphosis is seen. A flat thoracic spine may be a normal variant in young girls who otherwise have normal posture and may result from loss of this normal vertebral wedging. The optimal thoracic curve should be an even curve that extends from T1 to T12, with C7-T1 and T12-L1 being the transition points for the primary kyphotic curve as the spinal curves become the secondary cervical or lumbar curve, respectively. The apex of the thoracic curve should be at the level of T6-7. Common variations are seen: (1) Flattening of mid-dorsal kyphosis is more common in females than in males; (2) elongation of the thoracic primary curve into the lumbar spine, producing a short radius lumbar curve, is also common. Clinical experience suggests that these variations may well lead to symptoms or biomechanical stress that manifests as degenerative changes. Some variation in opinion is seen in the literature on what constitutes normal or optimal statics and dynamics, and because of our lack of knowledge, it is difficult to draw precise correlations between aberrant biomechanics and pathologic conditions and render a good theoretical basis for pathogenesis in this region of the spine. The anatomic shape of the vertebrae, as well as the muscular attachments and their postural functions, would in theory dictate concepts of optimal posture for the thoracic spine. Because few studies are available that establish normal and optimal posture for this region, we must rely on structural and functional integration to develop clinical models of optimal function.

Gray's Anatomy[11] holds that the cervical curve starts at C2 and ends at T2, the thoracic curve starts at T2 and extends to T12, and the lumbar curve starts at T12 and ends at L5. The normal apex of the thoracic curve is T7. The spine was normally seen to have a very slight lateral curve convexity to the right, thought to be caused by muscular development related to dominant right-handedness. Schmorl and Junghanns[12] reported that it was normal for 80% of spines to have a mild physiologic scoliosis, left in the cervical thoracic region and right in the thoracic and lumbar regions, whereas 20% of spines showed the reverse of this curve. These curves begin developing at 6 years of age; they were thought to be related to greater strength of right thoracic musculature caused by dominant right-handedness. It is interesting to note, however, that Figure 51 of their text, depicting these curves in a preparation by Virchow, is more representative of the four opposed rotational scolioses seen as normal and presented in chiropractic literature by Carver,[13] Beatty,[14] and Homewood.[15]

The Four Opposed Rotational Scolioses (Carver)

1. Right lower lumbar curve extending to L3; 3 transitional vertebrae
2. Left lumbar thoracic curve; apex at T12 and termination at T7-8, the transitional vertebrae
3. Right thoracic cervical curve; apex at T4, transition at C7-T1
4. Left cervical scoliosis, apex at C4, with a counteraction at C1-2, C1 right, C2 left

Carver's opinion was that the apex of the thoracic kyphosis was at T7-8, with the normal curve extending from T2-12. There appears to be some general agreement in the literature that the basic asymmetry of the body as well as dominant handedness produces mild rotational curves in the spine that develop in early childhood. A left cervical curve and a right thoracic curve may by all reports be a normal functional compensation for right-handed individuals and may account in part for the common low right shoulder seen in right-handed individuals. It is surprising how often in clinical practice one encounters a spinally healthy individual with the mild curves Carver considered as optimal—the four opposed rotational scoliosis. The key factor in a functional spine seems to be symmetry of mobility and balanced compensation rather than strictly alignment. The most important clinical factors in assessing the statics of the spine would be (1) the curves should be smooth and even, and each individual vertebra should participate uniformly in the configuration; (2) the apex and transitions of the curves should be at the levels just stated; and (3) the spine should fall so that the center of gravity passes through the center of the body of C7 and the center of the body of T12 with only a mild deviation (scoliosis) presented on postural analysis. Dynamic motion should be equal to each side, and the curve should be uniform; that is, each motion segment should participate smoothly and somewhat equally, reaching the end point of the motion with uniform rhythm.

Dynamics of the Thoracic Spine

The thoracic spine is the longest region of the spine but the least mobile. This lack of mobility is caused primarily by the fact that the height of the disc is approximately 20% to 25% that of the height of the thoracic vertebral body, a ratio that is the lowest in the spine. Additionally, the rib cage with the double posterior and anterior costosternal attachments limits rotation and lateral flexion. When the sternum is removed, the stiffness of the thoracic spine imparted by the rib cage is negated.[4] These movements are slightly less limited in the lower thoracic region, where the elasticity of the costal cartilages allows for a slightly greater degree of mobility in certain ranges. The thoracic vertebral facet facings limit flexion and extension to some degree but do little to impede rotation and lateral flexion of the thoracic segment, which is mainly limited by the ribs. During extension the facets are seen to make contact, which limits movement along with the anterior longitudinal ligament. All motion in the thoracic spine is accompanied by movement in the ribs, which at times amounts to only a few millimeters of translational motion. Thoracic biomechanical dysfunctions, whether vertebral or costovertebral, are intimately related because of the osseous structural arrangement and the muscular attachments. When correcting dysfunction, concern for static alignment, joint motion, and the extrinsic forces that block the movement are of importance. White and Panjabi[16] emphasized six degrees of freedom in the thoracic motion segment similar to the findings in the lumbar spine: (1) anterior/posterior motion or translation along the Z axis; (2) lateral to medial motion around the X axis; and (3) superior to inferior motion around the Y axis. The traditional descriptors flexion, extension, lateral flexion, and rotation do not conform to the actual movements in the spine because all movements are combined or coupled movements. The primary coupled motion is easily detected on a motion study plain film radiograph, and it is well understood that lateral flexion is combined with rotation and vice versa. It is important to note that tertiary motions in translation, flexion or extension, or motion along the Y axis also accompany these main motions. Clinicians often believe that when the tertiary motion is lost in a motion segment (joint blockage or subluxation), the neurologic reflex changes that take place are the most significant to the patient and explain some of the dramatic results obtained by the dynamic adjustive thrust when evaluation demonstrates little static or dynamic change other than the restoration of the paraphysiologic or tertiary motion. Panjabi et al.[17] showed that the average intervertebral translation motion was 1 mm in the sagittal plain. This amount of motion can be felt only through the end feel challenge method and clinically can be appreciated as altered after a dynamic adjustive correction. At times the palpable restoration of motion may represent restoration of tertiary motion, paraphysiologic motion, or translatory motion that may prove sometimes to be the same motions.

The axis of motion for rotation and lateral flexion is located in the center of the body of the vertebra and under normal circumstances very little shearing or translatory motion of the disc takes place. The axis of motion for flexion-extension is located in the center of the disc of the vertebra below and does not allow or require much shearing or translation. Clinically, anterior disc lipping and degeneration are common radiographic findings in middle age.[18,19] One cause of these pathologic changes is probably a shift of the axis of motion posteriorly and laterally caused by alteration in muscular activity that results in hypermobility of the anterior body during movement with resultant increased shearing force to the disc and stress and strain to all of the intrinsic structures. The alteration of movement or function produces a change in structure, resulting in the degenerative changes commonly seen in the anterior body of the thoracic spine and the osteophytic changes at the costotransverse joints.

The musculature of the thoracic spine is dealt with in detail in most anatomy texts. The action is usually described on a kinesiologic basis with such descriptions as extensors/rotators or lateral flexors of the spine. For the clinician involved in spinal correction, the specific attachment of these muscles and their individual actions and effects on the motion and biomechanics of the individual vertebra are important. Some of the discussion in this area must be theoretical at this stage because of limited experimental research and technology to validate our opinions; however, speculation based on structure, function, and observation is an important first stage. The Quiring and Warfel series[20,21] on musculature is a very good reference source for the clinician to use for the details of origin, insertion, nerve supply, and motor points. The detailed drawings allow us to speculate on the biomechanical action these muscles exert on the individual motion segment.

It is interesting to note that the trapezius, latissimus dorsi, and rhomboids, which always receive much attention from clinicians in clinical and legal reports on spinal dysfunction, are listed in these texts as extremity muscles, and in my opinion, rightly so. Under normal circumstances these mus-cles have little effect on spinal posture or movement biomechanics except when the upper limb is active or load bearing. As such, these muscles are not very often causative of spinal subluxation, whereas the deeper layers of spinal muscles are much more important and should capture the attention of clinicians.

It would appear that the reason the trapezius gets so much of our attention is because of its broad origin from the external occipital protuberance superior nuchal line, nuchal ligament, spinous processes, C7, and spinous process of all 12 thoracic vertebrae. The insertion is into the lateral third of clavicle, spine of scapula, and acromion. Palpable tenderness and spasm in the back musculature is often mistakenly related to this muscle, resulting in neglect of the more important deep muscles.

The latissimus dorsi arises from the lower six thoracic spinous processes, the lumbosacral fascia, the crest of the ilium, and the lower three or four ribs. The insertion is into the bicipital groove of the humerus. Rib fixations related to this muscle are common with sports or activities that require torsion and arm motion. Treatment is difficult because of the ease of trauma on returning to the sports activity. Rehabilitation of the patient with lower back or lumbodorsal problems, who must return to lifting tasks, should strengthen this muscle to stabilize the back.

The rhomboids arise from the ligamentum nuchae, the spinous process of C7, and the spinous processes of T1-5. They insert into the medial border of the scapula. In the prone position, elevation of the scapula and palpation of these muscles as well as of the trapezius can help determine if hypertonicity is present in these more superficial muscles or the deep muscles of the back.

The main muscles that control thoracic biomechanics are the trunk muscles, the erector spinae, and the transversospinal group (Figure 23-6).

The erector spinae group is made up of the (1) iliocostalis, (2) longissimus, and (3) spinalis.

1. Iliocostalis
The lumborum inferior portion arises from the sacrum, crest of ilium, and spinous processes of

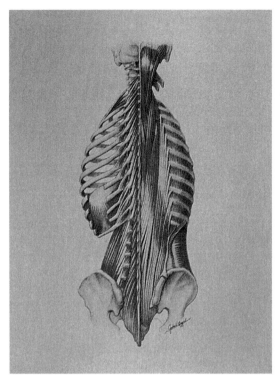

Figure 23-6 Erector spinae and transversospinal muscles. *(From Seeley RR, Stephens TD, Tate P. Anatomy and physiology. 3rd ed. St. Louis: Mosby; 1995.)*

T11-12 and all lumbar processes. Insertion is into the angle of the lower six to seven ribs. Origin of the medial lumbar portion is the angle of the lower six ribs. Insertion is into the upper medial portion of the angles of ribs T1-6. Origin of the upper portion is the angles of T3-6 ribs, with insertion into transverse processes of C4-6.

2. Longissimus Portion
a) Thoracic portion origin of transverse processes of lumbar spine and the lumbodorsal fascia; insertion into the transverse processes of the lower 9 or 10 ribs
b) Cervicis portion originates from upper fourth to fifth thoracic transverse processes with an insertion into the transverse processes of C2-6
c) Capitus portion originates from transverse processes of the upper four to five thoracic and

articular processes of lower three to four cervical vertebrae; insertion is into the posterior margin of the mastoid of the occiput

3. Spinalis Portion
a) Thoracic portion arises from spinous processes T11-12, L1-2; insertion is the fourth through the eighth thoracic spinous processes
b) Cervicis portion arises from spinous processes of T1-2, C7, and ligamentum nuchae; insertion is spinous processes of C2-4
c) Capitus portion originates from transverse processes of the upper six to seven thoracic vertebrae and articular pillars of C4-7 cervical vertebrae. Insertion is between inferior and superior nuchal lines on the occiput. It should be noted by the clinician at this point that much of the attachment of these muscles is devoted to attachments to the ribs. These attachments help to stabilize the head of the rib into the thoracic transverse processes.

The nerve supply for these is the posterior primary rami branching from each segment; therefore this muscle tends to act as individual slips and can produce dysfunction. Examples are occiput to cervical or thoracic, cervical to thoracic or rib, and thoracic to lumbar. Careful static palpation and motion can assist in differentiating specific fixations and determining the related regions of the spine, both of which may need correction.

Transversospinal Muscles
The most important muscle in this group is the semispinalis, which has three portions. Semispinalis thoracis has its origin from the transverse processes of the lower six thoracic vertebrae and the insertion into the spines of T1-4 and C6-7. Semispinalis cervicis has its origin from the transverse processes of T1-6 and the articular pillar of C4-7 with the insertion into the spinous processes of C2-5 cervical vertebrae.

Semispinalis capitus has its origin from the transverse processes of T1-6 and C7 as well as articular pillar C4-6 and the insertion into the occipital line between superior and inferior nuchal line. Multifidus is a segmental muscle not as well developed in the thoracic region as in the lumbar spine or the cervical spine. The origin is from the spinous process of the vertebra above; the insertion is into the transverse processes of vertebra below and extending as far down as three to four segments. The rotational components of the thoracic segments are further supported by rotatory muscles, which lie deep to the multifidus in pairs and are present only in the thoracic spine. The origin is from the transverse process of one vertebra and the insertion is into the lamina of the vertebra above. Segmental motion is further supported by the interspinales muscles and intertransversarii muscles, which are very small or even nonexistent in some thoracic spines. Clinically these latter muscles may have little significance.

The serratus posterior superior is a broad thin muscle that arises from the ligamentum nuchae C7, T1-4 spinous processes, and it inserts lateral to the angle of T2-5 ribs. The serratus posterior/inferior, also broad and thin, arises from spinous processes of T11-12, L1-2, and lumbar fascia and inserts into inferior borders of the lower four ribs. Nerve supply is anterior primary rami for these latter muscles; therefore the whole muscle tends to act as a unit.

Kinematics of the Thoracic Spine

Kapandji[22] reports movement of the spine as a whole. His diagrams demonstrate 45 degrees of flexion-extension, 20 degrees of lateral flexion to each side (total of 40 degrees), and 35 degrees of rotation to each side (total of 70 degrees). Gregerson and Lucas's study[23] of normal medical students using Steinmann's surgical pins inserted into the spinous processes showed an average segmental rotation of 6 degrees. They showed a slight difference between sitting and standing, with sitting showing less motion in the lower thoracic vertebrae. They reported a total range of motion similar to the figures suggested by Kapanji[22] (37 degrees to one side, or a total of 74 degrees of rotation). In this same study, rotation during gait was observed. During normal walking, T7-8 was seen to stay relatively stable and formed the transition point for total body rotation developed by the pelvis, opposed to the counter-rotation seen in the

shoulders with normal arm swing. With each step, the gross rotation motion of the body at the sacrum is approximately 8 degrees, which reduces to 0 degree at T7-8. The arm swing and shoulder motion produce an opposite rotation of 6 degrees at T2. Therefore T7-8 would show the most rotation segmentally during normal walking (approximately 2.5 degrees). The segmental rotation at T11-12 and T1-2 during walking amounts to about 0.5 degree. These biomechanical observations would lend logical support to the concept that T7 should be the optimal apex of the thoracic kyphosis. The most definitive study of the biomechanics and the range of segmental motion in the thoracic region comes from White and Panjabi[24] (Table 23-1).

Flexion-Extension Range of Motion: Sagittal Plane Rotation

Median figures are 4 degrees of motion for the upper thoracic segments, 6 degrees for the mid-thoracic segments, and 12 degrees of motion each for the T11, T12, and L1 segments. White and Panjabi[25] suggested that the instantaneous axis of motion for flexion is located in the anterior one third of the superior aspect of the vertebral body of the vertebra below; for extension, the location is in the anterior one third of the inferior aspect of the vertebra of the superior motion segment (Figure 23-7).

Lateral Flexion Range of Motion: Frontal Plane of Motion

As in other areas of the spine, lateral flexion is accompanied by a coupled motion; the main coupled motion is rotation in the sagittal plane. Lateral motion totals approximately 52 degrees to each side with intersegmental movement of approximately 5 to 6 degrees in the upper segments and 8 to 9 degrees in the lower segments. During lateral flexion the instantaneous axis of motion is located in the body of the vertebra below. Lateral flexion on plain film radiographs demonstrates that the primary coupled motion, generally in the upper thoracic vertebrae, is similar to a cervical

Table 23-1

Segmental Motion in the Thoracic Spine

Interspace	Flexion/extension Limits of ranges (degrees)	Flexion/extension Representative angle (degrees)	Lateral bending Limits of ranges (degrees)	Lateral bending Representative angle (degrees)	Axial rotation Limits of ranges (degrees)	Axial rotation Representative angle (degrees)
T1-T2	3-5	4	5	6	14	9
T2-T3	3-5	4	5-7	6	4-12	8
T3-T4	2-5	4	3-7	6	5-11	8
T4-T5	2-5	4	5-6	6	4-11	8
T5-T6	3-5	4	5-6	6	5-11	8
T6-T7	2-7	5	6	6	4-11	8
T7-T8	3-8	6	3-8	6	4-11	8
T8-T9	3-8	6	4-7	6	6-7	7
T9-T10	3-8	6	4-7	6	3-5	4
T10-T11	4-14	9	3-10	7	2-3	2
T11-T12	6-20	12	4-13	9	2-3	2
T12-L1	6-20	12	5-10	8	2-3	2

From White AA III, Panjabi MM. Spine 1978;3:12.

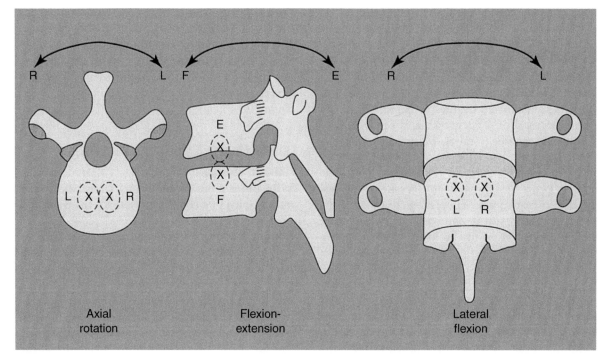

Axial rotation   Flexion-extension   Lateral flexion

Figure 23-7   Instantaneous axis of motion (flexion-extension, rotation, lateral flexion).

motion segment in that the spinous processes rotate to the convexity (type 2 motion). In the lower thoracic vertebrae, the normal behavior is similar to that of a lumbar segment; the spinous processes rotate to the concavity (type 1 motion). My own clinical observations of coupling patterns suggest that the optimal or normal pattern for the upper thoracic segment is a type 2 pattern and for the lower thoracic segment a type 1 pattern, the transition point being T6-7. The typing of motion patterns was developed in the lumbar spine and reported by Grice,[26,27] Cassidy,[28] and Gitelman.[29] These observations can be clinically produced by a radiographic study that places the seated patient with the dorsal spine against the bucky and laterally flexioning the patient, keeping the spine in contact with the bucky. Deviations from this pattern are common and in my opinion are clinically significant on a long-term biomechanical basis. White and Panjabi[4] discuss the disagreement about coupling patterns in the thoracic region and suggest that the complexity of the motion along with variation in techniques of study may be the reason. They go on to observe that abnormal coupling patterns are seen in scoliotic deformities.

Rotation Range of Motion: Motion in the Horizontal Plane

Rotation in the thoracic spine also produces coupled motions, the prime motion being that of lateral flexion. These patterns of coupled motion, as in the case of lateral flexion, can be altered voluntarily by postural change. Vertical axial rotation of the thoracic spine to the right results in lateral flexion to the left, particularly in the lower thoracic region. Clinically, it must be remembered that there is an additional coupled motion in the sagittal plane during rotation. In the lower thoracic region, this motion appears to be extension, whereas in the upper thoracic region it appears to be flexion. The coupled pattern in the upper thoracic region can be altered by slight flexion, producing lateral flexion on the same side. The transition point for these movements in the transverse and sagittal plane is approximately T6-7. This transition point and T5-6 are often clinically found to demonstrate

marked spinous tenderness and subluxation. A flattening, or saucer effect, also may occur in the region of the spine and is usually related to the extensor group of thoracic muscles being overactive.

The rotation range of motion for the whole thoracic spine is 41 degrees. Each vertebral segment in the upper half of the thoracic spine moves approximately 4 degrees to each side with a total of 8 to 9 degrees, whereas the lower three thoracic segments move only about 2 degrees to each side.[4]

Biomechanics of the Rib Cage

Very little has been added to the literature about rib motion.[30] The vertebral sternal attachments of the typical true ribs T2-7 and T1 form the basis for the concept of the bucket handle type of motion. These ribs from their double vertebral attachments extend outward, then forward, downward, and inward to their medial attachments on the sternum. Kapandji[22] states that the double vertebral body transverse process attachment acts as a swivel for the rib, the angle of which controls the movement of the distal sternal end of the rib. This concept alters the bucket handle concept by demonstrating that one handle of the bucket being more rigidly fixed becomes the axis of motion around which the more flexible chest cage moves, therefore controlling the nature of the motion of the opposite handle of the bucket at the distal attachment. The result is that on inspiration the distal portion of the rib elevates, thus causing the chest to rise. Steindler[31] states that the double anchorage of the rib into the vertebra limits the motion to 1 degree at the spine attachment.

The elasticity of the chondral cartilages forms the basis for the concept of the caliper motion seen in the vertebral chondral ribs 8, 9, and 10, as well as 11 and 12, the floating rib. The double vertebral attachment serves to intimately connect thoracic vertebral motion to rib motion. Any type of rib resection results in excessive rotation and lateral flexion of the involved vertebrae, resulting in instability and scoliosis of the spine. To properly analyze any spinal dysfunction, palpation of the rib cage and the thoracic spine is necessary.

Many of the muscles that produce subluxations/fixations in the thoracic spine also cause costovertebral dysfunction or subluxation; that is to say, primary thoracic vertebral fixation may result in costovertebral or costal-costal fixations, or primary costal fixations may produce costovertebral or vertebral-vertebral fixations. This is caused by their biomechanical interaction or the muscular forces that interlock these segments. As in other parts of the body, when somatic dysfunction arises and pain is produced, the body compensates. This may result in control of the pain or, in the case of decompensation, stress or strain may increase. Further pain may arise and result in further compensations. In any case, a lesion may result in a wide variety of responses that often cloud the primary cause or condition. Nowhere in the body can it be more difficult to distinguish the major or initial problem than in the thoracic spine, probably because of the number of structures and joints located in this region and the complex interactive functions between these related structures. In many cases, successful treatment may not revolve around determining a major or minor lesion, but rather an organized progressive correction of each distortion pattern should be systematically addressed.

One of the primary functions of the rib cage is respiration. The alteration of breathing mechanics can be an important cause of spinal or rib cage dysfunction. As previously stated, Wyke[6] drew attention to the fact that the rhythmic sensory input from the costovertebral joints is necessary to stimulate normal respiration; when the rib articulation was anesthetized, respiration ceased. He stressed that this sensorimotor feedback loop was an essential function to normal respiration. This factor may explain why patients with sleep apnea respond to postural changes and corrective changes in the musculoskeletal holding elements of the thoracic spine and ribs. Angina patients with fixed or arthritic dorsal spines may trigger attacks by poor posture or sleeping on their backs; often, they must sleep in a semi-sitting position.

Kapandji[22] further explains mechanics of motion of the ribs during respiration by showing that the costovertebral-costotransverse angle causes the upper ribs to raise on the anterior aspect during inspiration. In the upper ribs, as the bucket at the spine handle rolls over in inspiration, the distal handle elevates and the sternum as a whole rises. This movement can be simulated on one side to some degree by laterally flexing the thoracic spine and neck. Evaluation of the biomechanics explains why movement and deep breathing can produce the same anterior chest pain when biomechanical problems exist. The costovertebral-costotransverse angle in the lower ribs is about 45 degrees in the sagittal plane. Coupled with the downward angulation of the ribs as the rib moves laterally and anteriorly, the lower ribs elevate on inspiration, exaggerating the bucket handle concept in the mid-dorsals. Steindler[31] suggests that the horizontal angle of the ribs as they move forward laterally is 50 degrees for the first rib, 43 degrees for the fourth rib, and 42 degrees for the seventh rib. The elasticity of the chondral cartilages allows the caliper-type motion in the lower rib cage. This motion can be simulated by deep inspiration or by rotation. Rotation to the right increases the AP and lateral dimensions of the rib cage on the right and causes a decrease or concavity of the rib cage on the left side. Gross thoracic motion such as rotation and lateral flexion, when combined with inspiration and expiration, can help to locate costovertebral lesions and determine whether the problem muscles are primarily postural muscles or respiratory muscles.

Segmental palpation of the thoracic spine and ribs should take into consideration not only spinal motion but also respiration. Basmajian[32] discussed the mechanisms in respiration, stating that during quiet breathing, thoracic mobility is minimal and the diaphragm is the main muscle of respiration. The diaphragm contracts as a unit during inspiration and causes the ribs to move upward and outward. Clinically, a patient presenting with anxiety and stress shows a tendency toward this type of flaring of the lower ribs and has poor vital capacity. The diaphragm is a tripartite muscle with right and left costal portions and a central crural portion. The muscle develops from eight slips: one or two from the sternum, two to seven from the costal and lumbar areas, and eight from the crus. When active, the muscle functions as a unit. Continuous overcontraction of the diaphragm causes a typical lower dorsal/lumbar fixation, which is often present in the anxious patient and usually involves the lower ribs and lower dorsal lumbars.

Basmajian[32] describes in detail the activity of muscles during breathing, suggesting that complex variations in the pattern are possible. For our purposes, it is sufficient to extract that the diaphragm, as well as the upper intercostals and scaleni muscles, are constantly active during quiet inspiration, producing an increase of the thorax cavity in a vertical direction as well as in the AP and lateral dimensions. Quiet expiration is a passive nonmuscular phase of breathing.

Accessory Muscles of Respiration and the Biomechanical Effects

The quadratus lumborum has been shown to act with the diaphragm, particularly during deep breathing, and it serves to stabilize the lower ribs. When a person is under stress, the scaleni and quadratus lumborum muscles become important causes of fixation of the ribs and spine; this should be addressed in all patients suffering from stress.

During quiet breathing, the first intercostals are always active and the second are active occasionally; with greater inspiration the intercostal activity progresses to successively lower intercostal levels. Forced expiration shows a slight carryover of rhythmicials contraction that seems to assist in expiration when the rhythmic relaxes; the lower intercostals from the eleventh and twelfth pairs are more important in assisting expiration. The scaleni muscles are considered by Basmajian to be primary muscles of respiration and have been shown in quiet breathing to elevate and anchor the first and second ribs. In forced inspiration, they became far more active and, in conjunction with normal neck posture, assist in elevating the anterior chest. Adjustment of this fixation pattern for the cervical spine has been described[33]; however, special attention to the upper ribs is important when the scaleni are involved.

The sternocleidomastoideus is active only during deep breathing. The suprahyoid muscles also are found to be active except during deep sleep and with excessive activity can be involved in that so-called lump in the throat experienced during times of stress. The internal and external obliques, as well as the transverse abdominis, are accessory muscles of respiration that limit forced inspiration and help to produce forced expiration; when tight, they are thought to produce that feeling of "butterflies in the stomach."

The pectoral muscles were also shown to be accessory muscles of respiration. There are conflicting reports as to the function of the trapezius as an accessory muscle of respiration. Tenderness and hypertonicity of the pectorals seem to be more common in female patients and may cause neurovascular outlet signs and symptoms when hypertonic. Clinically, these muscles become important in patients who show stress and anxiety and are commonly seen as problems in acceleration/deceleration motor vehicle accident (MVA) patients. Steindler[31] discusses the effect of calcification of the costal cartilages, showing that the presence of signs in ribs and sternal region limits respiratory function.

Biomechanical Diagnosis of Thoracic Spine and Ribs

This discussion is limited to the evaluation of musculoskeletal dysfunction, recognizing that organic dysfunction can produce pain patterns that simulate musculoskeletal disorders and vice versa, and may require differential diagnosis. A careful history, a physical examination, and the use of pain drawings can go a long way toward making a differential diagnosis. This should be routinely done, particularly when spinal dysfunction is limited or inconclusive.

Beal,[34] in a summary article, reviewed visceral somatic reflexes and their effects on the spine. Beal[35] and Cox et al.[36] showed that somatic dysfunction patterns can relate to underlying cardiovascular and coronary artery disease. Beal and Morlock[37] showed that somatic dysfunction patterns can also have a relationship to pulmonary disease. Beal and Kleiber[38] showed that somatic dysfunction can be an important predictor of coronary arterial disease. Johnston et al.[39] showed a relationship between somatic dysfunction and hypertension. Sato[40] demonstrated somatoautonomic reflexes that related cardiac function to gastrointestinal function and urinary tract function. Haldeman[41] presents a concept of multicausal factors in the production of pain in the lumbar spine and emphasizes the interrelationships of many factors in the manifestation of pain syndromes. The concepts discussed would be attributable to thoracic pain as well and should alert the clinician to multicausal factors in thoracic pain processes or diseases. His presentation discussed factors related to hyperesthesia, spinal problems, and pain, and explained why multiple approaches and a multidisciplinary approach may in fact be beneficial for a number of patients.

To assess a patient completely, a multiple model of approach may be necessary. If one attempts to marry the medical pathologic model with the functional model to expand our understanding of the lesion, as has been attempted in the lower spine by Cassidy[42] and by Haldeman,[43] it becomes apparent that an organized functional diagnostic analysis is a more important part of the diagnosis of the patient. This part of diagnosis has been largely neglected by the medical physician and possibly overused by the chiropractic physician.[44]

Classification of Pain in the Thoracic Spine

Love and Kiefer[45] in 1949 were two of the first to review and report protrusion of the thoracic disc and its production of a variety of symptoms. Pain, a common symptom, was often diagnosed as pleurodynia, rhythmicials neuralgia, or rhythmicials neuritis and fibrositis rather than discal protrusion. They were among the earliest to suggest that thoracic pain and rib cage pain were probably more attributable to musculoskeletal origin than to organic visceral origin, a fact that organized medicine struggles with even today. They further suggested that the upper thoracic vertebrae were more likely to produce these types of musculoskeletal neuralgic pain in the back, whereas the

lower thoracic vertebrae were more likely to produce radicular pain projected to the abdomen and groin. More often, they emphasized that intraabdominal disease was suggested rather than what they considered important—discal protrusion. That thoracic lumbar dysfunction can produce lumbar and pelvic pain has been reviewed and the mechanism suggested.[46] Costosternal dysfunction of T5-7 ribs also has been seen not only to produce local pain but pain and muscle spasm remote from the articulation, in the lower abdomen, the groin, and upper leg, as well as the lumbosacral region.[47] A number of other authors reported chest pain caused by costovertebral joints, rhythmicials, and posterior spinal muscles.[48-52]

Scheuermann's disease can produce an increased thoracic kyphosis and has also been seen clinically as a source of thoracic spinal pain. Bradford et al.[53] reported the use of spinal fusion with Harrington instrumentation and demonstrated some improvement in pain but related that because of the incidence of complications, conservative measures should be used for such patients, except in cases of unrelenting pain or spinal cord compression. Burke and Murray[54] reported that conservative management with rest and rehabilitation in cases of severe spinal injury with neurologic involvement produced comparable results to surgical procedures, and that the likelihood of developing postsurgical chronic pain was lessened.

In their text, *The Adult Spine*, Skubic and Kostuik[1] present a typical medical classification of thoracic pain syndromes:
I.   Thoracic Pain Syndromes without Neurological Deficit
II. Thoracic Pain with Neurologic Deficit
III. Postthoracotomy Pain Syndromes (See Classification Boxes 23-1 and 23-2.)

Medical Model of Pain: Emphasis on Pathologic Factors

1. Intervertebral Disc:
   • Herniation
   • Degeneration
   • Inflammation

BOX 23-1 ■ Classification of Pain in the Thoracic Spine

I.   Thoracic pain syndromes without neurologic impairment
   A. Viscerogenic and miscellaneous
   B. Costospondylogenic
      1. Costochondral
      2. Costovertebral
      3. Facetal
      4. Discogenic
   C. Neoplastic
   D. Infectious
   E. Structural
      1. Scoliosis
      2. Kyphosis
         a. Scheuermann's
         b. Posttraumatic
         c. Osteoporotic
   F. Cervical spondylogenic
II. Thoracic pain syndromes with neurologic impairment
   A. Neoplastic
      1. Extradural
         a. Primary
         b. Metastatic
      2. Intradural-extramedullary
      3. Intramedullary
   B. Infectious
   C. Thoracic disc herniation
III. Postthoracotomy syndrome

BOX 23-2 ■ Classification of Pain in the Thoracic Spine

I.   Intrathoracic
   A. Cardiovascular
      1. Angina pectoris
      2. Myocardial infarction
      3. Mitral valve prolapse
      4. Pericarditis
      5. Aortic aneurysm
   B. Pulmonary
      1. Pneumonia
      2. Carcinoma
      3. Pneumothorax
      4. Pleurisy
      5. Infarction, embolus
   C. Mediastinal
      1. Esophagitis, tumor
      2. Mediastinal tumors
II. Intraabdominal
   A. Hepatobiliary
      1. Hepatitis
      2. Abscess
      3. Cholecystitis, biliary colic
   B. Gastrointestinal
      1. Peptic ulcer disease
      2. Hernia—hiatal, inguinal, other
      3. Pancreatitis
III. Retroperitoneal
   A. Pyelonephritis
   B. Ureteral colic
   C. Aneurysm
   D. Tumor
IV. Miscellaneous
   A. Herpes zoster
   B. Polymyalgia rheumatica
   C. Hyperventilation syndrome
   D. Rib fracture, neoplasm

2. A. Vertebral body:
     • Spondylosis
     • Osteoporosis
  B. Rib:
     • Pathology
     • Exostosis
3. Posterior joint:
   • Instability
   • Congenital abnormality
   • Osteoarthritis
   • Rheumatoid arthritis

4. A. Soft tissue:
     • Ligamentous instability
     • Ligamentous, muscle contracture
  B. Costicartilage:
     • Calcification
     • Inflammation

5. Nerve tissue:
   • Inflammation
   • Compression or stretch
6. Visceral pathology

Chiropractic Model of Pain

Functional Factors: Mechanical Disorders

1. Posterior joint dysfunction, axis motion change
2. Discal dysfunction, internal or external strain, disruption
3. Costovertebral altered motion or respiratory dysfunction
4. Costochondral or sternal altered motion or respiratory dysfunction
5. Ligamentous strain
6. Muscular:
   • Postural fatigue
   • Hypertonicity
   • Imbalance or inappropriate action
7. Visceral-somatic dysfunction
8. Commonly accepted psychosocial factors:
   • Chronic pain syndrome
   • Psychologic factors, depression, hysteria
   • Malingering

Sources of Pain in the Thoracic Spine

The sources of pain in the thoracic region are thought to be similar to the structures in the lumbar and cervical spine. These structures gain their nerve supply from the sinuvertebral nerve and thoracic dorsal ramus. Wyke[55,56] reviewed the pain-sensitive structures in the thoracic spine. He described pain-sensitive nerve endings occurring in plexuses as free-ending of unmyelinated nerve fibers, which he found present in the following:

1. Fibrous capsules of the apophyseal joints, similar to fibrous capsules of all synovial joints
2. The interspinous ligaments and ligament flava, particularly more dense in the posterior ligaments
3. The periosteal coverings, fascias, and tendons
4. The dura, epidural fatty tissue
5. The blood vessels supplying the joints and cancellous bone of the vertebrae
6. The epidural and paravertebral veins

Branches of the sinuvertebral nerve innervate the thoracic vertebrae, the dura mater, the epidural blood vessels, and the posterior longitudinal ligaments. The sinuvertebral nerve is composed of an autonomic branch and a recurrent somatic branch that comes off the anterior superior surface of the thoracic root and passes back into the IVF (intervertebral foramina). The autonomic branch arises from gray ramus communicans at each segmental level or from the sympathetic ganglia near the nerve root. The thoracic dorsal rami supply the posterior thoracic muscles and the costotransverse joints. The proximal portion of the ribs is supplied by the sinuvertebral nerve, and the distal portion of the ribs is supplied by the sinuvertebral nerve. The zygapophyseal joints are innervated by the medial branch of the thoracic dorsal rami. It is likely that the thoracic disc is innervated by the sinuvertebral nerve, and it has been demonstrated to penetrate the disc along with blood vessels. Discs under repair have increased density of free nerve endings, as well as increased numbers of nerve fibers within the disc that are thought to arise as a result of increased vascularity stimulated by repair process.

Bogduk and Valencia[57] describe these neurologic relationships but remind us that, although it is likely that thoracic pain is caused by disorders of the thoracic synovial joints and muscles, no actual experimental evidence exists in the thoracic spine to confirm this conclusion. Wyke[55] is of the opinion, however, that because the mechanism is the same in the lumbar and cervical spine, it is likely that the mechanism is the same in the thoracic region, and therefore further experiments will find similar observations to the evidence found in these regions.

In the foregoing we have outlined a medical classification of pain related to the thoracic spine, demonstrating the emphasis on pathology. By reviewing Wyke's[56] and Bogduk's[57] tissue sources of pain and the suggested neurologic basis for the fact that pain can arise from nonphysiologic function of the thoracic spine, the muscular system, and the rib cage, the clinician must recognize the importance of spinal functional diagnosis and correction for control of pain. The clinician must also recognize the possibility that dysfunction of somatic structures has important reflex effects on the visceral organs as well as the cardiovascular and respiratory systems, reviewed elsewhere in this text, in some of the references in this chapter, and by Bronfort.[58] The examination and correction of spinal biomechanics should include careful monitoring of the effects of that correction as well as evaluation of the related organ systems. The osteopathic profession has over the years been most diligent in researching the relationship between spinal function, the autonomic nervous system, and visceral function. Homewood[15] outlined the theory of somatovisceral functional relationships, and Haldeman[59,60] gave some scientific basis for the theory of somatovisceral dysfunction. Clinical practice, however, demonstrates that the differential diagnosis of somatovisceral, viscerosomatic relationships, and organ pathology are difficult to assess.

Many authors have attempted to bridge these models, including Gatterman,[2] Schafer,[61,62] Dobrusin,[63] Bergmann et al.,[64] and Plaugher.[65] The integration of the medical model is an attempt to be certain that chiropractors will not neglect this model in their functional diagnostic approach. Overemphasis on the medical model has resulted in some instances in the total lack of the graduate's ability to understand the functional chiropractic model or its significance.

Diagnosis of musculoskeletal complaints in the thoracic region should include postural analysis, gross motion analysis, and static and motion palpation analysis assisted by other procedures when clinically indicated. Johnston[66-68] in a three-part series stressed the importance and interexaminer agreement on the diagnostic procedure to elicit somatic dysfunction and imbalance. Kobrossi and Steiman[69] reported on the use of thermography in dorsal and abdominal pain syndromes. Stillwagon et al.[70] suggest that thermography can be helpful as a diagnostic and assessment tool for the subluxation complex. Case studies on skin temperature have been reported by others, showing relationships between temperature changes and functional pathologies.[71,72] Plaugher et al.[73] studied interexaminer-intraexaminer reliability and para-

spinal skin temperature in the thoracic spine and reported substantial agreement of intraexaminer reliability and a significant association with skin temperature changes and palpation findings.

Kent and Gentempo[74] report that initial investigations using surface electromyelography (EMG) have shown an indication that it may be a reliable tool for the quantitive assessment of paraspinal muscle activity; therefore it is a recommended outcome assessment tool for chiropractic care. Sweat gland activity also has been associated with somatic dysfunction and reflex alteration.[75] Skin sensitivity[76] using skin rolling technique[77] and pressure algometry[78,79] have also been shown to be helpful in diagnosing spinal dysfunction and response to treatment. Radiographic assessment can assist in evaluation of posture and bony position, pathologic conditions, spinal dynamic alteration, and segmental alteration of motion.[80-82] Cox et al.[83] reported that osteophytic lipping of the thoracic spine was more prevalent in gallbladder disease, gastrointestinal disorders, and diabetes mellitus, and in a nonspecific study, coronary heart disease. Macones et al.[84] demonstrated hyperostosis as a result of mechanical forces at the costovertebral junctions, which they related to the iliocostalis muscle. This was shown to relate to occupation, the male sex, and dominant handedness. Osteophytic outgrowths also have been reported to produce compression on the sympathetic trunk.[85,86] As stated before, the thoracolumbar junction with its increased stress is an important site for degenerative change.[87,88]

The main diagnostic approach to developing an understanding of mechanical disorders is palpation. Fligg[89] outlined a classification of palpation. Schafer and Faye[3] discussed the importance of static palpation to elicit information about the tissues related to the manipulative lesion, such as tissue texture, bony alignment, skin temperature (inflammation), vascular change, and muscular tonicity. Sweat gland activity and skin hydration should be added to this list and have long been of interest to our profession.

Observation both follows and accompanies a good history. Observation of thoracic motion should be assessed during gait to evaluate arm swing, rhythm and amplitude, as well as postural change and gross spinal motion. Gross spinal motion in all its ranges—flexion/extension, lateral flexion, and rotation—should be assessed with the patient both standing and sitting. These postural dynamic tests start with observation of the static posture, the alignment of the head, shoulders, and pelvis, scapular position symmetry of muscle contraction for PA and AP, as well as the lateral posture. The degree of kyphosis and the overall postural balance and alignment for efficiency are important.[90,91]

Johnston[92] showed a high level of agreement in interexamination testing in gross passive range of motion. Sportelli and Tarala[90] presented a brief overview of physical examination of the spine, showing an integrated postural orthopedic neurologic approach.

Lateral flexion before a double plumbline should show an even curve from T1 to T12 and symmetry of motion to each side. Rotation should be assessed for symmetry; full trunk rotation is best used to assess the motion from T6 to T12, whereas full neck rotation is best suited to analyze motion from T1 to T6. Flexion-extension is limited in the thoracic spine and is best analyzed with the patient in a seated posture, where observations of the thoracic muscular function can be more easily assessed. Coupling of the general techniques of static palpation and springing vertebral challenge in the thoracic spine elicits more information about individual segments and does not depend on symmetry of spinal structures, which may be a problem, rendering false information, because bent spinous processes are a common finding in the thoracic spine.[93]

Faye[3] developed and taught the techniques initiated and presented by Gillet, who also had lectured to the profession and had prepared a series of lectures notes called the Belgian Chiropractic Research Notes.[94] Liekens, a colleague of Gillet's, was credited with developing a more precise movement-oriented procedure for spinal palpation that has been developed by Grice and, later, Fligg at the Canadian Chiropractic College; presented in class notes since 1980; and published in other sources.[29,30,33,95-100]

Dynamic Palpation of the Thoracic Spine

General Principles Related to Palpation

Patient's Concerns

1. Place your hands on a patient with respect and concern for his or her comfort. To examine the thoracic spine, have the patient cross hands across the chest, locking the upper body into a unit for ease, control, and precision of motion.
2. Educate the patient as to the purpose of your test and effect a trial run within the patient's tolerance and pain concerns.
3. Control the movement to provide for a smooth motion that allows you to focus an end-feel challenge of each segment.

Examiner's Concerns

1. Protect your posture from strain and fatigue and attempt to keep your body still, moving only your arms and hands to produce the motion.
2. Control the patient's active/passive motion with the indifferent hand throughout the movement, producing a rhythmic motion with minimal muscular effort, using your larger muscles.
3. Palpatory fingers should be stable and comfortable throughout the motion, and able to exert a comfortable challenge at the end of the motion.
4. Visualization of the anatomic structures and their motion throughout the test is helpful in appreciating the dynamics.

Fligg[89] reviewed the various motion palpation techniques: (1) static joint challenge, (2) joint play, (3) end joint analysis, and (4) dynamic motion palpation with the view of explaining the origin and application of each procedure.

Static joint challenge developed out of static palpation procedures and was so common to many practitioners that its origin is difficult to trace. The procedure is commonly used in the thoracic spine in the prone position. Fligg discussed the limitations of this procedure but pointed out that for acute pain it is often the palpatory procedure of choice.

Joint play was developed by Mennell[101] and was primarily used in peripheral joints for evaluating ranges of involuntary motion. This procedure was included in spinal examination and by some was known as end joint challenge, which had been used as a development of static joint challenge techniques.

Faye, in lectures and in a text,[3] popularized the generalized end joint spinal analysis procedures developed by Gillet and Liekens.[94] This procedure is very effective in the thoracic spine because our upright posture produces a thoracic spine in almost complete extension; therefore the extension challenge (see Figure 23-7) is easily performed. Reliability studies of motion palpation all have shown good intraexaminer reliability but in general not significant interexaminer reliability. Love et al.[102] studied the joint challenge technique in the thoracic spine and showed good intraexaminer reliability but not significant interexaminer reliability. They also reported a common finding that T9-10 was the most frequent level of fixation using this general joint challenge procedure. This lower dorsal area is commonly found subluxate using the prone movable table palpation challenge technique as well.

Dynamic motion palpation was developed out of Liekens' procedures, reported by Gillet and Liekens.[94] Our development of this technique attempted to correlate actual spinal dynamics and interpret what forces would limit the motions.[27,33] Gillet and Liekens[94] traditionally classified fixations as (1) muscular, (2) ligamentous, and (3) osseous. Schafer and Faye[3] discuss this classification in more detail, changing the third classification to an articular fixation that they describe as a more complete fixation that has developed adhesive changes. It is clinically important to note that fixations can be unilateral and fixing one facet can cause hypermobility at the opposite facet joint. If we carry this principle further, the clinician must realize that a motion segment may be hypermobile in one range of motion of the facet, and the holding elements can create hypermobility in another direction of motion within the same segment or facet. If a segment is blocked in motion at both facets, hypermobility might be established above

or below the joint, and these hypermobile joints should not be adjusted in the plane of that hypermobility. Dynamic palpation allows us to assess a number of planes of motion of these segments and, along with motion study radiography, deal more specifically with adjusting the direction of fixation and avoiding the direction or the segment of hypermobility.

Dynamic Motion Palpation of the Thoracic Spine

Basic Complete Screening Procedure
Flexion-Extension (Figure 23-8): Contact is in the interspinous space with three fingers or the thumb and index finger. Patient is controlled by having arms crossed in front with examiner's second hand on the elbows.

Motion: Patient is gently flexed and extended by force on the elbows and the palpating hand detects motion between the spinous process at each level. As each segment is brought into full extension, a slight challenge is given to detect end feel of each segment (Figures 23-9 and 23-10).

Lateral Flexion/Spinous Challenge
Because of the unusual change in the normal coupled motion at approximately T6-7, alteration of the technique for the upper thoracic vertebrae and lower thoracic spine is suggested.

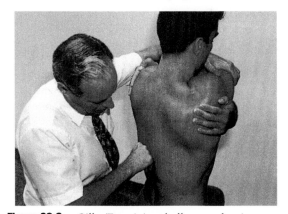

Figure 23-8   Gillet/Faye joint challenge palpation. Patient's arms are crossed in front with examiner's second hand on the elbows.

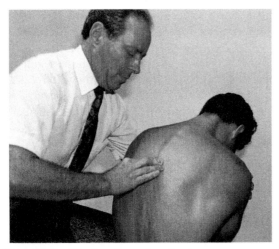

Figure 23-9   Flexion dynamic palpation.

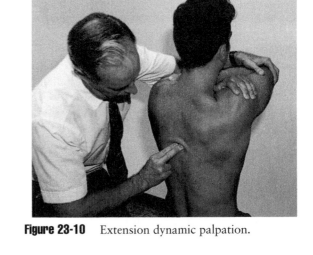

Figure 23-10   Extension dynamic palpation.

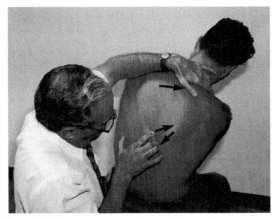

Figure 23-11   Dynamic palpation lower thoracic vertebrae. Normal spinous deviation to concavity T6-12.

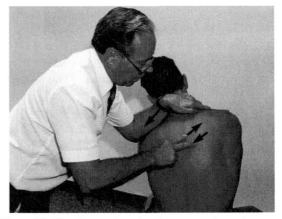

Figure 23-12   Dynamic palpation upper thoracic vertebrae. Normal spinous deviation to the convexity T1-6.

Contact of lower thoracic vertebrae: The spinous process of the vertebra below is hooked with the middle finger, while the index finger contacts the spinous process of the vertebra above, and the non-contact hand across the shoulders of the patient provides the leverage to laterally flex the patient from neutral to one side. Movement from T12 upward to T5-7 should show deviation of the spinous process toward the concave side. At the end of the motion, a slight challenge evaluates the motion, its character, and range. This test is done bilaterally using the opposite hands (Figure 23-11).

Palpation of upper thoracic from T6-8 up to T1 or above: Hook the spinous process of the inferior vertebra, and push the spinous process of the superior vertebra while the patient is flexed to the same side. In the upper thoracic region of the spine, the spinous processes should move to the convexity. The examiner's nonpalpating hand can be placed across the shoulders or on the head, using the head as a lever. This results in movement and control of cervical thoracic motion and thereby challenges cervical muscles that may be involved in cervicothoracic fixations (Figure 23-12).

Rotation

Students often experience difficulty in palpating this region because of the large muscles and tight spinous process overlapping. The indifferent hand is placed on the elbow or arm of the patient, who has arms crossed so that the contralateral arm is on top. This posture forms a good lever to control the rotation motion. The contact hand uses the thumb or the thumb and index finger on one or two adjacent spinous processes. Rotation to one side with an end point challenge is done by the indifferent hand controlling the rotation, and the palpating fingers exerting slight challenge as they walk up the spine testing rotation at each level (Figure 23-13).

Rib Palpation

Rotation Contact: Costovertebral fixations are best analyzed in the seated posture as in thoracic vertebral assessment, with the patient's arms folded across the body, a contact on the arm or elbow of the outside arm (similar to thoracic palpation), and the palpating fingers or thumb contacting the nonarticulating tubercle of the rib joint just lateral to the transverse process. At times, depending on the patient's musculature, the examiner must move more laterally to the angle of the ribs to gain the best springing rib palpation (Figure 23-14).

Analysis: Range of motion, resistance, and blockage of end feel is noted of this caliper-like motion.

Lateral Flexion

Contact Test I: Place the fourth finger on the lateral aspect of the lower rib, the third finger on the interspace, and index finger on the upper rib. Patient is laterally flexed using shoulder contact. Interspace motion is compared (Figures 23-15 and 23-16).

Contact Test II: With slight lateral flexion and the same finger contact, the respiratory function of

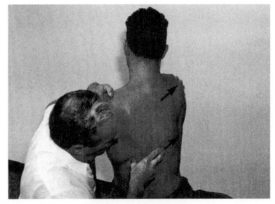

Figure 23-14 Rotation rib palpation.

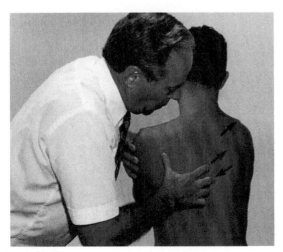

Figure 23-13 Rotation dynamic palpation.

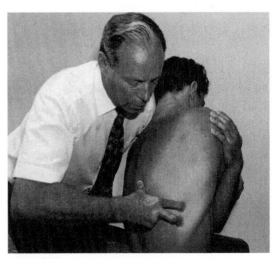

Figure 23-15 Rib palpation: bucket handle open.

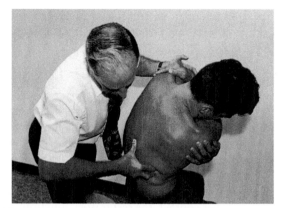

Figure 23-16   Rib palpation: bucket handle closed.

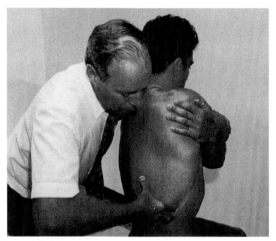

Figure 23-17   Respiratory function: inspiration, expiration.

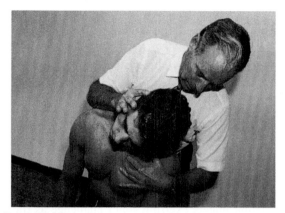

Figure 23-18   Anterior rib palpation: bucket handle and caliper motion.

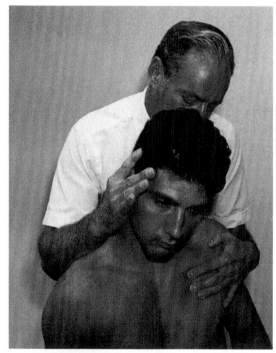

Figure 23-19   Upper ribs respiratory function: inspiration, expiration.

the ribs can be assessed by asking the patient to deeply inspire and expire (Figure 23-17).

Analysis: Free bucket-handle motion of the ribs should be felt during full lateral flexion and during respiratory functions. The upper ribs are protected by the arm and scapula; it is advisable to take an anterior chest contact for the upper ribs for this procedure.

Sternocostal fixations can be assessed by contacting the sternocostal junction with the fingers and producing posterior rotation and lateral flexion of the shoulders. Respiratory function of the shoulder also should be assessed with this same contact (Figures 23-18 and 23-19).

It must be realized that many individual techniques have been developed in spinal palpation. These methods allow for systematic assessment of dynamic thoracic motion and respiratory function of both the thoracic spine and ribs. Interpretation of the results gives the clinician some appreciation of the forces, particularly a clue to the muscles involved in producing the fixation patterns. Joint challenge and end feel challenge techniques are also of some value in assessing joint function at the multiple synovial joints of this region. The use of movable tables allows for motion procedures to assess spinal motion in a passive posture (Figure 23-20).

It should be stated at this point that fixations may be found singly or as a group pattern. Scoliosis and rotation deficits seen on radiograph often show a characteristic group of vertebrae involved in fixation along with the rib cage, particularly as these problems become more chronic or when patients become less physically fit.

In my opinion, the process of joint fixation begins with muscular tonicity alteration—spasm, inability to relax, or inappropriate excitability when at rest or when stress or activity takes place. Physiologically, if a muscle is under contraction for any sustained period, contraction or shortening of the muscle fibers takes place; thereby the body economizes on its energy expenditure. The result is, however, loss of motion in the opposite direction to the motion created by that muscle on contraction. Once a range of motion is lost the ligaments shorten, making the fixation more permanent. This process is said to take place starting within a few hours if motion does not occur and can develop some degree of measurable chronicity with days and weeks. Clinicians are of the opinion

that they can perceive the difference between muscular fixation and ligamentous fixation; no research has been undertaken to assess this position. Once there is a consistent loss of motion within a joint, articular and cartilaginous changes take place.

This final change is consistent with degenerative arthritis changes and demonstrates the importance of maintenance of spinal function and the management of fixation subluxations. The dynamic adjustive thrust has been shown to be the most effective tool for control of pain.[103] The reasons may be multiple, such as biomechanical, biochemical, or neurologic.[104] In the management of spinal dysfunction, one should recognize that there are stages of pathogenesis of any lesion, and our responsibility is to institute a total management program not only of adjustments but at some stage a rehabilitative exercise and educational program.

I am also of the opinion that in using the dynamic adjustive thrust, a more effective management approach is not only to elicit the direction of the fixation but also to attempt to elicit the muscular forces involved in producing the dysfunction and determine the stage of the pathogenic process; that is, muscular contraction or contracture, ligamentous and osseous changes, and to deliver the adjustment so that it affects these tissues as positively as possible. To make these decisions, one must integrate all of the physical examination procedures along with radiographic analyses including motion radiographic studies to develop a complete understanding of the lesion. Korr[105] suggested that much of the sensory input that alters reflex neurologic activity in somatic dysfunction may come from within the muscular system rather than from the joint proprioceptors. With this in mind, attention and treatment should be directed toward assuring that these muscular reflex patterns are altered in our treatment. Dynamic palpation allows for some appreciation of these muscular forces and an adjustive technique can be selected, not only to correct the fixation but also to introduce a dynamic stretch within the muscle that is preloaded or stretched before the thrust, thereby increasing the neurologic effectiveness of the adjustment. Empirical

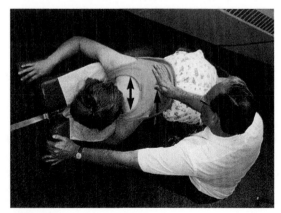

Figure 23-20   Adjusting table in motion: spinous challenge.

use of these procedures seems to improve results when this consideration is given. When thought is given to the specific muscle groups that are involved in the dysfunction or to the muscle groups that should be actively controlling optimal motion, an exercise and treatment program specific or appropriate for the muscle groups can be established.

Dynamic Motion Palpation Findings and Suggested Adjustive Correction

Serratus Posterior Superior

1. Lower thoracic
   Finding: Reversal of spinous in lateral flexion
   Adjustment: Spinous push (Figure 23-21)
   Sitting rib adjustment (Figure 23-22)

2. Upper thoracic
   Finding: Restricted anterior rotation upper ribs
   Restricted spinous rotation
   Adjustment: Thumb on spinous of thoracic, thenar contact on angle of rib (Figure 23-23)

3. Quadratus lumborum
   Finding: Restricted anterior rotation lower ribs
   Adjustment: Thenar contact on rib angle, sitting rotation adjustment (See Figure 23-22.)

4. Splenius cervicis and capitus
   Finding: Because this muscle allows normal mechanics in the upper thoracic vertebrae, palpatory findings are limited; anterior rotation of cervical spine and occiput and hypermobility

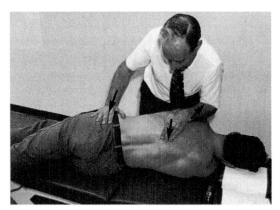

Figure 23-21   Reverse lumbar roll.

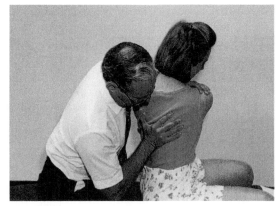

Figure 23-22   Sitting thoracic or rib adjustment.

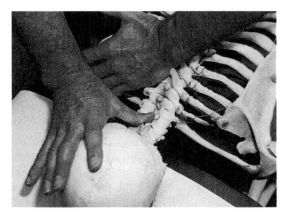

Figure 23-23   Spinous, transverse process, or rib contact. Head may be turned toward or away.

of flexion or excessive spinous deviation in lateral flexion of the thoracic spinouses may give an indication
Adjustment: Prone TM with cervical spine turned away from contact (Figure 23-24)
Secondary cervical fixation: Prone transverse process contact same position

Semispinalis Thoracis

This muscle is the major muscle in control of normal thoracic mechanics. Its attachment to the spinous processes of C6-7 and T1-4 in separate slips down to transverse process of T6-12 controls the normal mechanics of the thoracic spine in lateral flexion along with other muscle groups. Because this muscle controls normal mechanics, it is difficult to

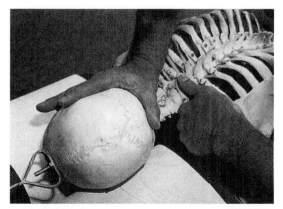

Figure 23-24   TM (thumb move) adjustment, head away from contact, traction by indifferent hand.

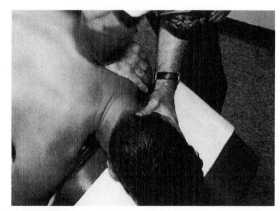

Figure 23-26   Transverse process or rib to occiput adjustment.

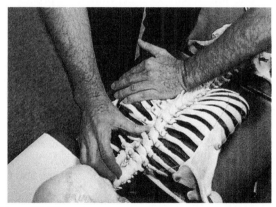

Figure 23-25   Thoracic spinous: transverse process or rib contact.

demonstrate palpation findings. The adjustment recommended is to take a spinous process contact with one hand and the transverse process–pisiform contact at the lower fixation involved. The spinous contact produces the traction; the head turned slightly toward the lesioned side with the pisiform on appropriate transverse process applies the thrust. Thrust is short amplitude and comes from a preload from superior to inferior distraction (Figure 23-25).

Semispinalis cervicis hypertonicity produces a superior pull on the transverse processes T1-6 and related spinous inferior C2-5. The combination

adjustment (thumb to spine opposite pisiform to transverse process, neck turned toward lesioned side, thrust from superior to inferior) is again indicated. The adjustment for semispinalis capitus is similar with contact on the occiput; the headpiece is lowered (Figure 23-26).

The iliocostalis lumborum muscle when hypertonic fixes the lower six ribs bucket handle down, caliper open. The secondary fixation involves the lumbar spine (type II fixation).[27] Two adjustive procedures are effective. First is the sitting rotation rib adjustment. (See Figure 23-22.) The contact hand is on the angle of the rib and the patient is positioned in rotation, slight lateral flexion away from side of contact. Thrust is given from inferior to superior. Second is the reverse lumbar roll. (See Figure 21-21.) The patient is placed in side posture, lesioned side up, shoulder forward, pelvis and leg backward. Contact is made with the forearm on the lower rib angles, fingers on the lumbar spinous process, thrust on rib angle superiorly and spinous processes are preloaded with a constant pressure from the superior, laterally; this preload pressure is reinforced by the second contact hand on the anterior ilium, which becomes the main preload force with a mild posterior thrust.

The iliocostalis thoracis portion is a main postural stabilizer of the thoracic spine, running from the upper six ribs to the lower six ribs at the angle of the ribs. Spasm or hypertonicity would produce in the superior ribs bucket handle down, and in the lower ribs bucket handle up. Any adjustment should be concerned with the direction of fixation. The thrust for the superior ribs should be inferior to superior (Figure 23-27), and the thrust for the inferior ribs should be from superior to inferior (Figure 23-28).

Prone rib contact adjustment: Superior rib correction subluxation is to the inferior. The crossed bilateral with contact on the angle of rib, second hand on opposite transverse process to stabilize the thoracic vertebra. Torquing thrust of shallow depth assists in the correction. (See Figure 23-28.)

Inferior rib correction: The rib is subluxated to the superior. Bilateral, noncrossed hands, contact hand thrusts from superior to inferior on angle of rib; support hand stabilizes opposite transverse process, same shallow torquing thrust.

Upper portion iliocostalis: Upper ribs elevated, bucket handle superior. Spinous processes of cervicals fixed toward side of lesion.

Double rib spinous contact (see Figures 23-25 and 23-26): Thrust on angle of rib from superior to inferior. The indifferent hand contacts the spinous process in the cervicals; patient's head is turned toward the side of contact.

Longissimus thoracic portion of sacrospinalis: This muscle is an important postural stabilizer, connecting transverse processes of lower 9 to 10 thoracic vertebrae and lumbar transverse processes. Fixation produces a posterior inferior fixation of thoracic vertebral transverse processes.

Prone adjustment: Contact transverse processes thrust from inferior to superior. In the lower thoracic, having the patient arch the back against the preload and slightly resist with just the back muscles assists in the comfort of this adjustment and helps protect the patient from painful extension and jamming of the facets. The thrust is of a lower amplitude and high velocity. Experience has shown that the procedure often taught (deep breath then breathe out and thrust), although it helps in patient relaxation, often leaves the patient without defense. This may result in trauma; therefore the procedure just described (Figures 23-29 and 23-30) is suggested.

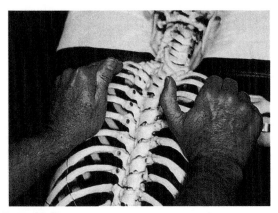

Figure 23-27   Inferior rib bilateral or unilateral.

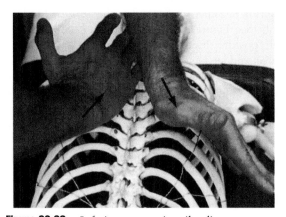

Figure 23-28   Inferior or superior rib adjustment. Thrust on either hand, opposite hand (indifferent) produces stabilization.

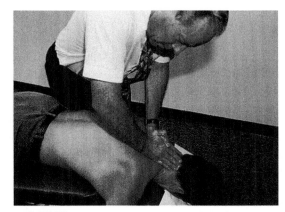

Figure 23-29   Transverse process or rib contact. Thrust may be from inferior to superior or from superior to inferior.

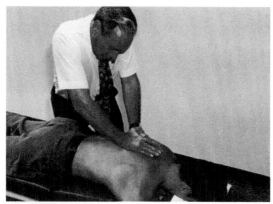

Figure 23-30   Lower thoracic bridge contact inferior to superior.

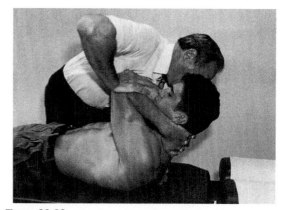

Figure 23-32   Supine upper thoracic or rib.

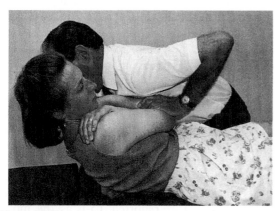

Figure 23-31   Supine lower thoracic or rib.

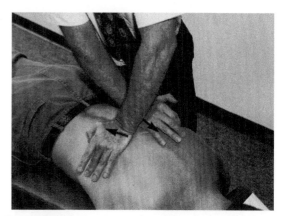

Figure 23-33   Crossed bilateral with torque. Transverse process or rib.

Supine: Anterior thoracic adjustment (Figure 23-31) described later is also effective.

Longissimus, Cervical Portion
Prone transverse process adjustment from superior to inferior with patient's head turned away from lesioned side is used. Secondary hand produces traction on cervical transverse processes. (See Figure 23-26.) Supine upper dorsal transverse process contact with patient's hands clasped around the neck assists in stretching this muscle and releasing fixation (Figure 23-32).

Longissimus Capitus Portion
Prone transverse process contact adjustment from superior to inferior, secondary hand on occiput,

head turned away from lesioned side; headpiece lowered slightly. (See Figure 23-26.) Deep segmental muscles, such as rotatores and multifidi, respond well to crossed bilateral pisiform contact with torque (Figure 23-33) or pisiform transverse process spinous thumb contacts, causing rotatory shearing between adjacent segments (Figure 23-34).

The supine anterior thoracic adjustment can be made specific if the contact hand is placed at the bend of the thoracic spine. The thrust is delivered headward while the arms lock the body as a unit. This creates a flexion separation of the segments involved and is very effective for segmental muscles. (See Figures 23-31 and 23-32.) Segmental fixations involving small muscles that produce extension of thoracic segments can be corrected by a spinous

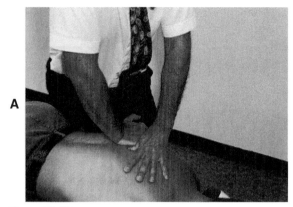

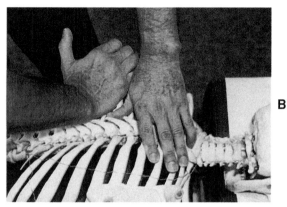

Figure 23-34   A, Transverse process/spinous segmental fix—small muscles; B, Transverse process/spinous segmental fix—larger muscles.

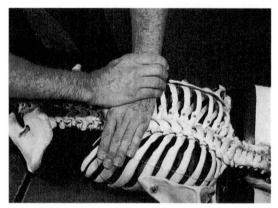

Figure 23-35   Drop centerpiece prone adjustment for use during pregnancy.

contact thrust from inferior to superior. (See Figures 23-31 and 23-32.)

General Adjustments

The longitudinal stretch for both cervical and thoracic segmental muscles is often helpful to release deep fixations. When traction is applied to the cervical spine with a short amplitude thrust, patients may feel release or stretch in the thoracic or even the lumbar spine. The standing thoracic lift is often used when a table is not available, when the thoracic vertebrae are rigidly fixed, or during pregnancy. The lift affords traction headward; the chest is the general contact. The key factor is that the thrust is directed longitudinally along the angle of the facets.

A drop centerpiece is helpful for prone adjustments when indicated, as in pregnancy (Figure 23-35).

The anterior thoracic adjustment has received much attention. Bergman, in lecture notes, asks the question, "Are anterior thoracics really anterior?" He explains the common appearance of a flattened or saucered mid-thoracic spine as caused by flexion of a thoracic vertebra, or by excessive activity of the spinal extensors causing an extension stacking of a group of segments above; hence the flat appearance.[106] The authors describe one method of a supine anterior thoracic, which is also described in detail by Fligg.[107] Fracheboud et al.[108] reported T5-6 as the most frequent site of involvement. Interscapular pain, respiratory problems, chest pain, and stomach complaints, in that order, were reported to be related. The paper also attempts to show the approach of various system techniques. My own observation would suggest that a muscle group such as the semispinalis thoracic, the spinalis cervicis, or possibly the multifidus, which attaches to the transverse process below and to the spinous processes of vertebrae above, would cause the lower vertebra to flex, particularly if bilateral contraction took place and the vertebrae above would extend. Other types of correction also are suggested in this case, and many other adjustive procedures are available to us for varying needs of the patient (Figure 23-36). These suggestions only serve to portray the thinking process in selecting the most effective correction.

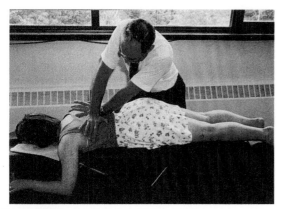

Figure 23-36   Knife-edge spinous adjustment.

Conclusion

This chapter was produced with the thought in mind to present an understanding of thoracic biomechanics that would stimulate thoughtful management of pain syndromes, pathomechanical states, and neurophysiologic effects related to subluxation/dysfunction of the thoracic spine and ribs. I have introduced a concept of not only considering joint position and joint mobility but also the holding elements: the muscles, ligaments, and discs. The suggestion has been made that the dynamic adjustment is probably the most effective tool in controlling pain and altering these intrinsic and extrinsic factors involved in aberrant biomechanical processes. Inherent in the discussion is the understanding of the pathokinesis that would allow us to develop other methods of treatment to benefit these intrinsic and extrinsic factors involved in the process and their reflex based or nonreflex-based relationship to the nervous system. Emphasis has been placed on the role of what would appear to be the most responsive tissue to treatment other than the nervous system involved in producing spinal biomechanical problems: the spinal musculature. An attempt was made to emphasize that there is an optimal neurologic pattern and therefore an optimal harmony of muscular control of the statics and dynamics of the spine. If the control or the harmony of muscular function is lost, the result is an alteration of joint dynamics or changes in the axis of motion of the motion segment, which causes excess wear and tear and sometimes pain. It is advisable for a clinician to address the kinesiopathogenesis of the spine in a systematic manner with an understanding of optimal function, degrees of abnormal function that may be present, and the demands of structural change (pathogenesis) that may occur. With this understanding of the problem, a more effective management program may be established. Such a program should deal with the acute reactive painful phase of treatment, the rehabilitative stabilization phase of treatment that involves patient responsibility, and, if necessary, the supportive maintenance phase of care. Total management of the patient not only addresses the intrinsic and extrinsic factors related to aberrant spinal biomechanics, but also the illness behavior and, finally, the wellness awareness and behavior of the patient. In the chiropractic model of care, the patient is approached on a physical basis with the view of not only relieving pain and dysfunction, but also of reestablishing neurologic balance and integrity to the system as a whole.

References

1. Skubic JW, Kostuik JP. Thoracic pain syndromes and thoracic disk herniation 1988. In: Frymoyer JW, editor. The adult spine: principles and practice. New York: Raven Press; 1991.
2. Gatterman MI, Panzer DM. Disorders of the thoracic spine. In: Gatterman MI. Chiropractic management of spine related disorders. 2nd ed. Baltimore: Lippincott Williams & Wilkins; 2003. p. 198-228.
3. Schafer RC, Faye LJ. Motion palpation and chiropractic technic: principles of dynamic chiropractic. Vol. 4, 1st ed. Huntington Beach, CA: The Motion Palpation Institute; 1989. p. 143-94.
4. White AA, Panjabi MM. Clinical biomechanics of the spine. Toronto: JB Lippincott; 1978.
5. Valencia F. Biomechanics of the thoracic spine. Vol. 14. In: Grant T, editor. Physical therapy of the cervical and thoracic spine. New York: Churchill Livingstone; 1988.
6. Wyke BD. Morphological and functional features of the innervation of the costovertebral joints. Folia Morph Prague 1975;23:296-305.
7. Andersson GB, Ortengren R, Herbertz P. Quantitative electromyographic studies of back muscle activity related to posture and body. Orthop Clin North Am 1977;8:85.

8. Andersson GB, Ortengren R. Myoelectric back muscle activity during sitting. Scand J Rehabil Med Suppl 1974;3:73.

9. Nachemson A. Lumbar intradiscal pressure, experimental studies on post mortem material. Acta Orthop Scand Suppl 43;1960:1-104.

10. Andriacchi T, Schultz A, Belytschko T, Galante J. A model for studies of mechanical interactions between the lumbar spine and rib cage. J Biomech 1974;7:497-507.

11. Gray H. Gray's anatomy: the classic collector's edition. New York: Crown Publishers; 1977.

12. Smorl G, Junghanns H. The human spine in health and disease. New York: Grune Stratton; 1971. p. 32-4.

13. Carver W. Carver's chiropractic analysis of chiropractic principles as applied to pathology, relatology, symptomatology, and diagnosis. Oklahoma City: Self-published; 1909.

14. Beatty HG. Anatomical adjustive technic. 2nd ed. Denver: Self-published; 1939.

15. Homewood HG. The neurodynamics of the vertebral subluxation. Toronto: Valkyrie Press; 1962.

16. White AA, Panjabi MM. Analysis of the mechanics of the thoracic spine in man. Acta Orthop Scand Suppl 1969;127:1-105.

17. Panjabi MM, Brand RA, White AA. Mechanical properties of lower thoracic spine as shown by three-dimensional load-displacement curves. J Bone Joint Surg 1976;58A:642.

18. Vasilev V, Ovcharov V, Malinor G. Age-related changes in the thoracic intervertebral disc of humans. Nauchni Tr Vissh Med Inst Sofia 1971;50:15-24.

19. Bastin JM, Thomes JD. Acquired blocks and vertebral fusions in cases of degenerative discopathy and of joint aging. Rev Rheum Mal Osteoartic 1973;40:443-6.

20. Quiring DP, Warfel JH. The head, neck, and trunk. Philadelphia: Lea & Febiger; 1969.

21. Quiring DP, Warfel JH. The extremities 2. Philadelphia: Lea & Febiger; 1967.

22. Kapandji IA. The physiology of the joints. Vol 11. The trunk and vertebral column. London: Churchill Livingstone; 1974.

23. Gregersen GG, Lucas DB. An in vivo study of the axial rotation of the human thoracolumbar spine. J Bone Joint Surg 1967;49A:247.

24. White AA, Panjabi MM. The basic kinematics of the human spine: a review of past and current knowledge. Spine 1978;3:12.

25. White AA, Panjabi MM. Spinal kinematics: the research status of spinal manipulative therapy. NINCDS Monograph No. 15:93. Washington, DC: U.S. Department of Health, Education, and Welfare; 1975.

26. Grice AS. Harmony of joint and muscle function in the prevention of lower back syndromes. J Can Chiro Assoc 1976;20:2.

27. Grice AS. Radiographic, biomechanical, and clinical factors in lumbar lateral flexion. Part 1. J Manipulative Physiol Ther 1979;2:26.

28. Cassidy JD. Roentgenological examinations of the functional mechanics of the lumbar spine in lateral flexion. J Can Chiro Assoc 1976;20:2-13.

29. Gitelman R. A chiropractic approach to biomechanical disorders of the lumbar spine and pelvis. In: Haldeman S, editor. Modern developments in the principles and practice of chiropractic. New York: Appleton-Century-Crofts; 1980.

30. Grice AS. A biomechanical approach to cervical and dorsal adjusting. In: Haldeman S, editor. Modern developments in the principles and practice of chiropractic. New York: Appleton-Century-Crofts; 1980.

31. Steindler A. Kinesiology of the human body under normal and pathological conditions. Springfield, IL: Charles C Thomas; 1955.

32. Basmajian JB. Muscles alive: their function revealed by electromyography. Baltimore: Williams & Wilkins; 1967.

33. Grice AS. Scalenus anticus syndrome: diagnosis and chiropractic adjustive procedure. J Can Chiro Assoc 1977;(Mar):3-10.

34. Beal MC. Viscerosomatic reflexes: a review. JAOA 1985;85:786-98.

35. Beal MC. Palpatory testing for somatic dysfunction in patients with cardiovascular disease. JAOA 1983; 82(11):73-82.

36. Cox JM, Gorbis S, Dick LM, Rogers JC, Rogers FJ. Palpable musculoskeletal findings in coronary artery disease: results of a double-blind study. JAOA 1983; 82(11):86-90.

37. Beal MC, Morlock JW. Somatic dysfunction associated with pulmonary disease. JAOA 1984;84(2):57-61.

38. Beal MC, Kleiber GE. Somatic dysfunction as a predictor of coronary artery disease. JAOA 1985;85(5):70-5.

39. Johnston WL, Hill JL, Sealey JW, Sucher BM. Palpatory findings in the cervicothoracic region: variations in normotensive and hypertensive subjects. A preliminary report. JAOA 1980;79(5):55-63.

40. Sato A. The importance of somato-autonomic reflexes in the regulation of visceral organ function. J Can Assoc 1976;20(4):32-8.

41. Haldeman S. Why one cause of back pain. In: Buerger AA, Tobis JS, editors. Approaches to the validation of manipulative therapy. Springfield, IL: Charles C Thomas; 1977.

42. Kirkaldy-Willis WH. Managing low back pain. 2nd ed. New York: Churchill-Livingstone; 1988. p. 4.

43. Haldeman S. The neurophysiology of pain. In: Haldeman S, editor. Principles and practice of chiropractic. 2nd ed. East Norwalk, CT: Appleton & Lange; 1992. p. 165-84.

44. Schafer RC. Clinical biomechanics: musculoskeletal actions and reactions. Baltimore: Williams & Wilkins; 1983.

45. Love JG, Kiefer EJ. Root pain in paraplegia due to protrusions of thoracic intervertebral disks. J Neurosurg 1950;7:62-9.

46. Maigne R. Low back pain of thoracolumbar origin. Arch Phys Med Rehabil 1980;(Sep):61.

47. Tichy J, Mojzisova L. The role of sternocostal articulations in low back pain. Manual Medicine 1986;2: 122-5.

48. Arroyo JF, Jolliet P, Junod AF. Costovertebral joint dysfunction: another misdiagnosed cause of atypical chest pain. Postgrad Med J 1992;68:655-9.

49. Chiacchi MS. The association of the serratus anticus and rhomboid major musculature in anterolateral thoracic pain syndromes: a synopsis. Dig Chir Econ 1991;34:50.

50. Fam AG. Musculoskeletal chest wall pain. Can Med Assoc J 1985;(Sep):379-89.

51. Raney FL. Costovertebral-costotransverse joint complex as the source of local or referred pain. J Bone Joint Surg 1966;48A:1451-2.

52. Maurer EL. The thoracic-costal facet syndrome with introduction of the margin line and the rib sign. ACA J Chiro 1976;10S:151-64.

53. Bradford DS, Moe JE, Montalvo FJ, Winter RB. Scheuermann's kyphosis. J Bone Joint Surg June 1975; 57A:4.

54. Burke BC, Murray DD. The management of thoracic and thoracolumbar injuries of the spine with neurological involvement. J Bone Joint Surg 1976;1B:58.

55. Wyke B. The neurological basis of thoracic spinal pain. Rheumatol Phys Med 1967;10(7):356-68.

56. Wyke BD. Articular neurology: a review. Physiotherapy 1972;58:94-9.

57. Bogduk N, Valencia F. Innervation and pain patterns of the thoracic spine. In: Ruth G, editor. Physical therapy of the cervical and thoracic spine. New York: Churchill-Livingstone; 1988.

58. Bronfort G. Effectiveness of spinal manipulation and adjustments. In: Haldeman S, editor. Principles and practice of chiropractic. 2nd ed. East Norwalk, CT: Appleton & Lange; 1992.

59. Haldeman S. Modern developments in the principles and practice of chiropractic. New York: Appleton-Century-Crofts; 1980.

60. Haldeman S. Principles and practice of chiropractic. 2nd ed. East Norwalk, CT: Appleton & Lange; 1992.

61. Schafer RC. Clinical chiropractic: the management of pain and disability. Upper body complaints. Huntington Beach, CA: The Motion Palpation Institute; 1991.

62. Schafer RC. Chiropractic and physical spinal diagnosis. Oklahoma City: Assoc Chirop Acad Press; 1980.

63. Dobrusin R. An osteopathic approach to conservative management of thoracic outlet syndromes. JAOA 1989; 89(8):1046-56.

64. Peterson DH, Bergmann TF. Chiropractic technique. 2nd ed. St Louis: Mosby; 2002.

65. Plaugher G. Textbook of clinical chiropractic: a specific biomechanical approach. Baltimore: Williams & Wilkins; 1993.

66. Johnston WL. Segmental definition. Part I. A focal point for diagnosis of somatic dysfunction. JAOA 1988; 88(1):99-105.

67. Johnston WL. Segmental definition. Part II. Application of an indirect method in osteopathic manipulative treatment. JAOA 1988;88(2):211-7.

68. Johnston WL. Segmental definition. Part III. Definitive basis for distinguishing somatic findings of visceral reflex origin. JAOA 1988;88(3):347-63.

69. Kobrossi T, Steiman I. Thermographic investigation of viscerogenic pain: a case report. JCCA 1990;34:3.

70. Stillwagon G, Stillwagon KL, Stillwagon BS, Dalesio DL. Chiropractic thermography. ICA Review 1992; Jan/Feb:3-8.

71. BenEliyahu DJ. Infrared thermal imaging of the vertebral subluxation complex. ICA Review 1992;Jan/Feb:14-7.

72. Diakow RP. Thermographic assessment of sacroiliac syndrome: report of a case. JCCA 1990;34:3.

73. Plaugher G, Lopez A, Melch PE, Cremata EE. The inter- and intra-examiner reliability of paraspinal skin temperature differential instrument. J Manipulative Physiol Ther 1991;14:6.

74. Kent C, Gentempo P. Paraspinal surface EMG and outcome assessment for subluxation-based chiropractic care. ICA Review 1992;Jan/Feb:19-23.

75. Adams T, Steinmetz MA, Heisey SR, Holmes KR. Physiological basis for skin properties in palpatory physical diagnosis. JAOA 1982;81:6.

76. Bryner P, Baxter AJ, Sherwood BF. Thoracic paraspinal tenderness in chronic pain sufferers. J Aust Chiro Assoc 1989;19:132-6.

77. Taylor P, Tole G, Vernon H. Skin rolling techniques as an indicator of spinal dysfunction. JCCA 1990;34:2.

78. Vernon H. Pressure pain threshold: evaluation on the effect of spinal manipulation on chronic neck pain. A case study. J Can Chiro Assoc 1988;32(4):191-4.

79. Vernon H, Aker P, Burns S, Valjakanen S, Short L. Pressure pain threshold evaluation of the effect of spinal manipulation in the treatment of chronic neck pain: a pilot study. J Manipulative Physiol Ther 1990; 13:13-6.

80. Hildebrandt RW. Chiropractic spinography and postural roentgenology. Part 11. Clinical basis. J Manipulative Physiol Ther 1981;4:191-201.

81. Howe JW. The role of x-ray findings in structural diagnosis. In: Goldstein M, editor. The research status of spinal manipulative therapy. NINCDS Monograph No. 15. 1975;15:239-47.

82. Winterstein JF, Leverone RA. Full spine radiography: its methods and value. Digest Chiro Econ 1974;17: 26-30.

83. Cox JM, Gideon D, Rogers FJ. Incidence of osteophytic lipping of the thoracic spine in coronary heart disease: results of a pilot study. JAOA 1983;82(11):93-4.

84. Macones AJ, Fisher MS, Locke JL. Stress-related rib and vertebral changes. Radiology 1989;170:117-9.

85. Hilel N. Osteophytes of the spine compressing the sympathetic trunk and splanchnic nerves in the thorax. Spine 1987;12(6):527-32.

86. Lipschitz M, Bernstein-Lipschitz L, Hilel N. Thoracic sympathetic trunk compression by osteophytes associated with arthritis of the costovertebral joint: anatomical and clinical considerations. Acta Anat 1988;48-54.

87. Singer KP, Giles LG, Day RE. Influence of zygapophyseal joint orientation on hyaline cartilage at the thoracolumbar junction. J Manipulative Physiol Ther 1990; 13(4):207-14.

88. Singer KP, Giles LGF. Manual therapy considerations at the thoracolumbar junction: an anatomical and functional perspective. J Manipulative Physiol Ther 1990; 13:83-8.

89. Fligg DB. The art of motion palpation. JCCA 1984; 28(3):331-4.

90. Sportelli G, Tarola GA. The history and physical examination. In: Haldeman S, editor. Principles and practice of chiropractic. 2nd ed. East Norwalk, CT: Appleton & Lange; 1992.

91. Grice AS. Posture and posture mechanics. JCCA 1970; (Jul):19-21.

92. Johnston WL, Elkiss ML, Marino RV, Blum GA. Passive gross motion testing. Part II. A study of interexaminer agreement. JAOA 1982;81(5):304-8.

93. Lewit K. Deviation of the spinous processes. Br J Radiol 1957;30(351):162-4.

94. Gillet H, Liekens ME. Belgian chiropractic research notes. 10th ed. Brussels; 1973.

95. Fligg DB. Sacroiliac cross fix adjustment. JCCA 1983;27:4.

96. Fligg DB. Lumbar closure adjustment. JCCA 1983;27:2.

97. Fligg DB. Lower cervical spine motion palpation (C2-7). JCCA 1984;28:1.

98. Fligg DB. Upper cervical technique. JCCA 1985;29:2.

99. Fligg DB. The anterior thoracic adjustment. JCCA 1986;30:4.

100. Fligg DB. Lateral recumbent rib adjustment. JCCA 1984;28:2.

101. Mennell SM. Joint pain, diagnosis in treatment using manipulation techniques. Boston: Little, Brown, and Co; 1964.

102. Love RM, Brodeur RR. Inter- and intra-examiner reliability of motion palpation for the thoracolumbar spine. J Manipulative Physiol Ther 1987;10(1):1-4.

103. Manga P, Angus D. The effectiveness and cost-effectiveness of chiropractic management of low back pain. University of Ottawa, Canada: Author; 1993.

104. Leach RA. The chiropractic theories: a synopsis of scientific research. 2nd ed. Baltimore: Williams & Wilkins; 1986.

105. Korr IM. Proprioceptors and somatic dysfunction. JAOA 1975;74(7):173-5.

106. Zachman ZJ, Bolles S, Bergman TF, Triana AD. Understanding the anterior thoracic adjustment (a concept of a sectional subluxation). Chiropractic Technique 1989;1(1):30-3.

107. Fligg DB. The anterior thoracic adjustment. JCCA 1986;30(4):211-13.

108. Fracheboud R, Kraus S, Choiniere B. A survey of anterior thoracic adjustments. Chiropractic 1988;1(3):89-92.

Facet Subluxation Syndrome

David M. Panzer

Key Words   Facet subluxation syndrome, spinal zygapophyseal joints, meniscoids, tropism

After reading this chapter you should be able to answer the following questions:

Question 1   What is the primary function of the lumbar facet articulation?

Question 2   What is the pattern of referred pain from spinal facet joints?

Question 3   What are the 10 specific proposed effects that manipulation may have on spinal facet articulations?

Vertebral zygapophyseal (facet) joints have long been recognized as a source of spinal pain and dysfunction.[1-11] In 1933, Ghormley[12] introduced the term *facet syndrome,* but after the work of Mixter and Barr in 1934,[13] interest in intervertebral discs and irritated nerve roots overshadowed facet joints as a source of low back pain. In more recent years, the facet articulations have received much more attention. Kirkaldy-Willis and Burton[14] consider lumbar facet syndrome a "commonly occurring condition," and Cox[4] considers "facet subluxation syndromes probably the most common condition encountered in low back pain patients."

This chapter explores the role of facet joints in spinal pain and pathomechanics.

Facet Syndrome Defined

Facet syndrome may be broadly defined as pain or dysfunction arising primarily from the zygapophyseal joints and their immediately adjacent soft tissues. Earlier definitions include the following[10]:

1. The condition characterized by an overriding of the facets of adjacent vertebrae whereby the intervertebral foramina are narrowed from the superior to the inferior
2. A state of subluxation with tension, pressure, stretching, or irritation of the vertebral joint capsule as a result of postural strain or trauma but without narrowing of the related foramina
Specific diagnostic criteria for facet syndrome are discussed later in this chapter.

Facet Clinical Anatomy and Function

The lumbar spine has been the focus of most study relating to facet joint mechanics. A primary function of lumbar facet articulations is resistance to rotational and shear forces, thereby protecting the disc.[1,15] Lumbar facets also have a role in weight bearing. Normally they carry approximately one sixth of the total axial load of the vertebral motion segment.[1] Because of their relatively small surface area, this is roughly equivalent to 10 times the weight per square inch borne by the standing

knee joint.[4] Axial weight bearing is increased during extension and reaches up to 70% of the intervertebral compressive force in cases of degenerative disc narrowing.[1] Increased zygapophyseal weight bearing is often considered an important component of lumbar facet syndrome that can readily be measured radiographically.[4,10,16,17]

The innervation of the facet joints is well known. (See Chapter 3.) The joint capsule and adjacent tissues are innervated by twigs from the medial branch of the posterior primary rami, each facet receiving innervation from two spinal levels.[5,8-10,18,19] As the medial branch of the posterior primary ramus traverses inferior to the facet surfaces, it travels through a bony tunnel covered by the mammilloaccessory ligament.[8,9,19] Direct nerve entrapment is possible at this site as a result of overriding (imbrication) of facets that may occur with disc thinning or facet degeneration (Figure 24-1).[19]

Meniscoids

Intraarticular joint inclusions (synovial folds) have been described in all spinal zygapophyseal joints,[11,20] but most of the interest has centered on the lumbar spine. Typically, these structures consist of three parts: (1) a fibroadipose or loose connective tissue base arising from the joint capsule, (2) a highly vascularized synovial inclusion zone, and (3) a tip of dense connective tissue or cartilaginous tissue that projects between the articular surfaces[7,14,18,20-23] (Figure 24-2).

The primary functions of meniscoids are as follows[18,20,21]:

1. To fill space at the periphery of the joint surface
2. To increase surface area contact and therefore transfer load
3. To cover exposed articular surfaces and protect joint margins during flexion and extension
Mechanically, meniscoids have been implicated as a cause of the acute "locked back" or torticollis by becoming entrapped between the articular surfaces.* The success of spinal manipulative therapy directed at the facet joints may be explained by

---

*References 5, 7, 11, 14, 20-22, 24, 25.

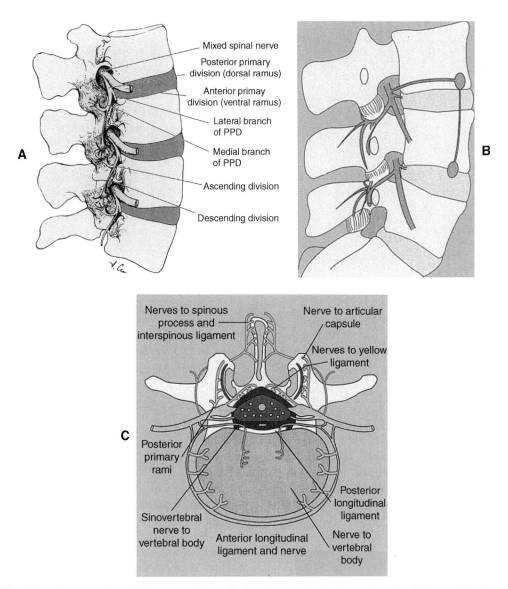

Figure 24-1   Facet innervation. **A,** Nerve supply to the lumbosacral spine from the side. **B,** Part of the lower spinal innervation showing the mammilloaccessory ligament *(arrow)*. **C,** A cross-sectional view of the spine. *(Figure 24-1, A, modified from Cramer D. Basic and clinical anatomy of the spine, spinal cord and ANS. St. Louis: Mosby; 1995. Figure 24-1, B, modified from Giles LGF. Anatomical basis of low back pain. Baltimore: Williams & Wilkins; 1989.)*

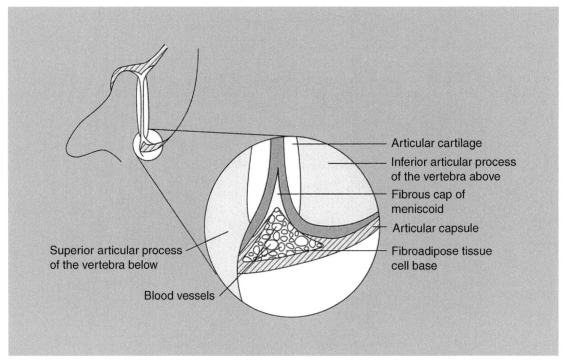

Figure 24-2   Diagrammatic representation of the fibroadipose meniscoid of a facet joint according to Engel and Bogduk. *(Modified from Bergmann T, Peterson D, Lawrence D. Chiropractic technique. Philadelphia: Churchill Livingstone; 1993.)*

this mechanism. Distraction of the articular surfaces may release the entrapped meniscoid and allow resolution of the consequent muscle spasm (Figures 24-3 to 24-5).* Other proposed mechanisms of meniscoid-related facet joint dysfunction include the following:

1. Entrapment of the meniscoid outside the joint surfaces in the capsular recess (see Figure 24-2)[18,27]
2. A free fragment of facet cartilage avulsed from the articular surface but still attached to the capsule[18]
3. Deformation of hyaline cartilage by presence of the meniscoid

---

*References 5, 7, 11, 20, 22, 24, 26.

Tropism

Normally, the upper lumbar facets are essentially sagittal in orientation and the lower lumbar joints are more coronal (Figure 24-6).[15,28] *Tropism* refers to an anomalous condition in which the articular facings are asymmetric.[4] Because the facets guide the motions of the lumbar spine,[1] it appears logical that asymmetric joint angles could disrupt normal biomechanics. Cyron and Hutton[15] have demonstrated unequal articular forces produced in tropism with consequent increase in pressure and arthrosis at the more oblique, that is, more sagittal facet (Figures 24-7 and 24-8). This results from rotational torsion occurring at the joint. Increased wear on the anulus of the disc is postulated to occur as a result of these same forces.[15] Cox[4] states that "patients with anomalous facet facings are at high risk for developing a disc lesion

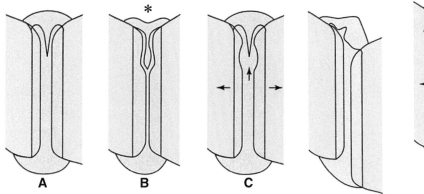

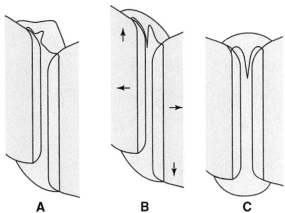

Figure 24-3 An illustration of the meniscoid entrapment theory. **A,** A meniscus with a firm fibrous apex but deformable fatty body projects into a zygapophysial joint from the rostral capsule. **B,** The apex deforms the articular cartilages forming a recess in which the apex becomes entrapped. Traction exerted through the body of the meniscus strains the joint capsule and evokes pain. **C,** A manipulation that separates the articular cartilages releases the trapped meniscus and relieves the capsular strain. *(Modified from Bogduk N, Jull G. Manual Med 1985;1:78-82.)*

Figure 24-4 Treatment of the meniscus entrapment syndrome by manipulation. **A,** The meniscoid lies impacted against the joint margin. **B,** Longitudinal distraction, or flexion, of the joint reduces the impaction. Separation of the joint surfaces by a rotary maneuver widens the joint space to encourage the meniscoid to reenter it. Capsular strain, and therefore the painful stimulus, is relieved. **C,** The joint is allowed to passively extend to its neutral position. If the meniscoid reenters the joint space, pain stays relieved and normal posture is restored. *(Modified from Bogduk N, Jull G. Manual Med 1985;1:78-82.)*

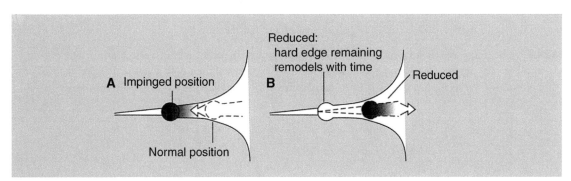

Figure 24-5 Entrapment of a meniscoid at the edge of a joint space according to the joint blockage theory of Wolf (1975). **A,** The meniscoid has moved between the joint facets and its hard edge has impinged. **B,** It has returned to normal position after treatment. A groove remains for a short time, but over time the articular cartilage will remodel. *(Modified from Bergmann T, Peterson D, Lawrence D. Chiropractic technique. Philadelphia: Churchill Livingstone; 1993.)*

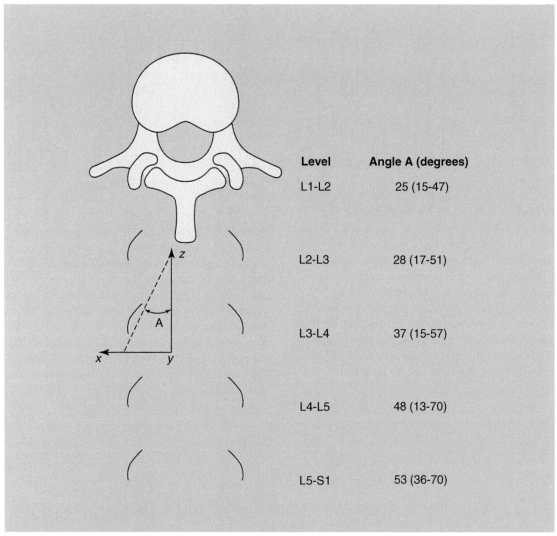

Level	Angle A (degrees)
L1-L2	25 (15-47)
L2-L3	28 (17-51)
L3-L4	37 (15-57)
L4-L5	48 (13-70)
L5-S1	53 (36-70)

Figure 24-6   The shape and inclination of the facets of the lumbar spine in the transverse plane *(xz plane)* are shown. The facet inclination with the sagittal plane increases toward the lower levels. *(Modified from White AA, Panjabi MM, Bogduk N, Twomey LT. Clinical anatomy of the lumbar spine. Edinburgh: Churchill Livingstone; 1987.)*

on rotation." Noren et al.[29] demonstrated that tropism was associated with an increased risk of disc degeneration. Other studies, however, have failed to find association between tropism and disc degeneration,[30] disc herniation,[31] and symptom reproduction by discography.[30]

It seems safe to conclude that tropism in the clinical context of a facet syndrome constitutes a potential complicating factor. Furthermore, the treating physician may wish to modify manipulative therapies to accommodate the alteration of facet joint planes.

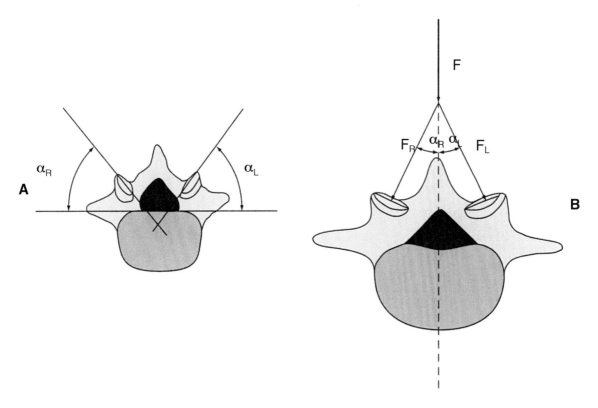

Figure 24-7   Tropism. **A,** Measurement of facet orientation. **B,** Forces *(F)* acting on symmetrically oriented superior articular facets. *(Modified from Cyron BM, Hutton WC. Spine 1980;5:171.)*

Facet versus Disc Degenerative Joint Disease

Degenerative joint disease (DJD) may occur at different rates in the discs and facets of the same motion segment. Ziv et al.[32] found severe fibrillation in histologic specimens of facets after the age of 30 years. Degeneration was more pronounced in the superior than in the inferior articular process. It was noted that even "young adults" showed ulceration or severe fibrillation, and that facet degeneration preceded disc degeneration. It was concluded that these facet changes were a likely source of back pain.

Beaman et al.[33] also demonstrated that facet DJD occurs with or without disc DJD. These findings support the presence of a clinical entity unique to the facet joints, which can occur inde-pendent of concurrent discal pathology or pathomechanics. They also counter previous studies that concluded that facet degeneration occurs only as a result of disc DJD.[34] It should be noted that disc and facet degeneration do often occur together, and either or both may be a primary pain source.

Facet Joint as a Source of Pain

Considerable evidence exists in support of the facet articulations as a source of pain, and innervation of the joint capsule and synovium have previously been described.* In addition to small-diameter nociceptive free nerve endings, the facet capsule and synovium have specific substance P–positive nerves,[22] as does the adjacent subchondral bone.[33]

---

*References 5, 8, 10, 18-20, 22, 23.

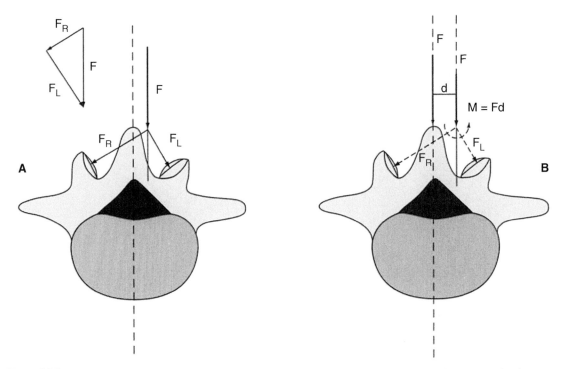

Figure 24-8   Tropism. Forces *(F)* acting on asymmetrically oriented superior articular facets. **A,** The force *(F)* acts at the point of concurrency and is distributed unevenly to the articular facets. **B,** The force is offset from the point of concurrency, and additional torsion is applied to the joint. *(Modified from Cyron BM, Hutton WC. Spine 1980;5:171.)*

Direct experimental evidence of the distribution of facet joint pain has been obtained by injection of hypertonic saline into the joint and mapping the pain produced. Mooney and Robertson[9] found that diffuse referred leg pain resulted from lumbar facet injection. They noted that the distance the referred pain radiated down the leg was dependent on the amount of facet irritation and the time involved. They described the pain referral pattern as matching the typical "lumbago and sciatica" distribution. McCall et al.[35] conducted similar experiments that also demonstrated diffuse (nondermatomal) pain referral patterns.

Facet pain patterns were found to be consistent enough in the cervical spine that examiners could predict the level of facet involvement in nine of nine patients based on pain distribution alone.[3] Confirmation was achieved with diagnostic medial branch nerve blocks. Facet pain was even found in patients who had undergone previous anterior cervical fusion. Bogduk and Marsland[3] concluded that cervical pain is frequently zygapophyseal in origin and because cervical zygapophyseal disorders are poorly understood, or not even considered in conventional practice, patients with this complaint are more likely to gravitate to a pain clinic, and thereby constitute an inordinate proportion of patients presenting with idiopathic neck pain.[3]

Other studies have taken the approach of injecting a local anesthetic or cortisone derivative into a specific facet joint believed to be causing pain. Relief confirms the facet articulation as the primary source of pain and is generally considered diagnostic of facet syndrome.[6,8,9,14,36] Helbig and Lee[6] showed that facets manifesting radiographic changes, especially marked DJD, responded best to facet injection. Kirkaldy-Willis and Burton[14] consider specific manipulation of a facet joint or precise facet injection to be the "most reliable way to make a specific diagnosis."

This view is not shared by Jackson,[37] who found that control injections of saline were as effective as a local anesthetic in relieving facet pain. He concluded a placebo effect was responsible. It is quite possible, however, that the saline control group actually received a therapeutic effect by stimulation of various articular receptors (e.g., proprioceptive, nociceptive). This effect may be similar to the pain-modulating mechanisms of manipulative therapy.[38,39] It is also possible that improved joint mobility and reduced intraarticular or periarticular adhesions resulted from the capsular distension caused by the saline injection.

Clinical Features of the Facet Syndrome

In addition to low back pain, classic lumbar facet syndrome includes the following symptoms[8]:
1. Hip and buttock pain
2. Cramping leg pain above the knee
3. Low back stiffness, especially in morning or after decreased activity
   Lippitt[8] also includes the following signs:
   1. Local paralumbar tenderness
   2. Pain on spine hyperextension
   3. Absence of neurologic deficit
   4. Absence of root tension signs
   5. Hip, buttock, or back pain with straight leg raising
Wood[25] describes the onset of "acute locked facet syndrome" as sudden, typically following a

trivial injurious force, often twisting or bending. He further describes "very marked immobility, out of proportion to the pain—both in range of movements and in the time taken to move—often feeling foolish, so marked is the immobility."

In an attempt to establish an objective and more accurate set of diagnostic criteria, Helbig and Lee[6] formulated a scorecard system in which clinical features are given points. Scoring is as follows:
- Back pain associated with groin or thigh pain: +30 points
- Well localized paraspinal tenderness: +20 points
- Reproduction of pain with extension-rotation: +30 points
- Significant corresponding radiographic changes (for example, facet asymmetry or DJD): +20 points
- Pain below knee: −10 points

All patients scoring 60 points or more (100 possible points) showed a positive and prolonged response to facet injection. It was concluded that this scoring system improves diagnostic accuracy and predictability of successful response to facet joint injection. These diagnostic parameters can readily be adopted by the chiropractic physician.

Radiographic features also may be helpful in the diagnosis of facet syndrome. Banks[17] found a significant increase in the lumbosacral angle (sacral base angle) of patients with facet syndrome compared with patients with disc herniation or normal controls (Figure 24-9). Similar results have been reported by Peters[10] and Cox.[4] These results are consistent with increased weight bearing forming an important component of facet syndrome. Cox[4] states that "any discal angle over 15° is a sign of severe facet syndrome." As previously mentioned, degenerative arthrosis, subchondral sclerosis, and tropism also may be significant radiographic features if they correspond to clinical findings.

Cervical pain of zygapophyseal origin has been described as having the following clinical features[18,40]:
1. Characteristic local and referred pain (occipital to interscapular, depending on vertebral level)
2. Abnormal end feel of facet joint capsule
3. Abnormal quality of resistance to motion

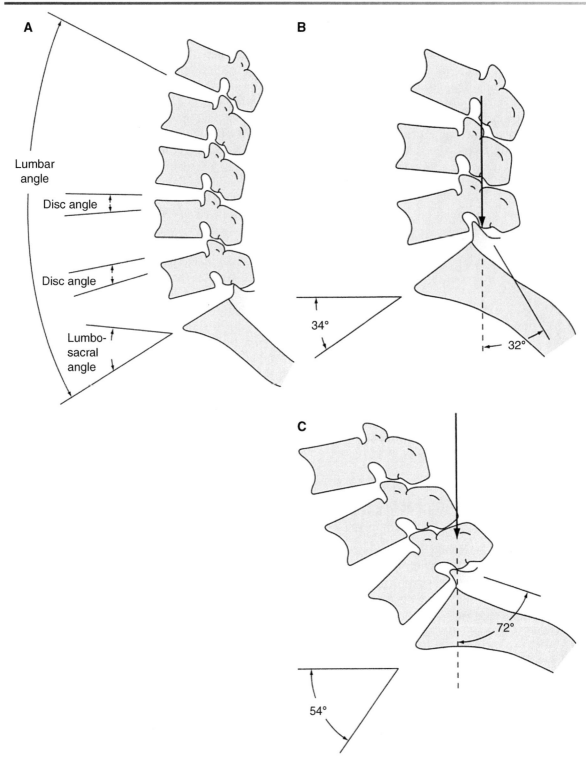

Figure 24-9 **A,** Lumbosacral, lumbar, and disc angles. **B,** Lumbosacral extension malposition (i.e., increased disc angle) increases facet loading. **C,** Lumbosacral facet orientation with excessively lordotic posture. *(Modified from Banks SD. J Manipulative Physiol Ther 1983;6:175-80.)*

4. Pain on palpation of segmental accessory movements
5. Confirmation possible with facet or medial branch nerve block

Thoracolumbar facet syndrome (Maigne's syndrome) also has been described, with pain typically referred to the iliac crest area. This pain is thought to be mediated by the cluneal nerves.[14]

Treatment of Facet Syndrome

Manipulation

Spinal manipulation directed to the facet articulations is generally considered the treatment of choice for facet syndrome.* Specific zygapophyseal manipulation is also used to confirm a diagnosis of facet syndrome.[14,45] It has even been postulated that the success seen in rotary manipulation for lumbar disc herniation is attributable to the relief of associated facet syndrome.[46] Because facet syndrome generally involves pain and joint dysfunction,[11,25,40] it seems logical to apply treatment that not only relieves pain but helps correct the underlying dysfunction. Posterior joint dysfunction appears to have a specific intraarticular origin and is not simply the product of segmental muscle spasm. This has been demonstrated by performing manipulation under anesthesia when the muscles are relaxed, yet the intrinsic joint dysfunction is still quite evident.[47,48] In fact, it has been noted that the joint dysfunction is rendered more obvious in the anesthetized patient.[47] It also has been observed that periarticular injection of a local anesthetic relieves the pain but not the immobility of acute locked facet syndrome.[25]

Below is a summary of specific proposed effects manipulation has on facet articulations:

1. Release of entrapped meniscoid†
2. Reduction in articular cartilage displacement by chronically entrapped meniscoid[26]
3. Pain relief by coactivation of various receptors[24,38]
4. Reduced weight bearing[4,10,16]

5. Reduction of intervertebral foramen stenosis caused by segmental hyperextension[4]
6. Reduced intracapsular or extracapsular adhesions[7,11,22]
7. Relief of abnormal tension on joint capsule[7]
8. Reduction of postimmobilization collagen cross-linking[11]
9. Reduction of local vascular stasis[22]
10. Release of osseous mechanical locking

Many studies have investigated the effectiveness of manipulation for low back pain, but few have focused on facet syndrome specifically.[49] Banks[16] demonstrated a normalization (reduction) of disc angle values after manipulation for radiographically verified facet syndrome. Cox et al.[41] reported excellent results in 69% and good or very good results in 15% of facet syndrome patients treated with manipulation.

Nonmanipulative treatment in acute incapacitating episodes may include brief periods of bed rest and medication. Overall, "the value of muscle relaxants and of anti-inflammatory drugs is doubtful."[14]

Facet Injection

Injection of facet joints or adjacent nerves with a local anesthetic or antiinflammatory agent has been described in this chapter. In addition to confirming the facet joint as a primary pain source, these techniques have been used to treat facet syndrome. If manipulation fails, Kirkaldy-Willis and Burton[14] recommend intraarticular injection of bupivacaine or xylocaine followed immediately by manipulation. Postinjection muscular relaxation may enhance the benefits of manipulation. They note that "facet injections nearly always relieve the pain for several hours. In approximately 50% of cases the patient is free of pain for weeks or months."

Lippitt,[8] in an uncontrolled retrospective study, reported the following results after 117 facet injections in 99 patients with low back and possible referred pain: excellent, 17%; good, 25%; fair, 9%; mediocre, 4%; and no change, 44%. It should be noted that these were primarily chronic patients; 20 had undergone previous discectomy and 4 had spinal stenosis, and they were not screened in advance for specific facet syndrome

---

*References 4, 7, 11, 14, 16, 22, 25, 41-45.
†References 5, 7, 11, 20, 22, 23, 26, 27.

criteria. When the previously mentioned facet syndrome "scorecard" was used to select patients for injection, Helbig and Lee[6] reported a 100% prolonged response in cases scoring high (60 points or more) for facet syndrome indicators. They also pointed out that the composite of multiple signs and symptoms is more predictive than a single indicator alone. The patients treated in their study had all been treated unsuccessfully with rest, anti-inflammatory medications, and physical therapy (heat, massage, transcutaneous electrical nerve stimulation [TENS], exercise) for two months before facet injection.

Even though he considered facet injection diagnostic rather than therapeutic because "any therapeutic effect is strictly coincidental...and ultimately transient," Murtagh[36] found a 94% short-term response (up to three months duration) and a 54% long-term response (lasting more than three months). He also found computed tomographic (CT) or fluoroscopic guidance helpful in placement of the needle.

Jackson[37] reported 85% of 390 low back patients injected experienced some relief. He observed that the greatest relief immediately after injection was in lumbar extension and rotation. He did not find these painful ranges of motion predictive of who would respond, however, and concluded that response to facet injection cannot be reliably predicted. He further concluded that facet joints are not commonly the single or primary source of low back pain, and he questions the existence of facet syndrome as a distinct clinical entity. He notes that further prospective, controlled, and randomized clinical studies are needed. A related form of treatment, facet denervation, was reviewed by Jackson,[37] who concluded that "facet denervation procedures generally provide inconsistent and frequently poor results, especially with time."

Predisposing Factors and Therapeutic Exercise

The occurrence of facet syndrome has been correlated to a postural increase in facet weight bearing, increased lumbar lordosis, or anterior sacral tipping.[4,10,16,17,42] It also has been observed that facet loading may cause the backache associated with prolonged standing, which is relieved by placing the foot on a step or by sitting.[1] In other words, flexion relieves the loading. With these factors in mind, the following measures are recommended to assist in the treatment of facet syndrome and its predisposing postural factors[10,42]:

1. Knee-chest (Williams) exercises
2. 90-90 positioning or traction (hips and knees 90 degrees)
3. Pelvic tilt exercises to decrease lumbar lordosis
4. Abdominal strengthening exercises
5. Weight reduction as appropriate
6. Avoidance of high heels

Conclusion

The facet joints are widely recognized as a source of spinal pain, and the facet subluxation syndrome is a relatively common clinical entity with well-defined features. Careful attention to clinical and radiographic indicators can enhance the accuracy of diagnosing this syndrome. Facet subluxation syndrome is generally amenable to conservative management with chiropractic manipulation and attention to predisposing factors. Such treatment helps address the important component of the manipulable subluxation.[50]

References

1. Adams MA, Hutton WC. The mechanical function of the lumbar apophyseal joints. Spine 1983;8:327-30.
2. Aprill C, Dwyer A, Bogduk N. Cervical zygapophyseal joint pain patterns. II. A clinical evaluation. Spine 1990;15:458-61.
3. Bogduk N, Marsland A. The cervical zygapophyseal joints as a source of neck pain. Spine 1988;13(6):610-7.
4. Cox JM. Low back pain mechanism, diagnosis, and treatment. Baltimore: Williams & Wilkins; 1990. p. 148-56, 437-66.
5. Giles LGF. Anatomical basis of low back pain. Baltimore: Williams & Wilkins; 1989. p. 27-40, 58-104.
6. Helbig T, Lee C. The lumbar facet syndrome. Spine 1988;13:61-4.
7. Jones TR, James JE, Adams JW, Garcia J, Walker SL, Ellis JP. Lumbar zygapophyseal joint meniscoids: evidence of their role in chronic intersegmental hypomobility. J Manipulative Physiol Ther 1989;12:374-85.
8. Lippitt AB. The facet joint and its role in spine pain. Spine 1984;9:746-50.

9. Mooney V, Robertson J. The facet syndrome. Clin Orthop 1976;115:149-56.
10. Peters RE. Facet syndrome. Eur J Chiro 1984;32:85-102.
11. Rahlmann JF. Mechanisms of intervertebral joint fixation: a literature review. J Manipulative Physiol Ther 1987;10: 177-87.
12. Ghormley RK. Low back pain with special reference to the articular facets with presentation of an operative procedure. JAMA 1933;101:1773-7.
13. Mixter WJ, Barr JS. Rupture of the intervertebral disc with involvement of the spinal cord. N Engl J Med 1934;211: 210-15.
14. Kirkaldy-Willis WH, Burton CV. Managing low back pain. 3rd ed. New York: Churchill Livingstone; 1992. p. 50-63, 122, 126, 137, 203, 211, 248.
15. Cyron BM, Hutton WC. Articular tropism and stability of the lumbar spine. Spine 1980;5:168-72.
16. Banks SD. Lumbar facet syndrome: spinographic assessment of treatment by spinal manipulative therapy. J Manipulative Physiol Ther 1983;6:175-80.
17. Banks SD. The use of spinographic parameters in the differential diagnosis of lumbar facet and disc syndromes. J Manipulative Physiol Ther 1983;6:113-16.
18. Bogduk N, Twomey LT. Clinical anatomy of the lumbar spine. New York: Churchill Livingstone; 1987. p. 30-2, 97-9, 140.
19. Sunderland S. The anatomy of the intervertebral foramen and the mechanisms of compression and stretch of nerve roots. In: Haldeman S, editor. Modern developments in the principles and practice of chiropractic. New York: Appleton-Century-Crofts; 1980. p. 62-4.
20. Giles LGF. Lumbosacral and cervical zygapophyseal joint inclusions. Manual Med 1986;2:89-92.
21. Bogduk N, Engel R. The menisci of the lumbar zygapophyseal joints: a review of their anatomy and clinical significance. Spine 1984;9:454-60.
22. Giles LGF. Pathoanatomical studies and clinical significance of lumbar zygapophyseal (facet) joints. J Manipulative Physiol Ther 1992;15:36-40.
23. Giles LGF, Taylor JR. Osteoarthrosis in human cadaveric lumbosacral zygapophyseal joints. J Manipulative Physiol Ther 1985;8:239-43.
24. Peterson DH, Bergmann TF. Chiropractic technique. 2nd ed. St. Louis: CV Mosby; 2002.
25. Wood L. Acute locked facet syndrome and its treatment by manipulation under local periarticular anesthesia. J Manipulative Physiol Ther 1984;7:211-17.
26. Lewit K. Manipulative therapy in rehabilitation of the locomotor system. Boston: Butterworth; 1985. p. 17-9.
27. Bogduk N, Jull G. The theoretical pathology of acute locked back: a basis for manipulative therapy. Manual Med 1985;1:78-82.
28. White AA, Panjabi MM. Clinical biomechanics of the spine. 2nd ed. San Francisco: JB Lippincott; 1990. p. 32.
29. Noren R, Trafimow J, Andersson GB, Huckman MS. The role of facet joint tropism and facet angle in disc degeneration. Spine 1991;16:530-2.
30. Vanharanta H, Floyd T, Ohnmeiss DD, Hochschuler SH, Guyer RD. The relationship of facet tropism to degenerative disc disease. Spine 1993;18:1000-5.
31. Cassidy JD, Loback D, Yong-Hing K, Tchang S. Lumbar facet joint asymmetry. Spine 1992;17:570-4.
32. Ziv I, Maroudas C, Robin G, Maroudas A. Human facet cartilage: swelling and some physiochemical characteristics as a function of age. Spine 1993;18:136-46.
33. Beaman DN, Graziano GP, Glover RA, Wojtys EM, Chang V. Substance P innervation of lumbar spine facet joints. Spine 1993;18:1044-9.
34. Butler D, Trafimow JH, Andersson GB, McNeill TW, Huckman MS. Discs degenerate before facets. Spine 1990;15:111-3.
35. McCall IW, Park WM, O'Brien JP. Induced pain referral from posterior lumbar elements in normal subjects. Spine 1979;4:441-6.
36. Murtagh FR. Computed tomography and fluoroscopic guided anesthesia and steroid injection in facet syndrome. Spine 1988;13:686-9.
37. Jackson RP. The facet syndrome: myth or reality? Clin Orthop 1992;279:110-21.
38. Gillette RG. A speculative argument for the coactivation of diverse somatic receptor populations by forceful chiropractic adjustments. Manual Med 1987;3:1-14.
39. Gillette RG. Personal communication, October 1993.
40. Jull G, Bogduk N, Marsland A. The accuracy of manual diagnosis for cervical zygapophyseal joint pain syndromes. Med J Aust 1988;148:233-6.
41. Cox JM, Fromelt KA, Shreiner S. Chiropractic statistical survey of 100 consecutive low back pain patients. J Manipulative Physiol Ther 1983;6:117-28.
42. Gatterman MI. Chiropractic management of spine related disorders. 2nd ed. Baltimore: Williams & Wilkins; 2003.
43. Hourigan CL, Bassett JM. Facet syndrome: clinical signs, symptoms, diagnosis, and treatment. J Manipulative Physiol Ther 1989;12:293-7.
44. Kirkaldy-Willis WH, Cassidy JD. Spinal manipulation in the treatment of low back pain. Can Fam Physician 1985;31:535-40.
45. Kirkaldy-Willis WH, Hill RJ. A more precise diagnosis for low back pain. Spine 1979;4:102-9.
46. Quon JA, Cassidy JD, O'Connor SM, Kirkaldy-Willis WH. Lumbar intervertebral disc herniation: treatment by rotational manipulation. J Manipulative Physiol Ther 1989;12:220-7.
47. Lewit K. The muscular and articular factor in movement restriction. Manual Med 1985;1:83-5.
48. Mennell JM. The validation of the diagnosis "joint dysfunction" in the synovial joints of the cervical spine. J Manipulative Physiol Ther 1990;13:7-12.
49. Bronfort G. Effectiveness of spinal manipulation and adjustments. In: Haldeman S, editor. Principles and practice of chiropractic. 2nd ed. San Mateo, CA: Appleton & Lange; 1992. p. 420-9.
50. Gatterman MI. Indications for spinal manipulation in the treatment of back pain. ACA J Chiro 1982;19(10):51-66.

Intervertebral Disc Syndrome

Doug Davison and
Meridel I. Gatterman

Key Words   Intervertebral disc syndrome, discogenic back pain, cauda equina syndrome, sciatica, somatic referred pain, radicular pain

After reading this chapter you should be able to answer the following questions:

Question 1   What is the contribution of disc herniation to spinal subluxation?

Question 2   Why is one type of treatment for all cases of intervertebral disc syndrome not in the best interest of the patient?

Question 3   What signs and symptoms associated with intervertebral disc syndrome suggest the need for referral for a neurologic evaluation?

Clinically, the symptoms associated with intervertebral disc syndrome can respond to the application of spinal manipulation.[1,2] Behavior of the spinal motion segment consistent with subluxation (altered alignment, movement integrity, and physiological function) is observed with disc degeneration and herniation. The interrelationship of the spinal three-joint complex[3] makes a precise diagnosis of low back pain difficult at best, and in many cases involves more than one component of the spinal motion segment.

When the intervertebral disc is affected, the posterior joints are also involved and vice versa. This means that even when the disc is the site of the main lesion, the posterior joints can be affected and contribute to the patient's symptoms. Conversely when the function of the posterior joints is abnormal, symptoms may also arise from the disc. This discussion of intervertebral disc syndrome explores the contribution of the intervertebral disc to motion segment subluxation and spinal dysfunction.

Historical Background

The publication in 1934 of a paper describing rupture of the intervertebral disc by Mixter and Barr[3] focused on the disc as the primary source of back pain. For the next 40 years, a period known as the "dynasty of the disc," spinal surgery was the primary treatment for disc lesions.

In 1964 Chrisman et al.[4] found that 51% of patients with sciatica improved clinically on side posture manipulation but that no changes in the myelographic appearance occurred, suggesting the possibility that the leg pain may not have been due solely to disc herniation. In 1974 Mathew and Yates[5] reported on the reduction in size of a disc herniation using epidurography pre- and post-manipulation. In 1979 Valentini reported that 171 of 194 patients with acute disc syndrome were successfully treated with side posture manipulation.[6]

Since that time, many studies have reported successful treatment of mechanical back pain with manipulation, including patients with disc lesions,[7] but there has not been a clear separation in most cases that identifies the contributing structures. Both side posture manipulation[1] and flexion-distraction[2] have been demonstrated to be effective in the treatment of intervertebral disc lesions. End-range lumbar extension exercise is another tool being used successfully in the treatment of these patients.

Anatomy of the Intervertebral Disc

Three distinct regions make up the structure of the intervertebral disc. They are the nucleus pulposus, anulus fibrosus, and cartilaginous end plates. The intervertebral discs are interposed between adjacent surfaces of the vertebral bodies, serving to unite as well as separate them.

Anulus Fibrosus

The anular fibers of the lumbar intervertebral disc form an outer ligament made up of fibrocartilaginous rings that restrain the nucleus. The outer anular fibers are more elastic. The enclosing fibers are arranged in successive layers overlapping in alternating oblique directions. The outermost fibers are attached to the periosteum and vertebral body just beyond the epiphyseal ring of cortical bone. The posterior and posterolateral parts of the anulus are much thinner, and there is less reinforcement from the thin posterior longitudinal ligament that narrows caudally from L1. It is less than half of the posterior disc margin by the time it reaches L5.

The differentiation between the inner fibers of the anulus and the nucleus pulposus is often described in ways that draw an image of a clear line of demarcation between the two. Analogies of a jelly donut or tire turned on its side insinuate that the nucleus resides in an open cavity, centered within well-organized walls of the inner anulus and the superior and inferior end plates. In actuality, the demarcation between anulus and nucleus pulposus can be difficult to discern because of a gradual transition from the fibrous network of the nucleus to the well-organized lamella of the anulus.[8]

The cervical disc has recently been shown to rely heavily on the posterior longitudinal ligament

(PLL) to support the nucleus pulposus posteriorly, because there is little or no anulus in that region. There is no layering of concentric rings of fibers lying at alternate angles; instead, there is a crescent-shaped collagen mass anteriorly that tapers laterally as it approaches the uncinate processes. There is a thin layer of posterior fibers supporting the disc between the uncinate processes and the lateral edge of the PLL, creating an inherent weakness in this region.[9]

Nucleus Pulposus

The nucleus pulposus is separated from the central parts of the vertebral bodies above and below by thin cartilaginous end plates. The nucleus is an avascular structure, and the end plates provide a permeable barrier between the nucleus pulposus and the vertebral bodies, permitting the transfer of tissue fluid that meets the nutritional demands of the disc.

The nucleus pulposus is a thick semifluid gel that makes up 40% of the intervertebral disc. It is composed of stellate cells sparsely scattered throughout a three-dimensional lattice gel of fine interlaced collagen fibrils that enmesh fibroblastic cells, and proteoglycans.[8] The nucleus is much more accurately thought of as a porous sponge filled with a thick, viscous material than as a well-demarcated fluid-filled space. Changes in the disc on maturation occur in the nucleus pulposus, with an increase in collagen fibers and breakdown of proteoglycans. This decreases the disc's ability to absorb fluid with resulting loss of disc height.

Cartilaginous End Plates

The outer end plate is a hard, bony ring with a larger central cartilaginous part that anchors the disc to the vertebral body. They are also important pathways for the diffusion of nutrients from the vascular spongiosa of the vertebrae into the central part of the disc. Ten percent of each bony vertebral end plate is perforated by small vascular buds that make contact with the cartilage plate.

The Disc and Spinal Motion

The spinal motion segment with its three joint complex is a marvel of function that combines both stability and flexibility. The intervertebral disc is central to the typical spinal motion segment. Each segment is composed of the anterior amphiarthrodial joint formed by the disc between the two vertebral bodies and two posterior (zygapophyseal) diarthrodial joints. In the cervical spine, the joints of Luschka on the lateral aspect of the vertebral bodies add additional stability. Whereas the intervertebral disc allows for six degrees of freedom (rotation around the three axes and translation along the three axes; see Chapter 11), the posterior joints guide and restrict motion. Segmental movement is determined by the direction of the facet planes that produces different patterns of movement in the various spinal regions. The contribution of the intervertebral disc to spinal motion is dependent on the discal turgor.

Intrinsic Equilibrium

Motion in the healthy spine is dependent on the elastic properties of the noncontractile structures that contribute to a comparatively stable mechanical unit. The forces acting on the typical spinal segment include the axial pressure of the nucleus pulposus against the vertebral end plates (that resist compression and separate adjacent vertebrae) and the tension exerted by ligaments holding each segment together. These forces form an intrinsic equilibrium that depends on the turgor of the nucleus pulposus and the integrity of the spinal ligaments that form a delicate balance mechanism.[10] This mechanism allows for erect posture with relatively little muscular force. Disruption of this balance mechanism occurs with disc degeneration. With reduced turgidity of the nucleus, segmental instability and subluxation result.

Pathology

Disc Degeneration

Unequivocal findings of disc degeneration in the form of cleft and radial tears in the central anulus fibrosus are abundant beginning at age 11 to 16 years. This is thought to be caused by a diminution of the blood supply to the disc through the end plate, which begins before age 2 but becomes most pronounced between the ages of 3 and 10 years.[11]

Three stages of disc degeneration in the cervical spine were described by Hall[12] in 1965. A transverse fissure was observed in the early stage with a slight increase in the apposition of the vertebrae. A second stage of degeneration was described, with a further decrease in disc height and a flaring of the joints of Luschka. In the later stage, a transverse fissure from one side of the intervertebral region to the other was noted with the uncus forming an oblique shelf with a flattened superior surface.

In 1971 Schmorl and Junghanns described loosening of the spinal motion segment.[13] Kirkaldy-Willis[14] in turn described the pathology and pathogenesis of the lumbar spine in 1978. He labeled the three phases of the spectrum of degenerative disc disease as dysfunction, the unstable phase, and late stage stabilization.[15] He noted that the changes in the stage of dysfunction are minor and perhaps reversible. Movement of the posterior joints may be restricted, and palpation at the level of the lesion may demonstrate that one spinous process is out of line with the next.[15]

Changes in the intervertebral disc as degeneration progresses are characterized by small circumferential tears and increasing laxity, which allows subluxation of the joint surfaces to occur. Manipulation of subluxated facet joints most likely brings relief at this stage.[16] Later these tears become larger and coalesce to become radial tears that pass from the anulus into the nucleus. Motion caused by an axial rotatory torque is increased by radial and transverse tears in the anulus more than motion caused by flexion, extension, or lateral bending.[17] Therefore one would expect to see increased rotational stresses in the three joint complex with significant radial or transverse anular tears.

These tears increase until there is complete internal disruption of the disc. The normal disc height is greatly reduced because of the loss of proteoglycans and water from the nucleus. The anulus becomes lax and bulges around the circumference. This bulge must be distinguished from disc herniation, which is a protrusion of nuclear material through the anulus and into the epidural space.

In the stabilization phase described by Kirkaldy-Willis,[14] the spinal motion segment becomes increasingly stiff due to facet joint fibrosis and the formation of osteophytes at the disc and vertebral body following disc resorption to create a stable spinal motion segment.[15] The stabilization of a spinal motion segment creates added stress and advances degeneration at least at the two levels immediately above the stabilized joint complex, creating findings similar to the findings immediately cephalad to a lumbosacral fusion.[18]

Disc Herniation

The mechanism of disc herniation may be a series of recurrent rotational injuries that produce circumferential and radial tears leading to disc bulge. In some cases the anulus is completely ruptured and the nucleus protrudes through the anulus. In severe cases, part of the nucleus breaks free and becomes sequestrated. The sequestrated fragment may move about, causing variations in symptoms from level to level and side-to-side.

A severe compression injury with the spine flexed may cause a sudden rupture of the anulus.[15] However, once the anulus is torn, the degree of flexion and the level of nucleus pulposus hydration are the two most influential factors with respect to whether or not the nucleus breaks loose and extrudes through the torn anulus. The rate of loading is not thought to be very important once the anular tear is present.[19] Disc herniation can compromise the nerve roots, and posterior herniation in the cervical spine can affect the spinal cord. Because the conus medullaris is superior to the lumbar spine, the cord is not affected by a central bulge or herniation in the lumbar spine.

Extremity pain can be the significant symptom of a patient presenting with a disc injury. Involvement of the nerve root is certainly one source of extremity symptoms in these patients. The nerve root is compressed by the extruded nucleus, or even by a focal bulge in the anulus, with the result being ischemic changes to the nerve root and possible long-term or even permanent neurologic damage. This type of mechanical compression of the nerve root causes true radicular signs and symptoms of pain in the dermatomal distribution of the affected nerve root, sensory changes (hyperesthesia, paresthesia, hypoesthesia, anesthesia) along the same dermatome, motor loss or weakness of muscles innervated in whole or part by the affected root, and a decrease in the deep tendon reflex of corresponding muscles.

Mechanical compression of nerve roots may not be the only cause of nerve root involvement in the clinical picture. The presence of nucleus pulposus material in the epidural space without compression of the root has been shown to produce nerve root inflammation and even irritation of the dorsal root ganglion, both of which can cause radicular signs and symptoms.[20] Epidural presence of nucleus pulposus has also been shown to reduce nerve root and DRG blood flow with a measurable reduction in nerve conduction velocity.[21]

There is a significant association between recent episodes of low back pain and disc degeneration demonstrable on MRI.[22] Even without the demonstrable presence of nucleus pulposus in the epidural space, patients may report buttock, hip, groin, or lower limb pain. Tears in the posterior anulus common to the degenerative disc have been shown capable of producing these symptoms with[22] or without[23] a posterior disc bulge.

Additionally, herniation can affect nonadjacent structures. For example, patients with documented lumbar disc herniations with back and leg pain have been found to have a high incidence of sacroiliac joint dysfunction, perhaps due to direct effects from the mechanical changes at the injured level or perhaps from changes in hamstring and iliopsoas muscle function as a result of nerve root irritation. These symptoms respond well to manual therapy of the SI joints.[24] (See Chapter 26.) This effect on a joint as complex and important to the totality of spinal motion as the sacroiliac joint demonstrates the importance of ensuring proper segmental motion on either side of a disc lesion as an important step to prevent secondary pain syndromes and biomechanical deficits throughout the kinetic chain.

Biomechanical changes associated with disc degeneration or herniation change the mechanics of adjacent vertebral three joint complexes, causing added or unusual stress and changes in function. These stresses may be expressed as a facet syndrome with referred pain patterns that mimic radicular pain in the extremity. This type of pain syndrome generally responds well to chiropractic adjustments.

Finally, a significant number of asymptomatic people have been shown to have disc bulges and, to a lesser extent, even herniations.[25] This supports the notion that the disc's effect on surrounding structures and the mechanics of the region may be as important as the direct effect on the nerve root.

Schmorl's Nodes

Protrusion of disc tissue into adjacent vertebral bodies is known as Schmorl's nodes.[13] At the centers of the cartilaginous plates are weak points where the notochord originally penetrated. Here herniation of the young fluid nucleus can penetrate into the spongiosa with little if any immediate adverse affect on functioning of the segment. However, it is thought that such damage to the end plate alters the distribution of stress through the anulus. Repeated loading following compressive damage to the end plate appears to cause buckling of the lamella of the anulus and subsequent tears.[26]

Clinical Findings

History

Patients presenting with disc herniation have frequently had prior episodes of low back pain. They may relate a precipitating event such as lifting, twisting, or heaving a heavy object but may only recount a minimal provocation incident.[27] It is not unusual to hear "I just bent over to pick up the soap in the shower" or "I just bent down to tie my shoe."[27]

Signs and Symptoms

The patient with a herniated disc may complain of back pain, back and leg pain, or leg pain alone. The pain is typically increased by activity and relieved by rest.[28,29] If inflammation is present from muscle strain or chemical irritation of the anular fibers, pain may be present at rest. It is usually less severe than when the patient is upright and active.[30] Coughing, sneezing, straining, and prolonged sitting aggravate the pain. Relief is often obtained when lying supine or on one side. Discogenic lower back pain is usually moderate to severe and described as a deep dull ache or burning pain.[31-33] The patient may have difficulty getting in and out of a vehicle and returning upright from bending forward, and pain often causes the patient to grab the lower back followed by the use of the hands walking up the thighs to return to the upright position (Minor's sign).[27]

Leg Pain

Somatic referred leg pain (also referred to as sclerotomic or pseudoradicular pain) is often less intense than discogenic low back pain. It is usually mild to moderate and is described as a dull ache that is characteristically difficult to localize.[31] The mechanism has been described as afferent impulses from the disc, activating neurons in the central nervous system (CNS) that converge on afferents from the leg. Stimulation of these CNS neurons by impulses from the disc results in the perception of pain in the leg, although there is no signal actually emanating from the leg.[31] Somatic referred leg pain is known as intervertebral disc syndrome without radiculopathy, because there are no sciatica symptoms, nerve tension signs, or neurologic deficits. Sciatica is defined as pain in the distribution of a lumbar nerve root and is often accompanied by neurologic deficit. Sciatica without neurologic deficit is also known as irritative radiculopathy, because it is thought that the sciatica symptoms and nerve tension signs are caused by nerve root irritation. Sciatica with neurologic deficit is also known as compressive radiculopathy, because the weakness, diminished sensation, and diminished reflexes are attributed to nerve root compression. Radicular pain is sharp, well localized, and often described as an electric shock-like pain. Referred pain into the lower extremities must not be interpreted as a radicular pain from nerve root compromise[27] (Table 25-1).

Examination

Patients with lumbar disc herniation commonly have an antalgic list with all movements restricted. Straight-leg raising is frequently markedly diminished. Passive straight-leg raising affects numerous tissues; recording the results of a straight-leg raising test as either positive or negative gives little guidance to the clinician.[27] In addition to neuromeningeal tension, passive straight-leg raising stretches the hamstring muscles, the tissues of the buttock, and the posterior facet joints, as well as stressing the sacroiliac joints.[27]

Straight-leg raising in the presence of sciatica caused by nerve-root pressure produces severe pain in the back, in the sciatic distribution of the affected leg, or in both (Figure 25-1). To confirm that the nerve root is the source of the pain, the involved leg is raised to the point of pain and then lowered a few degrees. Nerve-root stretch is then produced by forced dorsiflexion of the ankle[27] (Bragard test; Figure 25-2) or by firm pressure applied to the popliteal fossa over the posterior tibial nerve (Bowstring test).[34] If the pain is reproduced by either of these tests, altered root tension is indicated. Pain that occurs with less than 30 degrees of straight-leg raising is strongly indicative of disc herniation. Pain in the sacroiliac joints is usually elicited on straight-leg raising past 70 degrees in patients with a sacroiliac syndrome. (See Chapter 26.)

If the sciatic pain is reproduced on internal rotation of the femur after the straight leg is lowered a few degrees, it is indicative of irritation of the sciatic nerve by the piriformis muscle rather than a sign of nerve-root tension, and it is known as a positive piriformis sign. Trigger points in the piriformis muscle remain the most unrecognized cause of sciatica. Patients with this syndrome complain of pain and or paresthesia in the distribution of the sciatic nerve that is frequently misdiagnosed as nerve root compression.[35] Palpation of a trigger point deep in the belly of the piriformis muscle that produces radiation down the course of the sciatic nerve is confirmation that the piriformis muscle is a factor in the patient's sciatica and treatment should be directed to the involved muscle.[35] Centrally located protrusions tend to produce low back pain and leg pain. Leg pain is commonly produced only by laterally located protrusions. When pain is elicited in the affected

Table 25-1

Distinguishing Referred Pain from Radicular Pain in Disc Herniation

	Referred pain	Radicular pain
Symptoms	Deep, boring, ill-defined pain, poorly localized	Sharp, well-localized, electric shock-like pain
Radiation	Distant from origin in posterior joints, sacroiliac joints or muscles (i.e., gluteus medius and piriformis); pain may radiate to groin, posterolateral thigh or calf, rarely to foot	Most common presentations follow sciatic nerve root distribution from the back of the posterolateral thigh and calf to the foot or femoral nerve root distribution to the anterior thigh
Sensory alteration	Rare; occasional hyperesthesia	Frequent; follows a dermatomal distribution
Motor weakness	May have subjective weakness but objective weakness or atrophy is rare	Frequent objective weakness and atrophy with prolonged duration of symptoms
Reflex deficit	Rare; reported with posterior joint syndrome	Frequent
Nerve-root tension signs	Absent; straight-leg raising may cause increased low back pain at posterior joint or sacroiliac joint or may reveal tight hamstring muscles	Straight-leg raising produces pain in sciatic distribution, sciatic notch tenderness, popliteal and perineal nerve tenderness; hip extension with knee flexion produces pain in femoral distribution down anterior thigh

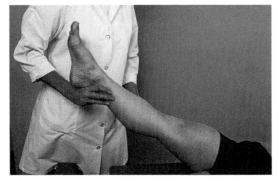

Figure 25-1   Straight-leg raise test.

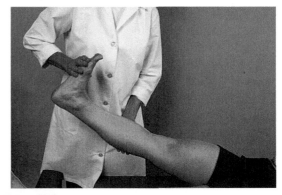

Figure 25-2   Bragard reinforcement test.

extremity by straight-leg raising of the opposite leg (Fajersztajn's sign or the well-leg-raising test),[27] it is strongly suggestive of a disc herniation, usually lying medial to the root within the "axilla" between the dura and the exiting root sleeve.[36]

To traction the femoral nerve, the patient lies on the unaffected side with the unaffected limb flexed slightly at the hip and the knee (Figure 25-3). The patient's back is kept straight (not hyperextended), and the neck is slightly flexed.

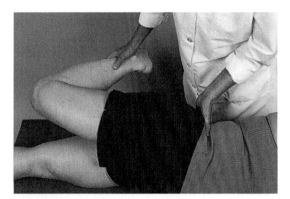

Figure 25-3   Femoral nerve traction.

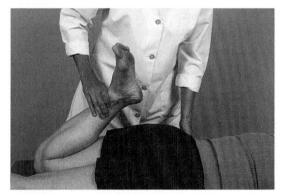

Figure 25-4   Nachlas test.

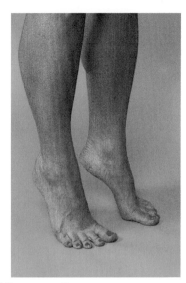

Figure 25-5   Toe walk.

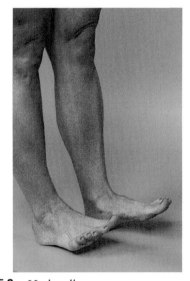

Figure 25-6   Heel walk.

The doctor grasps the patient's affected (painful) limb and extends the knee while gently extending the hip to approximately 15 degrees. The knee is then flexed, which further stretches the femoral nerve.[37] Alternatively, the patient may be placed in a prone position and the affected knee bent (Nachlas test; Figure 25-4),[34] with hip extension added if needed. Pain radiating to the anterior thigh indicates stretching of the femoral nerve. Pain in the groin and hip that radiates along the anterior medial thigh is indicative of an L3 nerve root lesion, while pain extending to the mid-tibia indicates an L4 nerve root problem.[37]

Having the patient walk on heels and toes readily tests muscle weakness. The patient is asked to heel walk toward the examiner to determine foot extensor weakness.[35] Walking on the heels tests the strength of the tibialis anterior, extensor digitorum longus, and the hallucis longus muscles.

Weakness of this muscle group is consistent with L5 nerve-root compression (Figure 25-5).[34] The patient is asked to toe walk away from the examiner to determine plantar flexor weakness. If one heel drops closer to the floor, weakness of the gastrocnemius, soleus, and plantaris muscles is indicated. Weakness of this muscle group is consistent with S1 nerve root compression (Figure 25-6).[34]

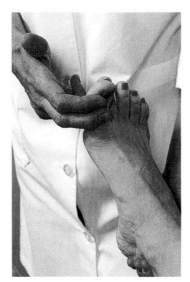

Figure 25-7   Great toe strength test.

Full squatting evaluates muscular strength and hip and knee function. If dysfunction is present, this movement usually produces pain at the site of pathology.[34] Weakness of the great toe should alert the examiner to the possibility of disc herniation affecting the L5 neurologic level, since this is often one of the first indicators (Figure 25-7). Commonly, numbness (hypoesthesia) can be detected over one dermatome on pinwheel testing.[34] The knee or ankle reflex may be markedly diminished or absent, depending on the level of herniation.[27]

Diagnostic Imaging

Most patients can be treated conservatively without confirmation of a disc abnormality on magnetic resonance (MR) or computed tomography (CT) imaging. Magnetic resonance imaging (MRI) has proven a valuable adjunct to computed tomography, providing markedly improved soft tissue contrast resolution of lumbar discs or neural elements and advanced imaging is a necessary part of a presurgical workup. Patients with bladder or bowel incontinence (cauda equina syndrome), foot drop, severe bilateral sciatica, or severe progressive neurologic deficit should be referred for an immediate neurologic consultation.

Chiropractic Management of Disc Herniation

Far too often patients with a disc disorder are routed into the surgical triage process without a fair trial of conservative treatment. In reality the only two reasons for surgical intervention in a case of disc lesion are *progressive* neurologic loss and the patient's inability to deal with the pain.

In the case of neurologic changes, it is important to differentiate between a neurologic deficit, such as a small area of paresthesia, and a more serious progressive loss of function, such as motor weakness. There is a danger that any nerve deficit caused by a disc lesion will be permanent but it is much more likely if the motor portion of the nerve is affected.

The pain experienced by a patient with a disc problem should never be underestimated. True radicular pain can be excruciating. Even at lesser intensities, the psychological effects of pain are cumulative. Over time they can be physically exhausting, cause emotional distress including anger and depression, and have a profound effect on relationships and the roles expected of the patient. At some point, the danger and negative aspects of spinal surgery can become acceptable risks for the patient looking for some escape from the pain sequelae.

It is much easier to approach the treatment of a disc patient with the goal of helping the body get to a point where it accommodates to the mechanical and spatial changes and begins to function more normally or at least less symptomatically than it is to try to cure the lesion. As we have already noted, patients with documented disc disease may well be asymptomatic as may patients with large osteophytes or other space occupying lesions that are slow to develop, thereby allowing the body time to accommodate as they progress. A major role of the chiropractor treating these patients is to deal with the mechanical and functional lesions (subluxations) caused by the changes in spinal mechanics and to minimize the symptoms associated with these changes. By controlling the patient's symptoms, chiropractic treatment can facilitate the body's compensation over time for the lesion.

A herniated disc does not preclude adjustive procedures. A conservative trial of intersegmental flexion-distraction technique or side-posture manipulation can help reduce the symptoms of disc herniation and should be employed in the absence of advancing neurological defects or cauda equina syndrome. Passive intersegmental flexion-distraction has been described in the osteopathic literature[38] and more recently the chiropractic literature.[2,39] Cox[2] recommends flexion-distraction manipulation for the treatment of lumbar disc protrusion, suggesting that this allows the intervertebral disc to resume its central position within the anulus and relieves irritation of the pain sensitive anular fibers. He describes the following mechanism of action:

1. Decompression of the neural structures and enlargement of the IVF
2. Centripetal force from posterior anular fibers and the posterior longitudinal ligament to push the nucleus anteriorly
3. Enhancement of disc nutrition through imbibition
4. Suction and traction
5. Deep muscle stretching and improved segmental mobility

Treatment consists of strapping the ankles of the prone patient to the caudal end of a table that is hinged to flex in the middle. Axial traction of the caudal half of the table is also used. With the patient positioned so that maximum flexion and traction occurs at the involved segment, the doctor uses a thenar contact on the spinous process, pushing cephalad in a pumping motion while the other hand flexes and pumps the caudal end of the table (Figure 25-8). Motorized tables may also be used. Care must be taken to monitor patient tolerance and to avoid excessive flexion, which may cause injury. Two inches of movement is commonly recommended.[2] The distal half of the table is also hinged to allow lateral flexion and/or rotational movements if necessary.[27] Benefits from flexion will be more likely in incomplete herniations, where the integrity of the posterior anular fibers and posterior longitudinal ligament have been preserved. In more severe cases, flexion may allow further posterior migration of nuclear mate-

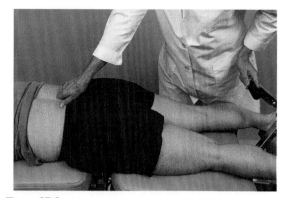

Figure 25-8   Flexion-distraction therapy.

rial with worsening of symptoms. Patient response must be carefully monitored to establish whether this form of therapy is appropriate.

Success with rotational manipulation in the treatment of disc herniation, particularly in cases of incomplete anular damage, has been reported by a number of authors.[1,27,38-43] Even when successful, this technique does not necessarily replace a displaced nucleus to its normal position but apparently moves it away from the neighboring nerve root, relieving radicular symptoms. Cassidy[1] has shown postmanipulative improvement of radiculopathy in patients who did and did not show CT changes in herniation size.

Aside from movement of the nucleus, other potential effects of manipulation may include improved disc hydrodynamics and nutrition, reducing anular tension, movement of the nerve root, improved motion segment dynamics, and optimized vascular exchange to allow dispersal of byproducts of inflammation.[27] Natural history should also be considered in the treatment of disc herniation. Herniations, especially larger ones, have been shown to "resorb" within as little as one year.[42,43]

Panzer et al.[27] notes that in order to minimize risk in the manipulation of patients with disc herniation, the patient should be carefully assessed before applying high velocity procedures. Examples of clinical findings useful in determining the appropriateness of rotational or other mobilization/manipulation include the following:

1. Antalgic position of patient (flexed antalgia without lateral lean) may indicate a more central herniation. A medial herniation with a positive well-leg raise test has a poorer prognosis for conservative (nonsurgical) care that a lateral herniation.[42]
2. Response of radicular symptoms to active and passive ranges of motion
3. Response of radicular symptoms to segmental motion palpation, "end play," and "overpressure" in specific vectors
4. Based on the above, simulate manipulative vector(s) with segmental mobilization to test the patient's response *before* thrusting.
5. Test various combinations of vectors (i.e. lateral bending, flexion, or extension) in combination with rotation to determine the vector(s) best tolerated. Vectors may change as the patient's condition evolves.

Side-posture rotational manipulation requires careful positioning for optimal results.[1] The patient is positioned in the side lying position with the sciatic leg on top (Figure 25-9). Contact is at the level of restricted motion and tenderness and the patient is taken to the point of tension. Contact is made on the mamillary or spinous process if a push thrust move is to be used or the spinous process if a pull move is preferred.[27, 40] If gentle mobilization aggravates the patient's leg or back pain on the set-up, then the position should be modified. When the patient tolerates the premanipulation set-up, a high velocity, low amplitude thrust is applied. Patients should be carefully monitored and any position, mobilization, or manipulation that increases the patient's sciatica or neurologic deficit should be avoided.

In contrast to flexion-distraction and rotational manipulation with the patient flexed, both extension manipulation and extension exercises are used to treat disc herniation. The rationale of this approach is that a disc injury almost invariably occurs during a flexed position, allowing the nucleus to migrate posteriorly due to anular damage.[16,27,44,45] Extension of the joint reverses this process, decompresses the disc, and may help shift the nucleus more anteriorly.* Quite commonly a disc lesion is associated with a vertebra fixed in a flexed position, and extension treatment may be the most appropriate and best tolerated by the patient.[27] The principle of extension can be applied with segmental manipulation in a prone, side-lying, supine, or knee-chest position. Even patients unable to extend actively when weight bearing may often quite easily be placed in this position passively when on their side and not weight bearing. Again, patient tolerance is an important guide, and previously described techniques to produce extension may be appropriate. Restoration of segmental mobility in extension by specific manipulative techniques may allow maximum benefit from McKenzie-type exercises to be realized.[42]

Extension exercises in the prone, standing, and even seated positions are useful in treating these patients.[6,42,45] Using MRI, Boumphrey[47] demonstrated that McKenzie extension exercises increased the disc height in normal and degenerated discs but did not have an effect on the position of the nucleus pulposus of normal, degenerated, or herniated discs. Passive extension as it increases facet weight bearing apparently distracts the vertebral bodies enough to enhance intradiscal imbibition.

Conclusion

Chiropractic manipulation is a well-recognized form of conservative treatment for intervertebral disc syndrome. When combined with exercise and

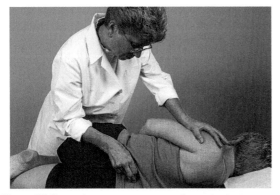

Figure 25-9   Side posture rotational manipulation.

*References 16, 40, 42, 44, 45, 46.

patient education, chiropractic manipulation can relieve pain, neurologic deficit, shorten the recovery period, and prevent the development of chronic pain and disability syndrome.

References

1. Cassidy JD, Theil HW, Kirkaldy-Willis WH. Side posture manipulation for intervertebral disc herniation. J Manipulative Physiol Ther 1993;16(2):96-103.
2. Cox JM, Hazen LJ, Mungovan M. Distraction manipulation reduction of an L5-S1disk herniation. J Manipulative Physiol Ther 1993;16(5):34-46.
3. Farfan HF. Mechanical disorders of the low back. Philadelphia: Lea and Febiger; 1973.
4. Chisman OD, Mittmacht A, Snook GA. A study of the results following rotatory manipulation in the lumbar intervertebral disc syndrome. J Bone Joint Surg 1964; 46A:517.
5. Mathew JA, Yates DAH. Treatment of sciatica. Lancet 1974;1:352.
6. Valentini E. Acute lumbar disc syndromes under chiropractic care: a statistical study. Annals Swiss Chiropractic Association 1981;7:67-83.
7. Gatterman MI, Cooperstein R, Perle S. Rating specific technique procedure for common low back conditions. J Manipulative Physiol Ther 2001;24:449-56.
8. Grignon B, Roland J. Can the human intervertebral disc be compared to a diarthrodial joint? Surg Radiol Anat 2000;22:101-5.
9. Mercer S, Bogduk N. The ligaments and anulus fibrosus of human adult cervical intervertebral discs. Spine 1999; 24:619-26.
10. Steindler A. Kinesiology of the human body under normal and pathological conditions. Springfield, IL: Charles C Thomas; 1973. p. 141-2.
11. Boos N, Weissbach S, Rohrbach H, Weiler C, Spratt KF, Nerlich AG. Classification of age-related changes in lumbar intervertebral discs. Spine 2002;27:23.
12. Hall MC. Luschka's joint. Springfield, IL: Charles C Thomas; 1965. p. 43-6.
13. Schmorl G, Junghanns H. The human spine in health and disease. 2nd ed. New York: Grune and Stratton; 1971.
14. Kirkaldy-Willis WH, Wedge J, Young Hing K, Reilly J. Pathology and pathogenesis of lumbar spondylosis and stenosis. Spine 1978;3:319-28.
15. Kirkaldy-Willis WH. Managing low back pain. 2nd ed. New York: Churchill Livingstone; 1988. p. 117-31.
16. Keim HA, Kirkaldy-Willis WH. Clinical symposia: low back pain. Summit, NJ: Ciba-Geigy; 1987;39:2-32.
17. Haughton VM, Schmidt TA, Keele K, An HS, Lim TH. Flexibility of lumbar spinal motion segments correlated to type of tears in the anulus fibrosus. J Neurosurg 2000;92:81-6.
18. Hambly MF, Wiltse LL, Raghaven N, Schneiderman G, Koening C. The transition zone above a lumbosacral fusion. Spine 1998;23:16.
19. Simunic DI, Broom ND, Robertson PA. Biomechanical factors influencing nuclear disruption of the intervertebral disc. Spine 2001;26:11.
20. Takebayashi T, Cavanaugh JM, Ozaktay AC, Kallakuri S, Chen C. Effect of nucleus pulposus on the neural activity of dorsal root ganglion. Spine 2001;26:940-5.
21. Otani K, Arai I, Mao GP, Konno S, Olmarker K, Kikuchi S. Nucleus pulposus-induced nerve root injury: relationship between blood flow and motor nerve conduction velocity. Neurosurgery 1999;45:3.
22. Luoma K, Riihimaki H, Luukkonen R, Raininko R, Viikari-Juntura E, Lamminen A. Low back pain in relation to lumbar disc injury. Spine 2000;25:4.
23. Saifuddin A, Emanuel R, White J, Renton P, Braithwaite I, Taylor BA. An analysis of radiating pain at lumbar discography. Eur Spine J 1998;7:358-62.
24. Galm R, Frohling M, Rittmeister M, Schmidt E. Sacroiliac joint dysfunction in patients with imaging-proven lumbar disc herniation. Eur Spine J 1998;7:450-3.
25. McCall IW. Lumbar herniated disks. Radiologic Clin of North Amer 2000;38:6.
26. Adams MA, Freeman BJC, Morrison HP, Nelson IW, Dolan P. Mechanical initiation of intervertebral disc degeneration. Spine 2000;25:13.
27. Panzer DM, Gatterman MI. Disorders of the lumbar spine. In: Gatterman MI, editor. Chiropractic management of spine related disorders. 2nd ed. Baltimore: Lippincott Williams & Wilkins; 2003. p. 150-97.
28. Deyo RA. Early diagnostic evaluation of low back pain. J Gen Intern Med 1986;1(Sept/Oct):328-38.
29. Deyo RA, Rainville J, Kent DL. What can the history and physical examination tell us about low back pain? J Am Med Assoc 1992;268:760-5.
30. Brown MD. The source of low back pain and sciatica. Sem in Arthritis Rheum Suppl 1989;18(4):67-72.
31. Bogduk N, Twomey LT, editors. Clinical anatomy of the lumbar spine. 2nd ed. Melbourne: Churchill Livingstone; 1991. p. 151-73.
32. Hall H. A simple approach to back pain management. Patient Care 1992;15:77-92.
33. Fast A. Low back disorders: conservative management. Arch Phys Med Rehab 1988;69:880-90.
34. Evans RC. Illustrated essentials in orthopedic physical assessment. 2nd ed. St. Louis: Mosby; 2001.
35. Gatterman MI, Blunt KL, Goe DR. Muscle and myofascial pain syndromes. In: Gatterman MI, editor. Chiropractic management of spine related disorders. 2nd ed. Baltimore: Lippincott Williams & Wilkins; 2003.
36. Finneson BE. Low back pain. 2nd ed. Philadelphia: JB Lippincott; 1980.
37. Magee DJ. Orthopedic physical assessment. 4th ed. Philadelphia: Saunders; 2002.

38. Stoddard A. Manual of osteopathic technique. London: Hutchinson; 1980.

39. Cox JM, Hazen LJ, Mungovan M. Distraction manipulation reduction of an L5-S1 disk herniation. J Manipulative Physiol Ther 1993;16:342-6.

40. Peterson DH, Bergmann TF. Chiropractic technique. St. Louis: Mosby; 2002.

41. Stoddard A. Manual of osteopathic technique. London: Hutchinson; 1980.

42. LeFebvre R, Panzer D, Agresta J et al. Herniated lumbar disc with radiculopathy. Portland, OR: Western States Chiropractic College Conservative Care Pathways; 1999.

43. Saal JA, Saal JS. Nonoperative treatment of herniated lumbar intervertebral disc with radiculopathy: an outcome study. Spine 1989;14:431-7.

44. McKenzie RA. The lumbar spine. Waikana, New Zealand: Spinal Publications; 1981. p. 16-7.

45. Donelson R, Aprill C, Medcalf R, Grant W. A prospective study of centralization of lumbar and referred pain. Spine 1997;22:1115-22.

46. Mooney V, Saal JA, Saal JS. Evaluation and treatment of low back pain. Ciba Clinical Symposia 1996;48:2-32.

47. Boumphrey F. The challenge of the lumbar spine (seminar notes). San Francisco; 1986.

Sacroiliac Subluxation Syndrome

Meridel I. Gatterman and
David M. Panzer

Key Words   Sacroiliac subluxation syndrome, track-based motion, closed kinetic chain

After reading this chapter you should be able to answer the following questions:

Question 1   What three joints make the pelvic ring an atypical spinal motion segment?

Question 2   How may the track-bound motion of the sacroiliac joints contribute to the sacroiliac subluxation?

Question 3   What single activity is most likely to aggravate the pain from sacroiliac subluxation syndrome?

Manipulation of the sacroiliac joints for the treatment of sacroiliac subluxation has been described in chiropractic literature since the earliest textbooks.[1-5] Ignored as a cause of back pain by traditional medicine after Mixter and Barr[6] focused attention on disc herniation and surgery in 1934, the sacroiliac joints until recently were not commonly considered to be mobile enough to cause significant dysfunction from restricted motion. It is now recognized that the sacroiliac joints are moving, weight bearing synovial joints that exhibit the same characteristic subluxation and joint dysfunction that plague other diarthrodial joints. They are subject to reversible joint blockage (manipulable subluxations) that occurs within their limited range of motion, frequently at the extreme of possible range of movement. They become irritated and have a tendency for hypermobility when motion at adjacent articulations is restricted. They are also prone to degenerative disease as are other synovial joints.

Sacroiliac Joint Motion

Although sacroiliac joint motion is commonly considered to be very slight, 3 degrees to 9 degrees of rotation has been demonstrated in both anatomic specimens and living subjects.[7-9] Walker[7] describes motion of the sacroiliac joint as a coupling of rotation and translation that provides 6 degrees of freedom with a change in the instantaneous axis of rotation. She found modal rotation to be 3 degrees and the average translation to be less than 3 mm.[7] Scmidt[8] reported the average oblique-sagittal motion to be 9 degrees in live subjects, with no gender differences. In fresh cadaver studies of elderly subjects, a mean of 7 degrees of rotation on the left and 8 degrees of rotation on the right was observed.[9] The range of translation was reported as 4 to 8 mm in each of the cardinal directions (vertical, mediolateral, and anteroposterior).

Several factors affect sacroiliac motion, including age, gender, and configuration of the joint surfaces that exhibit complementary ridges and depressions. The degree of sacroiliac motion decreases with age more rapidly in men than in women.

Female sacroiliac joints tend to be flatter with a wider retroarticular space and longer interosseous ligaments, all of which promote greater mobility.[10] Reversible ligamentous laxity attributed to the hormone relaxin has been observed with pregnancy and, to a lesser degree, during the menstrual cycle.[11] Both translation and rotation (see Chapter 11) have been described as normal motion in the sacroiliac articulations. The primary movement pattern has been described as track bound, with opposing joint surfaces moving along and directed by a convex ridge on the iliac surface that glides in a concave sacral depression (Figure 26-1).[12] The axis of this rotation has not been consistently described and may shift with minimal translatory movement. The slight translation has been described as giving the joint shock absorption capability.[13] The two posterior joints and the anterior symphysis pubis have been likened to an atypical motion segment with the sacroiliac joints guiding motion. The posterior facet joints and the symphysis pubis provide slight translation in a manner similar to the intervertebral discs.[14] This three-joint complex is a closed kinetic chain, with

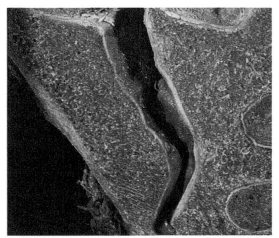

Figure 26-1   Motion of the sacroiliac joint primarily occurs in the oblique sagittal plane, with the axis of rotation centered around the iliac tubercle. The joint surfaces appear to move along the tram tail, the convex ridge of the iliac surface gliding in the sacral grooves. *(From S. Mior, Canadian Memorial Chiropractic College.)*

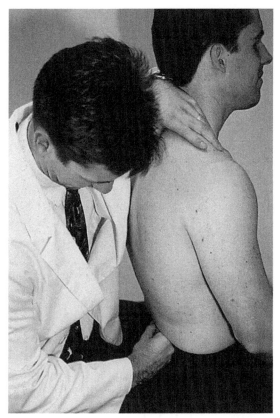

Figure 26-2   The screening method utilized by Gillet used the dorsum of the hand to challenge end feel.

each articulation having determinate relations with each of the other joints in the pelvic ring.[15] Gillet and Liekans[16] described the sacrum as floating within the pelvic ring, cushioning the slight amount of observed physiologic movement. They developed a method of monitoring this movement using palpation with the back of the hand to challenge end feel of the sacroiliac joints (Figure 26-2).

Sacroiliac Subluxation

Sacroiliac subluxation may take the form of simple joint locking or it may be accompanied by compensatory hypermobility in adjacent joints, especially in menstruating and pregnant females. Vleeming et al.[17] stated that it is theoretically possible that with abnormal loading, a sacroiliac joint may be forced into a new position where ridge and depression are no longer complementary. They note that this abnormal joint position may be regarded as a blocked joint (manipulable subluxation). It is thought that the resultant restriction of movement or aberrant motion that occurs from a shift in the normal axis of rotation then produces a sacroiliac subluxation syndrome. The characteristics of a sacroiliac subluxation have been described by Turek[18] as ligamentous stretching sufficient enough to permit the ilium to slip on the sacrum as an irregular prominence on one articular surface becomes wedged on another prominence of the other articular surface. He stated that this is consistent with surface irregularities that have been noted on examination of the sacroiliac joint surfaces.

Clinical Considerations

The clinical findings associated with sacroiliac subluxation syndrome are described by Turek[18] as intense muscle spasm accompanied by severe pain. The cause of sacroiliac subluxation is often indicated by the patient's history. Frequently, they describe a fall on the buttocks or a lifting injury that involved torsional stress. Stepping off of a curb or twisting such as getting out of bed have been reported.[14]

Pain Pattern

The pain of sacroiliac syndrome is typically located over the ipsilateral buttock, dull in character, and made worse by sitting. It occasionally may extend down the lateral and posterior calf as far as the ankle, foot, and toes (Figure 26-3). Sensory changes rarely occur but occasionally take the form of paresthesias in the ipsilateral lower extremity. Pain referred from the sacroiliac joints is experienced in the posterior dermatomal areas of L5, S1, and S2, radiating over the sacrum and into the buttocks. Pain referral from the anterior ligaments radiates into the anterior dermatomal areas of L2 and L3, particularly into the thigh region immediately below the groin.[19,20] Pain from a hypermobile sacroiliac joint also may be experienced in the ipsilateral hip because of contraction of the ipsilateral piriformis muscle, which originates at the sacrum and ilium (Figure 26-4).

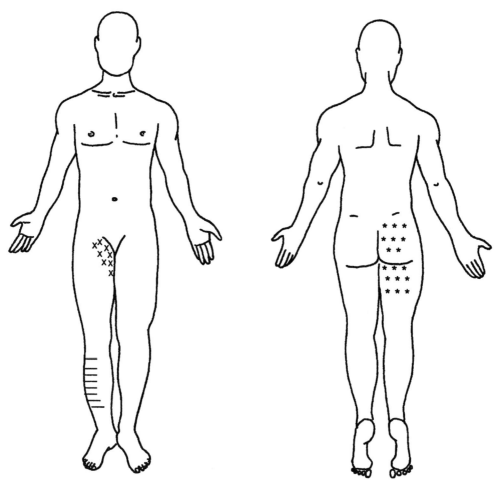

Figure 26-3   Pain pattern of a patient with a right sacroiliac syndrome (*, aching; x, burning; –, numbness). *(From Gatterman MI. Chiropractic management of spine related disorders. Baltimore: Williams & Wilkins, 1990.)*

A hypermobile joint generally stabilizes within three to six weeks when abnormal motion is restricted by a trochanteric support bandage (Figure 26-5). Localized tenderness is produced on palpation of the subluxated sacroiliac joint. The patient also may exhibit a limping gait to minimize pain on weight bearing.

Although localized pain and tenderness have demonstrated higher interrater reliability than other palpatory indicators such as motion palpation, misalignment palpation, and muscle tension palpation,[21] pain alone cannot be considered the major criterion for diagnosis of subluxations.

Nonmanipulable subluxations in which forceful manipulation is contraindicated may exhibit pain and tenderness from hypermobility and, in extreme cases, instability. (See Chapter 8.)

Tests for Sacroiliac Dysfunction

Sacroiliac dysfunction can be detected by a number of orthopedic tests. Like other areas of the spine, the manipulable subluxation is best detected through static and motion palpation and joint play testing. Other specific tests detect sacroiliac involvement, but give no indication as to whether

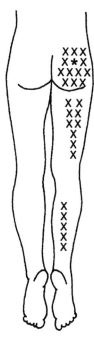

Figure 26-4   Piriformis syndrome. Trigger points *(*)* located near the belly and insertion of the piriformis muscle refer pain *(x)* in a characteristic pattern. *(From Gatterman MI. Chiropractic management of spine related disorders. Baltimore: Williams & Wilkins; 1990.)*

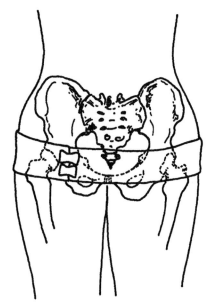

Figure 26-5   A hypermobile joint can be stabilized with a tight elastic trochanteric bandage. The sacroiliac joint is generally stabilized within three to six weeks with this form of continuous stabilization. *(From Gatterman MI. Chiropractic management of spine related disorders. Baltimore: Williams & Wilkins; 1990.)*

manipulation is indicated. Provocation tests are based on provoked sacroiliac joint pain as a sign of articular dysfunction but they do not differentiate the nature of the dysfunction. Toussaint[22] concluded that the consistency between three palpation tests was moderate to good and the percentage agreement acceptable. Laslett[23] found reasonable reproducibility and reliability with pain provocation tests employing distraction, compression, posterior glide, and pelvic torsion. In another study[24] the diagnostic value of 12 tests commonly used to detect sacroiliac joint pain was questioned. Using diagnostic joint block, the study found the most sensitive tests to be sacrosulcus tenderness, pain over the sacroiliac joint, buttock pain, and indication by the patient pointing to the PSIS (posterior superior iliac spine) as the main

pain source. This suggests the importance of carefully noting patients' perception of their pain source when evaluating pain provocation tests.

Pelvic Compression

Pain, especially in irritated or inflamed joints, can indicate sacroiliac involvement when compression is applied to the pelvis. Pressure can be applied to the iliac crests with the patient lying on the side or supine (Figure 26-6). Pain provoked in the sacroiliac regions indicates a positive test in any of these positions, but does not differentiate the exact nature of the sacroiliac problem or give an indication of the appropriate treatment.

Figure of Four (FABERE) Test

The acronym *FABERE* stands for *f*lexion, *ab*duction, *e*xternal *r*otation, and *e*xtension, which forms a figure of four when the thigh is passively

A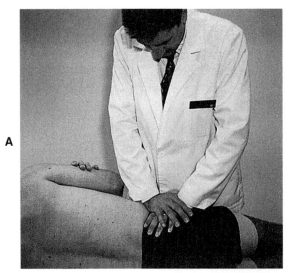

B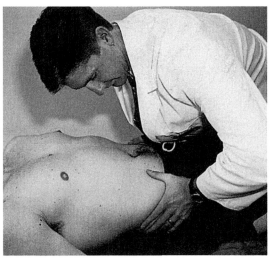

C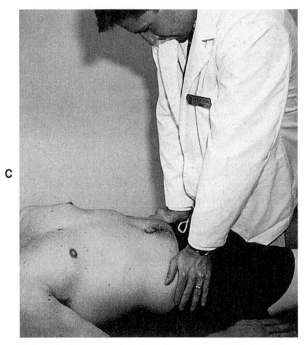

Figure 26-6   Compression applied to the iliac crest(s) with the patient side lying (**A**) or supine (**B**) may produce pain in irritated or inflamed sacroiliac joints. Sacroiliac involvement is also suspected if pain is produced when sacroiliac joint function is provoked by pressure applied to separate the iliac crests (**C**).

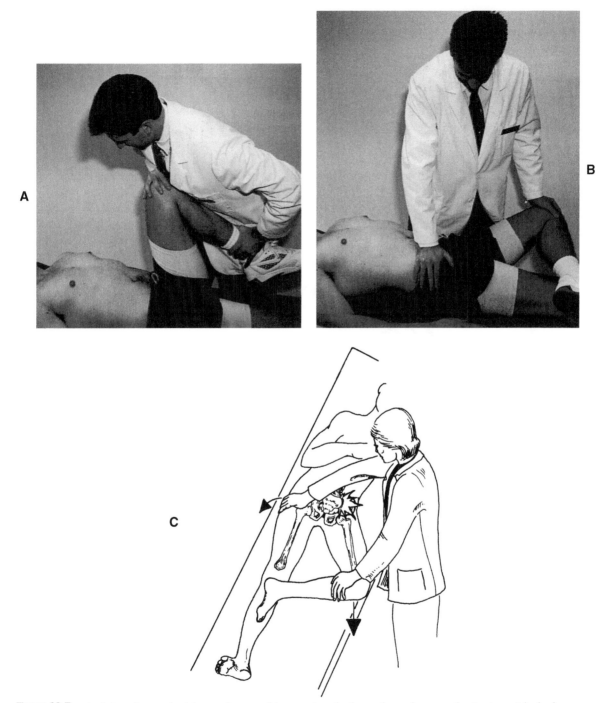

Figure 26-7   **A,** Joint play at the hip can be tested by moving the knee through an arc beginning with the knee and thigh flexed, adducted, and internally rotated, and **B,** ending with the thigh flexed, abducted, and externally rotated. C, Pain in the sacroiliac joint can be differentiated from hip pain by the Patrick FABERE test. *(Figure 26-7, C, from Gatterman MI. Chiropractic management of spine related disorders. Baltimore: Williams & Wilkins; 1990.)*

put through these movements (Figure 26-7). Pain can be localized to either the ipsilateral hip or sacroiliac joints by this test.

Straight Leg Raise (SLR, Lasègue's Sign)

The straight leg raise is used in detecting sciatic nerve irritation and also can indicate sacroiliac involvement when pain is localized to the ipsilateral articulation. Sciatic involvement generally produces pain when the straight leg is raised to less than 45 degrees, whereas the test becomes positive for sacroiliac dysfunction when pain is caused by raising the leg between 70 and 90 degrees (Figure 26-8).

Thigh Hyperextension (Yeoman's Test)

Yeoman[25] noted in 1928 that subluxation of the sacroiliac joint was a common diagnosis. He described a diagnostic test involving hyperextension of the hip with the patient prone. The doctor was instructed to grasp the patient's ankle with the knee flexed and the other hand placed over the sacroiliac joint to stabilize the pelvis. The hip was then hyperextended by lifting the knee off of the table. He stated that this procedure stretches the anterior sacroiliac ligament and elicits pain in the presence of a lesion in the sacroiliac joint. In the normal person he found the procedure to be pain-

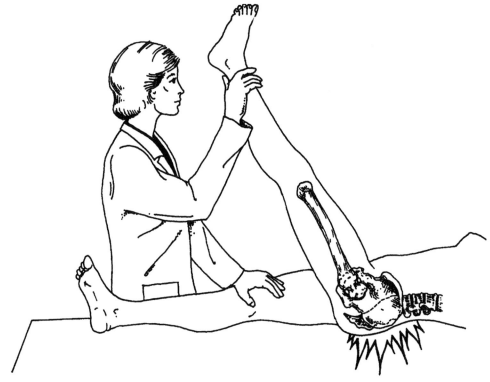

Figure 26-8   Normally the straight leg can be raised to 90 degrees without discomfort. Pain at 45 degrees or, less particularly, of the electric shock type that radiates into the feet, the back, or the opposite side indicates nonspecific irritation of the sciatic nerve or root. Pain produced from 70 to 90 degrees and localized to the sacroiliac joint is more indicative of a sacroiliac lesion. *(From Gatterman MI. Chiropractic management of spine related disorders. Baltimore: Williams & Wilkins; 1990.)*

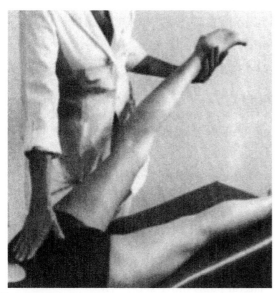

Figure 26-9 Hyperextension of the ipsilateral thigh produces pain with lesions of the sacroiliac joint. *(From Gatterman MI. Chiropractic management of spine related disorders. Baltimore: Williams & Wilkins; 1990.)*

to is immediately inferomedial to the posterior superior iliac spine within 1 cm and the procedure repeatable, then it is suggestive of sacroiliac dysfunction.[27] As with orthopedic tests that suggest sacroiliac involvement, these findings alone do not indicate whether the pain is due to restricted joint movement or a hypermobile state. Cibulka[28] found a cluster of sacroiliac joint tests useful in identifying sacroiliac dysfunction. The four procedures that he recommended are the standing flexion test, palpation of posterior-superior iliac spine heights while sitting, and the supine long-sitting and prone knee flexion tests. His criterion for a positive test on any of these four procedures was an observable difference estimated visually at a minimum of 2.45 cm between sides on bilateral comparison of bony landmarks.

It is important not to rely on a single procedure when making a diagnostic assessment. Although palpatory findings are most likely to determine the likelihood of success in the treatment of sacroiliac subluxation syndrome, provocation tests as well as pain localization can produce valuable information. A clinical trial of manipulation specifically directed to the sacroiliac joints can confirm the diagnosis of sacroiliac joint subluxation when it results in relief of the patient's symptoms.

Radiographic Findings
The sacroiliac joints are difficult to visualize radiographically and are best viewed with the beam passing posterior to anterior. Plain film radiographs cannot detect a manipulable subluxation, although several marking systems have been used to detect pelvic misalignment. Pelvic instability can be demonstrated by radiokinetic tests that stress the sacroiliac joints and the symphysis pubis (Figure 26-10, *A, B, C*). The patient stands on two blocks approximately 6 inches from the floor. The blocks are alternately removed to allow one leg to hang free.[29] A neutral view with inclusion of the sacroiliac joints in all views is recommended. Instability of the sacroiliac joints is confirmed by separation of the symphysis pubis in the vertical plane.[30]

less. Pain localized to the sacroiliac joint on hyperextension of the ipsilateral thigh indicates a test positive for sacroiliac involvement but does not differentiate the nature of the problem (Figure 26-9). Walsh[26] found that Yeoman's test was more responsive to sacroiliac pain than a battery of other tests for sacroiliac function. With a sacroiliac subluxation, the prone patient is often able to actively extend the leg much higher on the uninvolved side. Restricted sacroiliac joint motion in turn prevents full hyperextension of the ipsilateral thigh.

Pain Localization
Localization of the primary site of pain by the patient has been validated by Fortin with use of sacroiliac block injections. He recommended asking the patient to point to the region of pain with one finger. He noted that if the area pointed

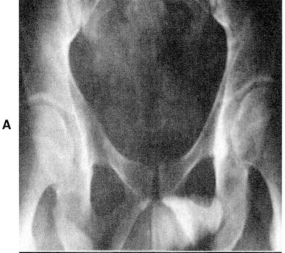

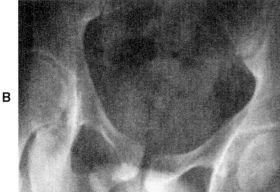

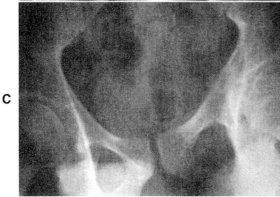

Figure 26-10 Pelvic instability can be demonstrated by radiokinetic tests that stress the sacroiliac joints and the symphysis pubis. In **A,** the patient is standing with the weight evenly distributed for the neutral PA view of the symphysis pubis. In **B,** the patient is standing on the left leg while the right leg hangs free. Note the superior sheer of the left pubic bone. In **C,** the patient is standing on the right leg while the left leg hangs free. The pubic bones are now aligned. *(From Gatterman MI. Chiropractic management of spine related disorders. Baltimore: Williams & Wilkins; 1990.)*

Mechanics of Sacroiliac Subluxation and Dysfunction

Because motion of the sacroiliac joint occurs largely in the sagittal plane[31] (flexion and extension[32]), it is not surprising that the plane of blocked sacroiliac joint motion is generally flexion or extension with accompanying malposition in this plane. The ilium fixed in a flexed position in relation to the sacrum has been termed a PI (posteroinferior) ilium, with the posterior superior iliac spine (PSIS) as the reference point.[33] The AS (anterosuperior) ilium describes an ilium fixed in an extended position. When the ilium flexes, the following actions occur[33]:

1. PSIS moves posteriorly and inferiorly
2. ASIS (anterior superior iliac spine) and ipsilateral pubis move superiorly
3. Acetabulum moves anteriorly, laterally, and slightly superiorly, causing functional shortening of the leg
4. Sacrum moves relatively anteriorly and interiorly on the ipsilateral side[32]

Opposite movements occur during iliac extension. Among the findings mentioned is the movement of the acetabulum. When the pelvis becomes locked in a torqued position with one ilium in extension and the other in flexion, the relative position of the acetabulae may be different enough to result in measurable difference in functional leg length (Figure 26-11). It is important to note that this phenomenon is quite distinct from anatomic leg length discrepancy[33] and is generally correctable with appropriate sacroiliac manipulation. Common postural features of functional and anatomic leg length discrepancies are unleveling of the greater trochanters and/or iliac crests while standing.

Alterations in the static alignment of anatomic landmarks may also assist in the diagnosis and classification of sacroiliac subluxation.[32] Table 26-1 gives examples of common palpatory characteristics that differentiate a flexion malposition (PI ilium) from an extension malposition (AS ilium).[32,33]

A survey of current texts used in chiropractic education shows a variety of dynamic examination procedures that are used in addition to the aforementioned static tests.[19,20,32,34,35] These dynamic

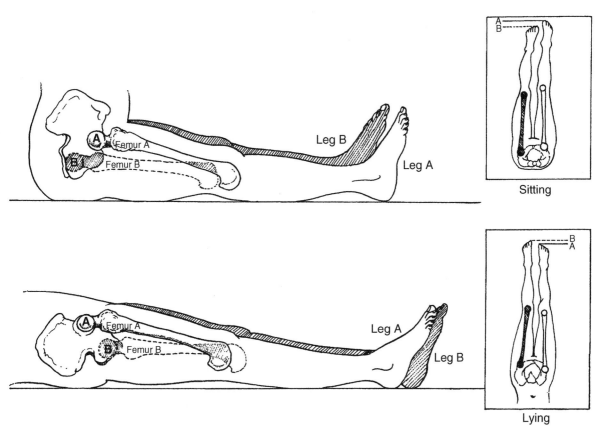

Figure 26-11 Relative changes observed in functional leg length during change from supine to sitting position when a simple sacroiliac subluxation/fixation is present. Leg A represents the side of the PI ilium (flexion malposition) and leg B the AS ilium (extension malposition). Because of the relative anterior displacement of the acetabulum resulting from the flexed ilium (and opposite for the extended ilium), the leg that is functionally short reverses as the patient sits and the hip joint is flexed to 90 degrees. *(From Gatterman MI. Chiropractic management of spine related disorders. Baltimore: Williams & Wilkins; 1990.)*

procedures are directed at the assessment of sacroiliac function. Perhaps the most widely used of these tests is the standing palpatory examination of comparative sacroiliac motion by palpating the relative motion between sacrum and ilium while the patient raises and lowers each leg (Figure 26-12). Although these standing motion tests are widely used, intraexaminer reliability has been shown to exceed interexaminer reliability, and the validity of these procedures has yet to be fully demonstrated.[35] Palpation of overall sacroiliac movement may be complicated by aberrant motion that may occur because of a shift of the axis of rotation caused by subluxation.

Another test for sacroiliac pathomechanics is the "sacral push." The doctor sits behind the seated patient with thumbs spanning the space between the PSIS and the sacral base (across the sacroiliac joint). As the patient extends the torso, the sacral base glides anteriorly and can be followed by the doctor's thumbs.[32] Motion in the oblique coronal plane can be monitored by having

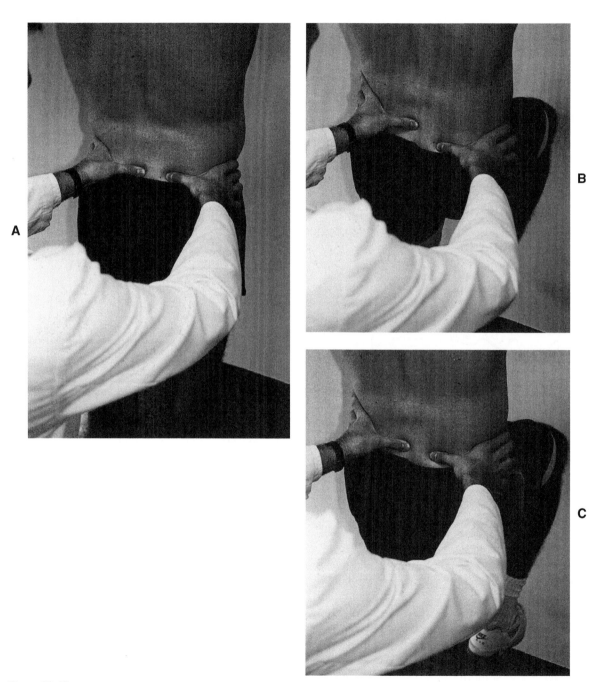

Figure 26-12   A, Relative motion of the left sacroiliac joint is palpated with the thumb placed over the second sacral tubercle and the other over the posterior superior iliac spine (PSIS). B, With normal motion, the PSIS moves downward 1 to 2 cm as the leg is raised. C, If the joint is fixed, the PSIS does not move downward.

Table 26-1

Common Palpatory Characteristics
That Differentiate a Flexion Malposition
(PI Ilium) from an Extension Malposition
(AS Ilium)

PI	AS
1. Prominent and inferior PSIS	1. Less prominent and superior PSIS
2. Superior positioned ASIS	2. Inferior positioned ASIS
3. Functionally shorter leg supine, prone, and standing	3. Functionally longer leg supine, prone, and standing
4. Functionally longer leg sitting (see Figure 26-11)	4. Functionally shorter leg sitting (see Figure 26-11)
5. Lower iliac crest (standing)	5. Higher iliac crest (standing)

PSIS, Posterior superior iliac spine; *ASIS,* anterior superior illiac spine.

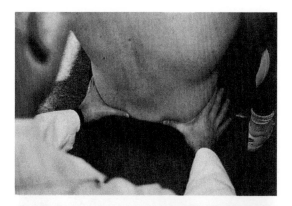

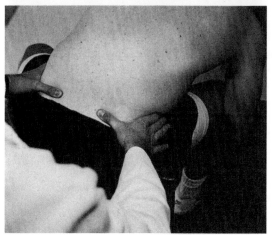

Figure 26-13   Relative motion in the oblique coronal plane can be monitored by having the patient flex and laterally bend to each side as if to tie his or her shoe.

the patient flex and laterally bend to each side as if to tie his or her shoe. Restricted motion in this plane is most easily restored by using a sacral contact (Figure 26-13).

The preceding tests are examples of tests that evaluate sacroiliac range and quality of motion. Another dynamic palpatory procedure used in evaluation of sacroiliac joint function is joint play examination. Joint play motions are completely passive in nature; that is, they are produced entirely by the doctor without active movement of the patient. These movements can be produced with the patient sitting, prone, or lying on one side and are thoroughly described in current chiropractic procedural texts.[32] Joint play tests seek to detect abnormal resistance to specific gliding movements or the presence of increased pain to identify potential sacroiliac dysfunction.[32]

Treatment of Sacroiliac Subluxation Syndrome

The treatment of choice for sacroiliac subluxation syndrome is specific manipulative therapy (Figure 26-14) directed at the sacroiliac articulations.[14,19,20,32] Prospective clinical studies have shown a successful response in more than 90% of patients receiving daily manipulation over a 2- to 3-week period for chronic disabling sacroiliac syndrome.[19] Mobilizing and stretching techniques, as well as exercises, also can be helpful in the management of this condition (Figure 26-15).[36] Accompanying muscle syndromes should be addressed when present.[37]

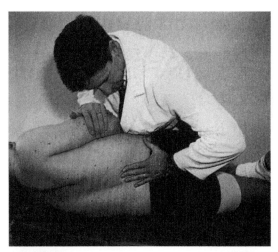

Figure 26-14   The patient with a sacral rotational fixation is positioned in side posture, with the side of fixation involvement placed down. The hand contacts the upper portion of the sacrum, and with a scooping motion the thrust is delivered anteriorly, away from the locked joint.

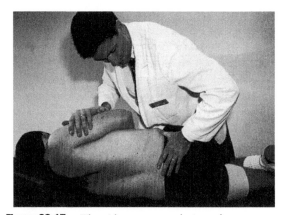

Figure 26-15   The side posture technique for manipulation of a right superior sacroiliac joint fixation has the doctor's stabilizing hand tractioning the patient's superior shoulder while the thrusting hand contacts the affected ilium. The manipulative thrust is directed through the ilium, down the thigh, and the long axis of the patient's flexed leg. The patient's superior leg is tractioned with the doctor's inferior thigh, and a body drop is simultaneously instituted as the thrust is delivered.

References

1. Smith OG, Langworthy SM, Paxson MC. Modernized chiropractic. Vol 2. Cedar Rapids, IA: Lawrence Press; 1906. p. 217-73.
2. Palmer BJ. An exposition of old moves. 2nd ed. Davenport, IA: Palmer School of Chiropractic; 1911. p. 121-2.
3. Gregory AA. Spinal treatment: auxiliary methods of treatment. 2nd ed. Oklahoma City: Palmer-Gregory College; 1912. p. 545-9.
4. Carver W. Carver's chiropractic analysis of chiropractic principles as applied to pathology, relatology, symptomatology, and diagnosis. 3rd ed, Vol 1. Oklahoma City: Paul O Parr; 1921.
5. Forester AL. Principles and practices of spinal adjustment. Chicago: National School of Chiropractic; 1915. p. 374-5.
6. Mixter WJ, Barr JS. Rupture of the intervertebral disk with involvement of the spinal canal. N Engl J Med 1934;211:220.
7. Walker JM. The sacroiliac joint: a critical review. Physical Therapy 1992;72:903-16.
8. Smidt GL, McQuade K, Wei SH, Barakatt E. Sacroiliac kinematics for reciprocal straddle positions. Spine 1995;20(9):1047-54.
9. Smidt GL, Wei SH, McQuade K. Sacroiliac motion for extreme hip positions. Spine 1997;22:2073-82.
10. Bowen V, Cassidy JD. Macroscopic and microscopic anatomy of the sacroiliac joint from embryonic life until the eighth decade. Spine 1981;6:620-8.
11. Maclennan AH. The role of the hormone relaxin in human reproduction and pelvic girdle relaxation. Scand J Rheumatol 1991;S88:7-15.
12. Kapandji IA. The physiology of the joints: the trunk and vertebral column. Vol 3. New York: Churchill Livingstone; 1974. p. 59.
13. Wilder DG, Pope MG, Frymoyer JW. The functional topography of the sacroiliac joint. Spine 1980;5:575-9.
14. Gatterman MI. Disorders of the pelvic ring. In: Gatterman MI. Chiropractic management of spine related disorders. 2nd ed. Baltimore: Williams & Wilkins; 2003. p. 129.
15. Brunstrum S. Clinical kinesiology. 3rd ed. Philadelphia: FA Davis; 1979. p. 11.
16. Gillet H, Liekans M. Belgium chiropractic research notes. 4th ed. Huntington Beach, CA: Motion Palpation Institute; 1981. p. 9.
17. Vleeming A, Volkers ACW, Snijders CJ, Stoeckert R. Relation between form and function in the sacroiliac joint. Part II. Biomechanical aspects. Spine 1990;15(2):133-5.
18. Turek SL. Orthopedics principles and their application. 3rd ed. Philadelphia: JB Lippincott; 1977. p. 1469.
19. Cassidy JD, Mierau DR. Pathophysiology of the sacroiliac joint. In: Haldeman S, editor. Principles and practice of chiropractic. 2nd ed. San Mateo, CA: Appleton and Lange; 1992. p. 211-24.
20. Kirkaldy-Willis WH, Burton CV. Managing low back pain. 3rd ed. New York: Churchill Livingstone; 1992. p. 123-6.

21. Keating JC, Bergmann TF, Jacobs GE, Finer BA, Larson K. Interexaminer reliability of eight evaluative dimensions of lumbar segmental abnormality. J Manipulative Physiol Ther 1990;13:463-70.

22. Toussaint R, Gawlick CS, Rehder U, Ruther W. Sacroiliac joint diagnostics in the Hamburg construction workers study. J Manipulative Physiol Ther 1999;22:139-43.

23. Laslett M, Williams M. The reliability of selected pain provocation tests for sacroiliac joint pathology. Spine 1994;19:1243-9.

24. Dreyfus P, Michaelsen M, Pauza K. The value of medical history and physical examination in diagnosing sacroiliac joint pain. Spine 1996;21:2594-602.

25. Yeoman W. The relation of the sacroiliac joint to sciatica, with analysis of 100 cases. Lancet 1928;Dec:1119-22.

26. Walsh MJ. Evaluation of orthopedic testing for the low back for nonspecific lower back pain. J Manipulative Physiol Ther 1998;21:232-6.

27. Fortin JD, Falco FJE. The Fortin finger test: an indicator of sacroiliac pain. Am J Orthop 1997;26:477-80.

28. Cibulka MT, Koldehoff R. Clinical usefulness of a cluster of sacroiliac joint tests in patients with and without low back pain. J Orth Sports Phys Ther 1999;29:83-93.

29. Ballinger PW. Merrill's atlas of radiographic positions and radiologic procedures. 5th ed, Vol 1. St. Louis: Mosby; 1982. p. 247.

30. Dihlman W. Diagnostic radiology of the sacroiliac joints. Chicago: Year Book; 1980. p. 12-16.

31. White AA, Panjabi MM. Clinical biomechanics of the spine. 2nd ed. San Francisco: JB Lippincott; 1990. p. 112-5.

32. Peterson DH, Bergmann TF. Chiropractic technique. 2nd ed. St Louis: Mosby; 2002. p. 315-35.

33. Panzer DM, Fechtal SG, Gatterman MI. Postural complex. In: Gatterman MI. Chiropractic management of spine related disorders. Baltimore: Williams & Wilkins; 1990. p. 278-81.

34. Walters PJ. Pelvis. In: Plaugher G, editor. Textbook of clinical chiropractic. Baltimore: Williams & Wilkins; 1993. p. 153-61.

35. Herzog W, Read LJ, Conway PJW, Shaw LD, McEwen MC. Reliability of motion palpation procedures to detect sacroiliac joint fixations. J Manipulative Physiol Ther 1989;12(2):86-92.

36. Don Tigny RL. Mechanics and treatment of the sacroiliac joint. J Manual Manipulative Ther 1993;1(1):3-12.

37. Gatterman MI, Blunt KL, Goe DR. Muscle and myofascial pain syndromes. In: Gatterman MI. Chiropractic management of spine related disorders. 2nd ed. Baltimore: Lippincott Williams & Wilkins; 2003. p. 319-69.

Coccygeal Subluxation Syndrome

John P. Mrozek

Key Words   Coccydynia, luxation, hypermobility

After reading this chapter you should be able to answer the following questions:

Question 1   What is the correlation between coccygeal angulation and coccydynia?

Question 2   What procedures may be used for treatment of coccygeal syndrome?

*C*occygeal *subluxation syndrome*, also referred to as *coccygodynia* or *coccygalgia*, is a term used to describe pain in and around the coccyx that does not radiate and is made worse by sitting or by standing up from a seated position.[1-3] For the purposes of this chapter the term *coccydynia* will be used. While treatment of the coccyx is taught in undergraduate chiropractic programs, chiropractic research and case reporting on clinical considerations involving this area is limited. Perhaps this chapter will contribute to a greater interest in research on this challenging clinical presentation.

Coccydynia, first described as a pathologic entity by Petit in 1726 and later clinically by Simpson in 1859,[1,4,5] is part of the urogenital and rectal pain syndromes. As a group of syndromes, including rectal pain, perineal pain, and vulvodynia, they can be difficult to diagnose and often the etiology is not found.[3] Adding to this diagnostic challenge for the chiropractor is the relationship described by several authors between coccydynia and low back pain.[3,6,7] Malbohan[7] reported that the pelvic diaphragm was clinically involved in nearly all of the 1500 cases of low back pain that they studied. Postacchini and Massobrio[6] studied normal radiographic anatomy involving 120 symptomatic patients, including a retrospective review of 51 patients who had a partial or total coccygectomy. They noted that conflicting results have been reported regarding the effectiveness of surgical treatment of the coccyx and the presence of coexisting low back pain. In a study involving 50 patients, Wray[3] observed that "virtually all" of the patients with CT evidence of lumbosacral disc prolapse were "cured" by local treatment of the coccyx.

The coccygeal syndrome is part of a larger group of syndromes that can be described as occasionally controversial with questions ranging from whether they exist to whether they are purely psychosomatic.[5] The causes and best therapeutic approaches to coccydynia are the focus of renewed interest especially with regard to area of pain management.[1] However, only a small number of clinical series have been published and much of the information on coccydynia is scattered in various disciplines. Therefore the clinical approach to managing coccygeal pain remains challenging.

Anatomic Considerations

The coccyx consists of usually four rudimentary vertebrae. Variations in segments of one less or one more also exist. The shape of the coccyx was seen as beaklike by early observers. The term *coccyx* is derived from the Greek word for cuckoo. The three inferior coccygeal segments often fuse in middle age. In old age the first coccygeal segment often fuses to the sacrum.[8] The pelvic diaphragm and its immediate surroundings constitute the major muscular considerations when dealing with the coccyx. For general purposes the pelvic diaphragm is formed by the levator ani and coccygeus muscles (Figures 27-1 and 27-2).

Levator Ani

The levator ani muscles form the posterior two thirds of the pelvic floor, and the anterior one third is formed by the perineal membrane, which bridges the pubic rami inferior to the anterior fibers of the levator ani muscles. The levator ani is penetrated by the anal canal, and the perineal membrane is penetrated by the urethra in the man and by the urethra and vagina in the woman.

- Origin: Pelvic surface of the body of the pubis to the ischial spine
- Insertion: The central perineal tendon, the wall of the anal canal, the anococcygeal ligament, the coccyx
- Action: Raise the pelvic floor. This action assists the abdominal muscles in compressing the abdominal contents. This is important in coughing, vomiting, urinating, and trunk fixation during strong movements of the upper limbs such as lifting.
- Innervation: Third and fourth sacral nerves and the inferior rectal nerve

Coccygeus

This muscle forms the posterior and smaller part of the pelvic diaphragm.
- Origin: The ischial spine

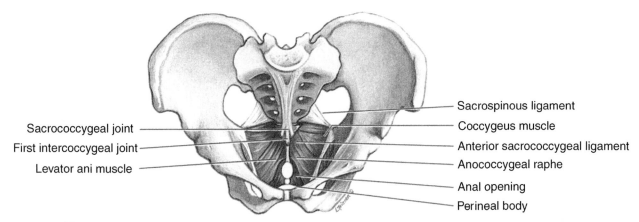

Sacrospinous ligament
Coccygeus muscle
Anterior sacrococcygeal ligament
Anococcygeal raphe
Anal opening
Perineal body

Sacrococcygeal joint
First intercoccygeal joint
Levator ani muscle

Figure 27-1   This illustration represents the relevant muscles and ligaments that pertain to the sacrococcygeal area from the posterior view. *(From Duckworth J, Friesen L.)*

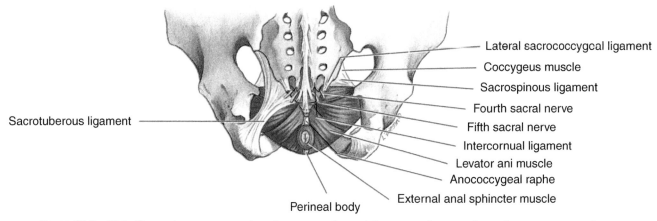

Lateral sacrococcygcal ligament
Coccygeus muscle
Sacrospinous ligament
Fourth sacral nerve
Fifth sacral nerve
Intercornual ligament
Levator ani muscle
Anococcygeal raphe
External anal sphincter muscle

Sacrotuberous ligament

Perineal body

Figure 27-2   This illustration represents the relevant muscles and ligaments that pertain to the sacrococcygeal area from the anterior view. *(From Duckworth J, Friesen L.)*

- Insertion: Lateral aspect of the fifth sacral vertebra and coccyx
- Action: Supports the coccyx and pulls it forward after defecation and childbirth
- Innervation: Fourth and fifth sacral nerves

The gluteus maximus also attaches to the coccyx. This anatomic reality must be taken into consideration when planning treatment of the coccygeal area. The gluteus maximus is the chief extensor of the thigh. The nerve supply is the infe-

rior gluteal nerve. Both the innervation and action must be assessed when formulating a treatment regimen.

The ligaments associated with the coccyx include the sacrotuberous, the sacrospinous, and the anococcygeal. In addition to their coccygeal attachments, the sacrotuberous and sacrospinous ligaments help resist sacral flexion (between the innominates) caused by gravitational effects of erect posture. Sandoz[9] refers to these structures as "check ligaments" of nutation. These two ligaments reinforce and add strength to the sacroiliac joint capsule.[10] The anococcygeal ligament is the median fibrous intersection of components of the levator ani muscle. It is located between the anal canal and the coccyx. (See Figures 27-1 and 27-2.) The actual configuration of the coccyx, particularly as seen on the lateral radiograph, shows an interesting pattern of variation including the fusion pattern of the coccygeal segments.

Diagnosis

Coccydynia occurs more frequently in women and elderly debilitated patients and may present as a single clinical entity or in combination with other painful presentations such as referred pain from lumbosacral spine, anus, rectum, pelvis, and genitourinary system.[1,5] The pain has been described as related to chronic trauma resulting from poor sitting positions, long car or plane rides, and snowmobiling. Idiopathic coccydynia is tail bone pain not associated with fractures, neoplasms, perineural cysts, or infectious diseases.[11] While a number of hypotheses have been put forward as to the cause of idiopathic coccydynia, none have been confirmed and controlled studies are few. As falls and childbirth are often associated with this clinical presentation, a mechanical basis of pain is likely. Owing to this observation, lesions of the sacrococcygeal or intercoccygeal discs have been hypothesized as the source of pain.[11]

Coccydynia can be classified according to the characteristics of the pain.[1] Somatic pain has mechanical characteristics associated with the bony, ligamentous, and muscular elements that attach to or make up the coccyx. Causes of somatic pain include idiopathic, hypermobility of the coccyx, luxation of the coccyx, myofascial syndromes, osteitis, and sacral hemangioma. Obesity, expressed as body mass index (BMI), has been found to have a significant relationship with coccydynia.[12]

Neuropathic pain-producing structures are generally not often known; however, nerve structures thought to be involved in this type of pain include those transmitting sympathetic stimuli and referred neuropathic pain related to dural irritation associated with lumbar disc herniation.[1] As noted earlier, this referred pain mechanism has been questioned by Wray.[1] Other conditions possibly giving rise to neuropathic pain include schwannomas of the sacral nerve roots, neurinomas, arachnoid cysts in cauda equina syndrome, and sacrococcygeal meningeal cysts.[1]

Further, De Andres and Chaves[1] noted that a mixed component pain presentation is associated with space-occupying lesions initially affecting bony and ligamentous structures generating somatic pain. Metastases involving the coccyx and chordomas are also associated with mixed component pain. Visceral somatic pain can refer to the coccyx arising from structures including the rectum, sigmoid colon, and genital system.

As the diagnosis of coccydynia is based largely on the clinical manifestations, the patient work-up must include a good history, physical examination, and focused diagnostic testing. Important factors in the history include the precipitating trauma, when it occurred, whether pain is encountered when passing from sitting to standing, and BMI. While personality and behavioral assessment are recommended with respect to anxiety and depression, severe coccydynia has not been correlated with the number of depressive signs.[1,3]

Maigne[12] noted that only the onset of coccydynia within a month from an accident or childbirth is likely to be traumatic in origin. With the exception of the one-month interval, "the time between the traumatic event and the onset of chronic coccydynia" does not seem to have a relationship to the lesion. Beyond the interval of a month, the number of patients with instability (luxation or hypermobility) did not differ significantly from those patients without a history of trauma lesion.

In addition to the consideration of trauma, Maigne[2] found in a study involving 208 consecutive patients that the higher the BMI, "the less his or her pelvis will rotate, and the steeper the angle between the coccyx and the seat" when going to the seated position. This produces luxation of the coccyges, an associated increase in coccygeal lesions, and predisposes the individual to greater risk of trauma to the coccygeal area.

Maigne, Guedj, and Straus[11] conducted a study involving 102 patients that included 51 patients with coccydynia and 51 as controls. They compared lateral films of the coccyx of the patient sitting with those of the patient in the lateral decubitus position. The films were compared by means of printing them on graph paper and superimposing them to measure saggital movement of the coccyx. The symptomatic group of patients then underwent discography. The researchers noted that abnormal movement of the coccyx in the sitting position was reduced in the lateral decubitus position. They concluded that coccygeal pain could come from the coccygeal disc. In addition, they proposed a classification of coccygeal mobility through the use of dynamic radiography. The classification is made up of four groups specified as luxation, hypermobility (exceeding 25 degrees of flexion when sitting), immobile coccyx, and normal mobility (movement of 5 to 25 degrees when going from a standing to a sitting position).

Maigne[12] also noted that patients who experienced pain passing from sitting to standing had a "very significantly" higher rate of coccygeal radiological abnormalities of all kinds than those who did not have such pain. Following on this observation, Maigne and Chatellier[13] modified the approach to classification of coccygeal mobility according to findings on dynamic radiography. The approach involved standing lateral radiographs taken in the neutral position and sitting views taken while in the painful position. The first radiograph was a standing film taken after that patient stood for 10 minutes. The second lateral radiograph was taken with the patient seated in the most uncomfortable position. The two radiographs were superimposed over a bright light, thus permitting measurement of the relative movement of the sacrum and coccyx. The angle of mobility was used as a sagittal measure of rotation of the coccyx with forward movement referred to as flexion and backward movement referred to as extension. In summary, Maigne[12] found that their radiological classification allowed for a high degree of lesion identification. Luxation and hypermobility are described as "culprit lesions,"

and increased BMI and trauma are noted as risk factors for luxation.

Postacchini and Massobrio[6] described four types of coccygeal configurations as seen on the lateral radiograph. Among their findings were that the sacrococcygeal and second intercoccygeal joints were found to be fused in approximately half of the symptomatic and asymptomatic patients; the first intercoccygeal joint was usually consistently present and well developed. This led to the observation that the first intercoccygeal joint is the "fulcrum of the movements of the coccyx." They also found "no qualitative differences in the configuration of the coccyx between symptomatic and asymptomatic" patients; however, they noted that coccygeal configurations with greater forward angulation were associated with increased symptomatology.

Treatment

A rectal approach allows for direct palpation of the coccyx and pelvic diaphragm. Palpating the coccyx by contacting it with a lubricated gloved index finger internally and thumb pressure applied externally allows for assessment of relative mobility. Patient position for the rectal examination should be prone with abdominal support or the lateral decubitus (Figure 27-3). The chiropractor must always be mindful of the patient's reaction to this pressure. This can best be monitored by having the patient turn the head to the side if in the prone position. In this position the chiropractor can view the facial response and observe for the patient's reaction to pain. One must be careful not to proceed beyond the patient's tolerance.

Maigne[14] noted that "coccygeal pain is very resistant to treatment." He further noted that massage of the levator ani muscle was not always successful. From his clinical experience, he observed that coccygeal pain occurring after a fall or childbirth is "practically always relieved" through manipulation of the coccyx. He described the maneuver consisting of placing the physician's free hand on the sacrum and maintaining pressure for 40 to 50 seconds, "pressing with all his weight

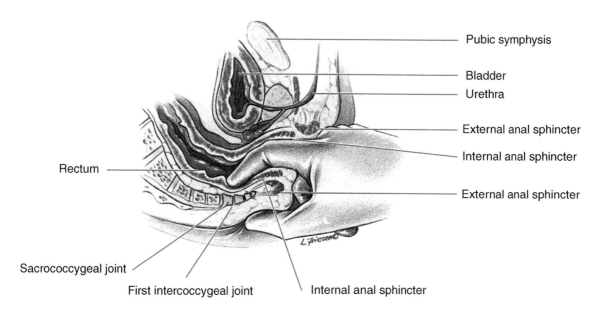

Pubic symphysis

Bladder

Urethra

External anal sphincter

Internal anal sphincter

External anal sphincter

Rectum

Sacrococcygeal joint

First intercoccygeal joint

Internal anal sphincter

Figure 27-3   The method of digital examination of the sacrococcygeal area as seen from the lateral view. *(From Duckworth J, Friesen L.)*

on the sacrum" while applying pressure with the finger of the other hand that has been introduced into the rectum, "simply maintaining the coccyx in hyperextension." He suggested that this maneuver should be performed several times. Maigne related that uncomplicated coccydynia should respond quickly to this type of treatment. Two or three treatments over a period of 7 to 10 days was stated as usually sufficient to achieve alleviation of symptoms.

In a pilot study involving 50 patients, Wray[3] found that coccygeal manipulation under general anesthesia combined with the injection of local anesthetics and corticoids had a success rate of 60% to 85%. The manipulation was performed by contacting the coccyx internally with the index finger and externally with the thumb and repeatedly flexing and extending the coccyx for approximately one minute.

Maigne and Chatellier[13] reported on a prospective pilot study with independent assessment and a 2-year follow-up to compare the efficacy of three manual coccydynia treatments. The classification of coccygeal mobility by means of dynamic radiography, as noted earlier, was performed on all

patients in this study. Patients with an immobile coccyx had the poorest results and patients with normal coccyx mobility had the best results. Patients with luxation and hypermobility had results between those patients with no mobility and those with normal mobility. In patients with a normally mobile coccyx, levator ani massage and stretch were more effective than joint mobilization. Patients who experienced pain while transitioning from the seated to standing position had better outcomes from manual treatment. However, with the six month posttreatment rate of satisfactory results at 25.7%, the need for a placebo-controlled study was indicated.

Notwithstanding the lack of conclusive evidence of the effectiveness of manual coccygeal treatments, a situation not unlike a number of therapeutic interventions, several manual approaches to the treatment of coccydynia are set out in the literature. Maigne and Chatellier[13] described three coccydynia treatment approaches including massage, mobilization, and stretch. The massage approach consists of massage of the levator ani and coccygeus; it was attributed by Maigne and Chatellier[13] to a description by Thiele in 1937.

This consists of the muscles massaged in the direction of their fibers on both sides of the coccyx. The procedure is reported as lasting 3 minutes per session while taking great care not to mobilize the coccyx.

The mobilization approach consists of grasping the coccyx between the external thumb and the internal index finger while the movements of flexion, extension, and rotation are applied. This is described as followed immediately with the treatment described by Maigne[14] noted earlier. This approach is applied for 30 seconds, twice per session. Care is taken not to contact the levator ani muscles.

The stretch approach consists of gradual stretching of the levator ani muscles using the internal index finger until contact with the coccyx is made. When contact is made, the finger is held in position for approximately 30 seconds. This approach does not involve mobilization of the coccyx and is performed 3 times per session.

Coccygectomy was indicated for approximately 20% of the patients in the study by Wray.[3] This was associated with a 20% relapse rate in patients who experienced initial relief with conservative treatment. In addition, the researchers found that if coccygectomy was eventually needed, the result of the surgery was not affected by prolonged conservative treatment. Postacchini and Massobrio[6] noted that coccygectomy is indicated when the symptoms are disabling and there is no evidence that the pain is psychogenic in nature. Maigne, Lagauche, and Doursounian[12] observed that good results for coccygectomy were confined to patients with instability that had not responded to conservative treatment.

In summary, although the differential diagnosis of coccydynia can be challenging, conservative measures are generally sufficient to result in significant pain relief.[5] As noted by Wray et al.,[3] a "striking feature" of their study was that patients were very grateful that their condition was taken seriously and treated sympathetically. A number of their patients had been in pain for a long period of time and felt that their symptoms had been "belittled." The chiropractor, owing to the skilled use of his or her hands, is well placed to offer considerable relief for this challenging syndrome.

References

1. De Andres J, Chaves S. Coccygodynia: a proposal for an algorithm for treatment. J Pain 2003;4(5):257-66.
2. Maigne JY, Doursounian L, Chatellier G. Causes and mechanisms of common coccydynia: role of body mass index and coccygeal trauma. Spine 2000;25:3072-9.
3. Wray CC, Easom S, Hoskinson J. Coccydynia: aetiology and treatment. J Bone Joint Surg Br 1991;73:335-8.
4. Kim NH, Suk KS. Clinical and radiological differences between traumatic and idiopathic coccygodynia. Yonsei Med J 1999;40(3):215-20.
5. Wesselmann U, Burnett AL, Heinberg LJ. The urogenital and rectal pain syndromes. Pain 1997;73(3):269-94.
6. Postacchini F, Massobrio M. Idiopathic coccygodynia: analysis of 51 cases and a radiographic study of the normal coccyx. J Bone Joint Surg 1983;65A:1116-24.
7. Malbohan IM, Mojzisova L, Tichy J. The role of coccygeal spasm in low back pain. Manual Med 1989;4:140-1.
8. Moore KL. Clinically oriented anatomy. Baltimore: Williams & Wilkins; 1980. p. 345-53, 620-2.
9. Sandoz RW. Structural and functional pathologies of the pelvic ring. Ann Swiss Assoc 1981;8:107.
10. Kirkaldy-Willis WH. Managing low back pain. 2nd ed. New York: Churchill Livingstone; 1988; p. 71.
11. Maigne JY, Guedj S, Straus C. Idiopathic coccygodynia. Lateral roentgenograms in the sitting position and coccygeal discography. Spine 1994;19:930-4.
12. Maigne JY, Lagauche D, Dousounian L. Instability of the coccyx in coccydynia. J Bone Joint Surg 2000;82B:1038-41.
13. Maigne JY, Chatellier G. Comparison of three manual coccydynia treatments: a pilot study. Spine 2001;26:E479-E483.
14. Maigne R. Orthopedic medicine. Springfield, IL: Charles C Thomas; 1972. p. 315-6.

Appendix A

Subluxation Syndromes

Subluxation Syndrome	Cervicogenic headache
Etiology	Subluxation of cervical articulations producing pain referral from articular and soft tissue structures; central sensitization from convergence of cervical and cranial afferents onto second order neurons; somatic, neurogenic, vascular, and autonomic components
History	Whiplash injury, postural overuse with static muscle loading, degeneration and trauma leading to joint misalignment, restricted motion and dysfunction
Signs and Symptoms	Neck and suboccipital pain with projections to forehead, temples vertex, and ears; pain may be increased with specific posture and movement
Exam Findings	Palpation reveals cervical motion segment misalignment, restricted motion, muscle hypertonicity, and/or tenderness
Imaging Findings	Segmental movement restriction on flexion-extension stress views
	Loss of cervical curve
Management	Adjustment, soft tissue therapy, and postural retraining; address pain-generating triggers
Differential Diagnosis	Rule out fractures, congenital anomalies, tumors, rheumatoid arthritis, and other arthritides

Subluxation Syndrome	Cervicogenic sympathetic syndrome
Etiology	Sympathetic dysfunction associated with cervical subluxation because of compromise of the cervical sympathetic ganglia that are in close association with vertebral bodies (C6-7 and T1 stellate ganglion, C5-6 middle cervical ganglion, C2 upper cervical ganglion)
History	Injury from motor vehicle accident, athletic injury, or cumulative microtrauma from repetitive use or sleeping positions that produce sympathetic involvement
Signs and Symptoms	Horner's syndrome (ptosis, miosis, and enopthalmus)
	Meniere's disease (vertigo, fluctuating hearing loss, fullness of ear, tinnitus)
	Numbness and tingling of the upper limb
	Barré-Liéou syndrome (suboccipital headache, vertigo, tinnitus with visual symptoms)
	Blurred vision
	Pain referral may be widespread and atypical
Exam Findings	Palpation reveals cervical motion segment misalignment, restricted motion, muscle hypertonicity, and/or tenderness. Special tests to measure cerebral blood flow and EEG used to evaluate neurologic function.
Imaging Findings	Segmental movement restriction on flexion-extension stress views
	Loss of cervical curve
Management	Adjustment, trigger point therapy, and postural retraining
Differential Diagnosis	Rule out fractures, infection, space-occupying lesions, and major nerve injury

Subluxation Syndrome	Whiplash injuries
Etiology	Acceleration/deceleration injury in which the head is whipped backward and forward
History	Motor vehicle accident, blow to the head, whiplike trauma to the head and neck, shaken baby syndrome
Signs and Symptoms	Neck pain and stiffness with decreased range of motion
	Weakness, numbness, or pain of arms and hands
	Cervical sympathetic syndrome
Exam Findings	Palpable muscle spasm, cervical motion segment misalignment, restricted motion, and/or tenderness
Imaging Findings	Segmental movement restriction on flexion-extension stress views
	Loss of cervical curve
Management	Cervical collar in early stages, adjustments, trigger point therapy, and postural retraining
Differential Diagnosis	Rule out fractures, congenital anomalies

Subluxation Syndrome	Cervicogenic dorsalgia
Etiology	Cervical trauma, static loading of the spine causing cumulative trauma disorder, and cervical spine subluxation and/or cervical disc disruption that irritate the medial branches of the dorsal primary ramus, producing pain in the dorsal region
History	Long hours working at a desk or computer, trauma or disk disease involving the cervical spine
Signs and Symptoms	Pain in the dorsal region with decreased range of motion in the cervical region; pain described as a deep and constant ache in the dorsal region that can radiate unilaterally or bilaterally to the arms; numbness or tingling in fingers bilaterally or unilaterally may be present
Exam Findings	Compression of the cervical spine in extension and rotation elicits the symptoms
	Palpable muscle spasm, cervical motion segment misalignment, restricted motion, and/or tenderness; anterior doorbell sign
Imaging Findings	Segmental movement restriction on cervical flexion-extension stress views
	Loss of cervical curve
Management	Primary therapy directed to the cervical spine with adjustment of subluxations, in the cervical region and thoracic region if present; soft tissue therapy; postural retraining to prevent recurrence
Differential Diagnosis	Rule out herpes zoster, cholecystic disease, visceral referred pain, rib or thoracic vertebra subluxation, musculoskeletal local or referred pain, malignancy, arthritides

Subluxation Syndrome	First rib subluxation
Etiology	Subluxation of the first rib from trauma or microtrauma, chronic postural asymmetry, and hypertonicity of the scalene muscles that can compromise the vascular and neural elements that pass through the thoracic outlet
History	Whiplash, trauma to the shoulder girdle, prolonged elevation of the upper extremity, and other static loading from dysfunctional posture
Signs and Symptoms	Paresthesia of the ipsilateral upper extremity including numbness, tingling, and vascular changes
Exam Findings	Elevation and movement restriction of first rib on palpation with the neck extended and laterally flexed to the ipsilateral side
Imaging Findings	Nondefinitive
Management	Adjustment, soft tissue therapy, and postural retraining
Differential Diagnosis	Lower cervical subluxation, scalene muscle spasm

Subluxation Syndrome	Thoracic subluxation syndrome
Etiology	Subluxation of a thoracic vertebra from trauma or microtrauma
History	Trauma to the chest, motor vehicle accident, sudden unguarded movement, cough, sneeze, can be secondary to scoliosis
Signs and Symptoms	Sharp stabbing pain in the thorax aggravated by movement, respiration coughing or sneezing
Exam Findings	Palpable muscle spasm, thoracic motion segment misalignment, restricted motion, and/or tenderness
Imaging Findings	Nondefinitive
Management	Adjustment, soft tissue therapy, and postural retraining
Differential Diagnosis	Fractures, anomalies, tumors, infection, metabolic disorders, degeneration, arthritides, and referred pain from visceral disorders

Subluxation Syndrome	Costovertebral subluxation syndrome
Etiology	Subluxation of a rib from trauma or microtrauma
History	Trauma to the chest, motor vehicle accident, sudden unguarded movement, cough, sneeze, can be secondary to scoliosis
Signs and Symptoms	Sharp stabbing pain in the thorax aggravated by movement, respiration coughing or sneezing
Exam Findings	Palpable muscle spasm, rib misalignment, tenderness, and loss of joint play at the costovertebral joint with failure of the rib to open and close palpated at the rib angle
Imaging Findings	Asymmetry of rib angle
Management	Adjustment, soft tissue therapy, postural retraining, and stabilization of excess motion with a rib belt if chronic
Differential Diagnosis	Fractures, anomalies, tumors, infection, metabolic disorders, degeneration, arthritides, and referred pain from visceral disorders

Subluxation Syndrome	Posterior joint (facet) syndrome
Etiology	Subluxation of a cervical or lumbar vertebra from trauma or microtrauma
History	Trauma, degeneration, postural overload, and lifting (lumbar spine)
Signs and Symptoms	Lumbar spine: Morning stiffness, low back and buttock pain that can refer to the groin and down the lower extremity to the knee; pain increased by hyperextension
	Cervical spine: Localized and referred pain ranging from the occiput to between the scapula and down the arm
Exam Findings	Provocation of pain on axial compression on extension and rotation; distraction relieves pain in the cervical spine. Palpable muscle spasm, motion segment misalignment, restricted motion, and/or tenderness
Imaging Findings	Lumbar spine: Facet imbrication with sclerosis in late stages
	Cervical spine: Segmental movement restriction on flexion-extension stress views
	Loss of cervical curve
Management	Adjustment, soft tissue therapy, and postural retraining
Differential Diagnosis	Intervertebral disc herniation, fractures, anomalies, degeneration, tumors, arthritides

Subluxation Syndrome	Intervertebral disc syndrome (The three joint complex of each motion segment involves both the disc and posterior [zygapophyseal] joint in all subluxation syndromes.)
Etiology	Disc herniation from anular tears that permits protrusion of nuclear material
History	Prior episodes of spine pain; traumatic or lifting incident can precede disc herniation
Signs and Symptoms	Pain from radicular involvement described as burning or stabbing down the involved extremity; loss of reflexes, and numbness in dermatomal pattern; pain increased by coughing, sneezing, and straining
	Lumbar spine: Back and/or leg pain
	Cervical spine: Neck and/or arm and hand pain
Exam Findings	In chronic cases, muscle weakness of the involved extremity
Imaging Findings	MRI confirms the diagnosis
Management	Adjustment, soft tissue therapy; patients may require pain medication if pain is severe
Differential Diagnosis	Facet syndrome, tumors, fractures, anomalies

Subluxation Syndrome	Sacroiliac syndrome
Etiology	Subluxation of the sacroiliac joint with misalignment and restriction of the track bound motion
History	Fall onto buttocks, misstep off of a curb, ligamentous loosening from premenstrual hormones, and pregnancy in the female
Signs and Symptoms	Dull pain in the ipsilateral buttock worsened by sitting; can refer into the medial thigh and lateral leg
Exam Findings	Motion palpation reveals restricted or aberrant motion, loss of joint play, and tenderness over the posterior superior iliac spine. Sacroiliac joint hypermobility produces trigger points in the belly of the piriformis muscle and at the insertion on the greater trochanter.
Imaging Findings	Nondefinitive
Management	Adjustment, soft tissue therapy, pelvic tilt and stretching exercises
Differential Diagnosis	Lumbar motion segment subluxation, tumor, fracture, infectious and inflammatory arthritis

Subluxation Syndrome	Coccygeal subluxation syndrome
Etiology	Subluxation from falling in a sitting position and childbirth in the female
History	Flexion injury or direct contusion to the coccyx; postpartum coccydynia
Signs and Symptoms	Unrelenting pain in the coccygeal region; can be aggravated during sitting, bowel movements, and intercourse
Exam Findings	Point tenderness at the coccyx with misalignment noted on palpation
Imaging Findings	Coccygeal displacement noted on radiographs
Management	Rectal adjustment of the coccyx; pressure applied to the sacrotuberous ligament
Differential Diagnosis	Fracture, tumor

Appendix B

Spinal Subluxation and Visceral Disorders

Brian Budgell

Virtually all chiropractors agree that the subluxation is a central concept in chiropractic. Perhaps because of this, in addition to more than one "consensus" definition, we are blessed with an overabundance of hypotheses about what this important lesion actually is. Indeed, this may be troublesome for readers of this text because they may feel obliged to wade through a morass of competing models in search of a clear vision of this elusive entity. The challenge of separating the "goats" from the "sheep" can be lightened and even made enjoyable by requiring that any robust definition or hypothetical model of the subluxation take into account clinical and laboratory observations, including the wealth of observations concerning visceral disease and visceral function in relation to subluxation.

To that end, and without depriving the reader of the pleasure of making his or her own judgments, we provide a list of observations, clinical and physiologic, in human subjects as they endured or were relieved of putative subluxations. Hence the scrutinizer of hypotheses may ask, "How is this model of the subluxation consistent with the observation that...?" The observations that we offer are segregated on the basis of organ system and therefore secondarily, physiologic function. This is a convenient strategy because human organ systems have well-characterized mechanisms of regulation, including neurologic control, which therefore give specific evidence of the effects of subluxation. We have selected evidence from a variety of research designs, taking account not only of the inherent strengths and weaknesses of different designs but also the *sine qua non* of quality of the report; that is to say, a poorly written report of an excellent experiment is no more useful than a well written report of a poor experiment.

This is most important considering the current stage of evolution of chiropractic research. Specifically, we must acknowledge that we are still trying to define the questions and may be getting ahead of ourselves by rushing into randomized clinical trials that may not address real-world clinical problems. Furthermore, in attempting to understand the subluxation, we must realize that clinical studies provide data concerning populations, while valuable insights into mechanisms of the subluxation are just as likely to arise from careful observation of individuals.

The Nervous System

With the above caveat in mind, a number of intriguing case studies and case series from Milne, Gorman, and more recently others deserve scrutiny. They have convincingly documented improvement in visual acuity in patients undergoing spinal manipulation and in several cases document the onset of visual symptoms coincident with biomechanical insult to the neck.[1-3] Their various patients do not generally seem to manifest symptoms related to neck position, which argues against mechanical compression of vessels or nerves as a cause of symptomatology. Patients report and the researchers document improvement either instantly or within very few treatments. These observations suggest a reflex effect on blood flow to the visual system, which would be consistent with numerous animal studies demonstrating influences of somatic stimulation on regional cerebral blood flow. The effects of spinal manipulation on visual function may therefore provide useful insights into the more sporadic reports of effects of spinal manipulation on other aspects of cerebral function.

The Cardiovascular System

Rather an impressive number of case studies and a few larger clinical studies[4-6] fail utterly to convince that spinal subluxation or its relief by spinal manipulation has any significant effect on blood pressure disorders. Conversely, a number of basic physiologic studies clearly demonstrate an influence on autonomic output to the heart and heart rate variability.[7,8] Furthermore, a handful of case studies suggest that spinal manipulation may relieve disorders of cardiac rhythm.[9] The astute student of physiology may deduce why it is relatively easy to demonstrate effects of spinal manipulation on cardiac rhythm but not on blood pressure. Blood pressure is the end product of a multiplicity of influences, including vascular tone throughout the body. All other factors being equal, if tone within one localized vascular bed is increased, compensation by various mechanisms makes a systemic effect on blood pressure unlikely. On the other hand, heart rate is strongly influenced by segmentally organized parasympathetic and sympathetic innervation and therefore is more likely to be significantly affected by localized spinal stimulation, as might occur with subluxation or adjustment.

The Respiratory System

Among the many respiratory disorders commonly seen in community-based practice, asthma seems particularly to have attracted the attention of chiropractors. Further, given the number and quality of reports available, it appears that in particular groups of patients spinal manipulation has a beneficial effect.[10-12] This level of evidence is not available for the many equally common or more common microbial disorders of the respiratory system. Therefore spinal manipulation appears to be far from a cure-all for respiratory complaints, but it may be beneficial in a specific subset of asthma patients. At this point, no investigators have come forth with a serious analysis of the underlying physiologic changes occurring in those patients who do experience improvement and so we can only speculate on whether effects are exerted through the nervous system, immune system, or other systems.

The Digestive System

While functional disorders of the digestive system are common and patients with such disorders are frequent visitors to chiropractic clinics, there is little convincing evidence that spinal manipulation provides relief of symptomatology attributable to the digestive system. A number of high-quality studies report benefits in infantile colic.[13,14] However, despite the traditional view that colic is the result of abdominal discomfort, there is no objective evidence to support this intuition. Some interesting observational studies link mid-thoracic and lower thoracic subluxation to dyspepsia[15,16] and gastric and duodenal ulcers.[17] On the other hand, we see no reports of any quality dealing with functional disorders of the small and large bowel. Esophageal and gastric functions are, of course, very much under the control of the sympathetic and parasympathetic nervous systems, whereas bowel function is much more dependent upon the relatively autonomous enteric nervous system. Hence a localized disturbance of the spinal column might well establish a reflex response in the nervous system that could potentially affect function of the upper digestive system. On the other hand, segmentally organized reflex effects on the lower digestive system seem less likely.

The Female Reproductive System

A case series and subsequent randomized trial have demonstrated that spinal manipulation is effective in the relief of symptoms attributable to premenstrual syndrome.[18,19] Beneficial effects have not been demonstrated for primary and secondary dysmenorrhea.[20] However, when one considers the technical and administrative difficulties of conducting studies of disorders associated with the menstrual cycle, it is quite remarkable that researchers have been able to demonstrate any effects at all.

Summary

Collectively, these results suggest that subluxation is associated with and spinal manipulation may provide relief of symptoms associated with functional disorders of a number of organ systems. These relationships are most readily explained by reference to neurophysiologic mechanisms rather than biomechanical mechanisms. In overview, the literature does not support the idea that subluxation is a pervasive or dominant cause of disease nor that spinal manipulation is a panacea. Rather, it appears that spinal subluxation is associated with specific syndromes. The relationships are most clear where the organs or functions of concern receive autonomic innervation from a specific level of the neuraxis. Hence studies of effects on heart rate and heart rate variability, for example,

have been quite productive, whereas studies of digestive disorders have been unimpressive. The hypothesis that particular disorders are associated with subluxation at particular levels of the spine does seem to be supported by clinical studies and has a sound neurophysiologic rationale. However, a number of studies also suggest that subluxation of the upper cervical spine (or relief of upper cervical subluxation) may also be relevant to the onset (or relief) of symptomatology in general and have a specific influence on certain syndromes. Hence upper cervical subluxation appears to have distinctive clinical qualities, which may therefore merit explanation by reference to distinct biomechanical and neurophysiologic characteristics.

References

1. Gorman RF, Anderson RL, Bilton D, Favoloro RJ, Pittorino AJ. Case report: spinal strain and visual perception deficit. Chiropr J Aust 1994;24:131-4.
2. Gorman R. Monocular visual loss after closed head trauma: immediate resolution associated with spinal manipulation. J Manipulative Physiol Ther 1995;18:308-14.
3. Stephens D, Pollard H, Bilton D, Thomson P, Gorman F. Bilateral simultaneous optic nerve dysfunction after pariorbital trauma: recovery of vision in association with chiropractic spinal manipulation therapy. J Manipulative Physiol Ther 1999;22(9):615-21.
4. Yates RG, Lamping DL, Abram NL, Wright C. Effects of chiropractic treatment on blood pressure and anxiety: a randomized, controlled trial. J Manipulative Physiol Ther 1988;11(6):484-8.
5. Goertz CH, Grimm RH, Svendsen K, Grandits G. Treatment of Hypertension with Alternative Therapies (THAT) Study: a randomized clinical trial. J Hypertens 2002;20(10):2063-8.
6. Morgan J, Dickey J, Hunt H, Hudgins P. A controlled trial of spinal manipulation in the management of hypertension. J Am Osteo Assoc 1985;85(5):308-13.
7. Fujimoto T, Budgell B, Uchida S, Suzuki A, Meguro K. Arterial tonometry in the measurement of the effects of innocuous mechanical stimulation of the neck on heart rate and blood pressure. J Autonomic Nerv Syst 1999;75:109-15.
8. Budgell B, Hirano F. Innocuous mechanical stimulation of the neck and alterations in heart-rate variability in healthy young adults. Autonomic Neuroscience: Basic and Clinical 2001;91:96-9.
9. Budgell BI, Igarashi Y. Case study: response of arrhythmia to upper cervical adjustment; monitoring by ECG with analysis of heart-rate variability. J Neuromusculoskeletal Syst 2001;9:97-103.

10. Nielsen NH, Bronfort G, Bendix T, Madsen F, Weeke B. Chronic asthma and chiropractic spinal manipulation: a randomized clinical trial. Clin Exp Allergy 1995;25:80-8.
11. Balon J, Aker P, Crowther E, Danielson C, Cox P, O'Shaughnessy D et al. A comparison of active and simulated chiropractic manipulation as adjunctive treatment for childhood asthma. N Engl J Med 1998;339: 1013-20.
12. Bronfort G, Evans R, Kubic P, Filkin P. Chronic pediatric asthma and chiropractic spinal manipulation: a prospective clinical series and randomized clinical pilot study. J Manipulative Physiol Ther 2001;24(6):369-77.
13. Klougart N, Nilsson N, Jacobsen J. Infantile colic treated by chiropractors: a prospective study of 316 cases. J Manipulative Physiol Ther 1989;12(4):281-8.
14. Wiberg JM, Nordsteen J, Nilsson N. The short-term effect of spinal manipulation in the treatment of infantile colic: a randomized controlled clinical trial with a blinded observer. J Manipulative Physiol Ther 1999;22(8):517-22.
15. Bryner P, Staerker PG. Indigestion and heartburn: a descriptive study of prevalence in persons seeking care from chiropractors. J Manipulative Physiol Ther 1996; 19(5):317-23.
16. Love Z, Bull P. Management of dyspepsia: a chiropractic perspective. Chiropr J Aust 2003;33:57-63.
17. Pikalov AA, Kharin VV. Use of spinal manipulative therapy in the treatment of duodenal ulcer: a pilot study. J Manipulative Physiol Ther 1994;17:310-3.
18. Walsh MJ, Chandraraj S, Polus BI. The efficacy of chiropractic therapy on premenstrual syndrome: a case series study. Chiropr J Aust 1994;24:122-6.
19. Walsh MJP, Barbara I. A randomized, placebo-controlled clinical trial on the efficacy of chiropractic therapy on premenstrual syndrome. J Manipulative Physiol Ther 1999; 22(9):582-5.
20. Proctor M, Hing W, Johnson T, Murphy P. Spinal manipulation for primary and secondary dysmenorrhoea. Cochrane Database Syst Rev 2004;3:CD002119.

Glossary

a priori From cause to effect, based on theory instead of experience.

adaptation The adjustment of an organism to its environment.

ADI Atlanto-odontoid-interspace.

adjustment Any chiropractic therapeutic procedure that utilizes controlled force, leverage, direction, amplitude, and velocity, and which is directed at specific joints or anatomical regions. Chiropractors commonly use such procedures to influence joint and neurophysiological function.

alignment To put in a straight line; arrangement of position in a straight line.

amplitude Greatness of size, magnitude, breadth, or range.

anecdotal procedure Includes categories and classifications of procedures, technologies, or equipment that have not received the benefit of the experimental method. Items included originate and depend upon experience and observation only.

autonomic The portion of the nervous system that is predominantly self-regulated and serves to control visceral function.

central sensitization A state where neurons activated by noxious mechanical and chemical stimulation became sensitized by this input, making them hyperresponsive to all subsequent stimuli delivered to their receptive fields.

cervicogenic headache Symptomatic head pain and cephalic dysfunction caused by subluxation of the spinal joint.

compensation Changes in structural relationships to accommodate foundation disturbances and maintain balance.

degrees of freedom The number of independent coordinates in a coordinate system required to completely specify the position of an object in space. One degree of freedom is rotation around or translation along one axis. The spine is considered to have six degrees of freedom because it has the capability of rotatory movement around three axes as well as translatory movement along three axes.

disc herniation Extrusion of the nucleus pulposus into a defect in the anulus fibrosus.

effleurage Form of massage employing slow, rhythmic stroking executed with minimum force and light pressure.

elastic deformation Any recoverable deformation.

elasticity Property of a material or structure that returns it to its original form following the removal of the deforming load.

end play (end feel) Discrete, short-range movements of a joint, independent of the action of voluntary muscles, determined by springing each vertebra at the limit of its passive range of motion.

enteric That portion of the autonomic nervous system that controls gastrointestinal activity.

facilitation Increase in afferent stimuli so that the synaptic threshold is more easily reached; thus there is an increase in the efficacy of subsequent impulses in that pathway or synapse. The consequence of increased efficacy is that continued stimulation produces hyperactive responses.

fibromyalgia A central sensitization syndrome characterized by chronic widespread musculoskeletal aching, pain, and stiffness as well as exquisite tenderness at consistent anatomical locations known as tender points.

friction massage   Deep, circular massage to irritate or stimulate a muscle or increase its tonus and/or its arterial perfusion, or express swelling by moving the skin over the subcutaneous tissue.

homeostasis   Maintenance of static or constant conditions in the internal environment; level of well-being of an individual maintained by internal physiologic harmony.

hypermobility   Excessive mobility of a motion segment that is not so severe as to be incapacitating, be life-threatening, or require surgery.

instability   Excessive mobility of a motion segment to the extent that there is potential for development of incapacitating deformities or pain as a result of structural changes in the articular holding elements.

intersegmental motion   Relative motion taking place between two adjacent vertebral segments or within a vertebral motion segment; described as the upper vertebra on the lower.

ischemic compression (trigger point therapy)   Application of progressively stronger painful pressure on a trigger point for the purpose of eliminating the point's tenderness; blanches the compressed tissue, which usually becomes hyperemic (flushed) on release of the pressure.

joint play   Discrete, short-range movements of a joint, independent of the action of voluntary muscles, determined by springing each vertebra in the neutral position.

listing (dynamic)   Designation of the abnormal movement characteristics of one vertebra in relation to subadjacent segments. Dynamic listing nomenclature: flexion restriction; extension restriction; lateral flexion restriction (right or left); rotational malposition (right or left).

manipulable subluxation   Subluxation in which altered alignment, movement, and/or function can be improved by manual thrust procedures.

manipulation   Manual procedure that involves a directed thrust to move a joint past the physiologic range of motion, without exceeding the anatomic limit.

manual therapy   Procedures by which the hands directly contact the body.

meric system   Treatment of visceral conditions through adjustment of vertebrae at the levels of neuromeric innervation to the organs involved.

mobilization   Movement applied singularly or repetitively or at the physiologic range of joint motion, without imparting a thrust or impulse, with the goal or restoring joint mobility.

motion segment   A functional unit made up of the two adjacent articulating surfaces and the connecting tissues binding them to each other.

motor unit   Functional unit of striated muscle comprised of the motor neuron and all the muscle fibers supplied by the neuron.

myofascial pain syndrome   Pain syndrome characterized by pain in regional muscles accompanied by trigger points that refer pain specifically to each muscle.

myofascial trigger point   Hyperirritable spot, usually within a taut band of skeletal muscle or in the muscle's fascia, that is painful on compression and that can give rise to characteristic referred pain, tenderness, and autonomic phenomena.

palpation   Act of feeling with the hands; application of variable manual pressure through the surface of the body for the purpose of determining the shape, size, consistency, position, inherent motility, and health of the tissues beneath.

motion palpation: palpatory diagnosis of passive and active segmental joint range motion.

static palpation: palpatory diagnosis of somatic structures in a neutral static position.

palpatory skills   Sensory skills used in performing palpatory diagnosis.

parasympathetic   The portion of the autonomic nervous system that functions to store, conserve, and replenish body energy.

petrissage   Same as kneading.

plastic deformation   Nonrecoverable deformation.

plasticity Property of a material to permanently deform when it is loaded beyond its elastic range.

post hoc, ergo propter hoc (Latin) After this, therefore, because of this (a false reasoning).

postganglionic A population of autonomic neurons located either in peripheral ganglia or the wall of specific viscera, which have axons innervating viscera.

preganglionic A population of autonomic neurons located in the central nervous system that have axons innervating postganglionic neurons located in the peripheral ganglia or viscera.

putative Supposed, reputed.

reflex Result of transforming an ingoing sensory impulse into an outgoing efferent impulse without the act of will.

reflex therapy Treatment that is aimed at stimulating afferent impulses and evoking a given response (i.e., neuromuscular).

resilience Property of returning to the former shape or size after distortion.

somatic Structures in the body wall and limbs are referred to as somatic structures.

somatogenic Produced by activity, reaction, and change originating in the musculoskeletal system.

somato-visceral reflex Reflex activation or inhibition of visceral function in response to somatic sensation.

spinal motion segment Two adjacent vertebrae and the connecting tissues binding them to each other.

splanchnic A descriptive term with reference to viscera (e.g., splanchnic nerves are autonomic nerves that innervate abdominal viscera).

stiffness Measure of resistance offered to external loads by a specimen or structure as it deforms.

stringiness Palpable tissue texture abnormality characterized by fine or string-like myofascial structures.

subluxation A motion segment in which alignment, movement integrity, and/or physiologic function are altered although contact between joint surfaces remains intact.

subluxation complex A theoretic model of motion segment dysfunction (subluxation) that incorporates the complex interaction of pathologic changes in nerve, muscle, ligamentous, vascular, and connective tissues.

subluxation syndrome An aggregate of signs and symptoms that relate to pathophysiology or dysfunction of spinal and pelvic motion segments or to peripheral joints.

substance P A peptide present in nerve cells scattered throughout the body and in special endocrine cells in the gut.

symmetry Similarity in corresponding parts or organs on opposite sides of the body.

sympathetic That portion of the autonomic nervous system that functions to regulate body functions in response to stress.

tapotement A tapping or percussing movement in massage; it includes clapping, beating, and punctuation.

tender points Local areas of hyperactivity found at consistent anatomic sites, which do not refer pain pressure but produce a pain response to light palpation. (See *fibromyalgia*.)

therapuetic Any treatment considered necessary to return the patient to a preclinical status or establish a stationary status.

thrust Sudden, manual application of a controlled directional force upon a suitable part of the patient, the delivery of which effects an adjustment.

traction Force acting on a longitudinal axis to draw structures apart.

visceral afferent Nerves that serve to conduct sensory information from the organs to the central nervous system are called visceral afferent nerves.

visceral efferent   Autonomic nerves that serve to increase organ function are called visceral efferent nerves.

viscerosomatic convergence   Convergent input to somatic neurons form visceral nociceptive afferents that project through the sympathetic chain, producing somatic pain from visceral disease.

viscerosomatic reflex   Reflex activation or inhibition or somatic function in response to visceral sensation.

viscoelasticity   Property of a material showing sensitivity to the rate of loading or deformation; two basic components are viscosity and elasticity.

viscosity   Property of materials to resist loads that produce shear.

Index

Page numbers followed by f indicate figures; t, tables; b, boxes.

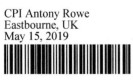